CARCINOGENESIS—
A COMPREHENSIVE SURVEY
VOLUME 7

Cocarcinogenesis and Biological Effects of Tumor Promoters

Carcinogenesis—A Comprehensive Survey

Carcinogenesis—
A Comprehensive Survey
Volume 7

Cocarcinogenesis and Biological Effects of Tumor Promoters

Editors

Erich Hecker, Ph.D.   N. E. Fusenig, M.D.
W. Kunz, M.D.   F. Marks, Ph.D.
H. W. Thielmann, M.D., Ph.D.

*Institute of Biochemistry, German Cancer Research Center,
Heidelberg, Federal Republic of Germany*

Raven Press ■ New York

Raven Press, 1140 Avenue of the Americas, New York, New York 10036

Made in the United States of America

Great care has been taken to maintain the accuracy of the information contained in this volume. However, Raven Press cannot be held responsible for errors or for any consequences arising from the use of the information contained herein.

Materials appearing in this book prepared by individuals as part of their official duties as U.S. Government employees are not covered by the above-mentioned copyright.

Library of Congress Cataloging in Publication Data
Main entry under title:

Cocarcinogenesis and biological effects of tumor promoters.

    (Carcinogenesis—a comprehensive survey; v.7)
    Selected papers from a symposium held
Oct. 13–16, 1980 in Schloss Elmau, Bavaria, Federal
Republic of Germany, and sponsored by the Deutsches
Krebsforschungszentrum Heidelberg, et al.
    Includes bibliographical references and index.
    1. Cocarcinogenesis—Congresses. 2. Cocarcinogens—
Congresses. I. Hecker, Erich, 1926– . II. Deutsches
Krebsforschungszentrum Heidelberg. III. Series.
RC268.5.C36   vol. 7   [RC268.52]   616.99′4071s   81-21044
89004-618-2   [616.99′4071] AACR2

Foreword

The very need for follow-up volumes on the topic of cocarcinogenesis and tumor promotion at relatively short intervals is a reflection of the amount of progress made in the field from so many different viewpoints. The subject is, in fact, no longer a matter of narrow interest for a small coterie of laboratory investigators: it is beginning to play a major role in contemporary speculations on tumor etiology and pathogenesis, and is likely to have a decided impact on future plans for the control of human cancer.

If I may for a moment introduce a personal note I could hardly have imagined, back in 1940, when investigating the peculiar properties of croton oil in relation to skin carcinogenesis in mice, that I was opening a kind of beneficial Pandora's box, and that 40 years later I would be introducing a book on the initiation/promotion principle related to those early experiments—but with all the added complexities brought about by recent developments.

The new, widespread interest in cocarcinogenesis, and more particularly in the promoting phase of carcinogenesis, came, as we all know, from two independent developments: (a) the availability of pure reagents, in the form of phorbol and many other polyfunctional diterpene esters, in the place of crude croton oil, which facilitated the study of mechanisms with far greater precision; and (b) the extension of the two-stage process from skin (in which it was first identified) to other organs and to tissue culture, and from animal to man.

I referred earlier to the fact that promoting action is nowadays being investigated from many different viewpoints. It is indeed very encouraging that most of the different approaches are well represented in this volume, as is evident from the chapter titles. Particularly important is presentation and interchange of results and ideas between researchers oriented etiologically or clinically and those oriented experimentally.

The solution to the most challenging problem—how promoting action operates—still eludes us, however, although there are so many good correlations, observed among a limited group of compounds, between potency of promoting activity in mouse skin and the multiplicity of biological or biochemical properties these compounds happen to possess. Perhaps one of the obstacles to a definitive conclusion is the previous overemphasis on *skin* promoters, which provided a rather one-sided picture.

In any case, rapid advancements in science often lead to growing complexity, with conflicting claims and some confusion. Fortunately, however, scientific issues are generally complicated only during the formative stages of research, and assume surprising simplicity once the level of final truth is reached.

Are we, then, approaching the stage of "simplicity" in our understanding of the mechanism of tumor induction? I would not hazard a guess. But the contents of this volume might indicate how near we are to reaching this goal.

With this expression of hopeful anticipation, I take pleasure in welcoming this volume.

I. Berenblum
The Weizmann Institute of Science
Rehovot, Israel

Preface

According to the International Agency for Research on Cancer (IARC) of the World Health Organization (WHO), approximately 700 solitary carcinogens have been reported. They are primarily of exogenous origin, and most of them were detected experimentally. Of these, only about 30 have been related beyond doubt to the etiology of human cancers. These findings support the idea stimulated by early observations of clinicians, such as Virchow and others, that, for many human cancers, a simple "unifactorial" relation between cause and consequence, i.e., *solitary carcinogenesis,* may be the exception rather than the rule. Indeed, as *carcinogenic risk factors,* solitary carcinogens have been shown to be involved primarily in occupational and iatrogenic cancers. The etiologies of most of the more common human cancers, however, may be considered the result of "multifactorial" exposure, mostly to carcinogenic risk factors unknown as yet. Indeed, it is only too likely that in the course of human life, depending on the individual *lifestyle,* a person might be exposed—either consecutively or simultaneously—to various categories of carcinogenic risk factors. Of these, the solitary carcinogens were for a long time the sole physicochemically well-defined class, and certain somatogenetic impact(s) was postulated as the source of their putative molecular mechanism of action.

An extension of the now classical concept of solitary carcinogenesis was particularly stimulated for the first time when the new, nonclassical toxicologic principle of *cocarcinogenesis* was determined experimentally and proclaimed independently by Rous and Shear in 1938. According to their concept, cocarcinogens are considered collectively as, per se noncarcinogenic, amplifiers of carcinogenesis. In the 1940s this idea was evaluated in greater depth, especially by Mottram, Berenblum, Rusch, Butenandt, and their associates, who investigated irritants or proliferation-stimulating hormones as cocarcinogens in various target tissues.

In 1947, using the skin irritant croton oil as a cocarcinogen and mouse skin as the target tissue, Berenblum and Shubik expressed their results in an especially precise way: if preceded by "tumor initiation," they concluded to have observed "tumor promotion" by exposure of mouse skin to the irritant, yet not strictly carcinogenic, croton oil. The former was achieved by subcarcinogenic exposure of the target tissue to a solitary carcinogen of the polycyclic aromatic hydrocarbon type. Thus, for experimental exploration of cocarcinogenesis, they were the first to propose a clearly defined prototype protocol known as "initiation/promotion." Indeed, it is only one of numerous possible combinations of doses and exposure times of the two types of carcinogenic factors.

In 1962, another well defined protocol of cocarcinogenesis known as "stimulated initiation/promotion" was introduced by Pound, again using mouse skin as the target tissue with urethane as "initiator," and employing croton oil, not only as a promoter but also as a stimulator of "initiation." (For the special protocol "stimulated initiation/promotion," some investigators also use the term "cocarcinogenesis," in contrast to the previous, and more general, definition of cocarcinogenesis given by Shear in 1938.) Yet, despite elaborate research all over the world, the new, toxicologic principle of cocarcinogenesis, i.e., amplification of carcinogenesis by noncarcinogens was not fully accepted for about 20 years. Some investigators even denied the possibility that, besides the solitary carcinogenic quality, a separate and defined cocarcinogenic in terms of a "tumor promoting" quality might exist.

Altogether, it turned out to be rather difficult to provide convincing experimental and/or epidemiologic evidence for multifactorial etiologies of cancer, especially for cocarcinogenesis. Thus, the new concept was not convincingly established until the late 1960s, when the tumor promoters present in croton oil became available as physicochemically well-defined partial esters of the polyfunctional diterpene phorbol. The chemical identification and the availability of this hitherto unknown class of molecular entities, particularly of the prototype promoter 12-O-tetradecanoylphorbol-13-acetate, known as TPA, allowed the rigorous biological, biochemical, and mechanistic characterization of highly active cocarcinogens *for the first time.* (Some suppliers and investigators refer to TPA as "phorbol-myristate-acetate" (PMA), which is a trivial name for the very same molecule.) Subsequently, many more most active promoters of the polyfunctional diterpene ester type originating from plant species have been detected and investigated. Together they have become prototype cocarcinogens, launching a true renaissance in the area of cocarcinogenesis. Furthermore, in an increasing number of target tissues other than skin, initiation/promotion has been investigated, including modifications in both its stages, *initiation and promotion.*

In this progressing new area of cancer research, a first international symposium was convened in 1977, as documented in volume 2 of the present series *Carcinogenesis—A Comprehensive Survey.* It proved to be an effective catalyst of research in cocarcinogens and particularly promoters, which would express, possibly by epigenetic mechanisms, phenotypes coined by the preceding impact of initiators on target cells. The revived field developed exponentially, it became possible to divide promotion itself into two defined stages and more and more relevant areas of general cell biology became involved owing to the plethora of cellular events stimulated by polyfunctional diterpene ester type cocarcinogens.

In 1980, the time was considered ripe to again discuss new data, to reexamine past hypotheses, and to integrate recent experimental observations of cell physiology into refined concepts of cocarcinogenesis, and particularly of initiation/promotion. Therefore, a second international symposium was convened, this time in the Federal Republic of Germany. This volume presents a careful selection of the most recent developments reported during the symposium, and their implications for cancer research. It is an update and extension of volume 2, which was published by Raven Press in the same series three years ago. The sections *Cocarcinogenesis and Tumor Promotion In Vivo, Epidemiologic Aspects,* and *Tumor Promotion In Vitro* contribute to clarify the truly basic problem—whether specific cocarcinogens are functioning as both promoters and stimulators of initiation, or if they do have only one of these capacities. Apart from their mechanistic validity, insights of this kind may be helpful in order to determine the degree of carcinogenic risk involved in exposure to cocarcinogens of whatever origin and nature. They are an undeniable prerequisite for differentiated risk/benefit evaluations aimed at implementing more sophisticated strategies of cancer prevention. Investigations reported in the sections *Effects of Tumor Promoters on Cell Proliferation and Differentiation, Membrane Interactions and Receptors, Effects on Intracellular Communication and Cell Metabolism,* together with *Viral and Immunologic Aspects,* extend present knowledge of the causes of cancer at the cell and molecular levels. They may help to introduce new preventive strategies and to stimulate refinements of therapeutic approaches in curing cancers.

It is my dedicated hope that in the years to come the contents of this volume will encourage multidisciplinary research on the fascinating etiologic, cell biologic, and molecular facets of cocarcinogenesis for the benefit of human beings.

Erich Hecker, Ph.D.
Deutsches Krebsforschungszentrum
Heidelberg, Federal Republic of Germany

Acknowledgments

The symposium "Cocarcinogenesis and Biological Effects of Tumor Promoters," on which this volume is based, was held from October 13th to 16th, 1980 in Schloss Elmau, Bavaria, Federal Republic of Germany. It was *patronized* by the International Agency for Research on Cancer (IARC, Director: J. Higginson), Lyon, France, and by the Deutsches Krebsforschungszentrum (DKFZ, Director: H. Neurath), Heidelberg, Federal Republic of Germany. The scientific program was arranged and the organization was performed and concluded by an International Program and Organizing Committee nominated jointly by IARC and DKFZ: E. Hecker, Chairman, DKFZ; N. E. Fusenig, Vice-Chairman, DKFZ; F. Marks, Vice-Chairman, DKFZ; W. Davis, IARC; E. Egenlauf, DKFZ; K. Goerttler, DKFZ; S. Herz, DKFZ; M. Hicks, UK; V. Kinzel, DKFZ; W. Kunz, DKFZ; J. Schweizer, DKFZ; T. J. Slaga, USA; H. Stamatiadis-Smidt, DKFZ; H. W. Thielmann, DKFZ; L. Tomatis, IARC; and H. Yamasaki, IARC.

Under the auspices of this committee, of the 161 presentations given during the symposium, 68 have been selected by the editors for publication in this volume.

The symposium was *sponsored* by: Deutsches Krebsforschungszentrum (DKFZ), Heidelberg, Federal Republic of Germany; The International Agency for Research on Cancer (IARC), Lyon, France; The Environmental Protection Agency (EPA), Research Triangle Park, North Carolina, USA; Deutsche Forschungsgemeinschaft (DFG), Bonn-Bad Godesberg, Federal Republic of Germany; and firms of the Pharmaceutical Industry in the United States and the Federal Republic of Germany.

On behalf of the committee, I wish to express our sincere appreciation for the moral and monetary support given by the patrons and by the sponsors. Thoughtful advice and efficient cooperation during all stages of the common task by the members of the committee is gratefully acknowledged. Publication of this volume would not have been possible without the excellent cooperation of Raven Press.

Erich Hecker, Ph.D.
Deutsches Krebsforschungszentrum
Heidelberg, Federal Republic of Germany

*This volume is dedicated to the memory of the distinguished
Prof. Dr. med., Drs. mult. hc. Karl-Heinrich Bauer,
initiator of the mutation hypothesis of carcinogenesis (1926)
and promoter of the Foundation of the Deutsches Krebsforschungszentrum
(1964).*

Contents

Nonepidermal Target Tissues

EPIDEMIOLOGIC ASPECTS

TUMOR PROMOTION IN VITRO

EFFECTS OF TUMOR PROMOTERS ON CELL PROLIFERATION AND DIFFERENTIATION

Epidermis

MEMBRANE INTERACTIONS AND RECEPTORS

EFFECTS ON INTERCELLULAR COMMUNICATION AND CELL METABOLISM

VIRAL AND IMMUNOLOGIC ASPECTS

Contributors

W. Adolf
Institute of Biochemistry
German Cancer Research Center
D-6900 Heidelberg, Federal Republic of
  Germany

F. Anders
Genetisches Institut
Justus-Liebig-Universität Giessen
D-6300 Giessen,
Federal Republic of Germany

Thomas S. Argyris
Department of Pathology
State University of New York
Upstate Medical Center
Syracuse, New York 13210

V. Armuth
Experimental Biology Unit
The Weizmann Institute of Science
Rehovot 76 100, Israel

C. L. Ashendel
McArdle Laboratory for Cancer Research
University of Wisconsin
Madison, Wisconsin 53706

Erle Astrup
McArdle Laboratory for Cancer Research
University of Wisconsin
Madison, Wisconsin 53706

Jerry A. Bash
Department of Microbiology
University of Cincinnati College of Medi-
  cine
Cincinnati, Ohio 45267

G. Bauer
Institut für Virologie
Zentrum für Hygiene
Freiburg, West Germany

C. Stuart Baxter
Department of Environmental Health
University of Cincinnati College of Medi-
  cine
Cincinnati, Ohio 45267

Sidney Belman
Institute of Environmental Medicine
New York University Medical Center
New York, New York 10016

I. Berenblum
Experimental Biology Unit
The Weizmann Institute of Science
Rehovot 76 100, Israel

David L. Berry
Toxicology Unit
United States Department of Agriculture
  Regional Research Center
Berkeley, California 94710

Stefan Bertsch
Institut für Biochemie
German Cancer Research Center
D-6900 Heidelberg, Federal Republic of
  Germany

J. R. Bickenbach
Dows Institute for Dental Research
The University of Iowa
Iowa City, Iowa 52242

Peter M. Blumberg
Department of Pharmacology
Harvard Medical School
Boston, Massachusetts 02115

Carmia Borek
Departments of Radiology, Pathology, Bio-
  chemistry and Medicine
Cancer Center/Institute of Cancer Re-
  search
Columbia University College of Physicians
  and Surgeons
New York, New York 10032

R. K. Boutwell
McArdle Laboratory for Cancer Research
University of Wisconsin
Madison, Wisconsin 53706

George T. Bowden
Department of Radiology
Division of Radiation Oncology
The University of Arizona Medical School
Arizona Health Sciences Center
Tucson, Arizona 85724

Yael Bromberg
Section of Immunology
Department of Human Microbiology
Sackler School of Medicine
Tel-Aviv University
Ranat-Aviv, Tel-Aviv, Israel

Kay Brune
Department of Pharmacology
Biozentrum
University of Basel
CH-4056 Basel, Switzerland

Michael Callaham
Biology Division
Oak Ridge National Laboratory
Oak Ridge, Tennessee 37830

M. Castagna
Institut de Recherches Scientifiques sur le
* Cancer*
Villejuif F-94800, France

Chia-cheng Chang
Department of Pediatrics and Human De-
* velopment*
Michigan State University
East Lansing, Michigan 48824

S. J. Cheng
Cancer Institute
Chinese Academy of Medical Sciences
Peking, China

I. Chouroulinkov
Institut de Recherches Scientifiques sur le
* Cancer*
94800 Villejuif, France

Leonard A. Cohen
American Health Foundation
Valhalla, New York 10595

Nancy H. Colburn
Laboratory of Viral Carcinogenesis
National Cancer Institute
Frederick Cancer Research Center
Frederick, Maryland 21701

J. Croop
Department of Anatomy
School of Medicine
University of Pennsylvania
Philadelphia, Pennsylvania 19104

Nicholas E. Day
Biostatistics Programme
Division of Human Cancer and Field Pro-
* grammes*
International Agency for Research on
* Cancer*
69372 Lyon Cedex 2, France

Joseph E. De Larco
Laboratory of Viral Carcinogenesis
National Cancer Institute
Frederick, Maryland 21701

K. Barry Delclos
Department of Pharmacology
Harvard Medical School
Boston, Massachusetts 02115

M. Deleers
Laboratory of Experimental Medicine
Brussels University
Brussels, Belgium

C. Delescluse
Institute of Biochemistry
German Cancer Research Center
D-6900 Heidelberg, Federal Republic of
* Germany*

Luigi M. De Luca
Differentiation Control Section
Laboratory of Experimental Pathology
National Cancer Institute
National Institutes of Health
Bethesda, Maryland 20205

L. David Dion
Laboratory of Viral Carcinogenesis
National Cancer Institute
Frederick Cancer Research Center
Frederick, Maryland 21701

J. A. DiPaolo
Laboratory of Biology
National Cancer Institute
Bethesda, Maryland 20205

A. Dlugosz
Department of Anatomy
School of Medicine
University of Pennsylvania
Philadelphia, Pennsylvania 19104

J. N. Doniger
Laboratory of Biology
National Cancer Institute
Bethesda, Maryland 20205

Cécile Drevon
International Agency for Research on
  Cancer
69372 Lyon Cedex 2, France

William G. Dunphy
Department of Pharmacology
Harvard Medical School
Boston, Massachusetts 02115

Rule T. Dzarlieva
German Cancer Research Center
Institute of Biochemistry
6900 Heidelberg, Federal Republic of Germany

C. H. Evans
Laboratory of Biology
National Cancer Institute
Bethesda, Maryland 20205

Thomas A. Ferguson
Department of Microbiology
University of Cincinnati College of Medicine
Cincinnati, Ohio 45267

S. M. Fischer
Biology Division
Oak Ridge National Laboratory
Oak Ridge, Tennessee 37830

Larry A. Fish
Department of Environmental Health
University of Cincinnati College of Medicine
Cincinnati, Ohio 45267

Paul B. Fisher
Division of Environmental Sciences and
  Cancer Center
Institute of Cancer Research and Departments of Medicine, Microbiology, and
  Pathology
Columbia University
College of Physicians and Surgeons
New York, New York 10032

D. James Fitzgerald
School of Biological Sciences
Flinders University
Bedford Park, South Australia 5042

Maya Freund
Sections of Immunology
Department of Human Microbiology
Sackler School of Medicine
Tel-Aviv University
Ranat-Aviv, Tel-Aviv, Israel

R. J. M. Fry
Biology Division
Oak Ridge National Laboratory
Oak Ridge, Tennessee 37830

H. Fujiki
National Cancer Center Research Institute
Tokyo 104, Japan

Gerhard Fürstenberger
Institute of Biochemistry
German Cancer Research Center
D-6900 Heidelberg, Federal Republic of
  Germany

Norbert E. Fusenig
German Cancer Research Center
Institute of Biochemistry
6900 Heidelberg, Federal Republic of Germany

Seymour J. Garte
Institute of Environmental Medicine
New York University Medical Center
New York, New York 10016

C. R. Geard
Departments of Radiology, Pathology, Bio-
chemistry, and Medicine
Cancer Center/Institute of Cancer Re-
search
Columbia University College of Physicians
and Surgeons
New York, New York 10032

K. Goerttler
German Cancer Research Center
Institute of Experimental Pathology
6900 Heidelberg, Federal Republic of Germany

S. Goldfarb
Pathology Department
University of Wisconsin
Madison, Wisconsin 53706

Bernard Goldstein
Department of Environmental and Com-
munity Medicine
Rutgers Medical School
Piscataway, New Jersey 08854

Tom Goldsworthy
McArdle Laboratory for Cancer Research
Departments of Oncology and Pathology
The Medical School
University of Wisconsin
Madison, Wisconsin 53706

Ellen Greenebaum
Division of Environmental Sciences and
Cancer Center
Institute of Cancer Research and Cancer
Research and Departments of Medicine,
Microbiology and Pathology
Columbia University
College of Physicians and Surgeons
New York, New York 10032

D. Grube
Division of Biological and Medical Re-
search
Argonne National Laboratory
Argonne, Illinois 60439

D. L. Guernsey
Departments of Radiology, Pathology, Bio-
chemistry, and Medicine
Cancer Center/Institute of Cancer Re-
search
Columbia University College of Physicians
and Surgeons
New York, New York 10032

Graeme R. Guy
School of Biological Sciences
Flinders University
Bedford Park, South Australia 5042

E. Hecker
Institute of Biochemistry
German Cancer Research Center
D-6900 Heidelberg, Federal Republic of
Germany

Charles Heidelberger
University of Southern California Compre-
hensive Cancer Center
Los Angeles, California 90033

Henry Hennings
In Vitro Pathogenesis Section
Laboratory of Experimental Pathology
National Cancer Institute
Bethesda, Maryland 20205

B. Hesse
German Cancer Research Center
Institute of Experimental Pathology
6900 Heidelberg, Federal Republic of Germany

R. Marian Hicks
School of Pathology
Middlesex Hospital Medical School
London W1P 7LD, England

Peter Hill
American Health Foundation
Valhalla, New York 10595

M. Hirota
Department of Food Science and Technol-
ogy
Faculty of Agriculture
Kyoto University
Kyoto 606, Japan

K. Holbrook
Department of Biological Structure
University of Washington
Seattle, Washington 98104

H. Holtzer
Department of Anatomy
School of Medicine
University of Pennsylvania
Philadelphia, Pennsylvania 19104

Yoshio Honma
Department of Chemotherapy
Saitama Cancer Center Research Institute
Saitama 362, Japan

Ann D. Horowitz
Division of Environmental Sciences and
  Cancer Center
Institute of Cancer Research and Depart-
  ments of Medicine, Microbiology, and
  Pathology
Columbia University
College of Physicians and Surgeons
New York, New York 10032

Motoo Hozumi
Department of Chemotherapy
Saitama Cancer Center Research Institute
Saitama 362, Japan

Eliezer Huberman
Biology Division
Oak Ridge National Laboratory
Oak Ridge, Tennessee 37830

Nobuyuki Ito
First Department of Pathology
Nagoya City University Medical School
Nagoya 467, Japan

Vesna Ivanovic
Division of Environmental Sciences and
  Cancer Center
Institute of Cancer Research and Depart-
  ments of Medicine, Microbiology, and
  Pathology
Columbia University
College of Physicians and Surgeons
New York, New York 10032

Eric A. Jaffe
Division of Hematology-Oncology
Department of Medicine
Cornell University Medical College
New York, New York 10021

Susan Jaken
Department of Pharmacology
Harvard Medical School
Boston, Massachusetts 02115

Anton M. Jetten
Differentiation Control Section
Laboratory of Experimental Pathology
National Cancer Institute
National Institutes of Health
Bethesda, Maryland 20205

Takashi Kasukabe
Department of Chemotherapy
Saitama Cancer Center Research Institute
Saitama 362, Japan

Yona Keisari
Section of Immunology
Department of Human Microbiology
Sackler School of Medicine
Tel-Aviv University
Ranat-Aviv, Tel-Aviv, Israel

R. Keist
Immunobiology Research Group
Institute for Immunology and Virology
University of Zurich
CH-8032 Zurich, Switzerland

R. Keller
Immunobiology Research Group
Institute for Immunology and Virology
University of Zurich
CH-8032 Zurich, Switzerland

Ann R. Kennedy
Laboratory of Radiobiology
Harvard University School of Public
  Health
Boston, Massachusetts 02115

Volker Kinzel
Institute of Experimental Pathology
German Cancer Research Center
D-6900 Heidelberg, Federal Republic of
  Germany

A. J. P. Klein-Szanto
Biology Division
Oak Ridge National Laboratory
Oak Ridge, Tennessee 37830

L. Kopelovich
Memorial Sloan-Kettering Cancer Center
and Cornell University Graduate School
of Medical Sciences
New York, New York 10021

P. Köppel
Immunobiology Research Group
Institute for Immunology and Virology
University of Zurich
CH-8032 Zurich, Switzerland

K. Koshimizu
Department of Food Science and Technology
Faculty of Agriculture
Kyoto 606, Japan

Molly Kulesz-Martin
In Vitro Pathogenesis Section
Laboratory of Experimental Pathology
National Cancer Institute
Bethesda, Maryland 20205

Werner Kunz
The German Cancer Research Centre
Institute of Biochemistry
D-6900 Heidelberg, Federal Republic of
Germany

René Lanz
Department of Pharmacology
Biozentrum
University of Basel
CH-4056 Basel, Switzerland

Lih-Syng Lee
General Electric Corporate Research and
Development Center
Schenectady, New York 12301

Lawrence Levine
Department of Biochemistry
Brandeis University
Waltham, Massachusetts 02254

R. D. Ley
Biology Division
Oak Ridge National Laboratory
Oak Ridge, Tennessee 37830

M. H. Li
Cancer Institute
Chinese Academy of Medical Sciences
Peking, China

Ulrike Lichti
In Vitro Pathogenesis Section
Laboratory of Experimental Pathology
National Cancer Institute
Bethesda, Maryland 20205

John B. Little
Laboratory of Radiobiology
Harvard University School of Public
Health
Boston, Massachusetts 02115

Jean M. Lockyer
Department of Anatomy
The University of Arizona Medical School
Arizona Health Sciences Center
Tucson, Arizona 85724

H. Loehrke
German Cancer Research Center
Institute of Experimental Pathology
6900 Heidelberg, Federal Republic of Germany

Joseph Lotem
Department of Genetics
Weizmann Institute of Science
Rehovot, Israel

I. C. Mackenzie
Dows Institute for Dental Research
The University of Iowa
Iowa City, Iowa 52242

Bruce E. Magun
Departments of Radiology
Division of Radiation Oncology and
Department of Anatomy
The University of Arizona Medical School
Arizona Health Sciences Center
Tucson, Arizona 85724

S. K. Major
Biology Division
Oak Ridge National Laboratory
Oak Ridge, Tennessee 37830

W. J. Malaisse
Laboratory of Experimental Medicine
Brussels University
Brussels, Belgium

M. Mamrack
Biology Division
Oak Ridge National Laboratory
Oak Ridge, Tennessee 37830

Friederich Marks
Institute for Biochemistry
German Cancer Research Center
D-6900 Heidelberg 1, Federal Republic of
Germany

Nicole Martel
International Agency for Research on
Cancer
69372 Lyon Cedex 2, France

Andrea M. Mastro
Department of Microbiology, Cell Biology,
Biochemistry and Biophysics
The Pennsylvania State University
University Park, Pennsylvania 16802

Lynn M. Matrisian
Department of Anatomy
The University of Arizona Medical School
Arizona Health Sciences Center
Tucson, Arizona 85724

J. Gabriel Michael
Department of Microbiology
University of Cincinnati College of Medi-
cine
Cincinnati, Ohio 45267

N. Mihailovich
Pathology and Radiology Departments
University of Chicago
Chicago, Illinois 60637

R. C. Miller
Departments of Radiology, Pathology, Bio-
chemistry and Medicine
Cancer Center/Institute of Cancer Re-
search
Columbia University College of Physicians
and Surgeons
New York, New York 10032

Sukdeb Mondal
University of Southern California Compre-
hensive Cancer Center
Los Angeles, California 90033

R. E. Moore
Department of Chemistry
University of Hawaii
Honolulu, Hawaii 96822

Susan Moran
McArdle Laboratory for Cancer Research
Departments of Oncology and Pathology
The Medical School
University of Wisconsin
Madison, Wisconsin 53706

M. Mori
National Cancer Center
Research Institute
Tokyo 104, Japan

David Moscatelli
Department of Cell Biology
New York University Medical Center
New York, New York 10016

G. C. Mueller
McArdle Laboratory for Cancer Research
University of Wisconsin
Madison, Wisconsin 53706

R. Alan Mufson
Division of Environmental Sciences and
Cancer Center
Institute of Cancer Research and Depart-
ments of Medicine, Microbiology, and
Pathology
Columbia University
College of Physicians and Surgeons
New York, New York 10032

Andrew W. Murray
School of Biological Sciences
Flinders University
Bedford Park, South Australia 5042

Keisuke Nakanishi
First Department of Pathology
Nagoya City University Medical School
Nagoya 467, Japan

M. Nakayasu
National Cancer Center Research Institute
Tokyo 104, Japan

K. Nelson
Biology Division
Oak Ridge National Laboratory
Oak Ridge, Tennessee 37830

M. Nemeč
J. Stefan Institute
E. Kardelj University of Ljubljana
61000 Ljubljana, Yugoslavia

G. Ohde
Institute of Toxicology and Pharmacology
3350 Marburg, Federal Republic of Germany

H. Ohigashi
Department of Food Science and Technology
Faculty of Agriculture
Kyoto University
Kyoto 606, Japan

M. Pacifici
Department of Anatomy
School of Medicine
University of Pennsylvania
Philadelphia, Pennsylvania 19104

R. Payette
Department of Anatomy
School of Medicine
University of Pennsylvania
Philadelphia, Pennsylvania 19104

S. Pečar
Department of Pharmacology and J. Stefan Institute
E. Kardelj University of Ljubljana
61000 Ljubljana, Yugoslavia

Karen G. Pepin
Department of Microbiology, Cell Biology,
Biochemistry and Biophysics
The Pennsylvania State University
University Park, Pennsylvania 16802

Carl Peraino
Division of Biological and Medical Research
Argonne National Laboratory
Argonne, Illinois 60439

Edgar Pick
Section of Immunology
Department of Human Microbiology
Sackler School of Medicine
Tel-Aviv University
Ranat-Aviv, Tel-Aviv, Israel

Henry C. Pitot
McArdle Laboratory for Cancer Research
Departments of Oncology and Pathology
The Medical School
University of Wisconsin
Madison, Wisconsin 53706

N. C. Popescu
Laboratory of Biology
National Cancer Institute
Bethesda, Maryland 20205

K. V. N. Rao
Pathology and Radiology Departments
University of Chicago
Chicago, Illinois 60637

Bandura S. Reddy
American Health Foundation
Valhalla, New York 10595

James Richards
Institute of Experimental Pathology
German Cancer Research Center
D-6900 Heidelberg, Federal Republic of Germany

Hartmut Richter
Institute of Biochemistry
German Cancer Research Center
D-6900 Heidelberg, Federal Republic of Germany

Daniel B. Rifkin
Department of Cell Biology
New York University Medical Center
New York, New York 10016

Leo Sachs
Department of Genetics
Weizmann Institute of Science
Rehovot, Israel

M. Sala
Institut de Recherches Scientifiques sur le
Cancer
94800 Villejuif, France

Joachim Sasse
Max-Planck-Institut für Biochemie
Department of Connective Tissue Research
D-8033 Martinsried bei München, Federal
Republic of Germany

M. Schara
Stefan Institute
E. Kardelj University of Ljublijana
61000 Ljubljana, Yugoslavia

A. Schartl
Genetisches Institut
Justus-Liebig-Universität Giessen
D-6300 Giessen, Federal Republic of Ger-
many

M. Schartl
Genetisches Institut
Justus-Liebig-Universität Giessen
D-6300 Giessen, Federal Republic of Ger-
many

Gerda Schaude
The German Cancer Research Center
Institute of Biochemistry
D-6900 Heidelberg, Federal of Republic
of Germany

R. Schmidt
Institute of Biochemistry
German Cancer Research Center
D-6900 Heidelberg, Federal Republic of
Germany

R. Schulte-Hermann
Institute of Toxicology and Pharmacology
3350 Marburg, Federal Republic of Germany

J. Schuppler
Department of Toxicology
Schering 1000
Berlin 65, Federal Republic of Germany

Manfred Schwab
Genetisches Institut der Justus-Liebig-
Universität
D-6300 Giessen, Federal Republic of Ger-
many

Michael Schwarz
The German Cancer Research Centre
Institute of Biochemistry
D-6900 Heidelberg, Federal Republic of
Germany

Jürgen Schweizer
German Cancer Research Center
Institute of Experimental Pathology
6900 Heidelberg, Federal Republic of Germany

John D. Scribner
Pacific Northwest Research Foundation
Seattle, Washington 98104

Norma K. Scribner
Pacific Northwest Research Foundation
Seattle, Washington 98104

M. Šentjurc
J. Stefan Institute
E. Kardelj University of Ljubljana
61000 Ljubljana, Yugoslavia

Mohammed Shoyab
Laboratory of Viral Carcinogenesis
National Cancer Institute
Frederick, Maryland 21701

Alphonse E. Sirica
McArdle Laboratory for Cancer Research
Departments of Oncology and Pathology
The Medical School
University of Wisconsin
Madison, Wisconsin 53706

Thomas J. Slaga
Biology Division
Oak Ridge National Laboratory
Oak Ridge, Tennessee 37830

J. E. Smith
Departments of Radiology, Pathology, Bio-
chemistry, and Medicine
Cancer Center/Institute of Cancer Re-
search
Columbia University College of Physicians
and Surgeons
New York, New York 10032

J. R. Smythies
The Department of Psychiatry and The
Neurosciences Program
The University of Alabama in Birming-
ham
Birmingham, Alabama 35294

Virenda Solanki
Biology Division
Oak Ridge National Laboratory
Oak Ridge, Tennessee 37830

B. Sorg
Institute of Biochemistry
German Cancer Research Center
D-6900 Heidelberg 1, Federal Republic of
Germany

E. Staffeldt
Division of Biological and Medical Re-
search
Argonne National Laboratory
Argonne, Illinois 60439

Fred J. Stevens
Division of Biological and Medical Re-
search
Argonne National Laboratory
Argonne, Illinois 60439

Michael Stöhr
Institute of Experimental Pathology
German Cancer Research Center
D-6900 Heidelberg, Federal Republic of
Germany

Donna Stone
Department of Environmental Medicine
New York University Medical Center
New York, New York 10016

Takashi Sugimura
National Cancer Center Research Institute
Chuo-ku, Tokyo, Japan

Masae Tatematsu
First Department of Pathology
Nagoya City University Medical School
Nagoya 467, Japan

Henk Tennekes
The German Cancer Research Center
Institute of Biochemistry
D-6900 Heidelberg, Germany

M. Terada
National Cancer Center Research Institute
Tokyo 104, Japan

I. Timmermann-Trosiener
Institute of Toxicology und Pharmacology
Pilgrimstein 2
3350 Marburg, Federal Republic of Germany

George J. Todaro
Laboratory of Viral Carcinogenesis
National Cancer Institute
Frederick, Maryland 21701

Y. Toyama
Department of Anatomy
School of Medicine
University of Pennsylvania
Philadelphia, Pennsylvania 19104

Walter Troll
Department of Environmental Medicine
New York University Medical Center
New York, New York 10016

James E. Trosko
Department of Pediatrics and Human De-
velopment
Michigan State University
East Lansing, Michigan 48824

Hiroyuki Tsuda
First Department of Pathology
Nagoya City University Medical School
Nagoya 467, Japan

Gen Tsushimoto
Department of Pediatrics and Human De-
velopment
Michigan State University
East Lansing, Michigan 48824

K. Umezawa
National Cancer Center Research Institute
Tokyo 104, Japan

Ajit K. Verma
McArdle Laboratory for Cancer Research
University of Wisconsin
Madison, Wisconsin 53706

S. D. Vesselinovitch
Pathology and Radiology Departments
University of Chicago
Chicago, Illinois 60637

Klaus von der Mark
Max-Planck-Institut für Biochemie
Department of Connective Tissue Research
D-8033 Martinsried bei München, Federal
Republic of Germany

Stephan T. Warren
Department of Pediatrics and Human De-
velopment
Michigan State University
East Lansing, Michigan 48824

Charles E. Weeks
Biology Division
Oak Ridge National Laboratory
Oak Ridge, Tennessee 37830

Jane Weeks
McArdle Laboratory for Cancer Research
Departments of Oncology and Pathology
The Medical School
University of Wisconsin
Madison, Wisconsin 53706

I. Bernard Weinstein
Division of Environmental Sciences and
Cancer Center
Institute of Cancer Research and Depart-
ments of Medicine, Microbiology, and
Pathology
Columbia University
College of Physicians and Surgeons
New York, New York 10032

John H. Weisburger
American Health Foundation
Valhalla, New York 10595

Edmund J. Wendel
Laboratory of Viral Carcinogenesis
National Cancer Institute
Frederick Cancer Research Center
Frederick, Maryland 21701

P. W. Wertz
McArdle Laboratory for Cancer Research
University of Wisconsin
Madison, Wisconsin 53706

Gisela Witz
Department of Environmental and Com-
munity Medicine
Rutgers Medical School
Piscataway, New Jersey 08854

Ernst L. Wynder
American Health Foundation
Valhalla, New York 10595

Aniela Yakubowski
Section of Immunology
Department of Human Microbiology
Sackler School of Medicine
Tel-Aviv University
Ranat-Aviv, Tel-Aviv, Israel

N. Yamamoto
Institut für Virologia
Zentrum für Hygiene
7800 Freiburg, West Germany

Hiroshi Yamasaki
International Agency for Research on
Cancer
69372 Lyon Cédex 2, France

Larry P. Yotti
Department of Pediatrics and Human De-
velopment
Michigan State University
East Lansing, Michigan 48824

Stuart H. Yuspa
In Vitro Pathogenesis Section
Laboratory of Experimental Pathology
National Cancer Institute
Bethesda, Maryland 20205

S. Zayed
Institute of Biochemistry
German Cancer Research Center
D-6900 Heidelberg, Federal Republic of
Germany

Harald zur Hausen
Institut für Virologia
Zentrum für Hygiene
7800 Freiburg, West Germany

Carcinogenesis, Vol. 7, edited by E. Hecker et al.
Raven Press, New York © 1982.

Mouse Skin: A Useful Model System for Studying the Mechanism of Chemical Carcinogenesis

R. K. Boutwell, A. K. Verma, C. L. Ashendel, and Erle Astrup

McArdle Laboratory for Cancer Research, University of Wisconsin, Madison, Wisconsin 53706

MODEL SYSTEMS

The earliest written reports associating a causative agent with carcinogenesis allude to what we recognize as cocarcinogenesis and tumor promotion (6). Today, the generality of these phenomena is widely recognized and extensively studied. Excellent reviews of these two models for the experimental production of tumors exist (4,6,8,19,36,41).

The first of these models involves the concurrent application of agents, one of which is an effective solitary carcinogen, whereas the other agent is weakly or not carcinogenic when administered to mouse skin alone. If concurrent administration results in many tumors, the second agent is said to be a cocarcinogen. This model is properly named cocarcinogenesis and will be discussed in detail later (44).

The other model involves the sequential application of first, a single, essentially noncarcinogenic dose of a carcinogen, most commonly 7,12-dimethylbenz[a]anthracene (DMBA). It is followed by repetitive applications to the same area of skin of one of a number of unique agents, capable of eliciting many tumors in this regimen, but which causes only a few tumors when applied alone. The latter agents are called promoting agents and their definition is based strictly on the operational protocol just described. This protocol constitutes the two-stage, or initiation-promotion, model of tumor formation (5,6,19,41,44). The promotion stage has been further subdivided into two different components (40).

The two-stage protocol has provided an excellent model system to pursue studies on the mechanism of carcinogenesis. A very important component of these studies is the availability of pure phorbol esters that vary greatly in promoting activity as shown by Hecker and by Van Duuren (41). The most potent ester, 12-O-tetradecanoylphorbol-13-acetate (TPA), promotes tumors at levels of 0.5 to 10 nmole per application in a volume of 0.2 ml acetone and causes responses in cultured cells at levels as low as 5×10^{-10} M. For example, Perchellet and Boutwell found that TPA at 10^{-10} M increased the levels of both cyclic adenosine monophosphate (cyclic AMP) and guanosine monophosphate (cyclic GMP) in cultured mouse epidermal cells within 2 min (30).

The concept of tumor progression is not to be confused with the initiation and promotion procedure. Progression, as defined by Foulds (14), is not an operational term as are initiation and promotion. Rather, it is a theoretical concept that refers to the total development of a neoplasm from the first precancerous change in a cell that underlies the appearance of a tumor through the series of qualitative and independent changes in the many characters of the tumor during its life history, without regard to etiological agents. Therefore, the processes called initiation and promotion contribute to tumor progression.

A number of criteria have been established over the years that, if demonstrable, provide evidence that the two-stage mechanism is operative (5,6,19,26,34,41). These include: (a) Tumors should not develop, or do so only rarely, over the lifetime of animals treated with an initiator at only the low, initiating dose. (b) The promoting treatment, when given in appropriate doses, should cause only a few tumors after a long induction time. (c) An initiating treatment followed by the promoting regimen should result in very many tumors after a short induction time. (d) Treatment with the initiator and promoter in reverse order should cause no more tumors than either agent alone. (e) The effect of the initiator must be shown to be relatively irreversible by allowing a time interval (at least several months) to elapse between initiation and promotion. (f) In contrast, extended intervals between applications of the promoter should result in decreased tumor response. Some of these criteria are in the process of being explored in staged carcinogenesis of tumors in organs other than skin (19).

Examples of agents capable of accomplishing initiation include all agents that are carcinogenic for the skin when applied at appropriately low doses in a specified volume of a volatile solvent such as acetone. Polycyclic hydrocarbons, particularly DMBA, are commonly used. In addition, ultraviolet radiation (10) and ionizing radiation (37) have been shown to initiate mouse skin. It should be emphasized that skin carcinogenesis by a carcinogenic hydrocarbon (in the absence of a promoter) occurs only after application directly to the skin. In contrast, utilizing the initiation-promotion protocol, the hydrocarbon is capable of accomplishing initiation by intragastric or intraperitoneal routes followed by promoter application to the skin (5). Other examples include the following: Ritchie and Saffiotti (33) reported that orally administered 2-acetylaminofluorene, a liver carcinogen, acted as an initiator of skin tumors when fed to mice subsequently promoted with croton oil. This observation is of importance because neither lifetime feeding of 2-acetylaminofluorene nor skin application of it causes skin tumors. Likewise, lifetime skin application of urethan does not cause skin tumors in mice, yet intraperitoneal injection, skin application, or intragastric administration initiates skin so that skin tumors are elicited by a promoter (3). More recently, Goertler and Loehrke have reported that an initiator (either urethan or DMBA) administered to a pregnant mouse is effective transplacentally; application of TPA to the skin of the mice born of the treated mice elicits not only skin tumors at the site of application but also tumors of several internal organs (16). Promotion of tumors of internal organs by skin application of TPA is a very interesting development in the two-stage format, and further exploitation is important.

Therefore, a general theory to explain the initial event in chemical carcinogenesis is that all chemical carcinogens that are not electrophilic reactants must be converted metabolically into a chemically reactive electrophilic form, either by the skin itself or, if that is not possible, at some other site in the body after systemic administration (25). The chemically reactive ultimate carcinogen may then react with some critical macromolecule in the skin, presumably deoxyribonucleic acid (DNA), to initiate carcinogenesis (23,25). At higher doses that are carcinogenic after repetitive application, reaction with non-DNA chromatin components may occur and act to elicit the tumor phenotype. Skin carcinogenesis resulting from systemic administration of a carcinogen has not been accomplished, perhaps because a sufficient level of the carcinogen to elicit the tumor cell phenotype can not be achieved by remote administration. It is essential to recognize that, in general, initiating agents are carcinogenic for the skin at higher doses; to be properly called initiating, the dose should be sufficiently low that no pleiotypic response is observed (38,39). All agents that are carcinogenic for the skin act only as initiators at low doses that do not cause tumors; there are no exceptions known, but an exhaustive investigation of this issue has not been made. Thus the DNA repair and mutation fixation systems, as well as gene activation and inactivation, may be major determinants not only of initiation but also of skin carcinogenesis by repetitive exposure to a single carcinogenic agent. Many of the differences between carcinogens, initiators, and promoters are summarized in Table 1 (56).

The most effective tumor-promoting agent is TPA. There are many other phorbol esters having varying degrees of promoting, inflammatory, and irritating properties (19,41). Other specific compounds known to have promoting activity include iodoacetic acid, anthralin and a number of other phenols, *d*-limonene, certain fatty acid esters, and several surface active agents (5,6).

If the criteria for initiation and promotion are fulfilled, it may be concluded that the biological effects of the agents are qualitatively different and that studies to understand how tumors are elicited are simplified. For example, because initiation is irreversible and no pleiotypic response is observed (19,21,41), it is likely that the result of the process is an initiated cell that has the genotype of a tumor cell but the phenotype of a normal cell and that, therefore, is not a dormant tumor cell (5). This possibility is strengthened by the fact that more than the stimulation of cell division is required to elicit tumors (24,32); in contrast, stimulation of proliferation is sufficient to elicit visible tumors from dormant tumor cells (11). Specific unknown mechanisms are responsible for promotion.

It is important to recognize, however, that lifetime treatment of mouse skin with promoting doses of TPA, the most commonly used tumor promoter, causes

TABLE 1. *A comparison of the biological properties of carcinogens, initiators, and promoters*

Carcinogens	Initiators	Promoters
1. Carcinogenic at higher levels; initiate at lower levels	1. Initiate at lower levels; carcinogenic at higher levels	1. Cause few tumors after prolonged treatment
2. More than one agent generally additive, regardless of order	2. To obtain synergism, initiator must precede promoter	2. To obtain synergism, promoter must follow initiator
3. Very large single exposure, but generally long continued exposure	3. Single, very small exposure adequate	3. Repeated exposure essential
4. Partially reversible	4. Irreversible	4. Effect is reversible if application intervals prolonged or in uninitiated cells
5. Individual doses additive	5. Additive even at subthreshold doses	5. A threshold exists
6. Electrophilic or metabolized to electrophiles; react with nucleophiles	6. Electrophiles or metabolized to electrophiles; react with nucleophiles	6. Need not be an electrophile (phorbol esters: no covalent reactions)
7. Mutagenic or metabolized to mutagen	7. Mutagenic or metabolized to mutagen	7. Not mutagenic
8. Alter gene expression: hyperplasia, enzyme induction	8. Do not alter gene expression at low, initiating dose; no altered morphology detectable	8. Alter gene expression: hyperplasia, enzyme induction, inhibit maturation, and eliminates metabolic cooperation
9. Many biochemical responses	9. DNA binding and resultant repair are detectable responses	9. Many biochemical responses

both benign and malignant tumors to appear in the absence of intentional exposure to a carcinogen (1,5,7,43). Thus the promoter may be regarded as a weak carcinogen, as emphasized by Astrup et al. (1). Even so, this fact does not detract from the value of the model. The tumor response in the mice that were both initiated and promoted is not attributable to a mere additive effect of two weak carcinogenic stimuli; rather it is a remarkable synergism. A synergism is *ipso facto* evidence that independent, qualitatively different mechanisms are involved. A likely explanation for the tumors resulting from treatment with the phorbol ester only is provided by Van Duuren (43) and Prehn (31). Spontaneous tumors occur, and one must assume that these must be preceded by latent tumors cells whose appearance would be hastened by phorbol ester treatment. Spontaneous transformation occurs in cells in culture. It is generally recognized that hereditarily stable variant cells of spontaneous origin exist in the tissues of animals, and it is to be expected that some of these may reveal themselves as tumors after phorbol ester treatment. In addition, it is impossible for living organisms to escape exposure to low levels of carcinogens which may cause initiation. For example, carcinogenic hydrocarbons, ionizing radiation, mold products, and carcinogenic plant tissue components are ubiquitous, and nitrosamines are formed within the intestinal tract. Thus one might employ tumor promoters to assay for the background level of initiation.

One factor contributing to skepticism about the validity of the two-stage mechanism for skin tumor formation is that the phenomenon appeared to be unique to mouse skin. Goerttler and co-workers reported, however, that both rats and hamsters do respond to the two-stage regimen (17,18) and that TPA effectively promotes tumor formation in tissues other than skin (16,19).

MODIFIERS OF CHEMICAL CARCINOGENESIS

Although, in so far as is known, all promoting agents are capable of acting as cocarcinogens, Van Duuren (41,43,44,45) has reported specific examples of agents capable of cocarcinogenic action but that show no promoting activity. Thus, not only is there a distinct operational difference between the two model systems, but there is, in many cases, a clear mechanistic difference as well. For example, cocarcinogens may modify the response to chemical carcinogens by facilitating metabolic activation of the carcinogen or by altering DNA repair mechanisms, whereas promoters may function by inducing cells to acquire some of the characteristics of the tumor cell phenotype (6). To quote from Van Duuren: "In cocarcinogenesis experiments on mouse skin, two agents are administered simultaneously and repeatedly and result in significantly higher tumor incidences than the carcinogen alone. The cocarcinogen is usually noncarcinogenic when applied alone. Thus there is an operational difference, and most likely a real difference in mode of action" between tumor promoters, which act when applied subsequent to the initiating agent, and cocarcinogens. "Hence the terms promoter and cocarcinogen should not be used interchangeably (45)."

Examples of compounds with cocarcinogenic activity when applied to mouse skin concurrently with benzo[a]pyrene include catechol, pyrogallol, decane, undecane, pyrene, benzo[e]pyrene, and fluoranthene. Examples of inhibitors when applied concurrently with benzo[a]pyrene (anticarcinogens) include (each of these inhibited completely) esculin, quercetin, squalene, and oleic acid; those that inhibited partially include phenol, eugenol, resorcinol, hydroquinose, and hexadecane. Of these compounds, 6 were tested for tumor promotion in the two-stage protocol, and Van Duuren reported that no correlation existed between the two activities.

In the case of human exposures, no generalization can be made with respect to mode of exposure. It is likely that people are exposed to carcinogens concurrently with other carcinogens, promoting agents, cocarcinogens, and anticarcinogens, as exemplified by the case of tobacco smoke (45). Perhaps endogenous hormones may be regarded as promoters working together with low levels of environmental carcinogens to facilitate the development of certain human cancers. Examples might include epidermal growth factor (35), estrogens, and other hormones causing a pleiotypic response. The exposure to agents in the well-defined, sequential manner of the initiation-promotion protocol may be rare in human beings.

THEORIES OF SKIN CARCINOGENESIS

As with all protocols to produce experimental cancer, be it liver cancer caused by aromatic amines (25) or skin cancer caused by repeated skin paintings with hydrocarbons (20), the two-stage system has given rise to a number of theoretical concepts. The terms used to describe the two stages have theoretical implications; that is, initiation starts a process that is brought to fruition by promotion. In any case, the fact that skin carcinogenesis is divisible into two, qualitatively different components has been particularly fruitful in facilitating the study of the mechanism of carcinogenesis and in formulating hypotheses. Because initiation can be accomplished by very low doses of alkylating agents (electrophiles) or agents capable of being metabolized to electrophiles, it is reasonable that an interaction with epidermal macromolecules occurs. Because of the irreversible nature of initiation, it is theorized that the critical macromolecular target is DNA. In contrast, the promoting agents cause a whole cascade of pleiotypic responses including increased turnover of phosphatidyl choline, increased synthesis of prostaglandins, and induction of ornithine decarboxylase, as well as the more general indicators of gene activation, namely increased ribonucleic acid (RNA), protein, and DNA synthesis followed by cell division (6,19,41). All of these correlate with tumor formation, and this is emphasized by the fact that agents blocking certain of the responses also block tumor formation. This has led to the formulation of the following theory to explain carcinogenesis. The promoting agent causes the epidermis to mimic tumor cells in a reversible manner. In those cells that have been previously initiated, however, it is hypothesized that the tumor cell phenotype resulting from the action of the promoter is not reversible due to the deletion of a regulatory gene in the initiated cell. Thus, according to this theory, the initiated cell is qualitatively different from the normal cells in its response to the promoting stimulus. For example, if the control mechanism that is responsible for the rapid decline in ornithine decarboxylase is lost, that aspect of the tumor cell phenotype will remain permanent (29). Although the effect of tumor promoters is reversible in normal tissue, the effect may not be reversible in a very few cells of initiated mice that have acquired the proposed genetic defect, since only 6 weeks of promoter treatment will elicit carcinomas in 15% of the mice 44 weeks after cessation of promotion (47). Most all tumors, whether spontaneous, of viral origin, chemically induced, or resulting from radiation, show elevated ornithine decarboxylase activity, and all of the promoting agents induce ornithine decarboxylase activity in normal tissue. Ornithine decarboxylase is the rate-limiting enzyme for the synthesis of the polyamines putrescine, spermidine, and spermine. These amines function in the control of DNA, RNA, and protein synthesis and appear to play a decisive role in cell division (15) and possibly cell maturation (58).

There is evidence that elevated polyamines are essential, but not sufficient, for tumor promotion; additional changes are also essential (22,27,54). Berenblum, in 1954, theorized that promoting action is essentially a process of delayed maturation, thereby allowing a sufficient number of undifferentiated daughter cells to accumulate so that a critical size colony is formed (2). Support for this theory is beginning to appear; TPA has been found to control differentiation, and hypotheses based on altered cell differentiation have been proposed recently by several investigators (8). Thus, promotion may involve at least two components: an inhibition of maturation of the basal cells, plus their increased proliferation. Both may be accounted for by increased levels of polyamines, a phenotypic characteristic that may be locked-in in those cells in which a regulatory gene(s) for this characteristic is lost.

Implicit in this theory is the concept that the keratinocyte is autonomous and that the host plays no role in epithelial carcinogenesis via the dermis, growth regulators originating in other tissues, or immune mechanisms. The role of factors originating outside the epidermis may be identified by studies utilizing *in vitro* systems in which the nature and level of exogenous factors may be controlled (19,41).

There are other properties of TPA that may be important to its mechanism of action. Normal cells are capable of exchanging essential nutrients by a phenomenon called metabolic cooperation. There is convincing evidence that metabolic cooperation is eliminated by TPA, and it is possible that this is an important component of the mechanism of tumor promotion (12,57). For example, if a regulatory gene product were deleted as a result of initiation, that product could be obtained by the defective cells via metabolic cooperation with neighboring competent (uninitiated) cells. However, the irreversible defect would be manifest by elimination of metabolic cooperation. Finally, it has been suggested that the formation of dark cells is a TPA-specific component of tumor promotion (22).

An extensive study of inhibitors of carcinogenesis has been done by Wattenberg (53). Because many of the agents tested are naturally occurring and because some of the inhibitors were shown to be inducers of hydrocarbon-metabolizing enzymes, it is important to extend this approach to skin systems and to investigate relevance to human cancer. For example, 7,8-benzoflavone applied to the skin of mice 30 min before a single carcinogenic dose of 3.6 μmole of DMBA completely prevented tumor formation (49). Because of the impossibility of complete elimination of carcinogens from the human environment, research emphasis on inhibitors of carcinogenesis including application to human beings should be given very high priority.

As pointed out earlier, TPA causes a pleiotypic response which includes early, reversible increases in several cellular components (21). Of these, two are of particular interest. The early increase in the prostaglandin E_1 (PGE_1) level in the epidermis is blocked by indomethacin. Indomethacin also blocks the induction of ornithine decarboxylase activity and tumor promotion, linking these two biochemical changes to the mechanism of tumor promotion by TPA (46). Further evidence linking a permanently elevated level of ornithine decarboxylase activity to the mechanism of promotion comes from the use of putrescine as an effective blocking agent for the induction of ornithine decarboxylase. Thus, since putrescine is rapidly cleared from mouse skin (28) and the induction of the enzyme is prevented by putrescine (54), a permanently increased level of the enzyme and its product putrescine was precluded by application of putrescine to the skin, 1 hr after TPA application. Therefore, inhibition of tumor formation by putrescine is not contradictory to the proposal that permanently elevated levels are essential to tumor formation. With this protocol in a tumor induction experiment, putrescine inhibited tumor promotion (54).

Yet another example of a regimen inhibiting both tumor formation and ornithine decarboxylase activity and the resultant elevation of polyamine levels arises from experiments utilizing retinoic acid. Thus, retinoic acid treatment of the skin at the site of TPA application in doses between 1.7 and 34 nmole inhibits both the induction of ornithine decarboxylase activity and tumor formation. The inhibition is almost complete at the high dose. The time of application of retinoic acid is critical; it must be within 1 hr before or after application of TPA to obtain maximum inhibition of both tumor formation and ornithine decarboxylase activity. Because such small doses of retinoic acid are quickly cleared from the skin, application of retinoic acid 24 hr or more before application of the tumor promoter has no inhibitory effect on tumor formation (52). At this time, there is no elevated ornithine decarboxylase activity to be blocked by retinoic acid, suggesting that retinoic acid is not acting through some mechanism other than inhibition of the induction of ornithine decarboxylase to accomplish tumor inhibition. Furthermore, there is a close correlation in the ability of about 30 different retinoid derivatives to inhibit ornithine decarboxylase activity and tumor formation (51). Finally, the fact that indomethacin and retinoic acid act synergistically to inhibit ornithine decarboxylase activity and tumor formation provides evidence that these agents act independently at different sites in the induction of ornithine decarboxylase. Because retinoids are known to maintain normal maturation of skin keratinocytes (42), this action, too, may contribute to the prophylactic action of retinoids, perhaps by maintaining polyamines at low levels (48).

In contrast to the dramatic inhibition of tumor promotion by retinoic acid, no evidence was found for interference with the initiating process (48). Possibilities included alteration of the metabolic activation of the carcinogen, interference with the interaction of the carcinogen metabolites with macromolecules, altered DNA repair, and a selective effect on initiated cells. It is concluded that retinoic acid exerts its prophylactic effect by interference with promotion by the phorbol ester.

Caution in the extrapolation of the prophylactic effect of retinoids is indicated by other studies, however. The first suggestion for caution arose from a report by Epstein (9), which was confirmed by Forbes et al. (13). In these studies, retinoic acid-treated mice that were exposed to ultraviolet light developed more skin tumors than the controls that were treated only with ultraviolet light. Moreover, retinoic acid applied to the skin of mice in conjunction with a carcinogenic regimen consisting of multiple applications of dimethylbenzanthracene did not inhibit tumor formation, but rather resulted in a small increment in tumors. The reality of this observation is emphasized by its repeatability and by the fact that the effect of retinoic acid was tested on tumor promotion and on complete carcinogenesis concurrently, so that the experiment was internally controlled; the dose of retinoic acid was the same, dispensed from the same solution (19,49). Thus, retinoic acid inhibits the promotion of skin tumors in the initiation-promotion regimen but may not with the repetitive applications of dimethylbenzanthracene and with photocarcinogenesis.

SUMMARY

Mouse skin has a long history as a useful model for the study of the mechanism of carcinogenesis (6). In particular, the availability of specific diterpene esters has made possible rapid progress in understanding the mechanism of tumor formation (4,6,8,19,36,41), although certain details may be unique to promotion by phorbol esters. Evidence is compatible with an essential role for elevated levels of polyamines in tumor promotion, but other components of phorbol ester action on mouse skin are also essential (27,40,54). These may include the production of dark cells (22), inhibition of maturation (2,19,41), and the elimination of metabolic cooperation (12,57). Factors modifying biochemical processes that are essential to tumor formation produce a parallel effect on tumor formation. Some of these inhibitors act synergistically to inhibit tumor formation (50,55), and knowledge of their action may lead to practical application for the prevention of human cancer.

REFERENCES

1. Astrup, E. G., Iversen, O. H., and Elgjo, K. (1980): The tumorigenic and carcinogenic effect of TPA (12-O-tetradecanoylphorbol-13-acetate) when applied to the skin of BALB/cA mice. *Virchows Arch. B.*, 33:303–304.
2. Berenblum, I. (1954): A speculative review: The probable nature of promoting action and its significance in the understanding of the mechanism of carcinogenesis. *Cancer Res.*, 14:471–477.
3. Berenblum, I., and Haran-Ghera, N. (1957): A quantitative study of the systemic initiating action of urethane (ethyl carbamate) in mouse skin carcinogenesis. *Br. J. Cancer*, 11:77–84.
4. Blumberg, P. M. (1980): *In vitro* studies on the mode of action of the phorbol esters, potent tumor promoters: Part I. *CRC Crit. Rev. Toxicol.*, 8:153–197.
5. Boutwell, R. K. (1964): Some biological aspects of skin carcinogenesis. *Prog. Exp. Tumor Res.*, 4:207–250.
6. Boutwell, R. K. (1974): The function and mechanism of promoters of carcinogenesis. *CRC Crit. Rev. Toxicol.*, 2:419–443.
7. Chouroulinkov, I., and Lazar, P. (1974): Actions cancerogene et cocancerogene du 12-O-tetradecanoylphorbol-13-acetate (TPA) sur la peau de souris. *C.R. Acad. Sci. Pris.*, ser. D., 278:3,027–3,030.
8. Diamond, L., O'Brien, T. G., and Baird, W. M. (1980): Tumor promoters and the mechanism of tumor promotion. *Adv. Cancer Res.*, 32:1–74.
9. Epstein, J. H. (1977): Chemicals and photocarcinogenesis. *Australas. J. Dermatol.*, 18:57–61.
10. Epstein, J. H., and Roth, H. L. (1968): Experimental ultraviolet light carcinogenesis. *J. Invest. Dermatol.*, 50:387–389.
11. Fisher, B., and Fisher, E. R. (1959): Experimental evidence in support of the dormant tumor cell. *Science*, 130:918–919.
12. Fitzgerald, D. J., and Murray, A. W. (1980): Inhibition of intercellular communication by tumor-promoting phorbol esters. *Cancer Res.*, 40:2,935–2,937.
13. Forbes, P. D., Urbach, F., and Davies, R. E. (1979): Enhancement of experimental photocarcinogenesis by topical retinoic acid. *Cancer Lett.*, 7:85–90.
14. Foulds, L. (1954): The experimental study of tumor progression: A review. *Cancer Res.*, 14:327–339.
15. Gaugas, J. M., editor (1980): *Polyamines in Biomedical Research.* John Wiley and Sons, New York.
16. Goerttler, K., and Loehrke, H. (1977): Diaplacental carcinogenesis: Tumor localization and tumor incidence in NMRI-mice after diaplacental initiation with DMBA and urethane and postnatal promotion with the phorbol ester TPA in a modified 2-stage Berenblum/Mottram experiment. *Virchows Arch. (Pathol. Anat.)*, 376:117–122.
17. Goerttler, K., Loehrke, H., Schweizer, J., and Hesse, B. (1980a): Positive two-stage carcinogenesis in female Sprague-Dawley rats using 7,12-dimethylbenz[a]anthracene (DMBA) as initiator and 12-O-tetradecanoylphorbol-13-acetate (TPA) as promoter. *Virchows Arch. (Pathol. Anat.)*, 385:181–186.
18. Goerttler, K., Loehrke, H., Schweizer, J., and Hesse, B. (1980b): Two-stage tumorigenesis of dermal melanocytes in the back skin of the Syrian golden hamster using systemic initiation with 7,12-dimethylbenz[a]anthracene and topical promotion with 12-O-tetradecanoylphorbol-13-acetate. *Cancer Res.*, 40:155–161.
19. Hecker, E. H., Fusenig, N. E., Kunz, W., and Marks, F., editors (1981): *Carcinogenesis, A Comprehensive Survey*, vol. 7. Raven Press, New York.
20. Heidelberger, C. (1964): Studies on the molecular mechanism of hydrocarbon carcinogenesis. *J. Cell Comp. Physiol.*, 64:129–148.
21. Hershko, A. V., Mamont, P., Shields, R., and Tomkins, G. M. (1971): Pleiotypic response. *Nature New Biol.*, 232:206–211.

22. Klein-Szanto, A. J. P., Major, S. K., and Slaga, T. J. (1980): Induction of dark keratinocytes by 12-O-tetradecanoylphorbol-13-acetate and mezerein as an indicator of tumor-promoting efficiency. *Carcinogenesis*, 1:399–406.
23. Lawley, P. D. (1980): DNA as a target of alkylating carcinogens. *Br. Med. Bull.*, 36:19–24.
24. Marks, F. (1976): Epidermal growth control mechanisms, hyperplasia, and tumor promotion in the skin. *Cancer Res.*, 36:2,636–2,643.
25. Miller, J. A., and Miller, E. C. (1976): The metabolism of chemical carcinogens to reactive electrophiles and their possible mechanisms of action in carcinogenesis. In: *Chemical Carcinogens*, edited by C. E. Searle, pp. 737–762. American Chemical Society Monograph 173.
26. Mottram, J. C. (1944): A developing factor in experimental blastogenesis. *J. Pathol. Bacteriol.*, 56:181–187.
27. Mufson, R. A., Fischer, S. M., Verma, A. K., Gleason, G. L., Slaga, T. J., and Boutwell, R. K. (1979): Effects of 12-O-tetradecanoylphorbol-13-acetate and mezerein on epidermal ornithine decarboxylase activity, isoproterenol-stimulated levels of cyclic adenosine 3'5'-monophosphate, and induction of mouse skin tumors *in vivo*. *Cancer Res.*, 39:4,791–4,795.
28. O'Brien, T. G. (1976): The induction of ornithine decarboxylase as an early, possibly obligatory, event in mouse skin carcinogenesis. *Cancer Res.*, 36:2,644–2,653.
29. O'Brien, T. G., Simsiman, R. C., and Boutwell, R. K. (1975): Induction of the polyamine-biosynthetic enzymes in mouse epidermis and their specificity for tumor promotion. *Cancer Res.*, 35:2,426–2,433.
30. Perchellet, J.-P., and Boutwell, R. K. (1980): Enhancement by 3-isobutyl-1-methylxanthine and cholera toxin of 12-O-tetradecanoylphorbol-13-acetate-stimulated cyclic nucleotide levels and ornithine decarboxylase activity in isolated epidermal cells. *Cancer Res.*, 40:2,653–2,660.
31. Prehn, R. T. (1964): A clonal selection theory of chemical carcinogenesis. *J. Natl. Cancer Inst.*, 32:1–17.
32. Raick, A. N. (1974): Cell differentiation and tumor-promoting action in skin carcinogenesis. *Cancer Res.*, 34:2,915–2,925.
33. Ritchie, A. C., and Saffiotti, U. (1955): Orally administered 2-acetylaminofluorene as an initiator and as a promoter in epidermal carcinogenesis in the mouse. *Cancer Res.*, 15:84–88.
34. Roe, F. J. C. (1959): The effect of applying croton oil before a single application of 9,10-dimethyl-1,2-benzanthracene (DMBA). *Br. J. Cancer*, 13:87–91.
35. Rose, S. P., Stahn, R., Passovoy, D. S., and Herschman, H. (1976): Epidermal growth factor enhancement of skin tumor induction in mice. *Experientia*, 32:913–915.
36. Scribner, J. D., and Süss, R. (1978): Tumor initiation and promotion. *Int. Rev. Exp. Pathol.*, 18:138–198.
• 37. Shubik, P., Goldfarb, A. R., Ritchie, A. C., and Lisco, H. (1953): Latent carcinogenic action of beta-irradiation on mouse epidermis. *Nature* (Lond.), 171:934–936.
38. Slaga, T. J., Bowden, G. T., Shapas, B. G., and Boutwell, R. K. (1973): Macromolecular synthesis following a single application of alkylating agents used as initiators of mouse skin tumorigenesis. *Cancer Res.*, 30:769–776.
39. Slaga, T. J., Bowden, G. T., Shapas, B. G., and Boutwell, R. K. (1974): Macromolecular synthesis following a single application of polycyclic hydrocarbons used as initiators of mouse skin tumorigenesis. *Cancer Res.*, 34:771–777.
40. Slaga, T. J., Fischer, S. M., Nelson, K., and Gleason, G. L. (1980): Studies on the mechanism of skin tumor promotion: Evidence for several stages in promotion. *Proc. Natl. Acad. Sci. USA*, 77:3,659–3,663.
41. Slaga, T. J., Sivak, A., and Boutwell, R. K., editors (1978): *Carcinogenesis, A Comprehensive Survey, Vol. 2: Mechanisms of Tumor Promotion and Cocarcinogenesis*. Raven Press, New York.
42. Sporn, M. B., Dunlop, N. M., Newton, D. L., and Smith, J. M. (1976): Prevention of chemical carcinogenesis by vitamin A and its synthetic analogs (retinoids). *Fed. Proc.*, 35:1,332–1,338.
43. Van Duuren, B. L. (1969): Tumor-promoting agents in two-stage carcinogenesis. *Prog. Exp. Tumor Res.*, 11:31–68.
44. Van Duuren, B. L. (1976): Tumor-promoting and cocarcinogenic agents in chemical carcinogenesis. In: *Chemical Carcinogens*, edited by C. E. Searle, pp. 24–51. American Chemical Society, Monograph 173.
45. Van Duuren, B. L., and Goldschmidt, B. M. (1976): Cocarcinogenic and tumor-promoting agents in tobacco carcinogenesis. *J. Natl. Cancer Inst.*, 56:1,237–1,242.
46. Verma, A. K., Ashendel, C. L., and Boutwell, R. K. (1980): Inhibition by prostaglandin synthesis

inhibitors of the induction of epidermal ornithine decarboxylase activity, the accumulation of prostaglandins, and tumor promotion caused by 12-O-tetradecanoylphorbol-13-acetate. *Cancer Res.,* 40:308–315.

47. Verma, A. K., and Boutwell, R. K. (1980*a*): Effect of dose and duration of treatment with the tumor-promoting agent 12-O-tetradecanoylphorbol-13-acetate on mouse skin carcinogenesis. *Carcinogenesis,* 1:271–276.

48. Verma, A. K., and Boutwell, R. K. (1980*b*): Inhibition of tumor promoter-induced mouse epidermal ornithine decarboxylase activity and prevention of skin carcinogenesis by vitamin A acid and its analogs (retinoids). In: *Polyamines in Biomedical Research,* edited by J. M. Gaugas. John Wiley and Sons, Chichester.

49. Verma, A. K., Conrad, E. A., and Boutwell, R. K. (1980*a*): Induction of mouse epidermal ornithine decarboxylase activity and skin tumors by 7,12-dimethylbenz[a]anthracene: Modulation by retinoic acid and 7,8-benzoflavone. *Carcinogenesis,* 1:607–611.

50. Verma, A. K., Conrad, E. A., and Boutwell, R. K. (1980*b*): Inhibition of mouse skin carcinogenesis by a retinoid, steroid, and protease inhibitor. *Proc. Am. Assoc. Cancer Res.,* 21:93.

51. Verma, A. K., Rice, H. M., Shapas, B. G., and Boutwell, R. K. (1978): Inhibition of 12-O-tetradecanoylphorbol-13-acetate-induced ornithine decarboxylase activity in mouse epidermis by vitamin A analogs (retinoids). *Cancer Res.,* 38:793–801.

52. Verma, A. K., Shapas, B. G., Rice, H. M., and Boutwell, R. K. (1979): Correlation of the inhibition by retinoids of tumor promoter-induced ornithine decarboxylase activity and of skin tumor promotion. *Cancer Res.,* 39:419–425.

53. Wattenberg, L. W. (1978): Inhibitors of chemical carcinogenesis. *Adv. Cancer Res.,* 26:197–226.

54. Weekes, R. G., Verma, A. K., and Boutwell, R. K. (1980): Inhibition by putrescine of epidermal ornithine decarboxylase activity and tumor promotion caused by 12-O-tetradecanoylphorbol-13-acetate. *Cancer Res.,* 40:4,013–4,018.

55. Weeks, C. E., Slaga, T. J., Hennings, H., Gleason, G. L., and Bracken, W. M. (1979): Inhibition of phorbol ester-induced tumor promotion in mice by vitamin A analog and anti-inflammatory steroid. *J. Natl. Cancer Inst.,* 63:401–406.

56. Weinstein, I. B., Lee, L.-S., Fisher, P. B., Mufson, A., and Yamasaki, H. (1979): Action of phorbol esters in cell culture: Mimicry of transformation, altered differentiation, and effects on cell membranes. *J. Supramol. Struct.,* 12:195–208.

57. Yotti, L. P., Chang, C. C., and Trosko, J. E. (1979): Elimination of metabolic cooperation in Chinese hamster cells by a tumor promoter. *Science,* 206:1,089–1,091.

58. Younglai, E. V., Godeau, F., Mester, J., and Baulieu, E. E. (1980): Increased ornithine decarboxylase activity during meiotic maturation in *Xenopus laevis* oocytes. *Biochem. Biophys. Res. Comm.,* 96:1,274–1,281.

Carcinogenesis, Vol. 7, edited by E. Hecker et al.
Raven Press, New York © 1982.

Is the Initiation-Promotion Regimen in Mouse Skin Relevant to Complete Carcinogenesis?

John D. Scribner and Norma K. Scribner

Pacific Northwest Research Foundation, Seattle, Washington 98104

Since the acceptance of initiation and promotion as a valid experimental model for tumor induction in a variety of tissues, the pendulum of opinion in carcinogenesis research has swung in the direction of considering all complete carcinogenesis by pure compounds to consist of a combination of initiation and promotion. In fact, this assumption had never been confirmed by experiment before our publication showing that the weak tumor initiator (0.001 times as potent as 7,12-dimethylbenzanthracene) 7-bromomethylbenz[a]anthracene (BMBA) can promote papillomas initiated by dimethylbenzanthracene (DMBA) (2). In this chapter we show that certain complete carcinogens lack promoting activity and present evidence that cancer induction in mouse skin is not a consequence of promotion.

In our initial report we showed that 90 nmole of BMBA applied twice weekly to the backs of female SENCAR mice initiated with 25 μg of DMBA gave a mean latent period for papilloma induction of 9 weeks, with a maximum average of 10 papillomas/mouse. More recently, we found that 90 nmole of BMBA given once a week produced tumors with a latent period of 10 weeks, with a maximum of 15 tumors/mouse (Fig. 1). Administration once every 2 weeks still resulted in a latent period of only 15 weeks and a maximum of 14 tumors/mouse. Thus, at an average weekly dose of 45 nmole, BMBA promoted papillomas with a relatively short latent period and in high yield. This dose compares favorably with the maximum tolerated dose of 12-O-tetradecanoylphorbol-13-acetate (TPA) in CD-1 mice, about 35 nmole/week. Dose-response experiments now in progress should enable an accurate comparison of potencies between the two agents.

We also showed in our earlier work that dibenz[a,c]anthracene (DBA) is as active an initiator as BMBA, but lacks promoting activity at a level of 180 nmole/week. Thus, a total of 6.7 μmole failed to produce any tumors by 1 year after the beginning of application. On the other hand, promotion by TPA beginning after cessation of DBA treatment (37 weeks after beginning) yielded eight papillomas/mouse, a figure not significantly different from the expected value (6.7) based on the tumor yield in a second group that had received a single dose of 2.5 μmole DBA, followed by TPA promotion begun after the 37-week resting period (Fig. 2). This experiment demonstrates that the effect

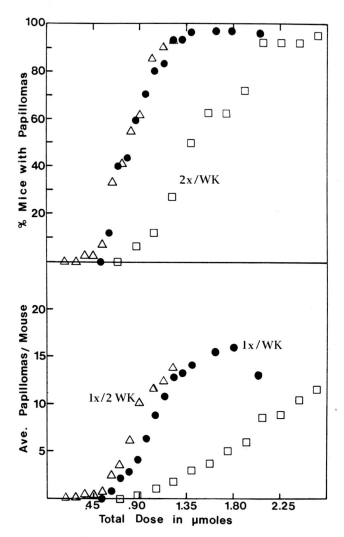

FIG. 1. Female SENCAR mice were obtained from the Carcinogenesis and Toxicology Program, Oak Ridge National Laboratory, at 6 weeks of age. At 8 weeks of age they were shaved. Animals showing no hair regrowth 2 days later were treated topically with 25 μg DMBA in 0.2 ml of acetone. Groups of 30 mice were treated topically with 90 nmole of BMBA in 0.2 ml of acetone beginning 1 week later, according to the regimen indicated in the figure.

of DBA is initiating only, and additive only. It may thus be called a pure initiator. Lijinsky, Garcia, and Saffiotti have shown, however, that a total dose of 40 μmole of DBA led to carcinomas in 50% of surviving mice, mice that were likely less sensitive than the SENCAR mice (1). Their weekly dose (611 nmole) was only three times the dose given in our experiment. Thus, there

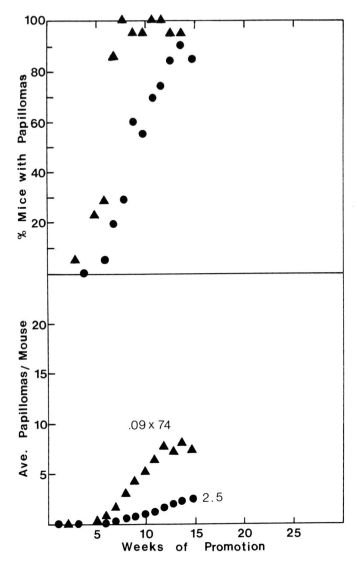

FIG. 2. Mice obtained and shaved as described in Fig. 1 were treated either with a single dose of 2.5 μmole DBA in 0.2 ml acetone (28 mice) or with 90 nmoles DBA in 0.2 ml acetone twice weekly beginning 1 week later (28 mice). Treatment of both groups with 2 μg TPA twice weekly in 0.2 ml acetone was begun after the second group had been treated for 37 weeks. One cage of 7 mice in the second group was not treated with TPA, and had developed no tumors when the experiment was terminated. Eighteen mice (of 21 originally) were still alive in the promoted group when the experiment was terminated.

seems to be strong evidence that DBA is a pure initiator which can produce cancer.

We have chosen a more potent initiator to determine whether or not promotion is required for carcinogenesis. 3-Methylcholanthrene (MC) initiation is reduced by dexamethasone, but its complete carcinogenicity is affected by dexamethasone to an extent that can be accounted for wholly by the reduction in initiating

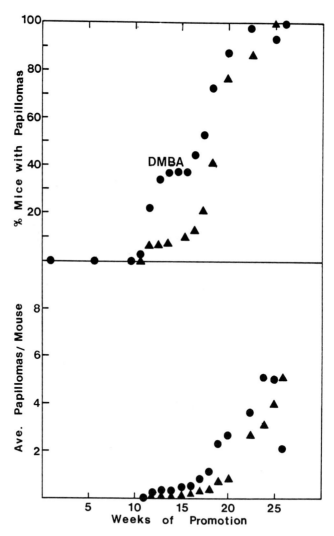

FIG. 3. Mice obtained and shaved as described in Fig. 1 were divided into two groups of 30. Two days after shaving, one group was treated with 25 μg of DMBA in 0.2 ml acetone. Both groups were treated with 90 nmole of MC in 0.2 ml acetone twice weekly, beginning 1 week after the DMBA treatment. (●): Treated with DMBA.

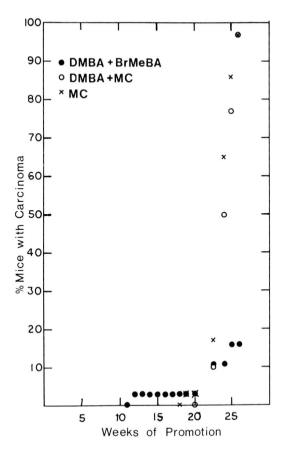

FIG. 4. As in Fig. 3, including a third group treated with a single dose of 25 μg DMBA in 0.2 ml acetone, followed by 90 nmole of BMBA in 0.2 ml acetone applied twice weekly. (●): DMBA + BrMeBA (BMBA). (O): DMBA + MC. (X): MC.

effects (3). This suggested that it should lack promoting activity when tested directly in a two-stage regimen. Figure 3 shows that, at a dose of 90 nmole two times per week, MC promoted papillomas in no more than 35% of the initiated mice, while without DMBA initiation, MC-induced papillomas appeared with a mean latent period of 19 weeks. Thus, this compound, which is 100 times more powerful than BMBA as an initiator, has minimal promoting activity, and induces papillomas with the same total dose as BMBA (2). In Fig. 4 we see the remarkable result that there is no difference at all between initiated and uninitiated mice in the rate at which MC induces cancer. Further, we see that the promoting compound BMBA lags in carcinoma induction, with an eventual mean latent period of 35 weeks (not shown). Thus, while promoting ability can compensate for low initiating activity in the induction of benign tumors, cancer induction clearly follows primarily as a consequence of initiating action. This conclusion agrees with the data obtained for DBA.

Further support for this position follows from the observation that, while the number of papillomas obtained from BMBA promotion is at least twice as high as that eventually obtained by BMBA or MC treatment without DMBA initiation, this is unrelated to the latent period of cancer induction, or the number of carcinomas seen. This result directly suggests that carcinomas do not arise as a direct consequence of promotion of papillomas. Indeed, it suggests that papillomas produced by the true two-step procedure are a form of differentiation in a direction other than toward cancer formation.

Thus, we conclude that cancer induction in mouse skin can be achieved without promotion of the type represented by TPA, and that it proceeds on a different developmental pathway from papillomas produced by a single dose of initiator followed by promotion. Further experiments at all levels of biology and chemistry are required to confirm this hypothesis, which may be crucial for understanding initiation and promotion in all experimental systems.

REFERENCES

1. Lijinsky, W., Garcia, H., and Saffiotti, U. (1970): Structure-activity relationships among some polynuclear hydrocarbons and their hydrogenated derivatives. *J. Natl. Cancer Inst.,* 44:641–649.
2. Scribner, N. K., and Scribner, J. D. (1980): Separation of initiating and promoting effects of the skin carcinogen 7-bromomethylbenz[a]anthracene. *Carcinogenesis,* 1:97–100.
3. Slaga, T. J., and Scribner, J. D. (1973): Inhibition of tumor initiation and promotion by antiinflammatory agents. *J. Natl. Cancer Inst.,* 51:1,723–1,725.

Carcinogenesis, Vol. 7, edited by E. Hecker et al.
Raven Press, New York © 1982.

Specificity and Mechanism(s) of Promoter Inhibitors in Multistage Promotion

T. J. Slaga, S. M. Fischer, C. E. Weeks, K. Nelson, M. Mamrack, and A. J. P. Klein-Szanto

Biology Division, Oak Ridge National Laboratory, Oak Ridge, Tennessee 37830

One of the best-studied models of multistep chemical carcinogenesis is the mouse skin system. Skin tumors can be induced by the sequential application of a subthreshold dose of a carcinogen (initiation phase) followed by repetitive treatment with a noncarcinogenic tumor promoter (promotion phase). The initiation phase requires only a single application of either a direct or indirect carcinogen at a subthreshold dose and is essentially irreversible, while the promotion phase is brought about by repetitive treatments after initiation and is initially reversible, later becoming irreversible. This system not only can be used to determine the tumor-initiating and -promoting activities of a compound but, if the agent is given repeatedly by itself, one can also determine if it is a complete carcinogen, i.e., if it has both tumor-initiating and -promoting activity. In addition, if the agent is given concurrently with a known complete carcinogen or a tumor initiator, one can also determine if the agent has cocarcinogenic or cotumor-initiating activity or even possibly anticarcinogenic activity. Likewise, if the agent is given concurrently with a known tumor promoter, one can determine if the agent has copromoting or antipromoting activity. Furthermore, like most carcinogenesis systems, skin carcinogens may have additive or synergistic effects. This system has provided an important model not only for studying carcinogenesis and for bioassaying carcinogenic agents but also for the study of modifiers of carcinogenesis.

TUMOR PROMOTION

Although the phorbol esters are the most potent of the mouse skin tumor promoters, a wide variety of other compounds have been shown to have skin tumor-promoting activity, as shown in Table 1. After the phorbol esters and dihydroteleocidin B, anthralin is the most potent tumor promoter known of the compounds listed in Table 1. Van Duuren and co-workers have reported a fairly extensive structure-activity study with anthralin and derivatives (48). Likewise, Boutwell and co-workers (10) have reported a structure-activity study of a number of phenolic compounds that are weak promoters in comparison to the phorbol esters and anthralin. Although several of the other compounds

TABLE 1. *Skin tumor promoters*

Promoters	Potency	References
Croton oil	strong	5, 8
Certain phorbol esters found in croton oil	strong	18, 44, 47
Some synthetic phorbol esters	strong	18
Certain euphorbia latices	strong	18
Anthralin	moderate	48
Certain fatty acids and fatty acid methyl esters	weak	1
Certain long chain alkanes	weak	48
A number of phenolic compounds	weak	10
Surface active agents (sodium lauryl sulfate, tween 60)	weak	8, 9
Citrus oils	weak	34
Extracts of unburned tobacco	moderate	7
Tobacco smoke condensate	moderate	49
Iodoacetic acid	weak	17
1-fluoro-2,4-dinitrobenzene	moderate	6
Benzo(e)pyrene	moderate	42
Benzoyl peroxide[a]	moderate	
Dihydroteleocidin β	strong	

[a] T. J. Slaga, manuscript in preparation.

shown in Table 1 have moderate to weak activity as tumor promoters, there have not been any extensive structure-activity studies performed. We have recently found that benzo(e)pyrene and benzoyl peroxide, as well as other free radical-generating compounds such as *m*-chloroperbenzoic acid and lauroyl peroxide, are relatively good tumor promoters (T. J. Slaga, *unpublished results*).

In addition to causing inflammation and epidermal hyperplasia, the phorbol ester tumor promoters and other promoters produce several other morphological and biochemical changes in skin, as listed in Table 2. Of the observed phorbol ester-related effects on the skin, the induction of epidermal cell proliferation, ornithine decarboxylase (ODC), and dark basal keratinocytes have the best correlation with promoting activity (27–30,41,44). In addition to the induction of dark cells which are normally present in large numbers in embryonic skin, there are many other embryonic conditions that appear in adult skin after treatment with tumor promoters (Table 2).

It is difficult to determine which of the many effects associated with phorbol ester tumor promotion are, in fact, essential components of the promotion process. A good correlation appears to exist between promotion and epidermal hyperplasia when induced by phorbol esters (44). Other agents that induce epidermal cell proliferation do not necessarily promote carcinogenesis, however (38). O'Brien et al. have reported an excellent correlation between the tumor-promoting ability of various compounds (phorbol esters as well as nonphorbol ester compounds) and their ability to induce ODC activity in mouse skin (27). However, mezerein, a diterpene similar to 12-O-tetradecanoylphorbol-13-acetate

TABLE 2. *Morphological and biochemical responses of mouse skin to phorbol ester and other tumor promoters*

Responses	References
Induction of inflammation and hyperplasia[a]	8, 44
Increase in DNA, RNA[b], and protein synthesis	2
An initial increase in keratinization followed by a decrease	28–30
Increase in phospholipid synthesis	35
Increase in prostaglandin synthesis	11
Increase in histone synthesis and phosphorylation	32, 33
Increase in ODC activity followed by increase in polyamines[a]	27
Decrease in the isoproterenol stimulation of cyclic AMP[c]	25
Induction of embryonic state in adult skin[a]	41
(a) Induction of dark cells (primitive stem cells)	21, 28–30
(b) Induction of embryonic proteins in adult skin	3, 26
(c) Induction of morphological changes in adult skin resembling papillomas, carcinomas, and embryonic skin	21, 28–30
(d) Decrease in histidase activity	12
(e) Increase in protease activity	46
(f) Decrease response of G1 chalone in adult skin	22
(g) Increase in cyclic AMP-independent protein kinase in adult skin resembling tumors and embryonic skin	23

[a] Events which appear to show a reasonable correlation with promotion.
[b] RNA, ribonucleic acid.
[c] cyclic AMP, cyclic adenosine monophosphate.

(TPA) but with weak promoting activity, was found to induce ODC to levels that were comparable to those induced by TPA (24). Raick found that phorbol ester tumor promoters induced the appearance of "dark basal cells" in the epidermis, whereas ethylphenylpropiolate (EPP), a nonpromoting epidermal hyperplastic agent, did not (28,31). Wounding induced a few dark cells, which seemed to correlate with its ability to be a weaker promoter (28–30). In addition, a large number of these dark cells are found in papillomas and carcinomas (28,29). Slaga et al. (21,40) reported that TPA induced about three to five times the number of dark cells as mezerein, which was the first major difference found between these compounds.

Inhibitors and Modifiers of Tumor Promotion

Various modifiers of the tumor promotion process have been very useful in our understanding of the mechanism(s) of tumor promotion. Table 3 lists the potent inhibitors of mouse skin tumor promotion by phorbol esters. The antiinflammatory steroid fluocinolone acetonide (FA) was an extremely potent inhibitor of phorbol ester tumor promotion in mouse skin (37). Repeated applications of as little as 0.01 μg almost completely counteracted skin tumorigenesis. FA also effectively counteracts the induced cellular proliferation associated with

TABLE 3. *Inhibitors of phorbol ester skin tumor promotion*

Inhibitors	References
1. Antiinflammatory steroids: cortisol, dexamethasone, and FA	37
2. Vitamin A derivatives	50
3. Combination of retinoids and antiinflammatory agents	50, 51
4. Protease inhibitors: tosyl lysine chloromethyl ketone (TLCK); tosyl arginine methyl ester (TAME); TPCK; antipain and leupeptin	46
5. Cyclic nucleotides	4
6. Phosphodiesterase inhibitors; IBMX[a]	
7. DMSO[a]	
8. Butyrate, acetic acid	4
9. BCG	36
10. Poly I:C	16
11. Prostaglandin synthesis inhibitors ETYA and RO-22-3582[a]	
12. Arachidonic acid	14
13. Polyamine synthesis inhibitor (DFMO)[a]	
14. BHA and BHT[a]	

[a] Unpublished results.

application of phorbol ester tumor promoters. Certain retinoids are also potent inhibitors of mouse skin tumor promotion (50). In addition, Sporn and co-workers have found that certain retinoids are potent inhibitors of lung, mammary, bladder, and colon carcinogenesis (45). Verma and co-workers (50) have shown that certain retinoids are potent inhibitors of phorbol ester-induced epidermal ODC activity. We have recently found that a combination of FA and retinoids produces an inhibitory effect on skin tumor promotion greater than that produced by each separately (51).

The work of Troll and Belman (4,46) has shown that protease inhibitors, cyclic nucleotides, dimethylsulfoxide (DMSO), and butyrate also inhibit mouse skin tumor promotion by phorbol esters. In addition to butyric acid, acetic acid also inhibits tumor promotion (38). The phosphodiesterase inhibitor isobutylmethylxanthine (IBMX) was also found to inhibit tumor promotion, which gives further support to the inhibitory effect of cyclic nucleotides (T. J. Slaga, *unpublished results*). Schinitsky and co-workers (36) reported the inhibitory effect of Bacillus Calmette-Guerin (BCG) vaccination on skin tumor promotion. It has been shown that polyriboinosinic-polyribocytidylic (Poly I:C) has an inhibitory effect on carcinogenesis and tumor promotion (16). This appears to be mediated by its inhibition of promoter- and carcinogen-induced cell proliferation (16).

Certain prostaglandin synthesis inhibitors also inhibit skin tumor promotion, which suggests that prostaglandins may be important in tumor promotion (S. M. Fischer, *unpublished results*). Although the mechanism is not presently understood, arachidonic acid at high doses is a potent inhibitor of tumor promotion (14). Difluoromethylornithine (DFMO), an inhibitor of polyamine synthesis, also inhibits tumor promotion, which suggests that polyamines are also important (C. E. Weeks, *unpublished results*). Although both butylated hydroxyanisole (BHA) and butylated hydroxyltoluene (BHT) are potent inhibitors of skin tumor promotion, their mechanism of action is currently not known (T. J. Slaga, *unpublished results*). It is possible that free radicals are important in tumor promotion; thus, these agents may prevent promotion by their free radical scavenging ability.

Table 4 lists a number of compounds that we have tested as modifiers of tumor promotion. Most of these compounds were examined because of their effect on either cellular polyamines, prostaglandins, or cyclic nucleotide levels. Although DFMO, an irreversible inhibitor of ODC, inhibited tumor promotion, α-methylornithine (αMO), a reversible inhibitor, either had no effect or a slight stimulatory effect (41). Putrescine, spermidine, and spermine were inactive as tumor promoters, but putrescine consistently was found to enhance TPA promotion, whereas spermine inhibited TPA promotion (41). The cyclooxygenase inhibitors indomethacin and flurbiprofen increased TPA tumor promotion (15), whereas 5,8,11,14-eicosatetraynoic acid (ETYA), which inhibits both the cyclooxygenase and lipoxygenase pathways, inhibited tumor promotion (S. M. Fischer, *unpublished results*). The thromboxane synthetase inhibitor RO-22-3382 was also found to inhibit TPA promotion (S. M. Fischer, *unpublished results*). It is of interest to point out that high doses of arachidonic acid inhibited tumor promotion, whereas linoleic acid had no effect (14). Prostaglandins E_1, E_2, and $F_{2\alpha}$ were inactive as tumor promoters, but E_2 and $F_{2\alpha}$, when given with TPA, increased its promoting ability, whereas E_1 inhibited tumor promotion by TPA (14).

Since polyamines have been implicated in the mechanism of tumor promotion, we were interested in determining the effects of various chemicals on epidermal

TABLE 4. *Modifiers of TPA promotion in mouse skin*[a]

Modifier (dose, μg)	Tumor response (% of TPA)	Modifier (dose, μg)	Tumor response (% of TPA)
FA (1)	2	Arachidonic acid (500)	15
RA (10)	10	Linoleic acid (500)	92
TPCK (10)	40	Prostaglandin E_2 (10)	140
DFMO (2,000)	65	Prostaglandin E_1 (10)	60
αMO (4,000)	125	Prostaglandin F_2 (10)	154
Putrescine (250)	160	IBMX (400)	45
Spermidine (200)	100	BHA, BHT (5,000)	20
Spermine (400)	60	DMSO and ethanol as	
Indomethacin (100)	145	solvent for TPA	40
Flurbiprofen (10)	140	Acetic acid (20,000)	10
ETYA (100)	55	A23187 (80)	180
RO-22-3582 (100)	45	Benzoyl peroxide (10,000)	200
		Mellitin (50)	120

[a] Mainly unpublished results.

ODC activity, polyamine levels, and tumor promotion. Table 5 shows that meze-rein is capable of increasing ODC activity and polyamine levels comparable to or greater than TPA, but is a weak tumor promoter (41). EPP, a hyperplastic agent with very weak promoting activity, increased ODC activity and polyamine levels, but to a much lesser degree than TPA or mezerein. FA, the very potent inhibitor of TPA promotion, only slightly decreased the TPA-increased ODC activity and polyamine levels. Although αMO caused a paradoxical increase in ODC activity induced by TPA, the level of putrescine was decreased. As shown in Table 5, αMO did not decrease TPA promotion. The irreversible inhibitor of ODC (DFMO), however, decreased the TPA-increased ODC activity, polyamine levels, and TPA promotion (41). The protease inhibitor tosyl phenylalanine chloromethyl ketone (TPCK) effectively inhibited tumor promotion but had very little effect on TPA-increased ODC activity. As previously shown by other investigators (50), retinoic acid (RA) inhibits TPA promotion as well as TPA-increased ODC activity and polyamine levels. Indomethacin was found to increase TPA promotion and to decrease TPA-increased ODC activity, whereas ETYA and RO-22-3582 inhibited TPA promotion but had no effect on TPA-increased ODC activity. IBMX was found to decrease TPA promotion, but had no effect on TPA-increased ODC activity. If all the data in Table 5 is taken into consideration, one would have to conclude that there is no direct relationship between changes in ODC activity and subsequent poly-amine levels and tumor promotion.

TABLE 5. *Effects of various chemicals on epidermal ODC activity, polyamine levels, and tumor formation[a]*

Compound (dose)	ODC activity (6 hr) (% TPA)	Putrescine (treated/control)	Tumor (% TPA)
TPA 1 μg	100[b]	3.2	100
2 μg	125	4.5	180
MEZ[c]1 μg	100	2.6	<2
2 μg	150	3.7	4
5 μg	—	6.5	8
EPP 3 mg	<5	1.2	1
30 mg	20	1.6	2
TPA 1 μg + FA 1 μg	60	2.7	5
TPA 1 μg + αMO 4 mg	200	2.1	125
TPA 1 μg + DFMO 2 mg	<10	0.7	65
TPA 2 μg + TPCK 10 μg	70	—	40
TPA 2 μg + RA 10 μg	10	0.8	20
TPA 1 μg + indomethacin 100 μg	40	—	145
TPA 1 μg + RO-22-3582 100 μg	95	—	45
TPA 1 μg + ETYA 100 μg	110	—	55
TPA 1 μg + IBMX 200 μg	100	—	45

[a] Unpublished results.
[b] Values are ratios 9 to 12 hr posttreatment.
[c] MEZ, mezerein.

Multistage Promotion

As previously discussed, mezerein, a diterpene similar to TPA (Fig. 1), was capable of causing most of the morphological and biochemical changes in skin and in cells in culture that TPA did, but TPA was at least 50 times more active as a tumor promoter (24). A comparison of these TPA and mezerein responses are shown in Table 6. Clearly, mezerein is as potent or more potent than TPA. This is especially true regarding the induction of epidermal ODC and epidermal hyperplasia. The effect of mezerein on ODC activity suggests that ODC induction is not a critical event in tumor promotion (24). It should be emphasized that this conclusion is also true for the other morphological and biochemical responses to mezerein.

Because of the many similarities in morphological and biochemical responses induced by TPA and mezerein, we felt that mezerein, although a weak promoter, would be a good candidate as a compound to be used in the second stage of a two-stage promotion protocol as originally reported by Boutwell (8). We re-

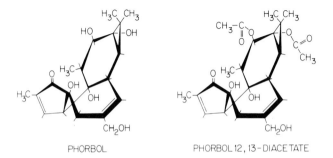

FIG. 1. A comparison of the structures of TPA, 4-0-me TPA, phorbol, phorbol 12,13-diacetate, and mezerein.

TABLE 6. *Comparison of cellular and biochemical responses to TPA and MEZ*

	Relative response[a]		
	TPA	MEZ	Reference
1. Enhancement of neoplastic phenotype	100	100	52
2. Promotion of neoplastic transformation (C3H-1OT 1/2)	100	80	19[b]
3. Induction of epidermal cellular proliferation	50	100	24, 44
4. Comitogenesis in lymphocytes	100	100	20
5. Inhibition of differentiation in Friend erythroleukemia cells	100	100	13, 50
6. Stimulation of DNA synthesis	50	100	24[c]
7. Stimulation of ODC activity	80	100	24[c]
8. Stimulation of plasminogen activator production	20	100	52

[a] For a comparative purpose, the maximum response of mezerein or TPA is expressed as 100. The values should only be considered as an approximation.

[b] S. Mondal and C. Heidelberger, personal communication.

[c] Manuscript in preparation by C. E. Weeks, S. M. Fischer and T. J. Slaga, "Comparative study on the effects of TPA and mezerein to induce epidermal DNA synthesis, ornithine decarboxylase, and polyamine *in vivo* and *in vitro.*"

cently reported that mezerein was a potent stage II promoter (39,40). Before these experiments are discussed in detail, a discussion of the original two-stage promotion protocol as reported by Boutwell (8) is needed. His results showed that promotion could be divided into two steps, conversion and propagation (8). After 7,12-dimethyl-benz(a)anthracene (DMBA) initiation, the conversion stage was accomplished by a limited number of croton oil treatments which, with no further treatment, only produced a few tumors. The propagation stage was accomplished by repeated treatment with turpentine, a nonpromoting hyperplastic agent (8). The three-stage protocol (initiation-conversion-propagation) produced a significant tumor response, but less than that observed when croton oil was given for the complete promotion stage (8). Although the above experiments were repeatable at that time, however, recent results suggest that nonpromoting hyperplastic agents such as turpentine, EPP, and acetic acid, when given repetitively after a few treatments with TPA, are not able to complete the promotion process as reported by Boutwell (30,31,38). In fact, Raick reported that turpentine and EPP gave fewer tumors in a three-stage system than when DMBA was followed only by limited TPA treatment (30,31). Similar results were reported by Slaga et al. (38) using acetic acid as a second step promoter. It should be pointed out that turpentine, EPP, and acetic acid do not induce many of the biochemical responses induced by TPA and mezerein, even though they are hyperplastic agents. It is possible that the variable response of turpentine as a stage II promoter may be related to the fact that it is a complex mixture which can vary from batch to batch (R. K. Boutwell, *personal communication*).

A summary of the results on the use of mezerein as a second stage promoter in two-stage promotion is shown in Table 7. As illustrated, TPA is about 50 times more active as a promoter than mezerein (compare experiments 1, 3, and 4). When 2 μg of TPA are given twice weekly for only 2 weeks after DMBA initiation, no tumors are induced, compared to twice weekly treatments of 18 weeks. When mezerein is given at a dose of either 1, 2, or 4 μg twice weekly after the limited TPA treatment, however, it induces a significant tumor response in a dose-dependent manner (compare experiments 5, 6, and 7 with 2). The ability of mezerein to act as a potent second stage promoter was repeated in 10 separate experiments (3,10,40,43). Also shown in Table 7 is the ineffectiveness of EPP as a complete promoter and as a second stage promoter. Table 8 shows that a good dose response exists for stage I of promotion. In addition, only a single application of TPA is necessary for stage I of promotion to be expressed after repeated applications of mezerein.

The effectiveness of some of the inhibitors of tumor promotion on two-stage promotion was recently reported by this laboratory (43). The effects of FA, RA, and TPCK on two-stage promotion are shown in Table 9. As shown in experiments 1 and 2 of Table 9, stages I and II of promotion separately do not cause tumors to develop after DMBA initiation when given under the treatment protocol shown. When stage I and II agents are given sequentially after DMBA initiation, however, a significant tumor response is observed (experiment 3). FA was a potent inhibitor of stage I and II of promotion, but to a greater degree for stage I than stage II. It should be emphasized that only four applications of FA with TPA were necessary to counteract the tumor response. RA was ineffective in stage I but was a potent inhibitor of stage II promotion, whereas TPCK specifically inhibited stage I but not stage II. These experiments were repeated several times and were very reproducible (40,43).

Since the only major morphological or biochemical difference between the effects of TPA and mezerein on the skin is the ability of TPA to induce a large number of dark basal keratinocytes (21,40), we were interested in determining the effects of various inhibitors of promotion on the appearance of these dark cells. We reasoned that if these dark cells are critical in the first stage of promotion, if FA and TPCK are potent inhibitors of stage I, and RA is an inhibitor of stage II, then FA and TPCK should counteract the appearance of these cells and RA should not. The results of FA, RA, and TPCK on the induction of dark basal keratinocytes by TPA are summarized in Table 10. As hypothesized, FA and TPCK were found to effectively counteract the appearance of the dark cells induced by TPA, whereas RA had no effect.

Since TPCK inhibited stage I of promotion but not stage II, and since TPCK counteracted the TPA-induced increase in the dark basal keratinocytes but did not have any effect on TPA-induced hyperplasia, we were interested in determining the effect of TPCK on TPA-induced ODC activity. As shown in Table 10, TPCK had very little effect on TPA- and mezerein-induced epidermal ODC activity (43).

TABLE 7. *Two-stage tumor promotion after DMBA initiation*[a]

Exp. no.	Treatment protocol 21 weeks[b]	Tumor response	
		pap/mouse	% of mice with tumors
1	DMBA $\xrightarrow{\text{1 wk}}$ TPA $\xrightarrow{\text{2×/wk for 20 wk}}$	8.2	100
2	DMBA $\xrightarrow{\text{1 wk}}$ TPA $\xrightarrow{\text{2×/wk for 2 wk}}$ acetone $\xrightarrow{\text{2×/wk for 18 wk}}$	0	0
3	DMBA $\xrightarrow{\text{1 wk}}$ MEZ 2 µg $\xrightarrow{\text{2×/wk for 20 wk}}$	0	0
4	DMBA $\xrightarrow{\text{1 wk}}$ MEZ 4 µg $\xrightarrow{\text{2×/wk for 20 wk}}$	0.2	18
5	DMBA $\xrightarrow{\text{1 wk}}$ TPA $\xrightarrow{\text{2×/wk for 2 wk}}$ MEZ 1 µg $\xrightarrow{\text{2×/wk for 18 wk}}$	2.1	60
6	DMBA $\xrightarrow{\text{1 wk}}$ TPA $\xrightarrow{\text{2×/wk for 2 wk}}$ MEZ 2 µg $\xrightarrow{\text{2×/wk for 18 wk}}$	4.0	90
7	DMBA $\xrightarrow{\text{1 wk}}$ TPA $\xrightarrow{\text{2×/wk for 2 wk}}$ MEZ 4 µg $\xrightarrow{\text{2×/wk for 18 wk}}$	7.1	100
8	DMBA $\xrightarrow{\text{1 wk}}$ acetone $\xrightarrow{\text{2×/wk for 2 wk}}$ MEZ 4 µg $\xrightarrow{\text{2×/wk for 18 wk}}$	0.1	10
9	DMBA $\xrightarrow{\text{1 wk}}$ EPP (14 mg) $\xrightarrow{\text{2×/wk for 20 wk}}$	0.1	10
10	DMBA $\xrightarrow{\text{1 wk}}$ TPA $\xrightarrow{\text{2×/wk for 2 wk}}$ EPP (14 mg) $\xrightarrow{\text{2×/wk for 18 wk}}$	0.2	12

[a] The mice were initiated with 10 nmole of DMBA, followed 1 week later by weekly applications of 2 µg of TPA for 2 weeks. Starting on the 3rd week of promotion, the mice received either twice weekly applications of various dose levels of MEZ, EPP, or only acetone. See ref. 39 for details.
[b] 95% or greater of the mice were alive at the end of the experimental period. The maximum percent standard deviation for the experiment was 16%.

TABLE 8. *Characteristics of two-state promotion[a]*

Stage I (No. of applications of TPA)	(Dose, μg)	Stage II (No. of applications of MEZ)	Tumor response (papillomas/mouse)
0	—	36	0
0	0	36[c]	0.2
1×	1	35	0.42
1×	2	35	1.40
1×	4	35	1.80
1×	6	35	2.20
1×	6	35[c]	3.40
2×	1	34	1.80
2×	2	34	2.50
2×	4	34	3.20
2×	6	34	3.60
2×	6	34[c]	4.60
4×	1	32	2.80
4×	2	32	4.10
4×	4	32	4.60
4×	4	—	0
4×	6	32	6.1
4×	6	—	0.2
4×	6	32[c]	8.4

[a] Unpublished results.

[b] Thirty mice per group were used. All the mice were initiated with 10 nmole of DMBA followed 1 week later by various dose levels and number of applications of TPA (stage I). Stage II was accomplished by twice weekly applications of 2 μg of MEZ after the last TPA treatment. Total promotion was continued for 18 weeks (36 applications).

[c] MEZ was applied twice weekly at 4 μg per application.

The antiinflammatory steroid FA not only counteracted the appearance of dark cells induced by TPA but also suppressed the hyperplasia induced by TPA (Table 10). In fact, the skins from FA plus TPA-treated mice appeared as untreated skin. This is in agreement with our previously reported observations on the inhibitory effect of FA on TPA-induced inflammation, hyperplasia, and deoxyribonucleic acid (DNA) synthesis (37). FA had very little effect on the TPA-increased ODC activity (Table 10), however, as compared to its effect on inhibition of promotion.

It is also of interest to point out that although RA inhibited stage II of promotion, it had no inhibitory effect on the TPA- or mezerein-induced hyperplasia (Table 10). However, certain retinoids have been found to be potent inhibitors of TPA- and mezerein-induced epidermal ODC activity (24,50). These data suggest that the induction of epidermal ODC activity followed by increased polyamines may be important in stage II of promotion. In this regard, FA and TPCK have either no effect or only a slight inhibitory effect on TPA- or mezerein-induced ODC activity (43). FA does, however, significantly decrease the TPA-induced spermidine levels in the epidermis (43). This effect, plus FA's

TABLE 9. *The effects of RA, FA, and TPCK on two-stage promotion after DMBA initiation*

Exp. No.	Treatment protocol 21 weeks[b]	Tumor response	
		Number of papillomas per mouse	% of mice w/tumors
1	DMBA $\xrightarrow{\text{1 wk}}$ TPA $\xrightarrow{\text{2×/wk for 2 wk}}$	0	0
2	DMBA $\xrightarrow{\text{1 wk}}$ acetone $\xrightarrow{\text{2×/wk for 2 wk}}$ MEZ $\xrightarrow{\text{2×/wk for 18 wk}}$	0	0
3	DMBA $\xrightarrow{\text{1 wk}}$ TPA $\xrightarrow{\text{2×/wk for 2 wk}}$ MEZ $\xrightarrow{\text{2×/wk for 18 wk}}$	4.2	92
4	DMBA $\xrightarrow{\text{1 wk}}$ TPA + FA (1 µg) $\xrightarrow{\text{2×/wk for 2 wk}}$ MEZ $\xrightarrow{\text{2×/wk for 18 wk}}$	0	0
5	DMBA $\xrightarrow{\text{1 wk}}$ TPA + FA (0.1 µg) $\xrightarrow{\text{2×/wk for 2 wk}}$ MEZ $\xrightarrow{\text{2×/wk for 18 wk}}$	0.4	26
6	DMBA $\xrightarrow{\text{1 wk}}$ TPA $\xrightarrow{\text{2×/wk for 2 wk}}$ MEZ + FA (1 µg) $\xrightarrow{\text{2×/wk for 18 wk}}$	0.8	35
7	DMBA $\xrightarrow{\text{1 wk}}$ TPA + RA (10 µg) $\xrightarrow{\text{2×/wk for 2 wk}}$ MEZ $\xrightarrow{\text{2×/wk for 18 wk}}$	4.0	88
8	DMBA $\xrightarrow{\text{1 wk}}$ TPA $\xrightarrow{\text{2×/wk for 2 wk}}$ MEZ + RA (10 µg) $\xrightarrow{\text{2×/wk for 18 wk}}$	0.8	34
9	DMBA $\xrightarrow{\text{1 wk}}$ TPA + TPCK (10 µg) $\xrightarrow{\text{2×/wk for 2 wk}}$ MEZ $\xrightarrow{\text{2×/wk for 18 wk}}$	1.0	40
10	DMBA $\xrightarrow{\text{1 wk}}$ TPA $\xrightarrow{\text{2×/wk for 2 wk}}$ MEZ + TPCK (10 µg) $\xrightarrow{\text{2×/wk for 18 wk}}$	3.8	87

[a] The mice were initiated with 10 nmole of DMBA and followed 1 week later by twice weekly applications of 2 µg of TPA for 2 weeks (stage I). Starting on the 3rd week of promotion, the mice received twice weekly applications of 2 µg of MEZ (stage II). In some experiments FA, RA, or TPCK were given simultaneously with either stage I or II. See ref. 43 for details.

[b] 98% or more of the mice were alive at the end of the experimental period. The maximum percent standard deviation for the experiment was 14%.

TABLE 10. *Effects of various inhibitors of tumor promotion on TPA- and MEZ-induced epidermal hyperplasia, dark keratinocytes, and polyamine levels*

Inhibitor	TPA-induced hyperplasia	Increased dark keratinocytes by TPA	Increased ODC and polyamine levels by TPA
FA	↓[a]	↓	—
RA	— or ↑[b]	—	↓
TPCK	—	↓	—

[a] ↓, Decreased.
[b] ↑, Increased.

inhibitory effect on TPA-induced hyperplasia, may be responsible for its inhibitory effect on stage II promotion.

CONCLUSIONS

The data presented from this laboratory suggest that at least two stages make up the promotion process, both of which can obviously be produced by repeated TPA treatment after tumor initiation. We believe that one of the important events in the first stage involves the induction of dark basal keratinocytes. The fact that mezerein is a potent second stage promoter, but only a weak complete promoter with much less ability to induce dark cells than TPA, and that FA and TPCK inhibit stage I and the induction of dark cells by TPA, suggest that the dark cells are important in stage I of promotion (Fig. 2). The dark basal keratinocytes are increased slightly by wounding, which correlates with its weak promoting ability. EPP, which is a nonpromoting hyperplastic agent, has no effect on dark cells (21,29–31). Furthermore, a large number of these dark cells are found in papillomas and carcinomas (29,30). These dark cells

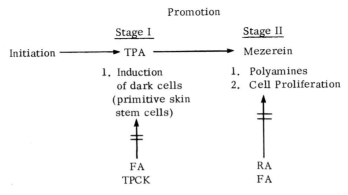

FIG. 2. A diagram of the various stages of skin carcinogenesis showing the important events in stages I and II of promotion and where FA, RA, and TPCK inhibit promotion.

may be primitive stem cells since we have found *(unpublished results)*, as have others (29,30), that they normally occur in large numbers in embryonic and newborn skin but are present only in very small numbers in adult skin. As stated earlier, we feel that the induction of ODC activity followed by increased polyamines and increased cellular proliferation are important events in stage II of promotion. Figure 2 depicts the various stages, the important events in each stage, and where the various inhibitors are effective. By seeking to divide the carcinogenic process into as many distinct stages as possible and finding specific inhibitors of each stage, we will have a greater opportunity of understanding the important events in carcinogenesis as well as possibly securing a rational and effective basis for the prevention of cancer.

ACKNOWLEDGMENTS

Research sponsored by the Office of Health and Environmental Research, U.S. Department of Energy, under contract W-7405-eng-26 with the Union Carbide Corporation.

REFERENCES

1. Arffman, E., and Glowind, J. (1971): Tumor-promoting activity of fatty acid methyl esters in mice. *Experientia,* 27:1,465–1,469.
2. Baird, W. M., Sedgwick, J. A., and Boutwell, R. K. (1971): Effects of phorbol and four diesters of phorbol on the incorporation of tritiated precursors into DNA, RNA, and protein in mouse epidermis. *Cancer Res.,* 31:1,434–1,439.
3. Balmain, A. (1976): The synthesis of specific proteins in adult mouse epidermis during phases of proliferation and differentiation induced by the tumor promoter TPA and in basal and differentiating layers of neonatal mouse epidermis. *J. Invest. Dermatol.,* 67:246–253.
4. Belman, S., and Troll, W. (1978): Hormones, cyclic nucleotides, and prostaglandins. In: *Carcinogenesis, Vol. 2: Mechanisms of Tumor Promotion and Carcinogenesis,* edited by T. J. Slaga, A. Sivak, and R. K. Boutwell, pp. 117–134. Raven Press, New York.
5. Berenblum, I. (1941): The cocarcinogenic action of croton resin. *Cancer Res.,* 1:44–50.
6. Bock, F. G., Fjelde, A., Fox, H. W., and Kelin, E. (1969): Tumor promotion by 1-fluoro-2,4-dinitrobenzene, a potent skin sensitizer. *Cancer Res.,* 29:179–182.
7. Bock, F. G., Moors, G. E., and Crouch, S. K. (1964): Tumor-promoting activity of extracts of unburned tobacco. *Science,* 145:231–234.
8. Boutwell, R. K. (1964): Some biological aspects of skin carcinogenesis. *Prog. Exp. Tumor Res.,* 4:207–250.
9. Boutwell, R. K., and Bosch, D. K. (1957): Studies on the role of surface active agents in the formation of skin tumors in mice. *Am. Assoc. Cancer Res.,* 2:190.
10. Boutwell, R. K., and Bosch, D. K. (1959): Tumor-promoting action of phenol and related compounds for mouse skin. *Cancer Res.,* 19:413–419.
11. Bresnick, E., Meunier, R., and Lamden, M. (1979): Epidermal prostaglandins after topical application of a tumor promoter. *Cancer Lett.,* 7:121–125.
12. Colburn, W. H., Lau, S., and Head, R. (1975): Decrease of epidermal histidase activity by tumor-promoting phorbol esters. *Cancer Res.,* 35:3,154–3,159.
13. Diamond, L., O'Brien, T., and Rovera, G. (1978): Tumor promoters inhibit terminal cell differentiation in culture. In: *Carcinogenesis, Vol. 2: Mechanisms of Tumor Promotion and Cocarcinogenesis,* edited by T. J. Slaga, A. Sivak, and R. K. Boutwell, pp. 335–341. Raven Press, New York.
14. Fischer, S. M., Gleason, G. L., Hardin, L. G., Bohrman, J. S., and Slaga, T. J. (1980): Prostaglandin modulation of phorbol ester skin tumor promotion. *Carcinogenesis,* 1:245–248.

15. Fischer, S. M., Gleason, G. L., Mills, G. D., and Slaga, T. J. (1980): Indomethacin enhancement of TPA tumor promotion in mice. *Cancer Lett.,* 10:343–350.
16. Gelboin, H. V., and Levy, H. B. (1970): Polyinosinic-polycytidylic acid inhibits chemically induced tumorigenesis in mouse skin. *Science,* 167:205–207.
17. Gwynn, R. H., and Salamon, N. H. (1953): Studies on cocarcinogenesis. SH-reactors and other substances tested for co-carcinogenic action in mouse skin, *Br. J. Cancer,* 7:482–488.
18. Hecker, E. (1978): Structure-activity relationships in diterpene esters irritant and cocarcinogenic to mouse skin. In: *Carcinogenesis, Vol. 2: Mechanisms of Tumor Promotion and Cocarcinogenesis,* edited by T. J. Slaga, A. Sivak, and R. K. Boutwell, pp. 11–42. Raven Press, New York.
19. Heidelberger, C., Mondal, S., and Peterson, A. R. (1978): Initiation and promotion in cell cultures. In: *Carcinogenesis, Vol. 2: Mechanisms of Tumor Promotion and Cocarcinogenesis,* edited by T. J. Slaga, A. Sivak, and R. K. Boutwell, pp. 197–202. Raven Press, New York.
20. Kensler, T. W., and Mueller, G. C. (1978): Retinoic acid inhibition of the comitogenic action of mezerein and phorbol esters in bovine lymphocytes. *Cancer Res.,* 38:771–775.
21. Klein-Szanto, A. J. P., Major, S. M., and Slaga, T. J. (1980): Introduction of dark keratinocytes by 12-O-tetradecanoylphorbol-13-acetate and mezerein as an indicator of tumor-promoting efficiency. *Carcinogenesis,* 1:399–406.
22. Krieg, L., Kuhlmann, J., and Marks, F. (1974): Effect of tumor-promoting phorbol esters and of acetic acid on mechanisms controlling DNA synthesis and mitosis (chalones) and on the biosynthesis of histidine-rich protein in mouse epidermis. *Cancer Res.,* 34:3,135–3,146.
23. Mamrack, M., and Slaga, T. J. (1981): Multistage skin tumor promotion: Involvement of a protein kinase. In: *Biological Carcinogenesis,* edited by M. A. Rich. Marcel Dekker, Inc., New York.
24. Mufson, R. A., Fischer, S. M., Verma, A. K., Gleason, G. L., Slaga, T. J., and Boutwell, R. K. (1979): Effects of 12-O-tetradecanoylphorbol-13-acetate and mezerein on epidermal ornithine decarboxylase activity, isoproterenol-stimulated levels of cyclic adenosine 3':5'-monophosphate, and induction of mouse skin tumors. *Cancer Res.,* 39:4,791–4,795.
25. Mufson, R. A., Simsiman, R. C., and Boutwell, R. K. (1977): The effect of the phorbol ester tumor promoters on the basal and catecholamine-stimulated levels of cyclic adenosine 3':5'-monophosphate in mouse skin and epidermis *in vivo. Cancer Res.,* 37:665–669.
26. Nelson, K. G., Stephenson, K. B., and Slaga, T. J. (1980): Tumor promoter-induced changes in mouse epidermal acidic proteins analyzed by two-dimensional gel electrophoresis. *Am. Assoc. Cancer Res.,* 21:115.
27. O'Brien, T. G., Simsiman, R. C., and Boutwell, R. K. (1975): Induction of the polyamine biosynthetic enzymes in mouse epidermis by tumor-promoting agents. *Cancer Res.,* 35:1,662–1,670.
28. Raick, A. N. (1973): Ultrastructural, histological, and biochemical alterations produced by 12-O-tetradecanoylphorbol-13-acetate on mouse epidermis and their relevance to skin tumor promotion. *Cancer Res.,* 33:269–286.
29. Raick, A. N. (1974a): Cell proliferation and promoting action in skin carcinogenesis. *Cancer Res.,* 34:920–926.
30. Raick, A. N. (1974b): Cell differentiation and tumor-promoting action in skin carcinogenesis. *Cancer Res.,* 34:2,915–2,925.
31. Raick, A. N., and Burdzy, K. (1973): Ultrastructural and biochemical changes induced in mouse epidermis by a hyperplastic agent, ethylphenylpropiolate. *Cancer Res.,* 33:2,221–2,230.
32. Raineri, R., Simsiman, R. C., and Boutwell, R. K. (1973): Stimulation of the phosphorylation of mouse epidermal histones by tumor-promoting agents. *Cancer Res.,* 33:134–139.
33. Raineri, R., Simsiman, R. C., and Boutwell, R. K. (1977): Stimulation of the synthesis of mouse epidermal histones by tumor-promoting agents. *Cancer Res.,* 37:4,584–4,589.
34. Roe, F. J. C., and Pierce, W. E. H. (1960): Tumor promotion by citrus oils: Tumors of the skin and urethral orifice in mice. *J. Natl. Cancer Inst.,* 24:1,389–1,392.
35. Rohrschneider, L. R., O'Brien, D. H., and Boutwell, R. K. (1972): The stimulation of phospholipid metabolism in mouse skin following phorbol ester treatment. *Biochim. Biophys. Acta,* 280:57–70.
36. Schnitsky, M. R., Hyman, L. R., Blazkovec, A. A., and Burkholder, P. M. (1973): Bacillus Calmette-Guerin vaccination and skin tumor promotion with croton oil in mice. *Cancer Res.,* 33:659–663.
37. Schwarz, J. A., Viaje, A., Slaga, T. J., Yuspa, S. H., Hennings, H., and Lichti, U. (1977):

Fluocinoline acetonide: A potent inhibitor of skin tumor promotion and epidermal DNA synthesis. *Chem. Biol. Interact.,* 17:331–347.

38. Slaga, T. J., Bowden, G. T., and Boutwell, R. K. (1975): Acetic acid, a potent stimulator of mouse epidermal macromolecular synthesis and hyperplasia but with weak tumor-promoting ability. *J. Natl. Cancer Inst.,* 55:983–987.

39. Slaga, T. J., Fischer, S. M., Nelson, K., and Gleason, G. L. (1980): Studies on the mechanism of skin tumor promotion: Evidence for several stages in promotion. *Proc. Natl. Acad. Sci. USA,* 77:3,659–3,663.

40. Slaga, T. J., Fischer, S. M., Weeks, C. E., and Klein-Szanto, A. J. P. (1980): Multistage chemical carcinogenesis. In: *Biochemistry of Normal and Abnormal Epidermal Differentiation,* edited by M. Seije and I. A. Bernstein, pp. 193–218. University of Tokyo Press, Tokyo.

41. Slaga, T. J., Fischer, S. M., Weeks, C. E., and Klein-Szanto, A. J. P. (1981): Cellular and biochemical mechanisms of mouse skin tumor promoters. In: *Reviews in Biochemical Toxicology,* vol. III, edited by E. Hodgson, J. Bend, and R. M. Philpot. Elsevier North-Holland, Inc. New York.

42. Slaga, T. J., Jecker, K., Bracken, W. M., and Weeks, C. E. (1979): The effects of weak or noncarcinogenic polycyclic hydrocarbons on 7,12-dimethylbenz(a)anthracene and benzo(a)pyrene skin tumor initiation. *Cancer Lett.,* 7:51–59.

43. Slaga, T. J., Klein-Szanto, A. J. P., Fischer, S. M., Weeks, C. E., Nelson, K., and Major, S. (1980): Studies on the mechanism of action of antitumor-promoting agents: Their specificity in two-stage promotion. *Proc. Natl. Acad. Sci. USA,* 77:2,251–2,254.

44. Slaga, T. J., Scribner, J. D., Thompson, S., and Viaje, A. (1974): Epidermal cell proliferation and promoting ability of phorbol esters. *J. Natl. Cancer Inst.,* 52:1,611–1,618.

45. Sporn, M. B., Dunlop, N. M., Newlon, D. L., and Smith, J. M. (1976): Prevention of chemical carcinogenesis by vitamin A and its synthetic analogs (retinoids). *Fed. Proc.,* 35:1,332–1,338.

46. Troll, W., Meyn, M. S., and Rossman, T. G. (1978): Mechanisms of protease action in carcinogenesis. In: *Carcinogenesis, Vol. 2: Mechanisms of Tumor Promotion and Cocarcinogenesis,* edited by T. J. Slaga, A. Sivak, and R. K. Boutwell, pp. 301–312. Raven Press, New York.

47. Van Duuren, B. L. (1969): Tumor-promoting agents in two-stage carcinogenesis. *Prog. Exp. Tumor Res.,* 11:31–68.

48. Van Duuren, B. L., and Goldschmidt, B. M. (1978): Structure-activity relationships of tumor promoters and cocarcinogens and interaction of phorbol myristate acetate and related esters with plasma membranes. In: *Carcinogenesis, Vol. 2: Mechanisms of Tumor Promotion and Cocarcinogenesis,* edited by T. J. Slaga, A. Sivak, and R. K. Boutwell, pp. 491–507. Raven Press, New York.

49. Van Duuren, B. L., Sivak, A., Langseth, L., Goldschmidt, B. M., and Segal, A. (1964): Initiators and promoters in tobacco carcinogenesis. *Natl. Cancer Inst. Monogr.,* 28:173–180.

50. Verma, A. K., Rice, H. M., Shapos, B. G., and Boutwell, R. K. (1978): Inhibition of 12-O-tetradecanoylphorbol-13-acetate-induced ornithine decarboxylase activity in mouse epidermis by vitamin A analogs (retinoids). *Cancer Res.,* 38:793–801.

51. Weeks, C. E., Slaga, T. J., Hennings, H., Gleason, G. L., and Bracken, W. M. (1979): Inhibition of phorbol ester-induced tumor promotion by vitamin A analog and antiinflammatory steroid. *J. Natl. Cancer Inst.,* 63:401–406.

52. Weinstein, I. B., Wigler, M., and Pietropaolo, C. (1977): The action of tumor-promoting agents in cell culture. In: *Origins of Human Cancer,* edited by H. H. Heatt, J. D. Watson, and J. A. Winsten, pp. 751–772. Cold Spring Harbor Laboratory.

Carcinogenesis, Vol. 7, edited by E. Hecker et al.
Raven Press, New York © 1982.

The Differential Effects of Retinoic Acid and 7,8-Benzoflavone on the Induction of Mouse Skin Tumors by the Initiation-Promotion Protocol and by the Complete Carcinogenesis Process

Ajit K. Verma

McArdle Laboratory for Cancer Research, University of Wisconsin, Madison, Wisconsin 53706

Mouse skin tumors can be induced by a single application of a large dose or repeated applications of a smaller dose of a carcinogen, such as the polycyclic hydrocarbon 7,12-dimethylbenz[a]anthracene (DMBA) (complete carcinogenesis) or repeated applications of a noncarcinogenic tumor-promoting agent, such as 12-O-tetradecanoylphorbol-13-acetate (TPA) to the initiated skin (two-stage model) (1,4,6).

It is not known if complete carcinogenesis consists of a combination of the initiating and promoting processes involving a promoting component with a mechanism analogous to that of TPA. We have shown that retinoic acid, which is a potent inhibitor of the induction of ornithine decarboxylase (ODC) activity as well as skin tumor promotion by TPA, fails to inhibit the induction of ODC activity and tumor formation by DMBA (6). This suggests that the nature of the promoting component in DMBA carcinogenesis differs from that of TPA promotion. We have further investigated the effect of retinoic acid and 7,8-benzoflavone on the induction of mouse skin tumors by the complete carcinogenesis process and by the initiation-promotion regimen to obtain clues about the mechanisms of these two tumor induction processes, and the results of these studies are summarized in this chapter.

RESULTS AND DISCUSSION

Effect of Retinoic Acid on Skin Tumor Formation

Application of retinoic acid at 1.7, 17, or 34 nmole-doses did not inhibit the appearance of tumors developed by repeated applications of DMBA, but did inhibit the formation of skin tumors when applied in conjunction with TPA to DMBA-initiated mouse skin (Fig. 1).

In a separate experiment, application of retinoic acid 1 hr before and 24 hr

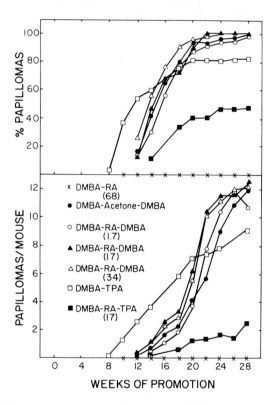

FIG. 1. Effect of RA on skin tumor formation by either DMBA or TPA. 0.2 μmole of DMBA in 0.2 ml acetone was applied to the shaved backs of CD-1 mice. After 2 weeks, mice were treated twice weekly with 68 nmole of RA only, acetone, or the indicated dose of RA 1 hr before once weekly applications of 0.2 μmole of DMBA, or twice weekly applications of 5 nmole of TPA.

after each weekly application of DMBA did not inhibit tumor formation but rather potentiated papillomas per mouse by 64%. Furthermore, 3.3 μmole of retinoic acid in corn oil given intraperitoneally 30 min before each topical application of 0.2 μmole of DMBA to mouse skin did not inhibit, but augmented the carcinogenic action of DMBA by 46% (Table 1).

The lack of effect of retinoic acid on DMBA carcinogenesis was not found to be due to a high dose of DMBA. Application of 34 nmole of retinoic acid 1 hr before twice weekly applications of 1, 10, or 50 nmole of DMBA failed to inhibit tumor formation by DMBA; but rather, some increase in yield as well as in incidence of skin tumors was observed (Table 1).

The inability of retinoic acid to inhibit complete carcinogenesis was not confined to that caused by DMBA. Topical application of retinoic acid at a 34 nmole-dose 30 min before each twice weekly application of 100 nmole of either

TABLE 1. *Effect of retinoic acid on the induction of mouse skin tumors by polycyclic aromatic hydrocarbons*

Experiment	Treatment	Papillomas/ mouse	% Carcinomas
1[a]	Acetone = 1 hr = DMBA = 24 hr = Acetone	11.43	71
	RA = 1 hr = DMBA = 24 hr = RA	18.72	83
2[b]	Corn oil = 30 min = DMBA	11.44	—
	RA in corn oil = 30 min = DMBA	16.75	—
3[c]	Acetone = 1 hr = DMBA (1 nmole)	0.00	0
	RA = 1 hr = DMBA (1 nmole)	0.00	0
	Acetone = 1 hr = DMBA (10 nmole)	0.21	4
	RA = 1 hr = DMBA (10 nmole)	1.37	8
	Acetone = 1 hr = DMBA (50 nmole)	6.76	33
	RA = 1 hr = DMBA (50 nmole)	9.92	48
4[d]	Acetone = 30 min = 3-MC	2.93	—
	RA = 30 min = 3-MC	2.63	—
	Acetone = 30 min = B[a]P	1.19	—
	RA = 30 min = B[a]P	2.85	—
5[e]	Acetone = 30 min = DMBA	8.33	33
	RA = 30 min = DMBA	12.75	33
	7,8-BF = 30 min = DMBA	1.75	0

[a] Experiment 1: 0.2 μmole of DMBA was applied to the shaved backs of mice 2 weeks before application of 17 nmole retinoic acid (RA) or acetone at the indicated times before and after application of 0.2 μmole of DMBA.

[b] Experiment 2: Mice were given intraperitoneally 0.2 ml of corn oil or 3.3 μmole of RA in 0.2 ml corn oil 30 min before each once weekly application of 0.2 μmole of DMBA in 0.2 ml acetone to the shaved backs of mice.

[c] Experiment 3: Acetone or 17 nmole of RA was applied 1 hr before twice weekly applications of DMBA.

[d] Experiment 4: Acetone or 34 nmole of RA was applied at the indicated times before each twice weekly applications of 100 nmole of 3-MC or B[a]P.

[e] Experiment 5: Acetone (0.2 ml), RA (34 nmole), or 7,8-benzoflavone (367 nmole) in 0.2 ml acetone was applied topically to the shaved backs of mice 30 min before each once weekly applications of 0.2 μmole DMBA in 0.2 ml acetone.

3-methylcholanthrene (3-MC) or benzo[a]pyrene (B[a]P) did not inhibit tumor formation (Table 1).

Application of a single 3.6 μmole-dose of DMBA to mouse skin led to tumor formation. Again, application of retinoic acid (0.17 to 68 nmole) in conjunction with DMBA failed to inhibit tumor formation (6). In contrast, topical application of 7,8-benzoflavone in conjunction with a single 3.6 μmole or once weekly 0.2 μmole-doses of DMBA inhibited tumor formation (6, Table 1).

Effect of Retinoic Acid on ODC Induction

As shown in Fig. 2, 17 nmole of retinoic acid, when applied 1 hr before treatment with 5 nmole of TPA, inhibited by about 90% the induction of ODC

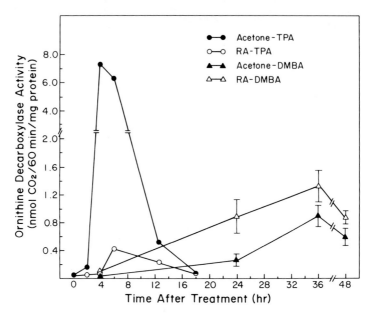

FIG. 2. Effect of RA pretreatment on the induction of ODC activity by TPA as well as by DMBA. Groups of mice were treated with 17 nmole of RA or acetone 1 hr before the application of 3.6 μmole of DMBA or 5 nmole of TPA. Epidermal ODC activity was determined at the indicated times following DMBA or TPA treatment (6). Each point represents the mean or the mean $\pm$ SE of determinations carried out from three groups of 3 mice each.

activity. In contrast, the application of retinoic acid 1 hr before the application of 3.6 μmole of DMBA failed to inhibit at any time point, but rather, paradoxically potentiated the induction of ODC activity at 24 hr ($p < 0.01$) after treatment. Even more extensive treatments with 0.017, 0.17, or 1.7 nmole of retinoic acid were ineffective; four applications of either dose at 3-hr intervals immediately preceding and four applications at 2-hr intervals immediately following 3.6 μmole of DMBA did not inhibit ODC induction. Furthermore, application of 17 nmole of retinoic acid 30 min before each 0.2 μmole of DMBA application failed to inhibit the induction of ODC activity at 28 hr after the seventh DMBA treatment. In contrast, 7,8-benzoflavone, which inhibits the metabolism of DMBA to proximate carcinogen(s), inhibited the induction of ODC activity by DMBA (6).

Retinoic acid, when administered in conjunction with an initiating dose of DMBA, had no apparent effect on the initiating potency of DMBA (5). Thus, it seems unlikely that this amplification by retinoic acid of DMBA carcinogenesis was the result of the effect of retinoic acid on enhancement of the metabolism of DMBA, its binding to deoxyribonucleic acid (DNA), or the inhibition of the DNA excision repair enzymes.

SUMMARY AND CONCLUSIONS

The biology of tumor formation by the initiation-promotion protocol differs from that of the complete carcinogenesis process. In the latter case, the latency period is longer and tumor yield is less, but carcinomas appear much earlier. Retinoic acid, a potent inhibitor of both the induction of ODC activity and tumor promotion by TPA, failed to inhibit both the induction of ODC activity and tumor formation by DMBA. 7,8-Benzoflavone, which did not inhibit the induction of ODC activity by TPA, inhibited the induction of ODC activity and tumor formation by DMBA.

The results indicate that: (a) mechanism of the induction of ODC activity and tumor formation by a complete carcinogen appears to be different from that of the tumor promoter TPA; (b) DMBA-induced ODC activity may be an important component of the mechanism of DMBA carcinogenesis; and (c) although there is a wealth of data that indicate the efficacy of the retinoids in the prevention of a variety of cancers in experimental animals, including mammary carcinogenesis by DMBA (3,5), the present results and those reported by others (2) are not in agreement with a universal effect of retinoic acid in the prevention of carcinogenesis.

ACKNOWLEDGMENT

The investigations were supported by grants CA-07175 and CA-22484 from the National Cancer Institute. The encouragement of Dr. R. K. Boutwell throughout the course of this work is gratefully acknowledged.

REFERENCES

1. Boutwell, R. K. (1974): The function and mechanism of promoters of carcinogenesis. *CRC Crit. Rev. Toxicol.,* 2:419–433.
2. Forbes, P. D., Urbach, F., and Davies, R. D. (1979): Enhancement of experimental photocarcinogenesis by topical retinoic acid. *Cancer Lett.,* 7:85–90.
3. Sporn, M. B., and Newton, D. L. (1979): Chemoprevention of cancer with retinoids. *Fed. Proc.,* 38:2,528–2,534.
4. Turusov, V., Day, N., Andrianov, L., and Jain, D. (1971): Influence of dose on skin tumors induced in mice by single application of 7,12-dimethylbenzanthracene. *J. Natl. Cancer Inst.,* 47:105–111.
5. Verma, A. K., Shapas, B. G., Rice, H. M., and Boutwell, R. K. (1979): Correlation of the inhibition of retinoids of tumor promoter-induced mouse epidermal ornithine decarboxylase activity and of skin tumor promotion. *Cancer Res.,* 39:419–425.
6. Verma, A. K., Conrad, E. A., and Boutwell, R. K. (1980): Induction of mouse epidermal ornithine decarboxylase activity and skin tumors by 7,12-dimethylbenz[a]anthracene: Modulation by retinoic acid and 7,8-benzoflavone. *Carcinogenesis,* 1:607–611.

Carcinogenesis, Vol. 7, edited by E. Hecker et al.
Raven Press, New York © 1982.

Further Exploration of Stages in Carcinogenesis

V. Armuth and I. Berenblum

Experimental Biology Unit, The Weizmann Institute of Science, Rehovot 76 100, Israel

An experiment on the influence of caffeine in skin carcinogenesis by the initiation-promotion technique is summarized in this chapter. A somatic mutation as the initiating phase in two-stage carcinogenesis has gained wide acceptance. According to current theory, the repair of deoxyribonucleic acid (DNA) damage plays a decisive role in mutation fixation, and thus in the establishment of initiated dormant tumour cells. Caffeine has been reported to enhance *in vitro* mutation and transformation frequencies by inhibiting postreplication DNA repair (1,2). *In vivo,* however, caffeine tends to decrease tumour induction by chemical carcinogens (3). In the present experiment, a single dose of caffeine was used as a possible gene-modulating factor during the carcinogenic process.

Young adult female ICR mice were injected s.c. with 25 mg urethan in 1 ml saline, followed 2 weeks later by twice-weekly topical applications of anthranil. Caffeine (100 μg/g body weight) was injected s.c. in the different experimental groups (see Table 1) to determine its influence in relation to late initiation and/or early promotion. Groups 8 to 12 were designed to explore any effect of caffeine treatment on the systemic carcinogenicity of urethan.

As shown in Fig. 1, a single caffeine injection 6 hr before urethan initiation,

TABLE 1. *Experimental groups*[a]

Group no.	Treatment				
(1)	Urethan				
(2)	Urethan	2 wk	Anthranil		
(3)	Caffeine	24 hr	Urethan	2 wk	Anthranil
(4)	Caffeine	9 hr	Urethan	2 wk	Anthranil
(5)	Caffeine	6 hr	Urethan	2 wk	Anthranil
(6)	Caffeine + urethan		2 wk	Anthranil	
(7)	Urethan	6 hr	Caffeine	2 wk	Anthranil
(8–12)	As groups 3–7, without subsequent Anthranil treatment (to be evaluated at autopsy)				
(13)	Untreated controls				

[a] 30 ICR female mice/group.

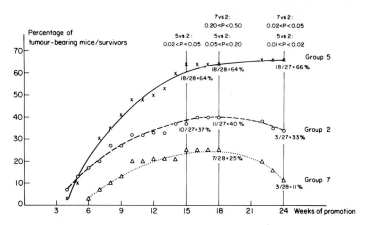

Fig. 1. Papilloma induction: Effect of caffeine, given 6 hr before or after urethan initiation. ○ - - - ○, group 2; x —— x, group 5; △......△, group 7 (See Table 1).

significantly increased the incidence of skin papillomas—most evidently by the 24th week from the beginning of promotion, when spontaneous regression in the control group (group 2) had already taken place. The importance of timing is reflected in the inhibitory effect of the same dose of caffeine, given 6 hr after urethan initiation, which no doubt accounts for the anticarcinogenic action of caffeine reported by others.

ACKNOWLEDGMENT

Supported by Grant 2R01-CA-21088, National Cancer Institute, DHEW.

REFERENCES

1. Donovan, P. J., and DiPaolo, J. A. (1974): Caffeine enhancement of chemical carcinogen-induced transformation of cultured Syrian hamster cells. *Cancer Res.,* 34:2,730–2,737.
2. Roberts, J. J., and Sturrock, J. E. (1973): Enhancement by caffeine of N-methyl-N-nitroso-urea-induced mutations and chromosome aberrations in Chinese hamster cells. *Mutat. Res.,* 20:243–255.
3. Rothwell, K. (1974): Dose-related inhibition of chemical carcinogenesis in mouse skin by caffeine. *Nature,* 252:69–70.

Carcinogenesis, Vol. 7, edited by E. Hecker et al.
Raven Press, New York © 1982.

Epidermal Tumor Promotion by Regeneration

Thomas S. Argyris

Department of Pathology, SUNY, Upstate Medical Center, Syracuse, New York 13210

Promotion is one of the principal stages of epidermal tumorigenesis in the skin of mice. The hallmark of promotion is the appearance of an epidermal hyperplasia. But epidermal hyperplasia is also characteristic of epidermal regeneration following damage of almost any kind (for review, see ref. 1). Therefore, some early investigators of epidermal carcinogenesis wondered if epidermal tumor promotion was not simply the production of a chronic, regenerative epidermal hyperplasia (for review, see ref. 1). Most investigators have argued, however, that epidermal tumor promotion could not be equated to the production of a chronic, regenerative hyperplasia because a number of hyperplasia-producing agents, such as acetic acid, cantharidin, and ethylphenylpropriolate, produce regenerative epidermal hyperplasias but do not promote epidermal tumorigenesis (for review, see ref. 5). A close inspection of the data clearly indicates that the above agents do act as promoters; but their efficiency for tumor promotion is much less than that of the optimal regimen of 12-O-tetradecanoylphorbol-13-acetate (TPA), the most powerful chemical tumor promoter known. Since the capability of these so-called "nonpromoters" to promote epidermal tumorigenesis has never been studied over a wide range of dosages, nor using different regimens, the possibility exists that these substances might prove to be potent tumor promoters if the proper dosage and regimen were found. Also, no thorough studies have been published of the nature of the epidermal hyperplasia produced during the chronic application of these substances that enable one to know if, in fact, the chronic application of these substances produces an epidermal hyperplasia similar to that produced by the optimal tumor-promoting regimen of TPA.

That regenerative epidermal hyperplasia may promote epidermal tumorigenesis is suggested by the experiments of several investigators who have shown that repeated full-thickness wounds made on the skin of mice appropriately initiated with dimethylbenzanthracene (DMBA) is a sufficient promoting stimulus for the production of epidermal papillomas (for review, see ref. 2). Indeed, if one takes into consideration the fact that the area promoted by a simple cut is much less than the area when TPA is applied, then wounding turns out to be as powerful a promoter as TPA if the number of tumors/unit area are determined (3). However, full thickness wounds, in addition to producing an epidermal hyperplasia, also produce marked connective tissue proliferation (2). To be certain that regenerative epidermal hyperplasia is a sufficient stimulus for promotion, we must show that it, by itself, can promote epidermal tumorigenesis. We have developed a technique for the production of a regenerative epidermal hyperplasia by abrading the skin of mice with a felt wheel mounted on a motor tool (2). This results in the removal of the epidermis. The epidermis regenerates from the cells of the underlying hair follicles. Under these conditions, very little connective tissue proliferation is seen.

Table 1 demonstrates that repeated abrasion, using either a felt or emery wheel, of skin of CD-1 female mice initiated with DMBA results in the appearance of papillomas. Therefore, a regenerative epidermal hyperplasia is a sufficient stimulus for promotion of papillomas. If one compares the number of tumors promoted by abrasion with that by TPA per unit area of epidermis, then abrasion does not appear to be as efficient a promoter as TPA. This is probably not due to a refractoriness of the skin to promotion produced by the repeated abrasions, because if initiated skin that has been repeatedly abraded is treated twice weekly with TPA, the number of tumors that appear is similar to the number of tumors that TPA would have promoted in initiated, but nonabraded, skin (Table 1). We believe that the reason the tumor yield is low is because repeated abrasion of the skin not only removes the epidermis, but inadvertently also removes many of the growing epidermal tumors.

Since a regenerative hyperplasia is a sufficient stimulus for promotion, the question may be raised if TPA-induced epidermal hyperplasia is a regenerative epidermal hyperplasia. To investigate this possibility, we applied 17 nmole of

TABLE 1. Epidermal tumors in CD-1 female mice initiated with 200 nmole of DMBA and promoted by repeated abrasion

Experiment	No. of mice	Treatment	Total no. of tumors	Tumors/ mouse
1	28	Initiated and felt wheel-abraded 5× + 36 days[a]	15	0.5
2	14	Initiated and emery wheel-abraded 4× + 35 days	6	0.5
3	16	Not initiated and felt wheel-abraded 11× + 35 days	0	0
4	13	Initiated and felt wheel-abraded 4× + 36 days, then 17 nm of TPA 2× weekly for 85 days	60	4.6
5	36	Initiated and 17 nm TPA 2× weekly for 70 days in an area 2.83 cm²	135	3.8

[a] Abrasions done approximately every 21 days.

TPA onto the backs of CD-1 female mice and took biopsy specimens at intervals from 3 hr to 10 days following the application of TPA. Within 24 hr after the application of 17 nmole of TPA, there is definite epidermal damage (Fig. 1B). The degree of damage is not uniform. It may consist of nuclear pyknosis, cytoplasmic vacuolization, separation of the epidermis from the dermis, and epidermal cell degeneration. Nuclear counts of the epidermis following TPA treatment (Table 2) show that there is a significant decrease in the number of basal nuclei/mm of interfollicular epidermis (IFE), which is consistent with the suggestion that the TPA has produced epidermal damage. Interestingly, the epidermal damage occurs concomitantly with epidermal growth, since, as Table 2 indicates, there is an increase in the total number of nuclei/mm IFE and in the number of nucleated cell layers at the time epidermal damage and the decrease in the number of basal cells are seen.

We next asked if a similar set of events occurs in CD-1 female mouse skin initiated with DMBA following a single application of 17 nmole of TPA. CD-1 female mice whose skin had been initiated with 200 nmole of DMBA had 17 nmole of TPA applied. Biopsy specimens were taken from the skin at intervals as described above. Figure 1C shows that, as in the case of normal skin, TPA produces epidermal damage within hours after its application. Again, the damage is not uniform, and there is a decrease in the number of basal nuclei/mm IFE. These events occur within hours after treatment, at a time when the epidermis is beginning to grow, as indicated by the increase in the total number of nuclei/mm IFE and the number of nucleated cell layers (Table 2). Thus TPA in initiated mouse skin results in epidermal damage that appears to be linked to the evolution of the epidermal hyperplasia. But, as we cautioned earlier (1), we do not know if continued treatment with TPA results in the same amount of epidermal damage, or indeed any damage at all, as the first application does, in either normal or initiated epidermis. Indeed, there is suggestive evidence that continued TPA treatment results in less damage to the epidermis, as if the epidermis becomes resistant to the toxic effects of TPA (1).

Thus we conclude that, for this one dosage of TPA tested, there is circumstantial evidence that the epidermal hyperplasia produced by one application of TPA is a regenerative hyperplasia. It now becomes important to determine if there is a correlation for varying doses of TPA between the amount of damage TPA produces, its ability to promote, and the production of an epidermal hyperplasia. It is also important to determine if such a correlation exists for promoters other than TPA.

Finally, if we are correct in assuming that tumor promotion is the production of a lasting regenerative hyperplasia, one should not conclude that tumor promotion is simply an increase in epidermal mitogenesis, or cell division, as often suggested. This is not the case. Indeed there is some suggestive evidence that an increase in epidermal mitogenesis alone, without the production of a noticeable epidermal hyperplasia, does not promote epidermal tumorigenesis in skin initiated with DMBA (for review, see ref. 2). Regenerative epidermal hyperplastic

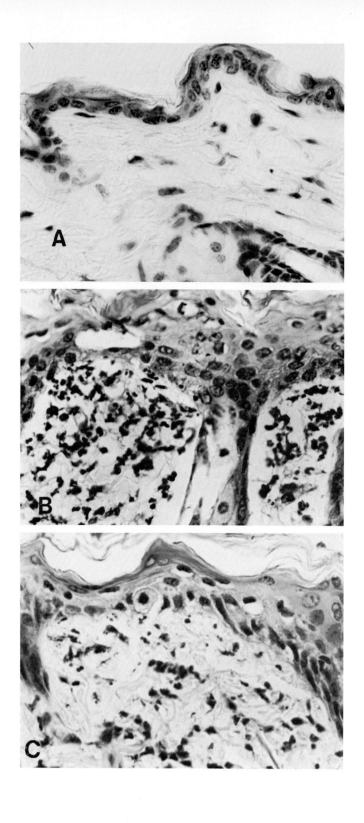

TABLE 2. *Nuclear counts and number of nucleated cell layers in normal or initiated mouse epidermis following treatment with TPA*

Days post-TPA treatment	No. of mice	Nuclear counts per mm IFE			No. of nucleated cell layers
		Normal Epidermis			
		Basal	Suprabasal	Total	
Normal	7	154 ± 5.8^a	64.3 ± 4.3	190 ± 7	2.0
1	7	99.7 ± 5.3	136 ± 17	235 ± 22	3.2 ± 0.2
2	6	110 ± 3.5	168 ± 17	278 ± 19	3.6 ± 0.2
3	7	126 ± 3.4	151 ± 8.9	277 ± 8.5	3.2 ± 0.2
4	7	146 ± 4.8	172 ± 19	318 ± 15	3.2 ± 0.3
5	8	139 ± 4.5	118 ± 7.6	256 ± 11	2.8 ± 0.2
10	4	143 ± 5.6	98 ± 6.9	241 ± 12	2.0
		Initiated Epidermis			
		Basal	Suprabasal	Total	
1	6	123 ± 5.6	175 ± 7.1	298 ± 11	3.2 ± 0.1
2	6	142 ± 6.7	199 ± 12	340 ± 19	3.6 ± 0.1
3	4	137 ± 5.5	196 ± 29	332 ± 24	3.6 ± 0.3
4	6	153 ± 5.0	199 ± 17	352 ± 14	3.6 ± 0.4
5	6	164 ± 2.1	171 ± 11	335 ± 12	3.2 ± 0.1
7	6	163 ± 4.8	146 ± 13	310 ± 15	2.8 ± 0.2
10	6	164 ± 5.6	137 ± 8.4	301 ± 12	2.3 ± 0.1

[a] Average $\pm$ SE of the mean.

growth is a complex developmental sequence. It does involve increased mitogenesis. But, in addition, it involves changes in the rates of epidermal differentiation characterized, for example, by an increased rate of cell loss, as evidenced by a decrease in the transit time, in spite of the fact that the epidermis is thickened (for review, see ref. 4). It also involves the appearance of a prominent stratum granulosum, an increase in the epidermal intercellular spaces, a marked enlargement of the epidermal cells, associated with a large increase in cellular ribonucleic acid (RNA) and protein, and an increase in the number of "dark" cells (for review, see ref. 4).

ACKNOWLEDGMENT

The author's research was supported by NIH Grant AM18219.

FIG. 1. **A:** Normal CD-1 female mouse epidermis. H&E, ×495. **B:** CD-1 female mouse epidermis 1 day after the application of 17 nmole of TPA. Compare to **A.** Note nuclear pyknosis and cytoplasmic degeneration. H&E, ×495. **C:** CD-1 female initiated mouse epidermis 18 hr after the application of 17 nmole of TPA. Compare to **A.** Note nuclear pyknosis and cytoplasmic vacuolization. H&E, ×495.

REFERENCES

1. Argyris, T. S. (1980*a*): Epidermal growth following a single application of 12-O-tetradecanoyl-phorbol-13-acetate in mice. *Am. J. Pathol.,* 98:639–648.
2. Argyris, T. S. (1980*b*): Tumor promotion by abrasion-induced epidermal hyperplasia in the skin of mice. *J. Invest. Dermatol.,* 75:360–362.
3. Argyris, T. S. (1980*c*): Tumor promotion by regenerative epidermal hyperplasia in mouse skin. *J. Cutaneous Pathol. (in press).*
4. Argyris, T. S. (1980*d*): The regulation of epidermal hyperplastic growth. *CRC Crit. Rev. Toxicol.* 9:151–200.
5. Scribner, J. D., and Suss, R. (1978): Tumor initiation and promotion. *Int. Rev. Exp. Pathol.,* 18:137–198.

Carcinogenesis, Vol. 7, edited by E. Hecker et al.
Raven Press, New York © 1982.

New, Most Active 1α-Alkyldaphnane-Type Irritants and Tumor Promoters from Species of the Thymelaeaceae

W. Adolf, S. Zayed, and E. Hecker

Institute of Biochemistry, German Cancer Research Center, D-6900 Heidelberg, Federal Republic of Germany

During the past 10 years, irritant principles of a large number of species of the plant families Euphorbiaceae and Thymelaeaceae have been isolated, structurally elucidated, and their irritant activity determined quantitatively on the mouse ear. They exhibit also vesicant activity in skin and sometimes are extremely toxic to eyes and mucous membranes (for recent reviews, see 2,3,4). Most, but not all, of the irritant principles also proved to be strong cocarcinogens of the tumor promoter type (5,6). The irritants (and promoters) from these plant families are polyfunctional, partially esterified derivatives of the diterpene parent hydrocarbons tigliane, ingenane, and daphnane, such as, for example, the well-known prototypes 12-O-tetradecanoylphorbol-13-acetate (TPA) (7), 3-O-hexa-decanoylingenol (1) and huratoxin (12), simplexin (10), or mezerein (11). The latter three are orthoesters, an otherwise rare class in naturally occurring compounds, and the latter two were isolated from Thymelaeaceae. Recently, in several species of the Thymelaeaceae family, we detected another structural type of diterpenoid orthoesters, derived from the parent hydrocarbon 1α-alkyl-daphnane (14). They exhibit extremely high irritant and tumor-promoting activities and may be considered especially helpful to clarify certain structure/activity relationships in this class of compounds for the benefit of mechanistic investigations (S. Pečar et al., *this volume,* and R. Schmidt and E. Hecker, *this volume*).

CHEMICAL STRUCTURE OF NEW 1α-ALKYLDAPHNANE-TYPE POLYFUNCTIONAL DITERPENES

Guided by the assay for irritant activity on the mouse ear, from leaves and roots of the Australian *Pimelea simplex F. Muell.,* besides simplexin, Pimelea factor S_7 was isolated exhibiting the same MW and molecular formula as simplexin (Fig. 1). Spectroscopic characterization indicates a daphnane-type orthoes-

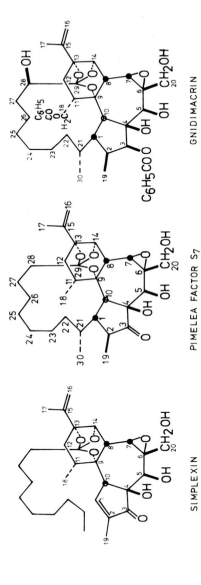

FIG. 1. Chemical structure of the new tumor promoter pimelea factor S₇, as compared to simplexin, both isolated from *Pimelea simplex* (Thymelaeaceae) and as compared to the antileukemic gnidimacrin, isolated from *Gnidia subcordata* (Thymelaeaceae).

ter as in simplexin. As compared to simplexin, however, clear evidence is provided for the absence of a 1,2-double bond. Instead, substitution at C-atom 1 may be deduced. Moreover, the presence of a saturated C-10 orthoester moiety including a branched methyl group and a C-C-double bond equivalent is apparent. The latter suggests a cyclic structure for the orthoester residue. Thus it may be concluded that, as in case of the highly antileukemic gnidimacrin (9) isolated from *Gnidia subcordata* (Meissn.) Engl. (Thymelaeaceae), the orthoester alkyl chain is covalently attached to position 1 of the daphnane skeleton, forming an ansa-like intramolecular bridge on the α-side of the diterpene moiety (see Fig. 1). The structure of gnidimacrin was fully established by X-ray diffraction analysis. The parent hydrocarbons of gnidimacrin and of Pimelea factor S_7 both represent the new 1α-alkyldaphnane skeleton. Like simplexin, Pimelea factor S_7 carries a 3-keto group in the diterpenoid parent. In both compounds, the 1α-alkyl residue, consisting of 10 carbon atoms, carries in the ω-position a carboxyl group. Together with the hydroxyl groups at C-atoms 9, 13, and 14, it is involved in the very stable orthoester group. The similarity and, hence, possible biogenetic relationship (2) of the structures of simplexin and Pimelea factor S_7 are evident.

From *Synaptolepis kirkii Oliv.,* another African species of the Thymelaeaceae, Synaptolepis factor K_1 was isolated (Fig. 2). It carries a 3-keto group as Pimelea factor S_7 does, but contains a C-16 1α-alkyl group with a double bond "conjugated" with the orthoester group. Two further highly irritant factors of the 1α-alkyldaphnane type, Pimelea factors P_2 and P_3, were isolated from both the New Zealandian *Pimelea prostrata Willd.* and the South American *Daphnopsis racemosa Griseb.* (14). Both factors carry, similar to gnidimacrin, a 3β-benzoyloxy group in the 3-position of the parent acid (see Fig. 2). From spectroscopic data it may be deduced that the factors P_2 and P_3 most probably are epimeric with respect to the secondary methyl group at C-atom 21 of the 1α-alkyl side chain.

IRRITANT AND PROMOTING ACTIVITIES OF THE NEW 1α-ALKYLDAPHNANE DERIVATIVES

Irritant Activities on the Mouse Ear

All of the new 1α-alkyldaphnane-type orthoesters exhibit on the mouse ear (7) low irritant doses 50 (ID_{50}), i.e. high irritant activities (see Table 1). The ID_{50} of Synaptolepis factor K_1 is one-fifth of that of TPA. The ID_{50} of Pimelea factors P_3 and S_7 is comparable with that of TPA. Pimelea factor P_2, most probably the 21-epimer of factor P_3, exhibits about one-third of the ID_{50} of the latter. Gnidimacrin (9), very similar in structure to Pimelea factor P_2, was not available to us and thus not tested so far *in vivo*.

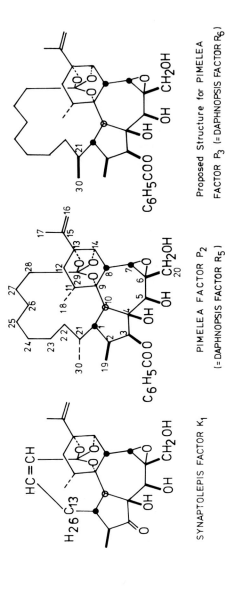

FIG. 2. Chemical structures of new tumor promoters of the 1α-alkyldaphnane type isolated from *Synaptolepis kirkii* (synaptolepis factor K₁), *Pimelea prostrata*, and *Daphnopsis racemosa* (pimelea factors P₂ and P₃).

TABLE 1. *Irritant activity on the mouse ear of the new tumor promoters of the 1-alkyldaphnane type as compared to TPA*

Factor	Isolated from	Irritant doses 50 (ID$_{50}$, nmole/ear)
P$_2$	*Pimelea prostrata* *Daphnopsis racemosa*	0.006
P$_3$	*Pimelea prostrata* *Daphnopsis racemosa*	0.02
S$_7$	*Pimelea simplex*	0.01
K$_1$	*Synaptolepis kirkii*	0.003
TPA	*Croton tiglium*	0.016
Gnidimacrin	*Gnidia subcordata*	not tested

Tumor-Promoting Activities on the Back Skin of Mice

The tumor-promoting activity in the standard assay on the back skin of mice (7) of most factors of the 1α-alkyldaphnane type is comparable to that of TPA in dose/response experiments with 10 nmole, 5 nmole, and even as low as 2.5 nmole per application, respectively (see Table 2). As does TPA, the new promoters show a clear dose response relation. The tumor rates and tumor yields of

TABLE 2. *Tumor rates and tumor yields of pimelea factors P$_2$ and P$_3$ and of Synaptolepis factor K$_1$ in various doses in the standardized assay on back skin of mice and compared to TPA after 12 and 24 weeks*[a]

Factor	Single dose p (nmole)	Tumor rates[b]		Tumor yields[c]	
		12 weeks	24 weeks	12 weeks	24 weeks
TPA	10	89	89	9.6	8.2
P$_3$	10	74	100	2.2	7.5
P$_2$	10	71	85	2.3	3.7
TPA	5	73	93	6.9	8.1
P$_3$	5	86	83	3.0	8.5
P$_2$	5	60	87	0.9	5.7
K$_1$	5	60	86	1.3	2.7
TPA	2.5	32	44	1.5	1.7
P$_3$	2.5	50	100	2.5	5.8
P$_2$	2.5	7	54	0.1	2.1
K$_1$	2.5	7	87	0.3	2.9
TPA	1.25	20	40	0.9	3.3
P$_3$	1.25	7	80	0.1	3.0
P$_2$	1.25	0	7	0	0.1

[a] Initiation: i = 0.1 μmole of DMBA; Promotion: twice weekly doses *p* of the promoters.
[b] Average tumor rate: number of tumor-bearing animals/number of survivors of the group in percent.
[c] Average tumor yield: number of tumors/number of survivors of the group.

Pimelea factor P_3, which exhibits less irritant activity than factor P_2 on the mouse ear, are definitely higher than those generated by factor P_2. In a dose of 2.5 nmole/application, the tumor rates and tumor yields of Pimelea factor P_3 appear to be even higher than those of TPA. With a lower dose of 1.25 nmole per application of TPA and Pimelea factor P_3 respectively, however, both exhibit similar low tumor rates and yields. With this dose and for the time interval of exposure chosen, factor P_2 does not produce any tumors (see Table 2). Pimelea factor S_7 could not be tested so far because of lack of compound. Gnidimacrin (9), which was not tested for tumor-promoting activity *in vivo*, was assayed for its capacity to induce plasminogen activator in human cell cultures (13). It was shown that, like tumor-promoting phorbol esters, gnidimacrin had a strong effect on the induction of this proteolytic enzyme. This may be considered a further example of molecules, such as mezerein showing tumor-promoting (4) as well as antileukemic activity (8).

The high tumor-promoting activities of the 1α-alkyldaphnane type orthoesters presented might introduce them as another new class of very potent tumor promoters. Their specific structure may make them especially helpful tools to sort out from the multiplicity of pleiotropic responses stimulated by diterpene ester-type promoters those parameters truly responsible for the biochemical mechanism of tumor promotion (S. Pečar et al., *this volume*, and R. Schmidt and E. Hecker, *this volume*).

ACKNOWLEDGMENT

The generous support of our investigations by the Wilhelm and Maria Meyenburg Foundation, Heidelberg (F. R. G.) is gratefully acknowledged.

REFERENCES

1. Adolf, W., and Hecker, E. (1975): On the active principles of the spurge family. III. Skin irritant and cocarcinogenic factors from the caper spurge. *Z. Krebsforsch.,* 84:325–344.
2. Adolf, W., and Hecker, E. (1977): Diterpenoid irritants and cocarcinogens in Euphorbiaceae and Thymelaeaceae: Structural relationships in view of their biogenesis. *Isr. J. Chem.,* 16:75–83.
3. Evans, F. J., and Schmidt, R. J. (1980): Plants and plant products that induce contact dermatitis. *Planta Med.,* 38:289–316.
4. Hecker, E. (1977): New toxic, irritant, and cocarcinogenic diterpene esters from Euphorbiaceae and from Thymelaeaceae. *Pure Appl. Chem.,* 49:1,423–1,431.
5. Hecker, E. (1978): Structure activity relationships in diterpene esters irritant and cocarcinogenic to mouse skin. In: *Carcinogenesis, Vol. 2: Mechanism of Tumor Promotion and Cocarcinogenesis,* edited by T. J. Slaga, A. Sivak, and R. K. Boutwell, pp. 11–48. Raven Press, New York.
6. Hecker, E. (1981): Cocarcinogenesis and tumor promoters of the diterpene ester-type as possible carcinogenic risk factors. *J. Cancer Res. Clin. Oncol.,* 99:103–124.
7. Hecker, E., and Schmidt, R. (1974): Phorbolesters—The irritants and cocarcinogens of *Croton tiglium* L. *Prog. Chem. Org. Natur. Prod.,* 31:377–467.
8. Kupchan, S. M., and Baxter, R. L. (1974): Mezerein: Antileukemic principle isolated from *Daphne mezereum* L. *Science,* 187:652–653.
9. Kupchan, S. M., Shizuri, Y., Murae, T., Sweeny, Y. G., Haynes, H. R., Shen, M. S., Barrick,

J. C., Bryan, R. F., van der Helm, D., and Wu, K. K. (1976): Gnidimacrin and Gnidimacrin-20-palmitate: Novel macrocyclic antileukemic diterpenoid esters from *Gnidia subcordata. J. Am. Chem. Soc.,* 98:5,719–5,720.

10. Roberts, H. B., McClure, T. J., Ritchie, E., Taylor, W. C., and Freeman, P. W. (1975): The isolation and structure of the toxin of *Pimelea simplex* responsible for St. George disease of cattle. *Aust. Vet. J.,* 51:325–326.

11. Ronlan, A., and Wickberg, B. (1970): The structure of mezerein, a major toxic principle of *Daphne mezereum* L. *Tetrahedron Letters,* 49:4,261–4,264.

12. Sakata, K., Kawazu, K., Mitsui, T., and Masaki, N. (1971): Structure and stereochemistry of huratoxin, a piscicidal constituent of *Hura crepitans. Tetrahedron Letters,* 16:1,141–1,144.

13. Weinstein, I. B., Wigler, M., and Pietropaolo, C. (1977): The action of tumor-promoting agents in cell culture. In: *Mechanisms of Carcinogenesis, Proceedings of the Cold Spring Harbor Conferences on Cell Proliferation,* Vol. 4, edited by H. H. Hiatt, J. D. Watson, and J. A. Winsten, pp. 751–772. Cold Spring Harbor Laboratory, Origins of Human Cancer, Cold Spring Harbor, New York.

14. Zayed, S., Adolf, W., Hafez, A., and Hecker, E. (1977): New highly irritant 1-alkyldaphnane derivatives from several species of Thymelaeaceae. *Tetrahedron Letters,* 39:3,481–3,482.

Carcinogenesis, Vol. 7, edited by E. Hecker et al.
Raven Press, New York © 1982.

Simple Phorbol Esters as Inhibitors of Tumor Promotion by TPA in Mouse Skin

R. Schmidt and E. Hecker

Institute of Biochemistry, German Cancer Research Center, D-6900 Heidelberg, Federal Republic of Germany

Tumor promotion by 12-O-tetradecanoylphorbol-13-acetate (TPA) in 7,12-dimethylbenz(a)anthracene(DMBA)-initiated mouse skin may be inhibited by a variety of compounds that differ in structure and mechanism of action. Among these are antiinflammatory steroids (13), prostaglandin synthetase inhibitors (11), retinoids (12), and protease inhibitors (6). Recently a "paradoxical" inhibiting effect on TPA-induced tumor promotion by anthralin (3) and by weakly or nonpromoting inflammatory agents (4) was reported.

For our search for more specific inhibitors, i.e., of inhibitors of early events in the TPA-induced biochemical cascade(s), the following hypothesis was postulated: for induction of their (promotion-?) specific biological activities, phorbol esters of the agonist-type (e.g., TPA) have to interact with acceptor/receptor site(s) in the target tissue and this interaction may be of a hydrophilic (diterpene part)/hydrophobic(long-chain ester)-type. Therefore it may be expected that TPA-induced tumor-promoting activity would be inhibited by certain structurally closely related phorbol esters as potential antagonists. Such phorbol esters may be selected by criteria derived from previous studies on structure/activity relationships—they should be marginally active or inactive as tumor promoters and as irritants, and they should carry an intact or only slightly modified phorbol moiety (5). Data will be presented to show that tumor promotion by TPA may be inhibited without dramatically altering the proliferative response of mouse skin.

METHODS AND RESULTS

Biological Experiments

Experimental Set-Up

The back skin of groups of 15 female NMRI mice was initiated at the age of 7 weeks with $i = 100$ nmole of DMBA. One week later, twice weekly treatments with either $p = 5$ nmole of TPA or TPA plus the amounts indicated of the respective inhibitor ($m \leq 40$ nmole) was started (see Figs. 1 to 3). Results

57

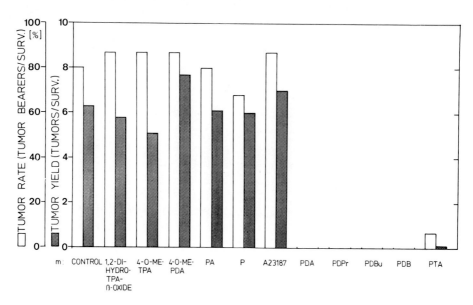

FIG. 1. Structure-activity relation of inhibition of tumor promotion. i = 100 nmole DMBA, p = 5 nmole TPA, m = 40 nmole, compounds as indicated. For structures, see Table 1. Data are shown for 12 weeks of treatment.

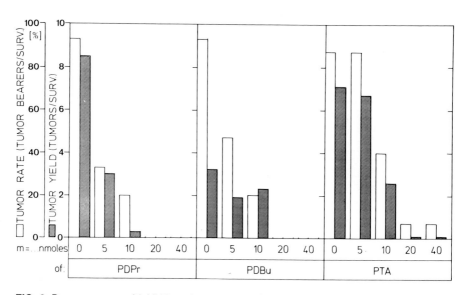

FIG. 2. Dose-response of inhibition of tumor promotion. i = 100 nmole DMBA, p = 5 nmole TPA, m = as indicated. For structures of compounds, see Table 1. Data are shown for 12 weeks of treatment.

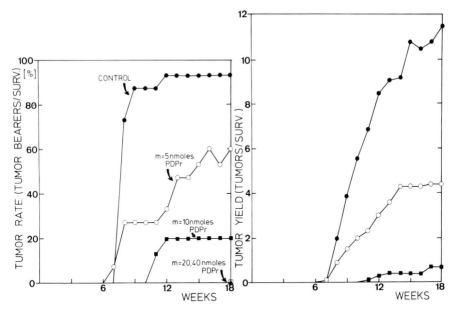

FIG. 3. Time course of dose-dependent inhibition by PDPr of tumor promotion by TPA. $i =$ 100 nmole DMBA, $p = 5$ nmole TPA, $m = \ldots$ nmole PDPr as indicated. For structures of compounds, see Table 1.

are expressed as average tumor rate (tumor bearing animals/survivors in %) and average tumor yield (tumors/survivors).

Inhibition of TPA-Promotion by Phorbol Derivatives In Vivo

Structure/activity correlation

(a) Compounds that inhibit promotion (Fig. 1): Promotion of tumors by 5 nmole of TPA alone gives rise to a high tumor rate and yield (Fig. 3). When applied concomittantly with TPA, the short-chain phorbol-12,13-diesters phorbol-12,13-diacetate (PDA), phorbol-12,13-dipropionate (PDPr), and phorbol-12,13-dibutyrate (PDBu), the ester-carrying aromatic acyl residues phorbol-12,13-dibenzoate (PDB), and the short-chain phorbol-12,13,20-triester (PTA) strongly inhibit tumor promotion at a dose level of $m = 40$ nmole. These derivatives have marginally to moderate irritating and, at the dose of 40 nmoles, no tumor-promoting activities (see Table 1).

(b) Compounds that have no inhibiting effect: Short- or long-chain phorbol esters, modified in the diterpene part, such as 4-O-methylphorbol-12,13-diacetate (4-O-MePDA), 4-O-methyl-12-O-tetradeconylphorbol-13-acetate (4-O-MeTPA), and 1,2-dihydroTPA-β-oxide (see Table 1) are without influence on

TABLE 1. Structures and comparative biological activities of various phorbol esters

Structures (I) and (II): OR^2, OR^3, OH (positions 12, 13), OR^1 (position 4), OR^4 (position 20); (II) with epoxide at positions 6, 7.

		Compounds				Biological activities		
Abbreviation	Formula	R^1	R^2	R^3	R^4	Irritation[a] ID_{50} nmole/ear	Promoting activity[b] (rel. potency)	Inhibition of promotion[c] (rel. potency)
P	I	H	H	H	H	>100	0	0
PA	"	"	H	Ac	"	40	0	0
TP	"	"	$CO(CH_2)_{12}CH_3$	H	"	>100	0	+
PDA	"	"	Ac	Ac	"	17.6	0^d	0
4-O-ME-PDA	"	CH_3	Ac	Ac	"	not tested	not tested	+
PDPr	"	H	$COCH_2CH_3$	$COCH_2CH_3$	"	2.6	0^d	+++
PDBu	"	"	$CO(CH_2)_2CH_3$	$CO(CH_2)_2CH_3$	"	0.7	0^d	+
PDB	"	"	COC_6H_5	COC_6H_5	"	0.24	0^d	+
TPA	"	"	$CO(CH_2)_{12}CH_3$	Ac	"	0.016	++++	0
4-O-ME-TPA	"	CH_3	"	"	"	2.3	$(+)^e$	0 (strong agonist)
PTA	II	H	Ac	"	Ac	not tested	$(+)^f$	+
1,2-DIHYDRO-TPA-β-OXIDE	"	"	$CO(CH_2)_{12}CH_3$	"	H	>100	0	0

[a] Irritant dose 50 (ID_{50}) on the mouse ear read 24 hr after administration (ref. 5).
[b] Initiation/promotion standard experiment with DMBA as initiator (ref. 5).
[c] Inhibitor (40 nmole) was administered together with TPA (5 nmole).
[d] $p = 40$ nmole of promoter.
[e] $p = 400$ nmole of promoter.
[f] $p = 2$ μmole of promoter.

promotion by TPA, as also is the case with the parent alcohol phorbol and the monoesters PA and TP. Interestingly the Ca^{2+}-Ionophore A23187, which is a strong skin irritant and hyperplasiogenic but not tumor promoting (9), does not interfere with TPA-promotion.

Dose/response relation

For the potent inhibitors PDPr, PDBu, and PTA, a dose-dependent inhibition was shown (see Figs. 2 and 3). It is obvious, that in the case of PDPr and PDBu, even at the 1:1 molar ratio of TPA versus inhibitor, both tumor rate and yield are significantly inhibited.

Biochemical Experiments

The following experiments were done by using female NMRI mice as above, treated with 5 nmole of TPA or the combination of 5 nmole TPA/40 nmole PDPr as indicated.

Thymidine Incorporation into Epidermal Deoxyribonucleic Acid

At various time intervals after treatment, mice were injected i.p. with 30 μCi ^{3}H-thymidine/30 g 1 hr prior to sacrifice. Skins were removed, epidermal scrapings were made from deep-frozen skin with a scalpel, deoxyribonucleic acid (DNA) was isolated, and radioactivity/DNA amount was determined by known methods (8). There was no significant difference in DNA labeling between the two treatments (TPA versus TPA/PDPr) (data not shown).

Metabolism and Clearance of ^{3}H-TPA from Epidermis

Mice were treated as outlined above, but with a ^{3}H-TPA preparation instead of nonlabeled TPA (7). Skins were removed at various times after treatment, epidermal scrapings were made at room temperature, homogenized in and extracted (five times) with chloroform/methanol (1:2) using a polytron PT 10 homogenizer (setting "6,45" for each extraction; ice-bath cooling). There was no significant difference between the ^{3}H-TPA and ^{3}H-TPA/PDPr treatment, with regard to quality (98% TPA, traces of PA) and quantity of radioactivity extracted, which were determined by radio-thin-layer chromatography (RTLC) on silica gel, diethyl ether/water saturated as solvent, and liquid scintillation counting of aliquots (data not shown).

Histology

Mice were treated once or eight times (4 weeks) with 5 nmole of TPA or 5 nmole TPA/40 nmole PDPr. Skins were removed, embedded in paraffin, and sections stained with hematoxylin/eosin (H/E). After the single application there was no difference between the two treatments with regard to hyperplasia. After eight treatments, however, the TPA-treated skins exhibited a slightly more intense hyperplasia than those treated with TPA/PDPr.

DISCUSSION

The results presented here show that it is possible to inhibit tumor promotion without dramatic influences on proliferation as measured by thymidine incorporation into DNA and histology. This observation is in agreement with the known fact that proliferation stimulation is not a sufficient (but probably a necessary) prerequisite for tumor promotion (5). The most effective inhibitors of TPA-promotion are short-chain phorbol-12,13-diesters (including the dibenzoate) and the short-chain 12,13,20-triester PTA.

It is remarkable that in attempts to modulate promotion induced by TPA, the long-chain analog 4-O-MeTPA (of marginal irritating and promoting, but strong hyperplasiogenic, activity (5)), 4-O-MePDA, the 1,2-dihydroTPA-β-oxide (no irritating and tumor-promoting activity (10)), and the structurally very different Ca^{2+}-Ionophore A23187, which is strongly irritating and hyperplasiogenic but not tumor promoting (9), are without effect. Similarly, the parent alcohol phorbol as well as PA proved to be noninhibitors.

Assuming that the inhibition by short-chain phorbol esters of TPA-mediated promotion works via a truly pharmacologic (and not merely by a toxicologic) interaction, this effect would support the concept that strong agonists like TPA have to interact in the target tissue with specific sites, or receptor(s). This interaction would then be inhibited (competitively ?) by marginally active analogs like PDA et al. It may be speculated that for a specific promoter/receptor interaction, primarily the diterpene part of the total molecule is the critical entity. For being a strong agonist (such as TPA), however, a certain lipophilicity as provided by the ester entity of the structure also appears to be necessary. Some other explanations may be considered as well: (a) the inhibitors studied might affect "down-regulation" of putative receptors; (b) they could modulate effects on "initiated cells" exerted, for example, by the immune surveillance system; or (c) they might have specific influences on the dermal reactions in response to TPA: irritation, activities of leukocytes, and so on. Nevertheless, short-chain phorbol esters offer to be promising tools for studying, out of the pleiotropic plurality of biochemical events well known from *in vitro* studies (for review, see refs. 1,2), the crucial biochemical mechanism of action of potent tumor promoters like TPA, including studies on possible receptor interactions. For interesting, however different, *in vivo* experimental approaches in the TPA receptor area, see W. Adolf et al. and S. Pečar et al., *this volume.*

REFERENCES

1. Blumberg, P. (1980): *In vitro* studies on the mode of action of the phorbol esters, potent tumor promoters: Part 1. *CRC Crit. Rev. Toxicol.,* 8:153–197.

2. Blumberg, P. (1981): *In vitro* studies on the mode of action of the phorbol esters, potent tumor promoters: Part 2. *CRC Crit. Rev. Toxicol.,* 8:199–234.

3. DeYoung, L. M., Helmes, C. T., Chao, W.-R., Young, J. M., and Miller, V. (1981): Paradoxical effect of anthralin on 12-O-tetradecanoylphorbol-13-acetate-induced mouse epidermal ornithine decarboxylase activity, proliferation, and tumor promotion. *Cancer Res.,* 41:204–208.

4. DiGiovanni, J., and Hoel, M. J. (1980): Inhibitory effects of weakly or nonpromoting inflammatory agents on skin tumor-promotion by TPA. *Proc. Am. Assoc. Cancer Res.,* 21:105.

5. Hecker, E. (1978): Structure-activity relationships in diterpene esters irritant and cocarcinogenic to mouse skin. In: *Carcinogenesis—A Comprehensive Survey, Vol. 2: Mechanisms of Tumor Promotion and Cocarcinogenesis,* edited by T. J. Slaga, A. Sivak, and R. K. Boutwell, pp. 11–48. Raven Press, New York.

6. Hozumi, M., Ogawa, M., Sugimura, T., Takeuchi, T., and Umezawa, H. (1972): Inhibition of tumorigenesis in mouse skin by leupeptin, a protease inhibitor from actinomycetes. *Cancer Res.,* 32:1725–1728.

7. Kreibich, G., and Hecker, E. (1970): On the active principles of Croton oil. X. Preparation of tritium-labeled Croton oil factor A_1 and other tritium-labeled phorbol derivatives. *Z. Krebsforsch.,* 74:448–456.

8. Krieg, L., Kühlmann, I., and Marks, F. (1974): Effect of tumor-promoting phorbol esters and of acetic acid on mechanisms controlling DNA synthesis and mitosis (chalones) and on the biosynthesis of histidine-rich protein in mouse epidermis. *Cancer Res.,* 34:3135–3146.

9. Marks, F., Fürstenberger, G., and Kownatzki, E. (1981): Prostaglandin E-mediated mitogenic stimulation of mouse epidermis *in vivo* by divalent cation ionophore A23187 and by tumor promoter 12-O-tetradecanoylphorbol-13-acetate. *Cancer Res.,* 41:696–702.

10. Schmidt, R., and Hecker, E. (1975): Biological activities of functional derivatives of the tumor promoter TPA. *3rd Meeting, European Association of Cancer Research,* Nottingham 23.9–25.9.1975, Abstracts, p. 63.

11. Verma, A. J., Ashendel, C. L., and Boutwell, R. K. (1980): Inhibition of prostaglandin synthesis inhibitors of the induction of epidermal ornithine decarboxylase activity, the accumulation of prostaglandins, and tumor promotion caused by 12-O-tetradecanoylphorbol-13-acetate. *Cancer Res.,* 40:308–315.

12. Verma, A. K., Slaga, T. J., Wertz, R. W., Mueller, G. C., and Boutwell, R. K. (1980): Inhibition of skin tumor promotion by retinoic acid and its metabolite 5,6-epoxyretinoic acid. *Cancer Res.,* 40:2367–2371.

13. Weeks, C. E., Slaga, T. J., Hennings, H., Gleason, G. L., and Bracken, W. M. (1979): Inhibition of phorbol ester-induced tumor promotion in mice by vitamin A analog and antiinflammatory steroid. *J. Natl. Cancer Inst.,* 63:401–406.

Carcinogenesis, Vol. 7, edited by E. Hecker et al.
Raven Press, New York © 1982.

Relation Between the Structures of Ingenol Esters and Their Ornithine Decarboxylase-Inducing Activities in Mouse Skin

*H. Fujiki, *M. Mori, *T. Sugimura, †H. Ohigashi, † M. Hirota, and †K. Koshimizu

*National Cancer Center Research Institute, Tsukiji 5-1-1, Chuo-ku, Tokyo 104; and
†Department of Food Science and Technology, Faculty of Agriculture,
Kyoto University, Kyoto 606, Japan

During studies on the induction of ornithine decarboxylase (ODC) activity in mouse skin by 12-O-hexadecanoyl-16-hydroxyphorbol-13-acetate and its derivatives including the 4-deoxycompound, we found that the structural requirements for ODC-inducing activity are similar to those for tumor-promoting activity (1). Hecker's group has reported the tumor-promoting activity of an ingenol ester, 3-O-hexadecanoylingenol, but the ODC-inducing activities of ingenol esters, including 3-O-hexadecanoylingenol, have not been investigated.

Previously, four new ingenol esters, 20-O-isobutyryl-3-O-propionylingenol, 20-O-isobutyrylingenol, 20-O-(S)-(2'-methyl)-butyryl-3-O-propionylingenol, and 3,20-di-O-isobutyrylingenol were isolated from dry leaves of *Euphorbia cotinifolia* L. as piscicidal constituents (2). We tested ODC induction of two of them, 20-O-isobutyryl-3-O-propionylingenol and 20-O-isobutyrylingenol (Fig. 1). Further, we synthesized five ingenol esters. This is a report of studies on the relationships between the structures of naturally occurring and synthetic ingenol esters and their ODC-inducing activities.

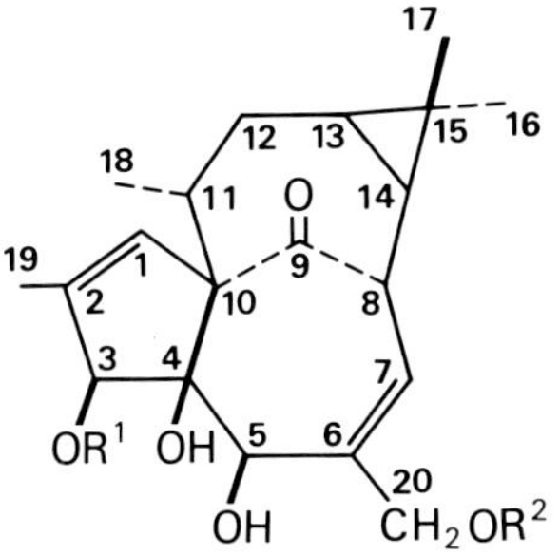

20-O-Isobutyryl-3-O-propionylingenol

$R^1 = COCH_2CH_3$
$R^2 = COCH(CH_3)_2$

20-O-Isobutyrylingenol

$R^1 = H$
$R^2 = COCH(CH_3)_2$

FIG. 1. Structures of new ingenol esters.

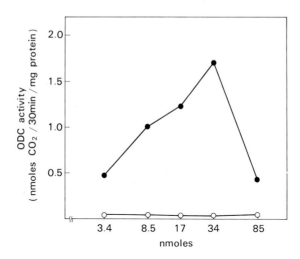

FIG. 2. Dose-response of ODC induction with 20-O-isobutyryl-3-O-propionylingenol and 20-O-isobutyrylingenol. ODC activity was determined in mouse skin, 4 hr after application of compounds. 20-O-isobutyryl-3-O-propionylingenol (●——●) and 20-O-isobutyrylingenol (○——○).

Induction of ODC activity in mouse skin occurred 3 to 5 hr after application of 20-O-isobutyryl-3-O-propionylingenol and was maximal at a dose of 34 nmole. In contrast, 20-O-isobutyrylingenol did not induce ODC activity at all (Fig. 2 and Table 1).

Results of ODC induction by synthetic ingenol esters are summarized in Table 1. 3,20-Di-O-tetradecanoylingenol and 3,20-di-O-decanoylingenol both induced ODC activity, their potencies being similar. However, ingenol esters acylated at C-5, i.e., 3,5,20-tri-O-acetylingenol and 3,5,20-tri-O-propionylingenol, caused no induction of ODC activity. The absence of ODC-inducing activity

TABLE 1. *Induction of ODC activity by naturally occurring and synthetic ingenol esters*

Compound (34 nmole)	Activity[a] nmole CO_2/30 min/mg protein
20-O-Isobutyryl-3-O-propionylingenol	1.70
20-O-Isobutyrylingenol	0.03
3,20-Di-O-tetradecanoylingenol	0.59
3,20-Di-O-decanoylingenol	0.69
3,5,20-Tri-O-propionylingenol	0.04
3,5,20-Tri-O-acetylingenol	0.04
Ingenol 3,4:5,20-diacetonide	0.01
Ingenol	0.03

[a] The ODC activity was measured 4 hr after their applications.

of these compounds seemed to be related to the esterification at C-5 of the ingenol ester rather than to a short fatty acid chain, because 20-O-isobutyryl-3-O-propionylingenol induced ODC activity. Furthermore, ingenol diacetonide did not induce ODC activity (Table 1).

These naturally occuring and synthetic ingenol esters may be useful in elucidating the role of the chain length of the acyl group attached to the oxygen at C-3, C-20, and C-5 in ODC induction and, possibly, also of tumor promotion.

ACKNOWLEDGMENTS

This work was supported in part by Grants-in-Aid for Cancer Research from the Ministry of Education, Science, and Culture and the Ministry of Health and Welfare of Japan, the Princess Takamatsu Cancer Research Fund, and the Research Foundation for Cancer and Cardiovascular Diseases.

REFERENCES

1. Fujiki, H., Mori, M., Sugimura, T., Hirota, M., Ohigashi, H., and Koshimizu, K. (1980): Relationship between ornithine decarboxylase-inducing activity and configuration at C-4 in phorbol ester derivatives. *J. Cancer Res. Clin. Oncol.*, 98:9–13.
2. Hirota, M., Ohigashi, H., Oki, Y., and Koshimizu, K. (1980): New ingenol-esters as piscicidal constituents of *Euphorbia cotinifolia* L. *Agric. Biol. Chem.*, 44:1,351–1,356.

Carcinogenesis, Vol. 7, edited by E. Hecker et al.
Raven Press, New York © 1982.

Teleocidin: New Naturally Occurring Tumor Promoter

*T. Sugimura, *H. Fujiki, *M. Mori, *M. Nakayasu, *M. Terada,
*K. Umezawa, and †R. E. Moore

National Cancer Center Research Institute, Chuo-ku, Tokyo 104, Japan;
and †Department of Chemistry, University of Hawaii,
Honolulu, Hawaii 96822

Investigations with 12-0-tetradecanoylphorbol-13-acetate (TPA), identified as the cocarcinogenic principle in croton oil, have provided much information on tumor promotion. Thinking that studies with other new and chemically different tumor promoters should open up new aspects of tumor promotion, we screened for new tumor promoters in our environment by measuring their effects in induction of ornithine decarboxylase (ODC) activity in mouse skin. We found that teleocidin, dihydroteleocidin B, lyngbyatoxin A, tetrahydrolyngbyatoxin A, and debromoaplysiatoxin induced ODC activity. Teleocidin was originally isolated from *Streptomyces mediocidicus* as a skin irritant in Japan. Dihydroteleocidin B was obtained by catalytic hydrogenation of the vinyl group of teleocidin. Lyngbyatoxin A and debromoaplysiatoxin, isolated from the marine blue-green alga *Lyngbya majuscula,* are known to be causative agents of "swimmers' itch" in Okinawa and Hawaii. Tetrahydrolyngbyatoxin A was prepared from lyngbyatoxin A by catalytic hydrogenation. The structures of these five compounds are shown in Fig. 1. Teleocidin, lyngbyatoxin A, and their hydrogenated derivatives are indole alkaloids and debromoaplysiatoxin is a polyacetate. All these compounds are chemically very different from phorbol esters.

Interestingly, the effective concentrations of teleocidin, dihydroteleocidin B, lyngbyatoxin A, tetrahydrolyngbyatoxin A, and debromoaplysiatoxin for induction of ODC activity in mouse skin were similar to that of TPA (1). Furthermore, the effects of these compounds in ODC induction were all markedly inhibited by 13-*cis*-retinoic acid, applied to the skin 1 hr previously. The ODC-inducing activities of teleocidin, dihydroteleocidin B, and lyngbyatoxin A were completely abolished by hydrolysis of these compounds with 6N hydrochloric acid containing 4% thioglycolic acid for 20 hr at 110°. The structural changes caused by hydrolysis of the lactam ring of these molecules might be responsible for the loss of biological activity.

The five compounds induced cell adhesion of human promyelocytic leukemia cells (HL-60) to flasks within 48 hr. They also induced differentiation of HL-

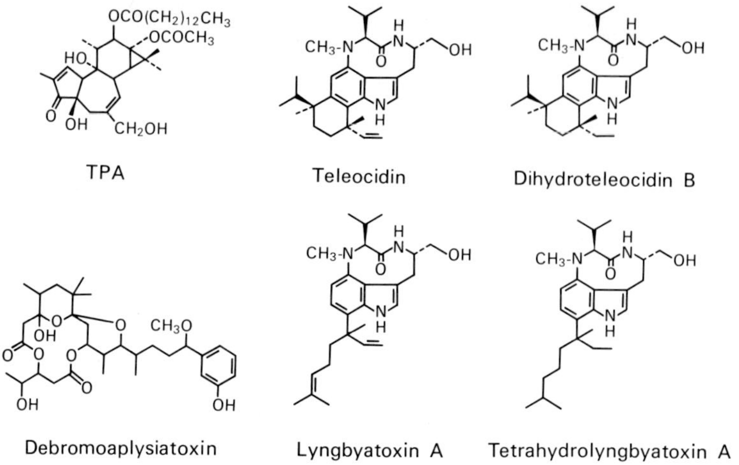

FIG. 1. Structures of TPA, teleocidin, dihydroteleocidin B, debromoaplysiatoxin, lyngbyatoxin A, and tetrahydrolyngbyatoxin A.

60 cells, characterized by the appearance of phagocytic and lysozyme activities, morphological changes, and loss of myeloperoxidase activity. Most of the differentiated cells showed the properties of macrophages. The effective doses of teleocidin and lyngbyatoxin A and their hydrogenated compounds for cell adhesion and differentiation of HL-60 cells were similar to that of TPA, but the effective dose of debromoaplysiatoxin was 100 times more.

These five compounds inhibited terminal differentiation of Friend erythroleukemia cells induced by dimethyl sulfoxide, which could be demonstrated by estimation of benzidine reactive cells. This effective dose of the first four compounds for this was also comparable to that of TPA.

We also studied the biological effects of teleocidin and dihydroteleocidin B *in vitro.* These compounds caused aggregation of human lymphoblastoid cells (3). Moreover, they induced increase of 2-deoxyglucose uptake, release of arachidonic acid, production of prostaglandins, inhibition of epidermal growth factor (EGF) binding, and competed with TPA for its receptor in 10T1/2 cells (K. Umezawa et al., *in preparation*). Therefore, teleocidin, dihydroteleocidin B, lyngbyatoxin A, and tetrahydrolyngbyatoxin A, like TPA, seem to possess strong tumor-promoting activities *in vivo.*

Tests on the effects of dihydroteleocidin B, teleocidin, and lyngbyatoxin A on mouse skin are being performed, based on the two-stage concept of carcinogenesis. Tests on dihydroteleocidin B are now finished. Carcinogenesis was initiated in the skin of female CD-1 mice (8 weeks old) with 100 μg of 7,12-dimethylbenz(a)anthracene (DMBA). Starting 8 days later, either 2.5 μg of dihydroteleocidin B or 2.5 μg of TPA was applied twice weekly. The doses of dihydroteleocidin B and TPA used were equivalent to the induction of ODC activity in mouse

TABLE 1. *Effects of dihydroteleocidin B and TPA on* in vivo *carcinogenicity tests on mouse skin*

	No. of survivors after 30 weeks	No. of mice with tumors	No. of tumors per mouse	No. of mice with carcinoma
DMBA + dihydroteleocidin B	19	17	4.6	11
DMBA + TPA	13	11	15.6	7
Dihydroteleocidin B	20	2	0.1	0
TPA	15	2	0.1	0
DMBA	14	0	0	0
Acetone	15	0	0	0

skin within 4 hr after their application. Four control groups treated for 30 weeks with only DMBA, dihydroteleocidin B, TPA, and acetone, respectively, were also included in this experiment. The tumor-promoting effects of dihydroteleocidin B and TPA in surviving mice after 30 weeks are summarized in Table 1 (2). The groups given DMBA plus dihydroteleocidin B or dihydroteleocidin B each consisted of 20 mice, while other groups consisted of 15 mice each. The percentages of tumor-bearing mice are shown in Fig. 2. Tumors of more than 1 mm in diameter were recorded every week. After 30 weeks, 90% of the mice treated with DMBA plus dihydroteleocidin B and 85% of those treated with DMBA plus TPA had tumors.

Quantitative differences were observed between these two groups, especially in the average number of skin tumors per mouse. The group treated with DMBA plus dihydroteleocidin B had 4.6 tumors per mouse, whereas the group given

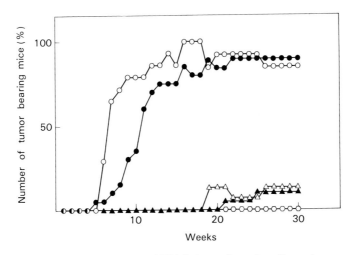

FIG. 2. Effects of dihydroteleocidin B and TPA in tumor formation. Percentages were calculated on the basis of the number of surviving mice. DMBA + Dihydroteleocidin B (●——●), DMBA + TPA (○——○), Dihydroteleocidin B (▲——▲), TPA (△——△), and DMBA (○——○).

TABLE 2. *Histological types of skin tumors*

Promoter	No. of skin tumors examined	Squamous cell carcinoma[a]	Papilloma[a]	Hyperplasia[a]
Dihydroteleocidin B	73	15	56	2
		(21)	(77)	(3)
TPA	132	11	117	4
		(8)	(89)	(3)

[a] Percent in parentheses.

DMBA plus TPA had 15.6 per mouse (Table 1). Moreover, the average diameter of tumors in the group given DMBA plus dihydroteleocidin B was 5.1 mm, whereas that in the group given DMBA plus TPA was 4.0 mm. The skin tumors in all groups were examined histologically. The numbers of mice bearing squamous cell carcinomas are shown in Table 1. The incidences of carcinomas were similar in the groups treated with dihydroteleocidin B and with TPA.

Histologically, the skin tumors were classified into three types: squamous cell carcinomas, papillomas, and hyperplasias. As shown in Table 2, 73 of the 87 tumors in the group treated with DMBA plus dihydroteleocidin B, and 132 of the 204 tumors in the group given DMBA plus TPA were examined. The percentage of incidences of squamous cell carcinomas and papillomas in the two groups were similar. Thus dihydroteleocidin B was as effective as TPA in production of malignancy.

Experiments now in progress show that teleocidin is also as potent as TPA *in vivo*. Because of the similarities in the chemical structure and biological actions of lyngbyatoxin A to those of dihydroteleocidin B, it seems very likely that this compound, too, is a tumor promoter. Debromoaplysiatoxin is of special interest, because its effective concentration for induction of ODC activity in mouse skin is similar to that of TPA, but its effective concentration for differentiation of HL-60 cells is comparable to that of 4-O-methyl-TPA, which is not a tumor promoter and does not induce ODC activity. The carcinogenicity of debromoaplysiatoxin remains to be investigated.

These findings support the idea that there may be other unknown promoters in our environment.

ACKNOWLEDGMENTS

This work was supported in part by Grants-in-Aid for Cancer Research from the Ministry of Education, Science, and Culture, the Ministry of Health and Welfare of Japan, and the Princess Takamatsu Cancer Research Fund. Work on the isolation of debromoaplysiatoxin and lyngbyatoxin A used in this study was supported by Grant CA12632-06 from the National Cancer Institute, Department of Health, Education, and Welfare of USA.

REFERENCES

1. Fujiki, H., Mori, M., Nakayasu, M., Terada, M., and Sugimura, T. (1979): A possible naturally occurring tumor promoter, teleocidin B from *Streptomyces. Biochem. Biophys. Res. Commun.,* 90:976–983.
2. Fujiki, H., Mori, M., and Sugimura, T. (1980): Experimental carcinogenesis by a new tumor promoter, dihydroteleocidin B. *Proc. Japanese Cancer Assoc.* pp. 24–25. 39th Annual Meeting, November (Tokyo).
3. Hoshino, H., Miwa, M., Fujiki, H., and Sugimura, T. (1980): Aggregation of human lymphoblastoid cells by tumor-promoting phorbol esters and dihydroteleocidin B. *Biochem. Biophys. Res. Commun.,* 95:842–848.

Carcinogenesis, Vol. 7, edited by E. Hecker et al.
Raven Press, New York © 1982.

Diterpene Ester-Mediated Two-Stage Carcinogenesis

K. Goerttler, H. Loehrke, J. Schweizer, and B. Hesse

*German Cancer Research Center, Institute of Experimental Pathology,
6900 Heidelberg, Germany*

The two-stage carcinogenesis experiment developed 40 years ago by Berenblum (2) and Mottram (21) has in no way diminished in importance for us today. It has, in fact, become even more important in the field of human pathology, since the possibility of multistage development of the most frequently occurring tumors in man has become more possible.

The classic experiment, consisting of an irreversible initiation phase that entails the single application of a subcarcinogenic dose of a carcinogen followed by a promotion phase during which hyperplasiogenic cocarcinogens are continuously applied, was originally performed on the back skin of mice. The isolated application of the same dosage of the carcinogen or of the cocarcinogen remains just as ineffectual as the temporal exchange of initiation and promotion.

The two-stage experiment has certain advantages. Only small amounts of carcinogen are necessary for tumor production, thus avoiding the possibility of side effects which accompany higher carcinogen doses. At the same time, tumor yields are increased and latent periods are drastically shortened. This also favors the recognition of weak carcinogens, such as urethane, which, due to their low tumorigenic potency and long latency periods, can easily escape detection. Furthermore, the high purity of chemically defined tumor-promoting diterpene esters offers excellent conditions for the conduction of experiments.

Criticism with respect to the applicability of the experiment has not been lacking. Following the investigation of Shubik (23), the effectiveness of the phorbol ester-mediated two-stage carcinogenesis experiment on other species came into question, in that positive results had been previously observed only with mice, and then only on back skin. It appeared then that a generalization of the two-stage experiment on other species, as well as in organs other than the skin, would be problematic.

This chapter deals with results obtained in our laboratory over the past 10 years with experiments related to diterpene ester-mediated two-stage carcinogenesis in different organs and species.

THE STANDARD TWO-STAGE CARCINOGENESIS EXPERIMENT
APPLIED TO VARIOUS MOUSE STRAINS

The standard two-stage experiment is performed in our laboratory on 12-week-old female NMRI mice with a single application of 0.1 μmole = 0.0256 mg/animal dimethylbenzanthracene (DMBA) in acetone on the shaved back skin, followed by promotion with 10 nmole = 0.00615 μg 12-0-tetradecanoyl-phorbol-13-acetate (TPA) applied twice weekly over a period of 26 weeks.

After 5 to 6 weeks the first papillomas appear, and after 12 weeks, the first carcinomas. The C3H mouse, when treated similarly, shows the same tumor spectrum (3). The C57Bl mice develop, in addition, small melanotic spots, but no independent melanomas *(unpublished results)*. In Swiss mice, an increase in the relatively high spontaneous leukemia rate can be observed *(unpublished results)*, similar to that seen after administration of phorbol to SWR-mice and thymectomized AKR mice as described by Armuth and Berenblum (1). Probably in Swiss mice a latent infection with leukemia viruses can manifest itself quite early through the addition of croton oil or TPA. It has not yet been investigated whether it is possible to also induce tumors through foregoing exogenic immuno-suppression followed by the addition of the tumor promoter TPA. Depending on the mouse strain, we must therefore take into account a variable sensitivity to tumor-promoting phorbol esters, which is especially apparent in the Sencar mouse strain used in some American laboratories (18,24).

If tumor manifestation can be directly promoted by TPA in noninitiated animals with high incidences of spontaneous tumors (Table 1), then we must consider the fact that not only latent infections with tumor viruses (such as leukemia viruses or herpetic viruses) but also genetically determined alterations may be a cause of neoplasia without any induction by an exogenous carcinogen (Table 1). Iversen's experiments on the tumorigenic action of TPA in hairless mice (Oslo strain of hr/hr-mice) is a case in point (17). These animals exhibit pathological alterations (5), especially cystic transformation of the skin append-ages, that may be interpreted as precancerous lesions that can be subsequently promoted by TPA.

The tumor yield resulting from the two-stage carcinogenesis standard experiment can be increased in the following manner (6). If a stationary hyperplasia is produced before initiation, and promotion is effected in the normal interval,

TABLE 1. *Two-stage carcinogenesis; possible variations at the level of initiation*

Exogenous initiation	—		Promotion = Tumor yield +	
Latent virus infection	—		Promotion = Tumor yield + (?)	
Endogenous or artificial predisposition	—		Promotion = Tumor yield + (?)	
Induced hyperplasia	—	Exogenous initiation	—	Promotion = Tumor yield + +

more tumors are produced earlier (Table 1). It will later be demonstrated that the promotion of epithelial tumors depends on whether or not a stationary noninflammatory hyperplasia can be produced in a distinct epithelium.

RESULTS OF THE TWO-STAGE EXPERIMENT ON BACK SKIN OF SPECIES OTHER THAN MOUSE

In 1950 Shubik (23) reported negative results of the two-stage experiments on rats, guinea pigs, and rabbits. This was to be treated as a key work and proof of the nontransferability of the two-stage experiment from mouse to other species. It appeared necessary to us to recheck the experiment, for there was a possibility that dose and length of the time with Shubik's application scheme was the reason for the failure, rather than the principle of nontransferability. We therefore initiated male Sprague-Dawley rats with 2.5 mg DMBA per animal and treated them three times weekly with 10 nmole TPA. This was carried out over 52 weeks (12).

By 12 weeks after the beginning of promotion, 63% of the rats treated with DMBA-TPA had already developed skin tumors, and the percentage of tumor-bearing animals increased to 95% with time. Animals treated with DMBA alone also produced tumors, which indicates a slight overdose of the initiator (12). More interesting than the positive results of this experiment, however, were pecularities in the histological tumor spectrum. The skin tumor morphology in the mouse is rather uniform, but in the rat we consistently observed several different tumors in the same animal. Besides fibroepitheliomas and squamous cell carcinomas, these tumors comprised adenomas and carcinomas of the sebaceous glands, trichoepitheliomas, basaliomas, and, surprisingly, also a wide spectrum of nonepithelial tumors such as fibromas, histiocytomas, spindle-cell sarcomas, angiosarcomas, and angioendotheliomas *(unpublished results)*.

This experiment gave us proof that the diterpene ester-mediated two-stage carcinogenesis experiment is also effective in the rat, provided the doses of the substances are varied accordingly. In addition, it seems clear that not only the epidermis, but also initiated cells of the subjacent nonepithelial dermal tissue, can be promoted after DMBA initiation with TPA.

In the same species we were also able to obtain similar results with a single application of the carcinogen diazoacetic ethyl ester (DAEE; 100 mg/kg body weight) in combination with TPA, although with a somewhat lower tumor yield *(unpublished results)*. TPA, by itself, remained ineffective.

Our positive results in the rat are certainly important with regard to a general validity of the two-stage carcinogenesis principle. The effectiveness found here is, however, bound to specific requirements and exhibits species-dependent variations. This may be related to the variable sensitivity to a certain carcinogen or to the promoter.

A two-stage experiment performed on guinea pigs yielded negative results. Although guinea pigs react to the application of 20 nmole TPA with a marked hyperplasia, the combination of 2 mg DMBA as initiator with up to 160 nmole TPA as promoting dose shows no tumor-producing effect. Possibly, the relative insensitivity of guinea pigs to DMBA may be the reason for the negative results (J. Schweizer et al. *manuscript in preparation*). In contrast, pilot experiments indicate that the DMBA-TPA-mediated two-stage skin carcinogenesis experiment is successfully applicable to the European hamster and to the rabbit *(unpublished results)*.

Experiments with the Syrian golden hamster led to the surprising result that the two-stage experiment was more effective in this animal than we expected (11). Our experimental methodology consisted of an intragastric initiation with 100 mg DMBA/kg body weight, followed by TPA treatment of the back three times weekly with 20 nmole TPA over 26 weeks. At the end of the experiment no skin papillomas were observed. Instead, however, melanotic melanomas of various sizes appeared. These melanomas developed from circumscribed perifollicular melanoses and sometimes reached down to the panniculus carnosus while still being encapsulated. They reacted clearly as benign tumors. When tumor material was removed and transplanted subcutaneously in syngeneic animals, however, malignant melanomas occurred that developed multiple metastases in the axillary lymph nodes and in the lungs (11).

In the Syrian golden hamster, the melanocytes consequently took over the function of the epidermal cells as target organs for the two-stage carcinogenesis. Detailed studies comprising determination of labeling indices in hamster epidermis after stimulation with various hyperplasiogens and tumor-promoting substances revealed that the epidermal cells did not react at all, even when TPA was given in doses of up to 160 nmole; that is, no cell proliferation or increase of deoxyribonucleic acid (DNA) synthesis was observed (14). This reaffirms that the promotion of initiated cells is not only connected to actual initiation, but also to promotion-induced hyperplasia. It should be emphasized, however, that the nonsensitivity of the skin of the back of the Syrian golden hamster in no way means that other epithelial organs of this species are not sensitive to diterpene ester-mediated carcinogenesis (11). Finally, the hyperplasiogenic effect of diterpene esters does not restrict itself only to rodents. TPA produces immediate desquamation and epithelial regeneration in *Xenopus laevis*. In chickens, the comb, just as the skin of the back, is TPA-sensitive *(unpublished results)*.

EFFECTIVENESS OF DITERPENE ESTER-MEDIATED CARCINOGENESIS ON ORGANS OTHER THAN BACK SKIN

The epidermis of the back skin offers optimal conditions in the pursuit of tumor development, but the morphological differentiation of back skin into interfollicular epidermis, hair follicles, and sebaceous glands always leads to the question of which cells, from the viewpoint of initiation and promotion, are particularly affected. On the other hand, the epithelial tissue of the digestive tract, the esophagus, and the forestomach offers a more uniform texture. We therefore treated C57B1 mice with DMBA at 50 mg/kg body weight applied orally, followed by twice weekly intragastric applications of TPA at 0.2 mg per animal (10). After 37 weeks we found a significant doubling in the number of papillomas of the forestomach in the DMBA-TPA-treated groups as compared to the DMBA group. These findings therefore demonstrated that the squamous epithelia as such, and not only specially differentiated epithelial cells such as the skin epithelial cells, are sensitive to two-stage carcinogenesis. Just as interesting was the observation that the adenomatous cells of the adjacent glandular stomach were absolutely refractory to the DMBA-TPA treatment (10).

Rodents have a keratinized squamous epithelium covering the forestomach, while, in man, such epithelia only exist in the esophagus. As a model closer to man, we therefore chose the vaginal epithelium of NMRI mice for an intravaginal variation of the two-stage model (9). Each animal received once, as a tampon inlay, 0.02 ml of 1% DMBA solution in sesame oil with a 24-hr application period. Over the next 52 weeks followed promotion treatment with twice weekly intravaginal instillation of 20 nmole TPA in sesame oil. The group treated solely with TPA showed only epithelial hyperplasias and an increased rate of leukemias as opposed to the untreated control group. The group treated only with DMBA showed dyskeratosis and dysplasias but no carcinomas. The DMBA-TPA-treated animals showed formations of carcinomas of the vaginal wall epithelium as well as papillomas, carcinomas, and even sarcomas of the entire vaginal area (9; Table 2).

The most positive aspect of this two-stage experiment in an epithelial organ other than the epidermis of the back is again the demonstration of the basic transferability of this model of carcinogenesis to other organs. The experiment revealed further information, however. As is known, all rodents lick their external sexual organs, and this leads, after application of DMBA and TPA, to a natural uptake of these substances into the digestive tract, with the result that we could additionally detect papillomas and carcinomas of the forestomach both in the

TABLE 2. *Intravaginal two-stage carcinogenesis; tumor spectrum and tumor localization*

Controls:	Spontaneous lung adenomas, leukemias
TPA promotion only:	Vaginal epithelial hyperplasia, hyperkeratosis, lung adenomas, leukemias
DMBA initiation only:	Vaginal dysplasia, forestomach papillomas, mammary carcinomas, granulosa cell tumors (ovary), lung adenomas, leukemias
DMBA initiation and TPA promotion:	Vaginal dysplasia, vaginal papillomas, carcinomas, sarcomas, forestomach papillomas, carcinomas, mammary carcinomas, granulosa cell tumors (ovary), lung adenomas, leukemias

DMBA group and in the DMBA-TPA group (Table 2). In the latter group, however, using the same number of experimental animals, the yield was threefold that after DMBA application alone (9). In our experiments with Syrian golden hamsters, we had a similar uptake of substances by licking with the same result as regards tumor formation in internal epithelia. Here we not only observed the reported melanomas, but also additional papillomas in the region of the upper digestive tract, i.e., tongue, esophagus, and forestomach (11).

The intravaginal two-stage experiment gave us further secondary findings. With both the DMBA group and the DMBA-TPA group, we observed a similar rate of formation of mammary carcinomas and granulosa cell tumors of the ovary, which suggests that for the formation of these tumors only the DMBA application is significant (9). The second additional finding is related to lung tumors and leukemias, both found in small numbers in the untreated control group. The incidence of these tumors was increased threefold in the TPA group, a little less in the DMBA group, and fivefold in the DMBA-TPA group as compared to the control group, the ratio of occurrence being 2:3 between the TPA group and the DMBA-TPA group (9). This further demonstrates that the existing ratio of spontaneous tumors can be increased in those organs producing spontaneous tumors with TPA alone or, more effectively, with a combination of DMBA and TPA. There is additional evidence that TPA certainly influences not only the locally treated epithelia but, via uptake into the blood vessels, other organs of the organism.

TRANSMATERNAL INITIATION AND POSTNATAL PROMOTION OF THE F_1 GENERATION

In 1971, Herbst et al. published observations on the appearance of vaginal adenocarcinomas in young women whose mothers had been treated with high doses of synthetic estrogens during early pregnancy because of the risk of abortion (15). These findings have in the meantime been confirmed from several sides and put in the right scale. Some years earlier, two German groups (16,20) had confirmed and extended the older observation of Larsen (19), which suggested the possibility of introducing carcinogens through the placenta into the fetus and thus to generate tumors in the F_1 generation. These findings led us to a modification of the classical application scheme of the two-stage carcinogenesis experiment in which the initiation step was performed in a mother animal and the promotion treatment in the F_1 generation.

In one of the first experiments in this series, we investigated if DMBA could be transferred to the weanling animals through the mother's milk (7). Indeed, when the grown-up F_1 animals were treated regularly with TPA, they developed a high incidence of skin tumors, thus indicating that they had taken up the carcinogen during the suckling period. Moreover, the tumor sensibility of the F_1 animals was found to be greater than the sensibility of the mother animals subjected to the same TPA treatment (7).

Two further experiments on a large scale in connection with diaplacental carcinogenesis yielded even more interesting results (8). When DMBA or urethane were applied diaplacentally as initiators at different stages and several times during fetal development, we obtained a large number of tumors, both of the back epidermis as well as in many other organs in the TPA-treated F_1 animals (8). The most interesting tumors in organs other than the skin were those of the brain and the vaginal tract (8). The latter tumors were particularly exciting in the light of the findings of Herbst et al. in humans (15). In order to use initiating doses better tolerated by the mother animals, we had initiated the fetuses diaplacentally several times and at different stages of embryonic development. A thorough investigation of the observed tumors revealed that both the overall tumor incidence and the tumor incidence in different organs varied in relation to the time of diaplacental application of the initiating agents (8). In order to better work out phases of special organ sensitivity to initiation, we subsequently reduced the initiation step to only 1 day of gestation, and therefore applied 60 mg DMBA/kg body weight by means of a stomach tube to pregnant mice on days 6 to 20 of gestation (13). After promotion of the F_1 animals with TPA, a gradual increase in the skin tumor incidence with advanced time of embryonic development was noticed. Both parameters reached their maximum after initiation at day 18 of fetal life (13). Numerous histological and biochemical investigations have shown that at embryonic day 18, the epidermis reaches its state of complete tissue differentiation (for reviews, see ref. 13). A time course of tumor development comparable of that of integumental skin was also found in the forestomach. Tumors of the Harderian gland developed in both sexes only after initiating during the late prenatal period, whereas the incidence of leukemias was highest when the fetuses where exposed to the initiator at days 10 and 11 of development *(unpublished results)*. These findings clearly indicate that in a developing organism, besides the well-known "teratogenic determination periods (22)," also exist "oncogenic determination periods (4)" that are obviously linked to the differentiation process of the organ under consideration. We recently examined this concept in a pilot experiment replacing the chemical carcinogen as initiator by a diaplacental infection with the Rauscher leukemia virus. Obviously the blood cells of the fetal organism can be affected by the virus only after infection at day 11. Seventy percent of the F_1 animals died within 6 months from leukemias after postnatal treatment with TPA *(unpublished results)*.

CONCLUSIONS

The efficiency of the two-stage carcinogenesis model by means of the standardized Berenblum-Mottram experiment is proven for most of the experimental animals. In general, both integumental and internal epithelia represent the most sensitive target organs in terms of tumor promotion. There is, however, a large body of evidence that other organs are also involved in diterpene ester-mediated

TABLE 3. *DMBA-TPA-mediated two-stage carcinogenesis*

Target organs:
  Back skin epidermis [mouse, mastomys natalensis (25), rat, European hamster, rabbit]

  Dermal melanocytes (Syrian golden hamster)

  Squamous epithelia of upper digestive tract (mouse, Syrian golden hamster)

  Squamous epithelia of vagina (mouse, rat)

  Dermal connective tissue (rat)

  Hematopoetic system (in strains with elevated spontaneous tumor and leukemia rate: mouse)

  Harderian gland (in strains with elevated spontaneous tumor rate: mouse)

  Lung (in strains with elevated spontaneous tumor rate: mouse)

Refractory organs:
  Mammary gland parenchyma (mouse)

  Ovary (mouse)

  Glandular epithelium of digestive tract (mouse)

---

two-stage carcinogenesis (Table 3). This is especially evident in the pigmentary system of the Syrian golden hamster and, after diaplacental initiation, in a variety of internal organs of the mouse. Only few organs have been found to be refractory to the combination DMBA/TPA (Table 3). The principle of two-stage and multistage carcinogenesis is probably also valid in man, at least as far as epithelial organs are concerned, and therefore is also of paramount importance for the human pathologist.

REFERENCES

1. Armuth, V., and Berenblum, I. (1972): Leukemogenic action of phorbol in intact and thymectomized mice of different strains. *Br. J. Cancer,* 34:516–522.
2. Berenblum, I. (1941): The mechanism of cocarinogenesis: A study of significance of cocarcinogenic action and related phenomena. *Cancer Res.,* 1:807–814.
3. Boukamp, H. (1974): Über den Effekt epidermaler Zellhyperplasie auf die Tumor-Initiierung bzw. Tumor-Promotion im Berenblum-Experiment an der Mäusehaut. M. D. thesis, University of Heidelberg.
4. Goerttler, K. (1968): Experimentell-teratologische Aspekte zur Onkologie. In: *Aktuelle Probleme aus dem Gebiet der Cancerologie.* vol. II, edited by H. Lettré and G. Wagner, pp. 34–41. Springer-Verlag, Berlin.
5. Goerttler, K., and Friedmann, W. (1970): Strukturelle Veränderungen der Rückenhaut haarloser hr/hr-Mäuse während des Lebens (Epidermocutanbild und histologische Befunde). *Arch. Klin Exp. Derm.,* 237:635–651.
6. Goerttler, K., and Loehrke, H. (1976): Improved tumor yields by means of a TPA-DMBA-TPA variation of the Berenblum-Mottram experiment on the back skin of NMRI mice. The effect of stationary hyperplasia without inflammation. *Exp. Pathol.,* 12:336–341.
7. Goerttler, K., and Loehrke, H. (1976a): Transmaternal variation of the Berenblum experiment with NMRI mice. Tumor initiation with DMBA via mother's milk followed by promotion of the phorbol ester TPA. *Virchows Arch. (Pathol. Anat.).,* 370:97–102.

8. Goerttler, K., and Loehrke, H. (1976*b*): Diaplacental carcinogenesis: Initiation with the carcinogens dimethylbenzanthracene (DMBA) and urethane during fetal life and postnatal promotion with the phorbol ester TPA in a modified 2-stage Berenblum-Mottram experiment. *Virchows Arch. (Pathol. Anat.)*, 372:29–38.

9. Goerttler, K., Loehrke, H., and Hesse, B. (1980): Two-stage carcinogenesis in NMRI mice: Intravaginal application of 7,12-dimethylbenz(a)anthracene as initiator followed by the phorbol ester 12-O-tetradecanoylphorbol-13-acetate as promotor. *Carcinogenesis*, 1:707–713.

10. Goerttler, K., Loehrke, H., Schweizer, J., and Hesse, B. (1979): Systemic 2-stage carcinogenesis in the epithelium of the forestomach of mice using 7,12-dimethylbenz(a)anthracene as initiator and the phorbol ester 12-O-tetradecanoylphorbol-13-acetete as promotor. *Cancer Res.*, 39:1,293–1,297.

11. Goerttler, K., Loehrke, H., Schweizer, J., and Hesse, B. (1980*a*): Two-stage tumorigenesis of dermal melanocytes in the back skin of the Syrian golden hamster using systematic initiation with 7,12-dimethylbenz(a)anthracene and topical promotion with 12-O-tetradecanoylphorbol-13-acetate. *Cancer Res.*, 40:155–161.

12. Goerttler, K., Loehrke, H., Schweizer, J., and Hesse, B. (1980*b*): Positive two-stage carcinogenesis in female Sprague-Dawley rats using 7,12-dimethylbenz(a)anthracene (DMBA) as initiator and 12-O-tetradecanoylphorbol-13-acetate (TPA) as promotor. Results of a pilot study. *Virchows Arch. (Pathol. Anat.)*, 385:181–186.

13. Goerttler, K., Loehrke, H., Schweizer, J., and Hesse, B. (1980*c*): Two-stage skin carcinogenesis by systemic initiation or pregnant mice with 7,12-dimethylbenz(a)anthracene during gestation days 6 to 20 and postnatal promotion of the F_1-generation with the phorbol ester 12-O-tetradecanoylphorbol-13-acetate. *J. Cancer Res. Clin. Oncol., 98:267–275.*

14. Hasper, F. (1981): Biochemische Untersuchungen zur Zellproliferation der Rückenepidermis des Syrischen Goldhamsters nach Kurz- und Langzeiteinwirkung von promotorischen und nicht promotorischen Hyperplasiogenen. M. D. thesis, University of Heidelberg.

15. Herbst, A., Ulfelder, L., and Poscanzer, D. C. (1971): Adenocarcinoma of the vagina. Association of maternal stilbestrol therapy with tumor appearance in young women. *N. Engl. J. Med.*, 284:878–881.

16. Ivankovic, S., Druckrey, H., and Preussmann, R. (1966): Erzeugung neurogener Tumoren bei den Nachkommen nach einmaliger Injektion von Ethylnitrosoharnstoff an schwangeren Ratten. *Naturwissenschaften,* 53:410.

17. Iversen, J. M., and Iversen, O. L. (1979): The carcinogenic effect of TPA (12-O-tetradecanoylphorbol-13-acetate) when applied to the skin of hairless mice. *Virchows Arch. (Zellpathol.,* 30:33–42.

18. Klein-Szanto, A.J.P., Major, S.K., and Slaga, T.J. (1980): Induction of dark keratinocytes by 12-O-tetradecanoylphorbol-13-acetate and mezereine as an indicator of tumor-promoting efficiency. *Carcinogenesis*, 1:399–406.

19. Larsen, C. D. (1947): Pulmonary-tumor induction by transplacental exposure to urethan. *J. Natl. Cancer Inst.*, 8:63–70.

20. Mohr, U., and Althoff, J. (1964): Mögliche diaplacentarcarcinogene Wirkung von Diethylnitrosamin beim Goldhamster. *Naturwissenschaften,* 51:515.

21. Mottram, J. C. A. (1944): Developing factors in epidermal blastogenesis. *J. Pathol. Bacteriol.,* 6:807–814.

22. Schwalbe, E. (1906): Allgemeine Missbildungslehre (Teratologie). Eine Einführung in das Studium der abnormen Entwicklung. Gustav Fischer, Jena.

23. Shubik, P. (1950): Studies on the promoting phase in the stages of carcinogenesis in mice, rats, rabbits, and guinea pigs. *Cancer Res.*, 10:13–17.

24. Slaga, T. J., Fischer, S. M., Nelson, K., and Gleason, G. L. (1980): Studies on the mechanism of skin tumor promotion. Evidence for several stages in promotion. *Proc. Natl. Acad. Sci. USA*, 77:3,659–3,663.

25. Wayss, K., Reyes-Mayes, D., and Volm, M. (1981): Two-stage carcinogenesis in the back skin of *Mastomys natalensis* (muridae) using topical initiation with 7,12-dimethylbenz(a)anthracene and topical promotion with 12-O-tetradecanoylphorbol-13-acetate. *Virchows Arch. (Pathol. Anat.) (in press).*

Carcinogenesis, Vol. 7, edited by E. Hecker et al.
Raven Press, New York © 1982.

Properties of Incomplete Carcinogens and Promoters in Hepatocarcinogenesis

Henry C. Pitot, Tom Goldsworthy, Susan Moran, Alphonse E. Sirica, and Jane Weeks

McArdle Laboratory for Cancer Research, Departments of Oncology and Pathology, The Medical School, University of Wisconsin, Madison, Wisconsin 53706

The complexities of the natural history of carcinogenesis were appreciated to some degree by histopathologists during the latter part of the 19th century and the beginning of the 20th. The experimental dissection of the natural history of neoplastic development began with the early studies of Rous and Kidd (35) and of Mottram (22). Subsequently the studies of Berenblum and Shubik (4) clearly demonstrated that epidermal carcinogenesis may be divided into at least two stages designated earlier by Rous and Kidd as initiation and promotion. Later studies by Boutwell (6), Hecker (13), and others (34,40,41,43) have confirmed and extended these earlier investigations.

The characteristics of the stages of initiation and promotion in the natural history of the development of epidermal cancer have been reviewed (6,13). The principal distinctions between the two processes are as follows. Initiation is irreversible and exhibits characteristics of "memory." Initiation is to some extent dependent on the cell cycle and, for those chemical carcinogens requiring metabolic activation, the metabolic capabilities of the target cell. In contrast, promotion is reversible and, as many have shown, capable of modulation by diet, hormones, and other environmental factors (5,6). The fact that repeated applications of a promoting agent such as tetradecanoylphorbol acetate (TPA) may lead to a low incidence of tumors has been suggested as indicating that known promoters are actually weak carcinogens. The fact that initiated cells may remain dormant for extended periods, however, even more than a year in mouse skin, suggests that efficient promoting agents may promote cells initiated by ambient environmental factors such as background radiation, dietary carcinogens, etc. (47). Unfortunately, no critical experiment to distinguish these two mechanisms for any particular promoting agent have thus far been reported. On the other hand, Salaman and Roe (36) demonstrated that the hepatic and pulmonary carcinogen urethane was capable of initiating cells in mouse skin but not of producing neoplasms. These investigators used the term incomplete carcinogen for such an agent, as contrasted with complete carcinogens that have the capability both of initiating and promoting neoplasia. Most known carcinogens appear to fall into this latter category of complete carcinogens.

TWO-STAGE CARCINOGENESIS IN LIVER AND OTHER EXTRAEPIDERMAL TISSUES

Although the large number and variety of "preneoplastic" lesions seen in human and experimental neoplasms suggested that the natural history of many, if not all, types of extraepidermal carcinogenesis did occur in stages, such a fact was not fully appreciated until the experiment of Peraino and his associates who demonstrated that initiation by a short feeding of 2-acetylaminofluorene in liver could be promoted to 100% tumor incidence by the subsequent administration in the diet of 0.05% phenobarbital (PB) (26). Some earlier studies demonstrating possible two-stage mechanisms in carcinogenesis of the mouse forestomach and rat thyroid were reported, but the vast majority of papers describing two-stage mechanisms in extraepidermal tissues have occurred during the last decade (31). These include such tissues as the bladder, colon, liver, lung, and mammary gland. Promoting agents found to be effective in these various tissues include saccharin in the bladder, bile acids in the colon, prolactin in the mammary gland, and butylated hydroxytoluene in the lung of the mouse. Since Peraino's original observation, several chemicals have been shown by his laboratory and others to be effective promoting agents when fed subsequent to the administration of low levels of acetylaminofluorene (24,25), azo dyes (16), or nitrosamines (30). In addition, several different model systems for demonstrating sequential steps in hepatocarcinogenesis have been described. That of Peraino and his colleagues (26) has been discussed above. Scherer and Emmelot (37,38) administered single small doses of diethylnitrosamine (DEN) following a 70% partial hepatectomy (PH) and monitored changes with qualitative histochemical strains for canalicular ATPase. In their studies, doses less than 30 mg/kg of the carcinogen given intragastrically induced only small enzyme-altered islands of cells in the liver and no hepatomas, the number of islands being directly proportional to the dose of carcinogen. At higher doses such proportionality was lost and animals developed hepatocellular carcinomas in addition. Ito and his co-workers (45) have employed a system similar to that of Peraino but for a much shorter period of promotion, monitoring only the induction of hyperplastic hepatic nodules. In addition, a PH was performed after 1 week of feeding the promoting agent.

A somewhat more complicated model has been devised by Solt and Farber and their associates. (44). In this instance, a single dose of DEN (200 mg/kg) is administered and 2 weeks later the feeding of a diet containing 0.02% acetylaminofluorene is begun. One week following this, PH is performed and the acetylaminofluorene diet continued for 1 week later. Within a relatively short time, usually within the week following the cessation of the acetylaminofluorene-containing diet, foci of cells appear that are basophilic and stain positive for the enzyme γ-glutamyltranspeptidase. Farber (9) has pointed out similarities between these various model systems, such as the necessity for cell proliferation during the stage of initiation, but the subsequent handling of the promotion phase differs significantly among the various systems. In our laboratory we have combined the system of Scherer and Emmelot, using only the lower doses of DEN with that of Peraino and his colleagues using PB as a promoter (29). It is the characteristics of this system that we will discuss in the remainder of this chapter.

CHARACTERISTICS OF AGENTS INDUCING, ENHANCING, OR MODIFYING HEPATOCARCINOGENESIS

Based on the pathogenesis of epidermal carcinoma, agents affecting and effecting the production of neoplasia of a specific histogenetic origin may be divided into three general categories for the purposes of this report, complete carcinogens, incomplete carcinogens (or pure initiating agents), and promoting agents. Complete carcinogens are those agents, chemical, physical, or biological, exhibiting the capability of inducing the neoplastic transformation in the absence of other enviornmental agents. Such agents exhibit the capacity both to initiate cells and to promote such initiated cells to neoplasia. An operational complication in identifying such agents unequivocally is the fact that many only exert their effects *in vivo,* where numerous other modifying environmental factors are always present, such as hormones and a variety of other small molecular and macromolecular compounds, many of which have been shown to act as promoting agents. In addition, although not to be discussed here, are other complicating factors such as cocarcinogens which permit rather than enhance the action of a complete or incomplete carcinogen and anticarcinogens which prevent the action of complete or incomplete carcinogens as well as promoting agents by a variety of mechanisms.

Prior to the pioneering experiments of Peraino, a number of workers, including Bannasch and Klinge (1), Goldfarb and Zak (12), and Farber (8), had suggested that specific lesions occurred within the liver prior to the appearance of hepatocellular carcinoma. These lesions ranged from foci of hepatocytes exhibiting abnormal glycogen storage (1) to the appearance of nodules of hepatocytes morphologically distinguishable from the normal liver structure (8,12). In addition Friedrich-Freska and his associates (11) more than a decade ago described the appearance of foci of hepatocytes exhibiting a deficient glucose-6-phosphatase activity as measured histochemically. The presence of such lesions and the hypothesis that they were somehow precursors to the final carcinoma implied the presence of stages during the process of hepatocarcinogenesis by complete carcinogens. It is only within the last 8 years, however, that such theories have borne fruit, making it now possible to investigate characteristics of individual stages of hepatocarcinogenesis and of agents selectively inducing the stages of initiation and of promotion.

CHARACTERISTICS OF INCOMPLETE CARCINOGENS (PURE INITIATORS) IN HEPATOCARCINOGENESIS

Studies of Salaman and Roe (36), as well as by Berenblum and Haran-Ghegra (3), demonstrating the incomplete carcinogenic, or pure initiating activity of urethane in mouse epidermal carcinogenesis serve as a model for the identification of incomplete carcinogens in hepatocarcinogenesis. If such existed, these agents should conform to certain theoretical criteria. These criteria are seen in Table 1. With the exception of point number 3 concerning the induction of enzyme-altered foci (EAF) which have been proposed as the immediate progeny of initiated cells in liver (11,29), the first two points also apply to epidermal carcinogenesis. If there were a mechanism to score or identify the immediate progeny of initiated cells in the epidermis, then presumably characteristic number 3 could also be satisfied in that tissue.

Studies from our laboratory have been directed in part towards identifying actual and potential incomplete carcinogens in hepatocarcinogenesis. Our initial study (18) demonstrated that the azo dye, 2-methyl-N,N-dimethyl-4-aminoazobenzene(2-Me-DAB), when fed for periods of 3 or 6 weeks to weanling rats, followed by 0.05% PB in the diet for 66 further weeks resulted in virtually all animals developing tumors, most of which were carcinomas. In contrast, controls given only the azo dye for comparable periods of time exhibited very few tumors and only one small carcinoma. Previous studies by Miller and Baumann (21) demonstrated that this material was not carcinogenic even when fed to adult rats for prolonged periods of time. Warwick reported, however, that a PH performed during the dye-feeding period did result in the production of hepatomas in most animals (48). Thus either PH or PB was capable of enhancing or promoting the formation of neoplasms following a relatively short time of administration of the azo dye (Peraino protocol). In addition, the administration of the agent with or without PB resulted in the production of a significant

TABLE 1. *Characteristics of initiators (incomplete carcinogens) and promoters in hepatocarcinogenesis*

Initiators (incomplete carcinogen)

1. Produce significant numbers of neoplasms in liver only when followed by administration of promoter. (Small nonnecrogenic doses of complete carcinogens may act as initiators.)
2. Mutagenic *per se* or may be metabolized to mutagenic form by liver.
3. A single dose following PH in the absence of a promoting agent induces a relatively small number of demonstrable EAF in liver.

Promoters

1. Produce no or a very few liver neoplasms on prolonged continuous administration.
2. Are not mutagenic in any form but do alter gene expression, especially xenobiotic metabolism, many acting via a receptor mechanism.
3. Prolonged administration following PH results in a relatively small number of EAF in liver, and serves to enhance the growth rather than the number of initiated foci.

---

number of EAF. Thus it does appear that cell proliferation occurring either normally at the age of the weanling animal or induced by PH or promotion with PB serves to complete the carcinogenicity of this compound. That 2-Me-DAB is mutagenic was recently shown by Rinkus and Legator (33). It would appear that 2-Me-Dab does satisfy the criteria in Table 1 for an incomplete carcinogen in liver carcinogenesis.

Last year we reported that the administration of dimethylbenz(a)anthracene (DMBA) (10 mg/kg) followed by the feeding of 0.05% PB for 6 months resulted in a marked increase in the number of EAF seen in the liver (38). Later studies (unpublished) showed that by maintaining animals for another 6 months on PB for a total of 1 year PB feeding resulted in most animals developing hepatocellular carcinomas. The data on the number of foci produced are seen in Table 2. It can be noted that administration of a single dose of DMBA alone, immediately following a PH also resulted in a significant number of EAF. This agent which is a complete carcinogen for epidermis is carcinogenic in the liver only when administered to the neonatal mouse, although Marquardt et al. (20) did report the induction of a single hepatoma in nine animals 300 days following the administration of an intravenous emulsion of 25 mg/kg DMBA 24 hr after a PH. More recently Kitagawa and his associates (17) have demonstrated the induction of hepatocellular carcinomas in seven of seven animals given benzo-(a)pyrene following a PH and PB-feeding for more than 50 weeks. In addition, the administration of the carcinogenic hydrocarbon alone following a PH resulted in a significant number of EAF (14). Both of these hydrocarbons are mutagenic in the Ames system (33) and thus conform to the criteria outlined in Table 1 for incomplete carcinogens for the liver.

That other incomplete carcinogens for liver exist is undoubtedly true. Tsuda, Lee, and Farber (46), using the protocal outlined above (11,44) with some modifications, demonstrated that dimethylhydrazine administration following a PH

TABLE 2. *The effect of PB (0.05%) in the diet on the number of EAF induced by DMBA following PH[a]*

	No. EAF/g liver	EAF % volume of liver
PH	11 ± 6	0.004
PH + DMBA (10 mg/kg)	102 ± 35	0.05 ± 0.01
PH + DMBA (10 mg/kg) + 0.05% PB	967 ± 175	1.2 ± 0.3

[a] 200 g female Sprague-Dawley rats were subjected to a 70% PH. DMBA was administered at the dose indicated by intubation in 1 cc mineral oil 24 hr later. Two months later, PB was added to the diet of the designated group at a level of 0.05% and feeding continued for 6 months further. Calculations of the numbers and volumes of EAF were carried out as described previously (29).

resulted in a significant number of EAF, as did several other mutagenic compounds not known to be hepatocarcinogenic. In preliminary experiments in our laboratory, the mutagen, proflavin, when fed to animals for 6 weeks during which time a PH was performed, resulted in a significantly increased number of EAF following 6-month feeding of PB. In none of these studies have hepatocellular carcinomas yet been produced, however. Thus the clear demonstration of other incomplete carcinogens for liver that conform to the criteria outlined in Table 1 must await further investigation.

PROPERTIES OF PROMOTING AGENTS IN HEPATOCARCINOGENESIS

In Table 1 are also listed characteristics of promoting agents in hepatocarcinogenesis. It is now clear, with the recent studies of Blumberg and his associates (7), that promoting agents in epidermal carcinogenesis conform to the first two characteristics listed. A possible exception may be their effect on xenobiotic metabolism, which may be peculiar to liver promotors, although this is by no means certain. Again, as with incomplete carcinogens, promotors appear to be associated with an increased number of EAF, but only on prolonged administration following PH, an effect quite different from that seen with the incomplete carcinogens that required only a single administration following PH in order to induce foci formation. The major differences between initiators and promotors are those related to mutagenesis, wherein promotors have not been found to be mutagenic. All promotors studied thus far alter gene expression, many through receptor mechanisms quite analogous to those seen with hormones. In fact, it is likely that all hormones are effective promoting agents in the genesis of one or another specific histogenetic neoplasm (2).

In our laboratory we have been principally concerned with the characteristics of hepatic promoting agents, initially using PB as the model promoting agent for this tissue. As we have reported earlier (29), administration of PB following an initiating dose of DEN 24 hr after PH resulted in a three- to fourfold increase in the number of EAF/g liver, while also inducing hepatocellular carcinomas. A summary of these investigations is seen in Table 3 with the appropriate controls. It can be seen that, in addition to increasing the number of foci, the size of these foci are markedly increased on promotion with PB. From this and other studies *(vide infra)* it would appear that PB administration stimulates the growth of EAF. Such a conclusion is further confirmed by the recent studies of Schulte-Hermann and his associates (39) demonstrating the enhancement of cell proliferation of enzyme-altered hepatocytes following the administration of PB, steroids, and other hepatic promoting agents. In fact, this characteristic of hepatic promoting agents can explain the fourfold increase in the number of foci seen after initiation and promotion as compared with initiation alone. The proposed mechanism is that PB stimulates proliferation of initiated cells that may lie quiescent in the absence of the promoting agent.

TABLE 3. *Promotion of DEN-induced EAF by PB following PH[a]*

Treatment	EAF/cm³ liver	% Liver volume occupied by EAF	No. animals with carcinomas
None	0	0	0/5
PH	11 ± 6	0.004	0/5
0.05% PB	54 ± 17	0.02	0/5
0.05% PB + PH	109 ± 22	0.1	0/5
DEN + PH	254 ± 65	0.4	0/6
DEN + PH + PB	874 ± 137	11.3	10/12

[a] See ref. 29 for details.

Such an effect of promoters can also explain other characteristics of two-stage hepatocarcinogenesis first reported by our laboratory. An example is the extreme degree of phenotypic heterogeneity seen in the EAF present in livers of animals initiated with DEN and promoted with PB (29). Using three biochemical markers, deficiencies of glucose-6-phosphatase, canalicular ATPase, and a positive marker, γ-glutamyl transpeptidase, our studies demonstrated that all seven possible combinations of the different phenotypes occur at significant frequencies in the livers of such animals. In the animals initiated with a PH followed by DEN (DEN/PH) (37), a majority (three-fourths) of the foci exhibited only a single enzyme abnormality. The phenotypes were divided equally among the three enzyme abnormalities. In animals initiated and then promoted with PB, there occurred a distinct shift in the distribution to foci exhibiting more than one enzyme abnormality, while at the same time, those exhibiting only a single defect in γ-glutamyl transpeptidase represented almost 45% of the total incidence.

When a fourth marker, that described by Hirota and Williams (15) and their associates (foci involving the inability of foci of hepatocytes to concentrate iron), was employed, foci in livers of initiated animals promoted with PB exhibited an even greater degree of heterogeneity. All 15 possible phenotypes were represented to varying degrees in these animals with γ-glutamyl transpeptidase being the principal marker (Fig. 1). The large focus exhibiting a defect in all four characteristics is an hepatocellular carcinoma.

The mechanism by which the phenotypic heterogeneity occurs is not clear. As we have pointed out earlier, it is quite analogous to the biochemical phenotypic heterogeneity seen in a variety of primary and transplanted hepatocarcinomas (29). An alternate explanation suggested by the earlier findings of Pugh and Goldfarb (32) is that the foci exhibiting single enzyme deficiencies progress to those with several abnormalities (23). Pugh and Goldfarb demonstrated that the thymidine-labeling index of foci having two or three enzyme abnormalities is significantly greater than those with only one. That such a progression does not appear to occur may be seen in Table 4. From the table it is apparent that no significant change in the frequency of occurrence of any of the seven

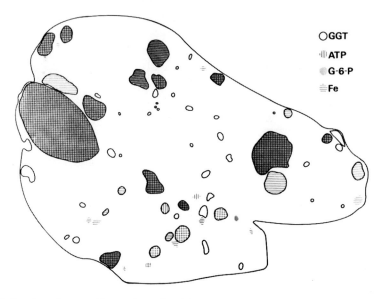

FIG. 1. Drawing of composite overlays of serial sections stained for γ-glutamyl transpeptidase (GGT), canalicular ATPase (ATP), glucose-6-phosphatase (G-6-P), and iron deficient foci (Fe). The technique utilized in compiling the composite has been published previously (29).

possible phenotypes occurs between 2 and 6 months of PB feeding. During this time, however, a significant growth of the foci occurs, which can be seen as a shift of the percent of total liver volume of the single abnormality phenotypes to the greater volume occupied by the double and triple abnormality phenotypes, especially the latter, after 6 months of PB feeding. This is to be expected since

TABLE 4. *Phenotypic heterogeneity of EAF after various periods of PB administration following DEN/PH*

	GGT[a]	ATP[a]	G6P[a]	GGT ATP	GGT G6P	ATP G6P	GGT ATP G6P
DEN/PH + PB for 2 mo	43(11)	26(23)	10(2)	11(18)	3(7)	2(18)	4(21)
DEN/PH ± PB for 3 mo	44 (8)	15(16)	10(5)	10(10)	4(3)	5(29)	23(23)
DEN/PH ± PB for 6 mo	42 (4)	21 (7)	9(4)	7 (6)	4(3)	6(16)	12(59)

[a] The abbreviations for the enzyme abnormalities are those seen in Fig. 1. In all cases, 0.05% PB feeding was begun 11 weeks following DEN/PH and continued for the times shown, at which time the animals were sacrificed. The data are the average from 3 to 8 rats at each point. The values are given as the percent of the total number of foci/cm^3 liver. The numbers in parentheses represent the volume of all foci of that phenotype as a percent of the total liver volume.

the latter have a higher rate of deoxyribonucleic acid (DNA) synthesis (32). Therefore we conclude that the hepatic promoting agent, PB and, by analogy, others as well, do not act to cause a progression from one phenotype to another but rather stimulate the growth and thus the appearance of all altered initiated cells through their clonal progeny.

In further substantiation of the independent and stable characteristic of each phenotype is the fact that transplantation of the cellular population of livers of animals exhibiting all seven phenotypes in abundance by the method of Laishes et al. (19), results in the appearance of all seven phenotypes after more than a year in the liver of the recipient animal (Table 5). This phenomenon suggests not only the stability of the phenotype but also its ability to exist as a "mechanical metastasis" indicative of its frank neoplastic nature.

A major question concerning promoting agents is if their effects are "reversible" in the sense that Boutwell had reported for tumor promotion in the mouse epidermis (5). In Boutwell's studies, administration of the total dose of promoting agent over a long period of time resulted in the production of no papillomas, while the same dose given over a much shorter time resulted in papilloma production. Studies from our laboratory (28) have clearly demonstrated the irreversiblity of the foci produced by the administration of PB following DEN/

TABLE 5. *Phenotypic heterogeneity of EAF resulting from intrahepatic inoculation of hepatocytes isolated from the liver of a rat initiated with DEN/PH and promoted with PB[a]*

Phenotype	Volume of foci as % total liver volume	No. foci cm³ liver	Mean volume of foci (mm)
GGT	0.23	80	0.025
ATP	0.615	151	0.035
G6P	0.14	40	0.015
G6T ATP	0.62	10	0.98
GGT G6P	0.28	2	0.92
ATP G6P	0.09	1	0.40
GGT G6P ATP	7.5	10	7.06
Total	9.46	294	0.5

[a] Hepatic cells from the liver of a Buffalo strain rat were cultured for 7 days initiated with DEN/PH followed by 0.05% PB promotion for 10 months using the technique of Sirica et al. (42). At the end of the culture period, cells were suspended by treatment with collagenase (42) and the cell suspension inoculated into the superior mesenteric vein of a Buffalo rat at the time of PH following the procedure of Laishes and Farber (19). 1 × 10⁶ cells were inoculated and the recipient host, beginning 2 weeks after inoculation, was maintained on 0.05% PB for 15 months. The host was then sacrificed and quantitation of the EAF carried out as described (30).

PH for as little as 2 months. Recently Peraino et al. (27) have shown that increasing the dose of dietary PB given over the same period of time results in an increasing yield of neoplasms, although there is clearly a characteristic plateau of the percentage of rats with tumors that occurs at each specific dose of the promoting agent.

Our first attempt to study the effect of intermittent administration as opposed to continuous administration of PB is seen in Table 6. One group of 24 rats beginning 2 weeks following DEN/PH was continuously given PB every 2 to 3 days at a dose equivalent to 0.01% PB in the diet. A second group of 19 animals followed the same regimen but were given PB either by injection or in the drinking water at a higher concentration every 2 weeks, such that the total dose over the 6-month period in the two groups was identical. As can be seen from the data in Table 6, the number of EAF/g liver in the group receiving continuous PB is more than twice that in animals receiving PB intermittently. Similarly, the volume of foci expressed as a percent of the total liver volume is less than half that in animals receiving intermittent PB. In this experiment, relatively few carcinomas arose in either group. Therefore, although these studies are preliminary in nature, they suggest that altering the frequency of administration of the promoting agent results in a significant decrease both in the number of foci produced and the growth rate of the foci as well.

If these studies can be confirmed, they have interesting implications not only as to the mechanism of tumor promotion in the liver and its complete congruence with that in skin, but also in designing whole animal bioassay tests for carcinoge-

TABLE 6. *Effect of altering the scheduling but not the total dose of PB on the number and volume of EAF following DEN/PH*

Experimental conditions		Volume of foci as % of total liver volume	No. enzyme foci/cm³ liver
1. PH/DEN (10 mg/kg) followed in 2 wks by continuous administration of PB for 6 mo[a]	(24)	5.40 ± 0.4	1,083 ± 100
2. PH/DEN (10 mg/kg) followed in 2 wks by fortnightly administration of PB for 6 mo	(19)	2.46 ± 0.3	388 ± 50

[a] The format of this experiment is essentially identical to that in Table 3, except for the method of PB administration. In group 1, PB was given either continuously in the drinking water at a level of 0.01% or injected every 3 days intraperitoneally at the same equivalent dose. In group 2, rats were either injected with five times the dose administered by the same method to group 1 every 2 weeks or were given 0.07% PB in the drinking water for a 2-day period every 2 weeks. The numbers in parentheses indicate the number of animals studied in each group. The quantitation of the number of foci and their volume was carried out as described previously (30).

nicity. If an agent produces neoplastic lesions upon continuous feeding for extended periods, is this true for intermittent feeding at the same total dose? If not, then risk estimations based on bioassay data must be significantly revised.

CONCLUSION

The two-stage mechanism of hepatocarcinogenesis is almost completely analogous to that seen in epidermal carcinogenesis. A comparison of the two-stage process of epidermal and hepatocellular carcinogenesis in the rat is seen in Table 7. Since time and space do not allow a complete discussion of this comparison, the reader is referred to the review by Pitot and Sirica (31) for more details. It is important to note, however, that the major remaining problem in understanding the biology of the two-stage process is related to the clear establishment of the reversibility of the effects of promoting agents and to the question of the promotion of cells already initiated by ambient environmental factors. This latter point is extremely important not only for our understanding of the mechanisms of carcinogenesis and tumor promotion but also in relation to the testing of chemical agents in animal species for their carcinogenicity and the extrapolation of these data to the environmental risks to the human population.

TABLE 7. *Comparison of two-stage process of epidermal and hepatocellular carcinogenesis in the rat*

Epidermis	Hepatocyte
Initiation:	
Irreversible.	Irreversible.
Initiated cells and their progeny not usually identifiable.	EAF probably represent progeny of initiated cells.
"Pure" initiator (incomplete carcinogen) causes no discernible change unless promoter applied.	Incomplete carcinogens induce EAF.
Dependent on cell cycle and, for many chemicals, on the metabolism of the cell.	Markedly enhanced by cell replication. Promoting agents administered with or before initiator inhibit initiation.
Promotion:	
Reversible, at least in early stages.	Reversibility appears to exist to some extent (Table 6). Promoting agents require a certain time of promotion for their full effect.
Papilloma resulting from promotion may regress.	Many hyperplastic nodules resulting from complete carcinogen administration regress on removal of carcinogenic stimulus.
Promoting agents may promote cells initiated by ambient environmental factors.	Promoting agents do appear to promote cells initiated by ambient environmental factors.
Promotion modulated by diet, hormonal, and other environmental factors.	Modulation of promotion not yet studied directly, but hepatocarcinogenesis is modulated by hormonal and dietary factors.

REFERENCES

1. Bannasch, P., and Klinge, O. (1971): Hepatocellulare glykogenose unt hepatombildung bein menschen. *Virchows Arch. Abt. A,* 352:175–184.
2. Berenblum, I. (1978): Established principles and unresolved problems in carcinogenesis. *J Natl. Cancer Inst.,* 60:723–726.
3. Berenblum, I., and Haran-Ghera, N. (1957): A quantitative study of the systemic initiating action of urethane (ethylcarbamate) in mouse skin carcinogenesis. *Br. J. Cancer,* 11:77–84.
4. Berenblum, I., and Shubik, P. (1947): The role of croton oil application associated with a single painting of a carcinogen in tumour induction of the mouse's skin. *Br. J. Cancer,* 1:379–391.
5. Boutwell, R. K. (1964): Some biological aspects of skin carcinogenesis. *Prog. Exp. Tumor Res.,* 4:207–250.
6. Boutwell, R. K. (1974): The function and mechanism of promoters of carcinogenesis. *Crit. Rev. Toxicol.,* 2:419–443.
7. Dunphy, W. G., Delclos, K. B., and Blumberg, P. M. (1980): Characterization of specific binding of [³H]phorbol 12,13-dibutyrate and [³H]phorbol-12-myristate-13-acetate to mouse brain. *Cancer Res.,* 40:3,635–3,641.
8. Farber, E. (1973): Hyperplastic liver nodules. *Methods Cancer Res.,* 7:345–374.
9. Farber, E. (1980): The sequential analysis of liver cancer induction. *Biochim. Biophys. Acta,* 605:149–166.
10. Farber, E., and Cameron, R. (1980): The sequential analysis of cancer development. *Adv. Cancer Res.,* 31:125–226.
11. Friedrich-Freksa, H., Gossner, W., and Borner, P. (1969): Histochemische Untersuchen der cancerogenese in der rattenleber nech dauergaben von diathylnitrosamin. *Z. Krebsforsch.,* 72:226–239.
12. Goldfarb, S., and Zak, F. G. (1961): Role of injury and hyperplasia in the induction of hepatocellular carcinoma. *J.A.M.A.,* 178:729–731.
13. Hecker, E. (1978): Co-carcinogene oder bedingt krebsauslosende faktoren. *Naturwissenschaften,* 65:640–648.
14. Hirakawa, T., Ishikawa, T., Nemoto, N., Takayama, S., and Kitagawa, T. (1979): Induction of enzyme-altered islands in rat liver by a single treatment with benzo(a)pyrene after partial hepatectomy. *Gann,* 70:393–394.
15. Hirota, N., and Williams, G. M. (1979): The sensitivity and heterogeneity of histochemical markers for altered foci involved in liver carcinogenesis. *Am. J. Pathol.,* 95:317–328.
16. Kimura, N. T., Kanematsu, T., and Baba, T. (1976): Polychlorinated biphenyls as a promotor in experimental hepatocarcinogenesis in rats. *Z. Krebsforsch.,* 87:257–266.
17. Kitagawa, T., Hirakawa, T., Ishikawa, T., Nemoto, N., and Takayama, S. (1980): Induction of hepatocellular carcinoma in rat liver by initial treatment with benzo(a)pyrene after partial hepatectomy and promotion by phenobarbital. *Toxicol. Lett.,* 6:167–171.
18. Kitagawa, T., Pitot, H. C., Miller, E. C., and Miller, J. A. (1979): Promotion by dietary phenobarbital of hepatocarcinogenesis by 2-methyl-N,N,-dimethyl-4-aminoazobenzene in the rat. *Cancer Res.,* 39:112–115.
19. Laishes, B. A., and Farber, E. (1978): The transfer of viable, putative preneoplastic hepatocytes to the livers of syngeneic host rats. *J. Natl. Cancer Inst.,* 61:507–512.
20. Marquardt, H., Sternberg, S. S., and Philips, F. S. (1970): 7,12-Dimethylbenz(a)anthracene and hepatic neoplasia in regenerating rat liver. *Chem. Biol. Interact.,* 2:401–403.
21. Miller, J. A., and Baumann, C. A. (1945): The carcinogenicity of certain azo dyes related to *p*-dimethylaminoazobenzene. *Cancer Res.,* 5:227–234.
22. Mottram, J. C. (1944): A developing factor in experimental blastogenesis. *J. Pathol. Bacterial.,* 56:181–187.
23. Ogawa, K., Solt, D. B., and Farber, E. (1980): Phenotypic diversity as an early property of putative preneoplastic hepatocyte populations in liver carcinogenesis. *Cancer Res.,* 40:725–733.
24. Peraino, C., Fry, R. J. M., Staffeldt, E., and Christopher, J. P. (1975): Comparative enhancing effects of phenobarbital, amobarbital, diphenylhydantoin, and dichlorodiphenyltrichloroethane on 2-acetylaminofluorene-induced hepatic tumorigenesis in the rat. *Cancer Res.,* 35:2,884–2,890.
25. Peraino, C., Fry, R. J. M., Staffeldt, E., and Christopher, J. P. (1977): Enhancing effects of

phenobarbitone and butylated hydroxytoluene on 2-acetylaminofluorene-induced hepatic tumorigenesis in the rat. *Fd. Cosmet. Toxicol.,* 15:93–96.

26. Peraino, C., Fry, R. J. M., Staffeldt, E., and Kisieleski, W. E. (1973): Effects of varying the exposure to phenobarbital on its enhancement of 2-acetylaminofluorene-induced hepatic tumorigenesis in the rat. *Cancer Res.,* 33:2,701–2,705.

27. Peraino, C., Staffeldt, E. F., Haugen, D. A., Lombard, L. S., Stevens, F. J., and Fry, R. J. M. (1980): Effects of varying the dietary concentration of phenobarbital on its enhancement of 2-acetylaminofluorene-induced hepatic tumorigenesis. *Cancer Res.,* 40:3,268–3,273.

28. Pitot, H. C. (1979): Drugs as promoters of carcinogenesis. In: *The Induction of Drug Metabolism,* edited by R. W. Estabrook and E. Lindenlaub, pp. 471–483. F. K. Schattauer Verlag, New York.

29. Pitot, H. C., Barsness, L., Goldsworthy, T., and Kitagawa, T. (1978): Biochemical characterization of stages of hepatocarcinogenesis after a single dose of diethylnitrosamine. *Nature,* 271:456–458.

30. Pitot, H. C., Goldsworthy, T., Campbell, H. A., and Poland, A. (1980): Quantitative evaluation of the promotion by 2,3,7,8-tetrachlorobenzo-*p*-dioxin of hepatocarcinogenesis from dimethylnitrosamine. *Cancer Res.,* 40:3,616–3,620.

31. Pitot, H. C., and Sirica, A. E. (1980): The stages of initiation and promotion in hepatocarcinogenesis. *Biochim. Biophys. Acta,* 605:191–215.

32. Pugh, T. D., and Goldfarb, S. (1978): Quantitative histochemical and autoradiographic studies of hepatocarcinogenesis in rats fed 2-acetylaminofluorene followed by phenobarbital. *Cancer Res.,* 38:4,450–4,457.

33. Rinkus, S. J., and Legator, M. S. (1979): Chemical characterization of 465 known or suspended carcinogens and their correlation with mutagenic activity in the *Salmonella typhimurium* system. *Cancer Res.,* 39:3,289–3,318.

34. Roe, F. J. C., and Clack, J. (1964): Two-stage carcinogenesis: Effect of length of promoting treatment on the yield of benign and malignant tumors. *Br. J. Cancer,* 17:596–604.

35. Rous, P., and Kidd, J. G. (1941): Conditional neoplasms and subthreshold neoplastic states. A study of tar tumors in rabbits. *J. Exp. Med.,* 73:365–374.

36. Salaman, M. H., and Roe, F. J. C. (1953): Incomplete carcinogens: Ethyl carbamate (urethane) as an initiator of skin tumour formation in the mouse. *Br. J. Cancer,* 7:472–481.

37. Scherer, E., and Emmelot, P. (1975*a*): Foci of altered liver cells induced by a single dose of diethylnitrosamine and partial hepatectomy: Their contribution to hepatocarcinogenesis in the rat. *Eur. J. Cancer,* 11:145–154.

38. Scherer, E., and Emmelot, P. (1975*b*): Kinetics of induction and growth of precancerous liver cell foci, and liver tumour formation by diethylnitrosamine in the rat. *Eur. J. Cancer,* 11:689–696.

39. Schulte-Hermann, R., Ohde, G., and Schuppler, J. (1981): Enhanced proliferation of putative preneoplastic cells in rat liver following treatment with tumor promoters phenobarbital, hexachlorocylohexane, steroid compounds, and nafenopin. *Cancer Res. (in press).*

40. Scribner, N. K., and Scribner, J. D. (1980): Separation of initiating and promoting effects of the skin carcinogen7-bromomethylbenz(a)anthracene. *Carcinogenesis,* 1:97–100.

41. Segal, A., Van Duuren, B. L., Mate, U., Solomon, J. J., Seidman, I., Smith, A., and Melchionne, S. (1978): Tumor-promoting activity of 2,3-dihydrophorbol myristate acetate and phorbol myristate acetate in mouse skin. *Cancer Res.,* 38:921–925.

42. Sirica, A. E., Richards, W., Tsukada, Y., Sattler, C. A., and Pitot, H. C. (1979): Fetal phenotypic expression by adult rat hepatocytes on collagen gel/nylon meshes. *Proc. Natl. Acad. Sci. USA,* 76:283–287.

43. Slaga, T. J., Fischer, S. M., Nelson, K., and Gleason, G. L. (1980): Studies on the mechanism of skin tumor promotion: Evidence for several stages in promotion. *Proc. Natl. Acad. Sci. USA,* 77:3,659–3,663.

44. Solt, D., and Farber, E. (1976): New principle for the analysis of chemical carcinogenesis. *Nature,* 263:701–703.

45. Tatematsu, M., Nakanishi, K., Murasaki, G., Miyata, Y., Hirose, M., and Ito, N. (1979): Enhancing effect of inducers of liver microsomal enzymes on induction of hyperplastic liver nodules by N-2-fluorenylacetamide in rats. *J. Natl. Cancer Inst.,* 63:1,411–1,416.

46. Tsuda, H., Lee, G., and Farber, E. (1980): Induction of resistant hepatocytes as a new principle for a possible short-term *in vivo* test for carcinogens. *Cancer Res.,* 40:1,157–1,164.

47. Van Duuren, B. L., Sivak, A., Katz, C., Seidman, I., and Melchionne, S. (1975): The effect of aging and interval between primary and secondary treatment in two-stage carcinogenesis in mouse skin. *Cancer Res.,* 35:502–505.
48. Warwick, G. P. (1967): The covalent binding of metabolites of tritiated 2-methyl-4-dimethylaminoazobenzene to rat liver nucleic acids and proteins, and the carcinogenicity of the unlabeled compound in partially hepatectomized rats. *Eur. J. Cancer,* 3:227–233.

Carcinogenesis, Vol. 7, edited by E. Hecker et al.
Raven Press, New York © 1982.

Effect of Tumor Promoters on Proliferation of Putative Preneoplastic Cells in Rat Liver

R. Schulte-Hermann, J. Schuppler, G. Ohde, and
I. Timmermann-Trosiener

Institute of Toxicology und Pharmacology, 3350 Marburg; and Department of Toxicology, Schering, 1000 Berlin 65, Federal Republic of Germany

Phenobarbital, hypolipidemic drugs, 2,2-di(*p*-chlorophenyl)-1,1,1-trichloromethane (DDT), hexachlorocyclohexane, nafenopin, and sex steroids, such as estradiol esters, mestranol, norethynodrel, and cyproterone acetate, at high dose levels, promote the development of neoplastic hepatic lesions in rats pretreated with initiating carcinogens (1,3,4,5). The purpose of our study was to investigate the effect of these compounds on islands of altered cells in rat liver that are believed to represent a preneoplastic cell population. Special attention was given to the proliferative ability of these island cells. Additionally, spontaneously occurring islands of altered cells in old rats were investigated to determine if a difference exists in comparison to islands produced by an initiating carcinogen.

In the rat, food consumption at the G_0- and R-stage in the hepatocyte mitotic cycle is a prerequisite for deoxyribonucleic acid (DNA) synthesis and cell division and constitutes a permissive factor for liver growth (2). In order to obtain further insight into the proliferative behavior of preneoplastic cells, and because neoplastic cells in culture often lack nutritional control of growth, we withdrew feed at the G_0- and R-stage and examined the ^{3}H-indices in putative preneoplastic and normal hepatocytes.

METHODS

Animals

Six-week-old female Wistar rats were generally used. To determine the effects of the promoters on spontaneous preneoplastic lesions, 2-year-old male rats of the same strain were used.

Induction of Preneoplastic Cells

Single oral doses of diethylnitrosamine (DENA, 75 or 150 mg/kg body weight) or N-nitrosomorpholine (NNM, 175 mg/kg body weight) were applied. The latent period between the initiating dose and the promoter was between 3 and 11 months.

Promotion

(a) By a single oral dose (24 to 30 hr before ^{3}H-thymidine):
   α-hexachlorocyclohexane (α-HCH, 200 mg/kg body weight),
   phenobarbital (50 mg/kg body weight),
   nafenopin (100 mg/kg body weight),
   16α-pregnenolone carbonitrile (PCN, 100 mg/kg body weight),
   cyproterone acetate, (CPA, 100 mg/kg body weight).
(b) By repeated weekly doses for 8.5 months:
   CPA (gavage, 100 mg/kg body weight) and progesterone (PRO, s.c. injection, 500 mg/kg body weight).

The latent period between initiation and start of promotion was 1 week in this part of the study.

Histological Identification of Putative Preneoplastic Cells

Arrangement in islands of γ-glutamyl-transpeptidase (γ-GT) positive cells.

Measurement of Cell Proliferation

(a) Determination of the ^{3}H-index as a measure of DNA synthesis, by injection of ^{3}H-thymidine (0.1 to 0.25 μCi/g body weight) and subsequent autoradiography.
(b) Determination of the mitotic index following injection of colchicine (2 $\times$ 1 mg/kg body weight).

Measurement of Island Size

By determination of the number of cells per island cross section.

Effect of Food Withdrawal on Cell Proliferation

In these studies the rats had been trained for 3 weeks to consume their daily food ration within 5 hr to elicit a more homogeneous effect when food was withdrawn. Food was withdrawn in the G_0- and R-stage and the effect of promoters on the proliferative ability of γ-GT positive islands and normal hepatocytes determined.

RESULTS

Islands of γ-GT-positive, presumably preneoplastic, hepatocytes appear in juvenile rats after a single dose of the initiating carcinogens. Irrespective of any stimulation by promoting compounds, these island cells show a 5- to 20-fold higher proliferative activity than normal (γ-GT-negative) hepatocytes. As shown in Table 1, however, the ^{3}H-index in island cells only attains a maximum value of about 6%.

A single dose of a promoting compound results in an increased proliferation of normal hepatocytes. This is an expected finding, since all the promoters listed stimulate liver growth. In comparison to normal hepatocytes, however, proliferation of putative preneoplastic cells is markedly enhanced (Table 1).

When the mitotic index was determined by blocking the mitosis in the metaphase with colchicine, the results of the count of the metaphase nuclei accurately reflect the situation occurring when the ^{3}H-index was determined, at least for the two compounds α-HCH and CPA. This shows that normal and preneoplastic hepatocytes not only synthesize DNA, but also appear to go through a regular mitotic cycle.

In 2-year-old male Wistar rats, γ-GT-positive preneoplastic islands occur spontaneously; morphologically they do not appear to differ from those induced by a carcinogen. Following a single dose of α-HCH or CPA, these islands also showed an enhanced rate of proliferation as measured by the strongly increased ^{3}H-index in comparison to the ^{3}H-index increase in the surrounding, normal hepatocytes (Table 2). These spontaneously occurring islands also show a higher ^{3}H-index in comparison to normal hepatocytes when no promoter is given. This implies that as far as proliferative activity following stimulation by a promoter is concerned, no significant difference exists between spontaneous and carcinogen-induced γ-GT-positive islands.

Repeated weekly dosing with CPA or PRO following a single dose of NNM resulted in an increase in the number of large islands after promotion for up to 8.5 months. Figure 1 gives the island size classes following promotion with

TABLE 1. *Effect of a single dose of a promoter on normal and γ-GT-positive hepatocytes in young female Wistar rats following a single dose of an inducing carcinogen*

| Promoter | Dose (mg/kg b.w.) | ^{3}H-Index[a] (%, X̄/SD) | | Mitotic index[b] (%, X̄/SD) | |
		Normal hepatocytes	γ-GT-positive hepatocytes	Normal hepatocytes	γ-GT-positive hepatocytes
— (controls)	Vehicle	1.5/0.1	6.5/0.1	0.1/0.1	1.4/0.3
α-HCH	200	3.2/1.9	13.7/4.1	0.7/0.2	6.9/1.9
CPA	100	7.4/1.5	25.0/5.2	4.3/1.2	18.8/8.1
PCN	100	8.8/5.4	17.8/2.3	—[c]	—
Nafenopin	100	3.7/1.8	17.1/4.4	—	—
Phenobarbital	50	3.0/1.0	12.6/1.8	—	—

[a] ^{3}H-index $= \dfrac{\text{Number of autoradiographically marked nuclei}}{\text{Total number of hepatocyte nuclei}} \times 100\%.$

[b] Mitotic index $= \dfrac{\text{Number of mitoses}}{\text{Total number of hepatocyte nuclei}} \times 100\%.$

[c] — = Not determined.

TABLE 2. *Effect of a single dose of a promoter on normal and γ-GT-positive hepatocytes occurring spontaneously in 2-year-old male Wistar rats*

Promoter	Dose (mg/kg b.w.)	³H-Index (%, X̄/SD)	
		Normal hepatocytes	γ-GT-positive hepatocytes
— (controls)	Vehicle	0.6/1.9	6.6/3.2
α-HCH	200	3.6/2.0	22.0/5.5
CPA	100	4.8/1.7	20.9/9.0

PRO and CPA for 5 months. In comparison to NNM alone without subsequent promotion, PRO and CPA cause a shift to large islands. Figure 1 is representative for the situation at 3, 6, 7.5, and 8.5 months.

Following the withdrawal of food in either the G_o- or R-stage of the mitotic cycle, both normal and γ-GT-positive liver cells show a lower ³H-index than when feeding occurred in both these stages. Similarly, if no food is offered in G_o or R, stimulation of proliferation by α-HCH and CPA is also reduced (Fig. 2).

DISCUSSION

As shown in Table 1, γ-GT-positive liver cells react much more strongly than normal hepatocytes to the proliferative stimulus of a promoter. This suggests

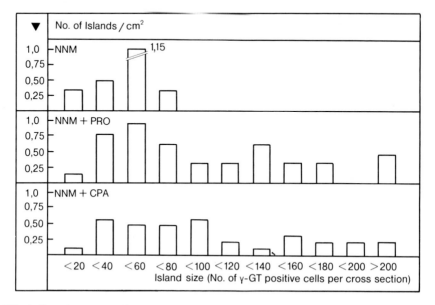

FIG. 1. Size classes of γ-GT-positive islands in rats given a single dose of NNM and weekly doses of the promoters CPA and PRO for 5 months.

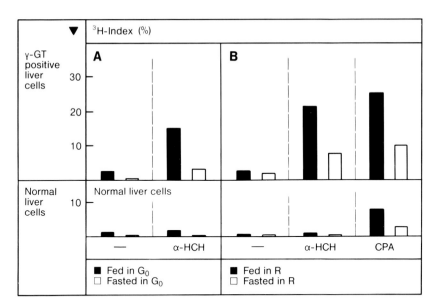

FIG. 2. The effect of food withdrawal in the G_o- or R-stage of the mitotic cycle on the proliferative activity of normal and γ-GT-positive hepatocytes.

that these putative preneoplastic cells have a defect in growth control which renders them much more susceptible to the mitogenic action of exogenous, and possibly endogenous, growth stimuli. It seems likely that multiplication of island cells has to some extent escaped homeostatic control.

The enhanced response of the putative preneoplastic cells to the mitogens tested appears to be a critical part of the tumor-promoting effect of these agents. This is underscored by the part of the study in which the promoters CPA and PRO were given weekly over a period of 8.5 months, in which the islands became much larger and were more frequent than in rats given the inducing carcinogen alone. These data present evidence that there appears to be no basic difference between the promoting activity of synthetic sex steroid hormones such as CPA and the naturally occurring gestagen PRO. It should also be noted that these effects were elicited at high dose levels of both hormones.

The fact that spontaneously occurring γ-GT positive islands in old rats react in a similar manner to those induced by an initiating carcinogen may explain the tumorigenic effects of the promoters when given for a long period of time at high dose levels without preceding initiation by a carcinogen. It may be supposed that the promoters act on spontaneous preneoplastic islands developing in the liver with the increasing age of the rat.

The use of altered feeding schedules shows that the γ-GT-positive islands still share (with normal hepatocytes) the restriction of their growth potential if food is removed at certain stages in the mitotic cycle. This suggests that island cells are still subject to some forms of control of proliferation. However, because of their enhanced proliferative activity following promotion, it appears that preneoplastic cells of γ-GT-positive islands are in a stage between homeostatic behavior and autonomy and are indeed preneoplastic with respect to growth control.

REFERENCES

1. Schulte-Hermann, R. (1974): Induction of liver growth by xenobiotic compounds and other stimuli. *Crit. Rev. Toxicol.,* 3:97.
2. Schulte-Hermann, R., (1977): Two-stage control of cell proliferation induced in rat liver by α-hexachlorocylclohexane. *Cancer Res.,* 37:166–171.
3. Schulte-Hermann, R., Ohde, G., and Schuppler, J. (1979): Proliferation präneoplastischer Leberzellen unter dem Einfluβ von Wachstumsreizen: *Verh. Dtsch. Ges. Path.,* 63:468–472.
4. Schulte-Hermann, R., Ohde, G., Schuppler, J., and Timmermann-Trosiener, I. (1981): Enhanced proliferation of putative preneoplastic cells in rat liver following treatment with the tumor promoters phenobarbital, hexachlorocyclohexane, steroid compounds, and nafenopin. *Cancer Res.,* 41:2556–2562.
5. Yager, J. D., and Yager, R. (1980): Oral contraceptive steroids as promoters of hepatocarcinogenesis in female Sprague-Dawley rats. *Cancer Res.,* 40:3,680–3,685.

Carcinogenesis, Vol. 7, edited by E. Hecker et al.
Raven Press, New York © 1982.

Development of a Model to Simulate the Characteristics of Rat Liver Tumor Promotion by Phenobarbital

Fred J. Stevens and Carl Peraino

Division of Biological and Medical Research, Argonne National Laboratory, Argonne, Illinois 60439

Studies in this laboratory first demonstrated that rats fed the hepatocarcinogen 2-acetylaminofluorene (AAF) exhibit a marked increase in the incidence of hepatic tumors when subsequently fed phenobarbital (3). The feeding of phenobarbital alone did not induce tumor formation (2) and phenobarbital inhibited tumorigenesis when fed simultaneously with AAF (3). These data suggest that hepatocarcinogenesis proceeds in qualitatively distinct sequential stages analogous to the initiation-promotion mechanism associated with tumor formation in mouse skin (1) and that phenobarbital may be considered a promoter of hepatic neoplasia. As reviewed recently (5), the following observations currently characterize the AAF/phenobarbital system of initiation and promotion in rat hepatic carcinogenesis:

(a) Initiated hepatocytes are persistent and can be promoted despite intervening time periods between the feeding of AAF and phenobarbital.
(b) Phenobarbital itself has no initiating activity.
(c) Phenobarbital increases tumor incidence but does not influence tumor growth or degree of differentiation.
(d) Tumor incidence is directly related to phenobarbital dosage.

MODEL

We are attempting to model the AAF/phenobarbital system of experimental hepatic tumorigenesis used in this laboratory. This model is based on current observations of the characteristics of liver tumor promotion by phenobarbital and is intended as a means of narrowing the range of possible mechanisms by which the promoting influence of phenobarbital is exerted. The present form of the model derives from the following assumptions based on observations originating from the above studies:

(a) Initiation occurs randomly and, therefore, initiated loci are randomly distributed throughout the liver population.

(b) Tumorigenesis can occur at any time after initiation.

(c) All livers have the same growth rate. The model can be reduced in scope to include only tumors of any particular "type," in which case this assumption becomes: all tumors of the same type have the same growth rate.

(d) A tumor that has not existed for sufficient time to accumulate a mass greater than the minimum required for observation will be unscored.

(e) Livers may be differentially vulnerable to initiation.

(f) Phenobarbital acts only through a direct effect at each initiated locus.

A computer program was developed that incorporated the above points in order to simulate the experimental system of hepatic tumorigenesis by initiation and promotion. This program is briefly described in the flow diagram depicted in Fig. 1. The terms used in this discussion are defined below:

N Number of initiated loci in total rat population—corresponds to AAF dose for whole population.

n_j Number of initiated loci in liver of rat j.

$P(n_j)$ Probability that rat j with n initiated loci will form a tumor.

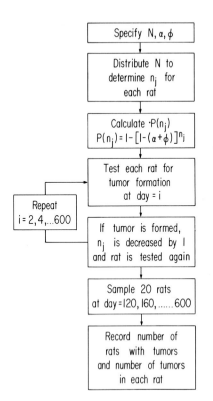

FIG. 1. Flow diagram for computer simulation of liver tumor formation by initiation and promotion.

α Probability that an initiated locus will form a tumor in the absence of phenobarbital.

ϕ Increment in the probability that an initiated locus will form a tumor in the presence of phenobarbital.

The first stage of the program distributes the total N initiated loci throughout the rat population. A random number generator that produces a number between 0 and 1 is used for this purpose. If the randomly generated number is less than an arbitrarily preselected criterion value, an initiation event is assigned to the rat. (This criterion value is a small number used for the sole purpose of producing a smooth distribution of loci throughout the population.) The entire rat population is repeatedly examined in this manner until the N events have been distributed. No assumptions are made regarding the specific nature of the initiation event; one or more events at the molecular level may be involved in the formation of the promotable locus.

The randomized distribution of initiated loci described above results in a Poisson distribution of these loci throughout the rat population. The program has the capacity to include heterogeneity of individual liver vulnerability to the action of AAF. In this case, a Poisson distribution is not achieved because the criterion level mentioned above is no longer the same for each rat.

The second stage of the program calculates the probability that each rat will form a tumor during the test interval. Since rat j with n_j initiated loci can form a tumor at any one of these loci

$$P(n_j) = 1 - [1 - (\alpha + \phi)]n_j,$$

where $(\alpha + \phi)$ represents the total probability that a locus will form a tumor during the 2-day test interval. (The values of α and ϕ are small; therefore, the cross product term $\alpha \cdot \phi$ may be neglected.)

The third stage of the program begins by testing each rat for tumor formation during the first test interval. A random number is generated and compared to $P(n_j)$. If the number is less than $P(n_j)$, a tumor is formed. Then, n_j is decreased by 1, $P(n_j)$ is recalculated, and the rat is retested for the formation of a second tumor. This process is repeated for each rat and the entire cycle is reiterated at 2-day intervals over the 500-day time course of the experiment (4).

Samples of 20 rats are selected during the course of the simulated experiment and the presence of tumors in these rats 100 days earlier is examined. This interval corresponds to a lag period incorporating postinitiation processes of transformation, and accumulation by the tumor of sufficient mass to be observed. The number of rats with tumors and the number of tumors in each rat is recorded. The program can also examine the entire rat population at each sampling period.

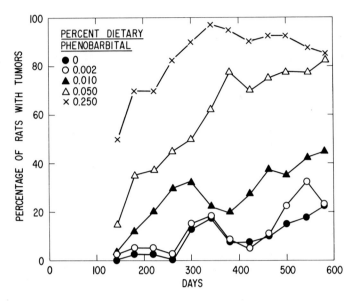

FIG. 2. Computer simulation of the effects of varying the dietary concentration of phenobarbital on its enhancement of 2-acetylaminofluorene-induced hepatic tumorigenesis using the initiation-promotion model diagrammed in Fig. 1. Parameters (see Fig. 1) are specified as follows: N = 500 and is distributed among 270 rats; α = 0.00050. "Phenobarbital dosages" are given to provide a basis for comparison with the experimental data (ref. 5, chart 2). For the zero phenobarbital dosage, ϕ was set at zero; for the 0.002% phenobarbital level, ϕ was set at 0.00020, as indicated above; subsequent ϕ values were successively incremented by factors of 5, as indicated. Each curve represents a separate simulation run. To faciliate comparisons of tumor incidence patterns, the curves were smoothed by a moving average procedure that involved averaging the data from two successive adjacent points on the curve and plotting the average at the mean interval between the points (4).

RESULTS AND DISCUSSION

The product of the current simulation is illustrated in Fig. 2 for a rat population homogeneous in vulnerability to the initiating effect of AAF. The results depicted in Fig. 2 compare favorably with experimental data presented earlier in terms of maximal percentage of rats with tumors and the suggestion of phenobarbital-dependent plateaus (5). By introducing a heterogeneity of AAF vulnerability into the rat population, the correspondence of simulated and experimental tumor frequency per liver was improved (not shown).

SUMMARY

Although development of the simulation is at a preliminary stage, certain general conclusions can be drawn.

(a) The model, derived from simple assumptions including random initiation and random promotion acting through a mechanism that increases the probability of expression of initiated loci, constitutes a reasonable first approximation of the experimental data as currently expressed.

(b) Comparison of the experimental data and the model suggests that rats are differentially vulnerable to initiation. The possibility of differential susceptibility to phenobarbital also exists.

(c) Relative to the current simulation, the full expression of phenobarbital's promoting effect under experimental conditions is apparently suppressed during the early stages of phenobarbital administration, even at dosages that do not affect growth rate (5), suggesting that phenobarbital may exert antipromoting, as well as promoting, activity.

(d) The greater definition of phenobarbital-dependent plateau levels observed experimentally relative to the simulated data suggests a possible refinement of the elementary probabilistic assumption of promoter action (5). For instance, the liver's susceptibility to phenobarbital promotion may decrease during the time course of the experiment.

Refinement of the model is in progress. Further development of the simulation will be based on more detailed analyses of the kinetics of tumor incidence and plateau appearance, distributions of tumor frequencies, and occurrences of different tumor types.

ACKNOWLEDGMENTS

This work was supported by the U. S. Department of Energy under contract No. W-31-109-Eng-38.

REFERENCES

1. Boutwell, R. K. (1964): Some biological aspects of skin carcinogenesis. *Prog. Exp. Tumor Res.,* 4:207–250.
2. Kunz, W., Schaude, G., and Thomas, C. (1969): The effect of phenobarbital and halogenated hydrocarbons on nitrosamine carcinogenesis. *Z. Krebsforsch.* 72:291–304.
3. Peraino, C., Fry, R. J. M., and Staffeldt, E. (1971): Reduction and enhancement by phenobarbital of hepatocarcinogenesis induced in the rat by 2-acetylaminofluorene. *Cancer Res.,* 31:1,506–1,512.
4. Peraino, C., Fry, R. J. M., and Staffeldt, E. (1977): Effects of varying the onset and duration of exposure to phenobarbital on its enhancement of 2-acetylaminofluorene-induced hepatic tumorigenesis in the rat. *Cancer Res.,* 37:3,623–3,627.
5. Peraino, C., Staffeldt, E. F., Haugen, D. A., Lombard, L. S., Stevens, F. J., and Fry, R. J. M. (1980): Effects of varying the dietary concentration of phenobarbital on its enhancement of 2-acetylaminofluorene-induced hepatic tumorigenesis. *Cancer Res.,* 40:3,268–3,273.

Carcinogenesis, Vol. 7, edited by E. Hecker et al.
Raven Press, New York © 1982.

Quantitative Aspects of Drug-Mediated Tumour Promotion in Liver and Its Toxicological Implications

Werner Kunz, Gerda Schaude, Michael Schwarz, and Henk Tennekes

The German Cancer Research Centre, Institute of Biochemistry, D-6900 Heidelberg, Germany

Tumour-promoting effects were first observed by Berenblum and his associates in carcinogenicity studies with the skin irritant croton oil (4,5). Ever since the isolation and characterisation of phorbol esters as active components (15), tumour promoters have proved to be useful model compounds in studies on the nature of critical steps in chemical carcinogenesis (7,15). Tumour-promoting effects of chemicals have subsequently been observed in a variety of organs, including the liver. In this latter organ, however, investigations were not focused primarily on the elucidation of the carcinogenic process, but rather on the assessment of the toxicological significance of drugs and environmental chemicals.

These investigations were initiated by the observation that exposure of animals to high doses of inducers of the microsomal monooxygenase system frequently resulted in pronounced liver enlargement (8,20,42). The general significance of this phenomenon is illustrated by a report showing that liver enlargement may occur in approximately 75% of chronic feeding studies with newly introduced and existing drugs or environmental chemicals (14).

EFFECTS OF INDUCERS OF LIVER ENLARGEMENT ON HEPATOCARCINOGENESIS

Detailed studies on the nature of drug-mediated liver enlargement revealed that although different initial events may trigger this response, it is invariably a result of a true growth response to meet increased functional demands (14, 20,22). At the cellular level, liver enlargement is usually characterised by pronounced cellular hypertrophy, polyploidization, and, to a lesser extent, by hyperplasia, i.e., cell multiplication (20,42).

This evidence raised the question as to whether the induction of liver enlargement by drugs might lead to enhancement of liver carcinogenesis. The results of ensuing studies showed that two principal effects of drugs on liver carcinogenesis had to be distinguished. Simultaneous treatment of rats with a liver carcinogen and a monooxygenase inducer, such as phenobarbital or 2,2-di-(*p*-chlorophenyl)-1, 1, 1-trichloroethane (DDT), resulted in inhibition of carcinogenic effectiveness (16,21,25,50). There is evidence that these effects are directly related to the influence of the inducer on the metabolic activation and/or inactivation of the carcinogen (1,19).

In contrast, exposure of animals to inducers of liver enlargement subsequent to carcinogen treatment, according to the initiation-promotion model employed in skin carcinogenicity experiments, resulted in enhancement of carcinogenic effectiveness. Pioneering studies on the latter effect of drugs have been conducted by Peraino and his associates, using 2-acetylaminofluorene and phenobarbital as model compounds (24,25,27,28,29).

Several other groups have obtained similar results with different carcinogens and a variety of drugs and hormones. At an earlt stage, Peraino advanced the concept that, in analogy to the effects of phorbol esters in skin, inducers of liver enlargement might act as tumour promoters (25). This contention has become subject of controversy, however, following reports that these substances may cause an increase in the incidence of liver tumours in certain rodent species without any previous exposure to liver carcinogens (17,26,46,47–49). These rodent strains generally show an unusually high incidence of "spontaneous" liver tumours, and it is difficult, therefore, to decide whether the observed increase in the occurrence of liver tumours is due to facilitation of the expression of preexisting oncogenic potential, i.e., tumour promotion, or to the action of a weakly carcinogenic agent. The latter mechanism of action, however, is not supported by experiments indicating that compounds such as phenobarbital, DDT, dieldrin, and clofibrate are devoid of mutagenic activity and fail to cause detectable damage to liver deoxyribonucleic acid (DNA), such as covalent binding or strand breakage (6,43,45,51). It has been argued, however, that current genotoxicity assays may not be appropriate for the prediction of carcinogenic hazards posed by chemicals.

There is general consensus that carcinogenic agents cause irreversible and cumulative effects in their target cells, whereas tumour promoters, almost by definition, do not; they can only function by amplifying carcinogen-induced initiating effects. Consequently, it is generally accepted that the effects of tumour promoters show a threshold in low dose regions and reach a maximum at high dose levels, the extent of which is dependent on the level of prior initiation. As a result, it would seem likely that phenomena such as tumour promotion and syncarcinogenesis exhibit different dose-time-response characteristics. Dose-time-response relationships observed with various liver carcinogens (9,10) applied in the current study are shown in Fig. 1. Model concepts of the dose-time-response kinetics of syncarcinogenesis and tumour promotion have been included in Fig. 1.

It should be possible in principle, therefore, to discriminate between tumour promoters and carcinogens on the basis of dose-time-response studies. In reality, however, this approach may not be feasible because tumour manifestation periods

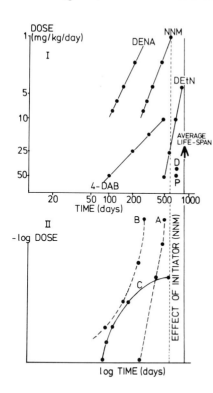

FIG. 1. Dose-time-response relationships of chemical carcinogenesis in liver. **I:** 50% tumour mortality in rats continuously exposed to DENA, 4-DAB, NNM, and diethanolnitrosamine (DEtN), as established by Druckrey (9,10) and in experiments reported in this chapter (NNM). *D* and *P* are indicative of the tumourigenic response of rodents to liver-enlarging drugs, such as phenobarbital or DDT (37). **II:** Model concepts of syncarcinogenesis and tumour promotion in a two-stage model of carcinogenesis. The curves have been based on the assumptions that carcinogens cause irreversible and cumulative effects, whereas the effects of tumour promoters show a threshold in low dose regions and reach a maximum at high dose levels, as described in the text. In this model, animals were assumed to have been initiated by daily administration of 20 mg NNM/kg for a period of 14 days. Curve *A* and *B* represent syncarcinogenic effects of compounds with different carcinogenic effectiveness. Curve *C* represents tumour promotion. The proposed dose-time-response relationship of tumour promotion is supported by observations made with TPA (E. Hecker and R. Schmidt, *personal communication*).

in low dose groups are likely to exceed the animal's average life-span (Fig. 1). This problem can only be overcome by the employment of a sensitive early marker of carcinogenic activity.

In recent years, evidence has accumulated that putatively preneoplastic areas in the liver may serve this purpose (2,11,12,13,40,44). These areas, commonly called islets, are deficient in enzymes such as ATPase or glucose-6-phosphatase, and may also show glycogen storage or a positive γ-glutamyl transferase reaction. It is not clear at present whether these cellular alterations are caused by somatic mutations, and, if so, whether these mutations are directly related to the carcinogenic process. There is, however, a strong quantitative correlation between carcinogen dose, the extent of enzyme-deficient areas, and the subsequent appearance of liver tumours (11,19,41). The development of an arbitrarily defined extent of ATPase-deficient areas in animals continuously treated with various levels of diethylnitrosamine (DENA) was found to show a dose-time-response relationship with characteristics identical to that observed for the induction of liver tumours (19).

Recently, this quantitative correlation has been confirmed for 4-dimethylaminoazobenzene (4-DAB, butter yellow) and N-nitrosomorpholine (NNM) (Fig. 2). It is evident from these data that islets are a sensitive marker of the effects of even very low doses of liver carcinogens well within the animals' average

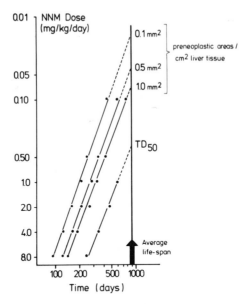

FIG. 2. Dose-time-response relationship for the induction of defined volumes of preneoplastic islets in rat liver by NNM and its quantitative correlation with the induction of liver tumours (33). Adult female Lewis rats were continuously exposed to the indicated levels of NNM. For every treatment group, the exposure time required for the induction of 0.1, 0.5, and 1.0% preneoplastic areas was determined on the basis of quantitative analyses of the preneoplastic response in a total of 20 animals, killed at different time intervals. These time periods were recorded versus dose in a double logarithmic plot and compared with the dose-time-response relationship observed for the induction of 50% liver tumour mortality (TD_{50}). The parallellism of both lines indicate an identical dose-time-response dependency, i.e., (dose) · (time)^n = constant.

life-span. Consequently, quantitative analyses of preneoplastic changes in liver may be particularly useful in dose-time-response studies on the effects of tumour promoters, for the reasons outlined above.

QUANTITATIVE STUDIES ON THE EFFECTS OF PUTATIVELY TUMOUR-PROMOTING DRUGS

In recent years investigations on preneoplastic areas in liver have played an increasingly prominent role in attempts to characterise stages in hepatocarcinogenesis (31,32,38,44; for review, see ref. 11). In most of these experiments, weanling animals were initiated with a single high dose of a liver carcinogen, usually combined with partial hepatectomy. This experimental design may be of particular advantage in a two-stage carcinogenesis model. It would appear to be less reliable in dose-response studies, however, since an application of a single dose of the carcinogen has been found to result in dose-response lines with a slope different from that seen after chronic exposure to low dose levels (11,38). Accordingly, in the current study, based on results of preliminary experiments (19), adult rats were pretreated for a period of 4 weeks with DENA or NNM at dose levels associated with relatively modest cytotoxic effects on hepatocytes, and with dose-time-response characteristics identical to those seen following continuous carcinogen treatment (36).

Figure 3 shows the time course of changes in number and size distribution of preneoplastic islets in livers of rats preexposed to three levels of DENA, followed or not by treatment with a constant dose of phenobarbital (0.1% in the drinking water).

Following discontinuation of carcinogen treatment, the number of preneoplastic islets in livers of controls continued to rise for a certain period of time and, after having reached a maximum, gradually decreased until a steady-state level was established. In accordance with results from cytokinetic studies on preneoplastic liver cells (34), the observed increase in islet number was not associated initially with a detectable shift in islet size distribution towards higher diameters. Enhanced islet growth became apparent only at later stages, when the cells appeared to have reached a more neoplastic state. Amplitude and time course of this process were found to depend on the dose level of the initiating carcinogen. Increased exposure levels led to an earlier appearance of maxima and steady-state at significantly higher levels (Figs. 3 and 4).

These characteristics of the preneoplastic response following cessation of carcinogen treatment have been observed by several groups (11,13,34,38,41) and were interpreted in various ways. Disappearance of enzyme-altered cells and steady-state levels are usually observed after a time period similar to the reported average life-span of hepatocytes. Accordingly, Friedrich-Freksa (13,39,41) has postulated that these enzyme deficiencies result from somatic, possibly recessive mutations, which may also become phenotypically manifest after cessation of carcinogen treatment, and which are subject to normal physiological turnover unless the cells assume a more neoplastic character. This explanation may be of considerable interest to the interpretation of the effects of tumour-promoting drugs.

Exposure of DENA-pretreated rats to phenobarbital resulted in pronounced enhancement of the preneoplastic response. During the initial stages of phenobarbital treatment, these effects were found to be due entirely to increases in the number of islets and not to any acceleration of islet cell growth (Fig. 3). Similar to the changes observed in control animals, a maximum was reached, followed by a decline, until the number of islets remained constant. Both maximum and steady-state were at considerably higher levels, however, and occurred at an earlier stage than in controls (Fig. 4). This acceleration of the preneoplastic process resulted in an early appearance of an increased number of islets with progressed neoplastic characteristics. This was evinced by the frequent appearance of cellular phenotypes, such as intermediate and basophilic cells, that are characteristic of later stages of hepatocarcinogenesis. Islet size distribution in phenobarbital-treated rats showed, at this time, a distinct shift to higher diameters (Fig. 3). It would seem likely, therefore, that the observed enhancement

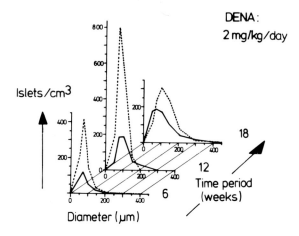

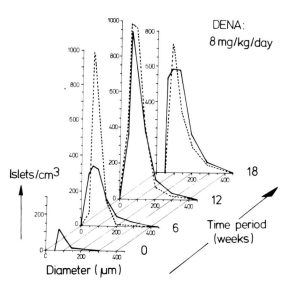

FIG. 3. The effect of phenobarbital treatment on number and size distribution of ATPase-deficient islets in livers of rats pretreated with different levels of DENA for 4 weeks. Adult Wistar rats were pretreated with DENA (per stomach tube) at the indicated dose levels and subsequently treated or not with phenobarbital (0.1% in drinking water). Groups of 5 animals were killed 6, 12, and 18 weeks after cessation of carcinogen pretreatment. Six sections per liver were morphometrically analyzed. Islet number per unit volume were estimated as described by Scherer et al. (39). (————): controls; (-------): phenobarbital. Data for 4 mg DENA/kg/day are not shown.

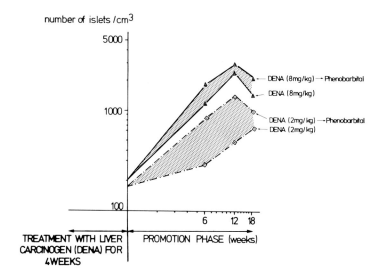

number of islets /cm³

5000

1000

100

6   12   18

DENA (8mg/kg) --Phenobarbital
DENA (8mg/kg)
DENA (2mg/kg) --Phenobarbital
DENA (2mg/kg)

TREATMENT WITH LIVER
CARCINOGEN (DENA) FOR
4 WEEKS

PROMOTION PHASE (weeks)

FIG. 4. The effect of phenobarbital treatment on the number of ATPase-deficient islets in livers of rats pretreated with DENA. Experimental details as in Fig. 3. The data observed in rats pretreated with 4 mg DENA/kg/day were omitted because of interference with the other curves. For the 4-mg DENA treatment group, control values were nearly identicial to that seen in the treatment group DENA (2 mg) + phenobarbital. Results observed in the treatment group DENA (4 mg) + phenobarbital were slightly higher than those seen in the DENA (8 mg) controls.

of islet growth at this stage resulted from an accelerated expression of neoplasmic character, and *not* from continuous growth stimulation by the promoting drug. The observation that islet number remained constant, even though phenobarbital treatment was continued, suggests that, in accordance with Friedrich-Freksa's postulation, (pre-)-neoplastic information had become maximally expressed at this stage.

The effectiveness of phenobarbital-mediated enhancement was found to be inversely related to the level of prior initiation, i.e., the effects of phenobarbital were most pronounced at the lowest exposure level of DENA (Fig. 3). This evidence suggests that the increase in the number of islets following discontinuation of DENA treatment is related to a promoting stimulus exerted either by the solitary carcinogen or by phenobarbital. Consequently, the extent to which a tumour promoter may facilitate the expression of carcinogenic potential may depend on the degree of promotion inflicted by the carcinogen. There is evidence that promoting effects of solitary carcinogens are dependent on the actual daily exposure level and correlate with the degree of carcinogen-induced cellular proliferation, which has also been found to be a concentration-dependent process (35).

Assuming that tumour promotion by drugs is also related to the induction of proliferative processes, it follows that intermittent treatment with liver-enlarging doses should produce effects similar to those seen after continuous treatment. In the case of phenobarbital, the effects on liver weight reach a plateau after approximately 1 week of treatment. Accordingly, rats initiated with DENA were treated with phenobarbital for 1 week at 6-weekly intervals for a period of 18 weeks, and results were compared with those obtained with rats treated

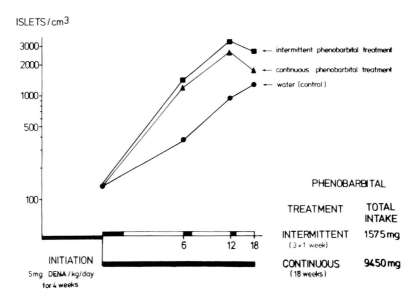

FIG. 5. The effect of intermittent and continuous phenobarbital treatment on the number of ATPase-deficient islets in livers of rats pretreated with DENA. Adult female Wistar rats were pretreated with DENA (50 ppm in the drinking water, equivalent to an uptake of 5 mg/kg/ day) for a period of 4 weeks. One group of carcinogen-pretreated animals was subsequently treated continuously with phenobarbital (0.1% in the drinking water) for 18 weeks, and a second group received this dose level for only 1 week at 6-weekly intervals. Remaining animals served as controls.

continuously. As shown in Fig. 5, intermittent exposure to phenobarbital resulted in similar, if not more pronounced, increases in the number of preneoplastic islets in liver.

The observation that a total phenobarbital dose of only one-sixth of that administered to continuously treated rats may exert similar enhancing effects on the preneoplastic response of liver sharply conflicts with the concept that phenobarbital acts as a weakly carcinogenic agent. The fact that tumour-promoting effects may even occur as a result of intermittent drug treatment, however, could raise considerable problems in terms of the assessment of drug safety in the human situation.

Since the doses of phenobarbital employed in animal carcinogenicity studies usually exceed the therapeutic dose by several orders of magnitude, the assess-

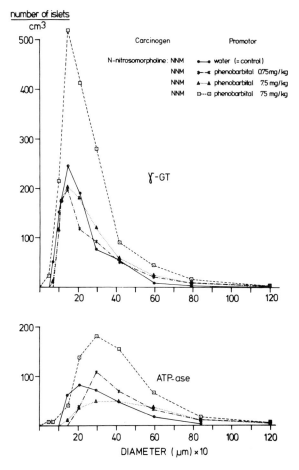

FIG. 6. The effects of varying doses of phenobarbital on the size distribution of the ATPase negative and γ-GT positive preneoplastic islets in livers of rats pretreated with NNM. Experimental details as in Table 1.

ment of the relevance of phenobarbital-mediated tumour-promotion to humans would seem to necessitate an evaluation of dose-response characteristics.

The results of dose-response studies indicated that significant tumour-promoting effects require the use of relatively high doses of phenobarbital. Quantitative analysis of number, total volume (Table 1), and size distribution of ATPase-negative and γ-glutamyl transferase-positive islets (Fig. 6) indicated that significant effects were associated with a phenobarbital dose of 75 mg/kg. Smaller exposure levels (7.5 and 0.75 mg/kg) caused limited effects within control range. None of the three phenobarbital exposure levels caused any effect in livers of noninitiated animals.

These results constitute additional evidence to indicate that the compound

TABLE 1. The effect of varying doses of phenobarbital on number and total volume of preneoplastic islets in livers of rats pretreated with NNM[a]

		Preneoplastic areas							
		ATPase-negative				γ-GT-positive			
		Number		Total volume		Number		Total volume	
Initiation	Promotion 18 weeks	n/cm³	Δ%	mm³/cm³	Δ%	n/cm³	Δ%	mm³/cm³	Δ%
NNM	water	288	100	8.2	100	780	100	8.3	100
NNM	Phenobarbital 0.75 mg/kg	270	92	8.4	103	657	84	9.2	111
NNM	Phenobarbital 7.5 mg/kg	285	99	10.2	124	720	92	10.6	115
NNM	Phenobarbital 75 mg/kg	612	213	21.4	261	1597	205	20.6	248
water	Phenobarbital 75 mg/kg	<10	0	<0.1	0	<10	0	<0.1	0
water	water	<10	0	<0.1	0	<10	0	<0.1	0

[a] Female Lewis rats, weighing approximately 200 g, were pretreated with NNM (120 ppm in the drinking water) for a period of 7 weeks. For details on histochemical assays, see ref. 19. Values indicate treatment mean (6 animals per group).

is devoid of carcinogenic activity. Our data are in full agreement with observations on the effect of phenobarbital dose on liver tumour incidence in rats pretreated with 2-acetylaminofluorene (30). Both of these experiments indicate that the phenobarbital dose levels usually employed in human therapy are associated with limited, if any, tumour-promoting action in rodents. The dose-response lines, when recorded as in Fig. 1, showed that in this dose region the effects approach zero. Even if a threshold dose were to be clearly defined on the basis of these studies, however, a risk assessment might remain problematic. In the case of tumour-promoting agents, extrapolation of animal data to man is complicated by a lack of evidence on the nature of the critical cellular events and the dose levels required to produce such effects in humans.

MECHANISTIC ASPECTS AND TOXICOLOGICAL IMPLICATIONS

Present evidence indicates that exposure to liver-enlarging drugs may lead to tumour promotion; it is by no means certain, however, that tumour promotion invariably requires significant organ growth. It can be envisaged that very discrete early events in the growth process are critical.

In the reported dose-response study with phenobarbital, induction of the microsomal monooxygenase system was noted in all treatment groups, followed by dose-dependent increases in liver weight. At dose levels associated with overt tumour-promoting action, an increase in microsomal formation of hydrogen peroxide and superoxide anions was observed. Interestingly, these effects have also been observed with the strongly tumor-promoting agents clofibrate and halothane, which trigger liver enlargement not by induction of microsomal monooxygenases, but via induction of particular enzymes involved in mitochondrial-cytoplastic hydrogen transfer. The formation of reactive oxygen species is presently discussed as a critical phenomenon in 12-0-tetradecanoylphorbol-13-acetate (TPA)-mediated tumour promotion, since this effect appears to be related to the stimulation of cell proliferation and, in particular, of cellular polyploidisation.

A marked increase in ploidy status is characteristic of drug-induced liver enlargement. Analyses of cytological parameters (Fig. 7) revealed that in the initial stages of liver enlargement, this phenomenon is due not only to DNA replication and endomitosis, but also to nuclear fusion within binuclear liver cells, as demonstrated by quantitative autoradiography and cytophotometrical DNA analyses. Following adaptation of the liver to the increased functional demands, and particularly after cessation of drug treatment, there is a decline in the extent of nuclear polyploidy; this is associated with an increase in the number of polynucleated cells. In the course of this process, there is no change in mitotic index, but dumbbell-like nuclear figures are frequently observed. It is conceivable that these nuclear figures, which have also been observed during carcinogen treatment, are a reflection of atypical nuclear division (23), which may be accompanied by an abnormal redistribution of genetic material. Under such circumstances, recessive mutations may become homozygous; in this manner recessive oncogenic information could be phenotypically expressed (18).

This concept is supported by all of the results of the current studies and provides an explanation for the observed increases in the number of islets for considerable periods of time after discontinuation of carcinogen treatment, and for the impact of tumour-promoting drugs on this process. The accelerated progression of the neoplastic character of islets may be similarly explained.

The induction of such critical events in rodent liver necessitates high exposure levels of tumour-promoting agents, which are considerably in excess of the therapeutic dose. Consequently, the toxicological relevance of drugs such as phenobarbital would appear to be very limited. It is conceivable, however, that some compounds may also induce these critical cytological disturbances in a more specific manner at dose levels that may be relevant to man (3).

These considerations may have important implications for the design and interpretation of animal carcinogenicity tests. Such experiments must address the question of whether tumorigenic effects are due to the action of a carcinogenic agent or to promotion of preexisting endogenous, viral, or environmental onco-genic factors in the animals. Since the primary hepatocellular effects of promoters

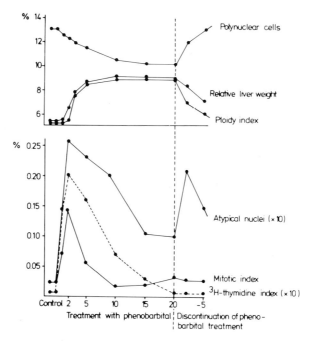

FIG. 7. Changes in hepatocellular parameters induced by phenobarbital. Adult female NMRI mice were continuously treated with phenobarbital (0.1% in the drinking water). All cytological parameters were quantified with light microscopy on liver sections. Ploidy histograms were measured in sections and, additionally, in isolated liver nuclei. ³H-thymidine autoradiography as described in ref. 34. DNA content of nuclei was determined by microscope fluorometry of Feulgen-stained material. Specific radioactivity in nuclei was determined using a Leitz microscope-photometer MPV.

are reversible, noncumulative and nonexistent below threshold levels, the risk associated with these compounds should be assessed on the basis of exposure levels relevant to man.

REFERENCES

1. Appel, K. E., Rickart, R., and Kunz, W. (1979): Influences of inducers and inhibitors of the microsomal monooxygenase system on the alkylating intensity of dimethylnitrosamine in mice. *J. Cancer Res. Clin. Oncol.,* 94:47–61.
2. Bannasch, P. (1968): The cytoplasm of hepatocytes during carcinogenesis. *Recent Results Cancer Res.,* 19, Springer Verlag, Berlin.
3. Barich, L. L., Swarz, J., Barich, D. J., and Horowitz, M. G. (1962): Oral griseofulvin: A cocarcinogenic agent to methylcholanthrene-induced cutaneous tumors. *Cancer Res.,* 22: 53–55.
4. Berenblum, I. (1941): The cocarcinogenic action of Croton resin. *Cancer Res.,* 1:44–48.
5. Berenblum, I., and Shubik, P. (1947): The role of croton oil application associated with a single pointing of a carcinogen, in tumor induction of the mouse's skin. *Br. J. Cancer,* 1:379–382.
6. Bidwell, K., Weber, E., Nienhold, I., Connor, T., and Legator, M. S. (1975): Comprehensive evaluation for mutagenic activity of dieldrin. *Mutat. Res.,* 31:314.
7. Boutwell, R. K. (1974): The function and mechanism of promoters of carcinogenesis. *Crit. Rev. Toxicol.,* 2:419–443.
8. Conney, A. H. (1967): Pharmacological implications of microsomal enzyme induction. *Pharmacol. Rev.,* 19:317–366.
9. Druckrey, H. (1967): Quantitative Aspects in Chemical Carcinogenesis. *U.I.C.C. Monographs,* 7:60–78.
10. Druckrey, H., Preussmann, R., Ivankovic, S., and Schmähl, D. (1967): Organotrope carcinogene Wirkungen bei 65 verschiedenen N-nitroso-Verbindungen an BD-Ratten. *Z. Krebsforch.,* 69:103–201.
11. Emmelot, P., and Scherer, E. (1980): The first relevant cell stage in rat liver carcinogenesis: A quantitative approach. *Biochem. Biophys. Acta,* 605:247–304.
12. Friedrich-Freksa, H., Gössner, W., and Börner, P. (1969): Histochemische Untersuchungen der Cancerogenese in der Rattenleber nach Dauergaben von Diäthylnitrosamin. *Z. Krebsforsch,* 72:226–253.
13. Friedrich-Freksa, H., Paradopulu, G., and Gössner, W. (1969): Histochemische Untersuchungen der Carcinogenese in der Rattenleber nach zeitlich begrenzter Verabfolgung von Diäthylnitrosamin. *Z. Krebsforsch.,* 72:240–253.
14. Golberg, L. (1966): Liver enlargement produced by drugs: Its significance. In: *Experimental Study of the Effects of Drugs on the Liver,* pp. 171–184. Excerpta Medica Foundation, Amsterdam International Congress Series No. 115.
15. Hecker, E. (1971): Isolation and characterization of the cocarcinogenic principles from croton oil. In: *Methods in Cancer Research,* edited by H. Busch. 6:439–484. Academic Press, New York.
16. Hoch-Legeti, G., Argus, M. F., and Arcos, S. C. (1968): Combined carcinogenic effects of dimethylnitrosamine and 3-methylcholanthrene in rat. *J. Natl. Cancer Inst.,* 40:535–550.
17. Ito, N., Nagasaki, H., Aoe, H., Sugihara, S., Miyata, Y., Arai, M., and Shirai, T. (1975): Brief communication: Development of hepatocellular carcinomas in rats treated with benzene hexachloride. *J. Natl. Cancer Inst.,* 54:801–805.
18. Kinsella, A. R., and Radman, M. G. (1978): Tumor promoter induces sister chromatid exchanges: Relevance to mechanisms of carcinogenesis. *Proc. Natl. Acad. Sci. USA,* 75:6,149–6,153.
19. Kunz, W., Appel, K. G., Schwarz, M., and Stöckle, G. (1978): Enhancement and inhibition of carcinogenic effectiveness of nitrosamines. In: *Primary Liver Tumours,* edited by H. Remmer, H. M. Bolt, P. Bannasch, and H. Popper, pp. 261–284. MTP Press, Lancaster, U.K.
20. Kunz, W., Schaude, W., and Siess, M. (1966): Stimulation of liver growth by drugs. In: *Proceedings of the European Society for the Study of Drug Toxicity,* VII, pp. 113–153. International Congress Series No. 115. Excerpta Medica, Amsterdam.

21. Kunz, W., Schaude, G., and Thomas, C. (1969): Die Beeinflussung der Nitrosamincarcinogenese durch Phenobarbital und Halogenkohlenwasserstoffe. *Z. Krebsforsch.,* 72:291–304.
22. Kunz, W., and Schnieders, B. (1970): RNA metabolism and induction of extramicrosomal enzymes during liver enlargement due to drugs. *Proc. IV, Int. Congr. Pharmacol.,* IV, pp. 326–340. Schwabe and Co. Publishers, Basel.
23. Masahito, P., Takayama, S., and Yamada, K. (1976): Early cytological changes induced in rat liver cells by chemicals. In: *Fundamentals in Cancer Prevention,* edited by P. N. Magee, pp. 103–111. University of Tokyo Press, Tokyo.
24. Peraino, C., Fry, R. J. M., and Grube, D. D. (1978): Drug-induced enhancement of hepatic tumorigenesis. In: *Mechanisms of Tumor Promotion and Cocarcinogenesis,* edited by T. J. Slaga, A. Sivak, and R. K. Boutwell, pp. 421–432. Raven Press, New York.
25. Peraino, C., Fry, R. J. M., and Staffeldt, E. (1971): Reduction and enhancement by phenobarbital of hepatocarcinogenesis induced in rat by 2-acetylaminofluorene. *Cancer Res.,* 31:1,506–1,512.
26. Peraino, C., Fry, R. J. M., and Staffeldt, E. (1973): Enhancement of spontaneous hepatic tumorigenesis in C3H mice by dietary phenobarbital. *J. Natl. Cancer Inst.,* 51:1,349–1,350.
27. Peraino, C., Fry, R. J. M., and Staffeldt, E. (1977): Effects of varying the onset and duration of exposure to phenobarbital on its enhancement of 2-acetylaminofluorene-induced hepatic tumorigenesis. *Cancer Res.,* 37:3,623–3,627.
28. Peraino, C., Fry, R. J. M., Staffeldt, E., and Christopher, J. P. (1975): Comparative enhancing effects of phenobarbital, amobarbital, diphenylhydantoin, and dichlorodiphenyltrichloroethane on 2-acetylaminofluorene-induced hepatic tumorigenesis in the rat. *Cancer Res.,* 35:2,884–2,890.
29. Peraino, C., Fry, R. J. M., Staffeldt, E., and Kisieleski, W. E. (1973): Effects of varying the exposure to phenobarbital on its enhancement of 2-acetylaminofluorene-induced hepatic tumorigenesis in the rat. *Cancer Res.,* 33:2,701–2,705.
30. Peraino, C., Staffeldt, E. F., Haugen, D. S., Lombard, L. S., Stevens, F. J., and Fry, R. J. M. (1980): Effects of varying the dietary concentration of phenobarbital on its enhancement of 2-acetylaminofluorene-induced hepatic tumorigenesis. *Cancer Res.,* 40:3,268–3,273.
31. Pitot, H. C., Borsness, L., Goldsworthy, T., and Kitagawa, T. (1978): Biochemical characterisation of stages of hepatocarcinogenesis after a single dose of diethylnitrosamine. *Nature,* 271:456–458.
32. Pitot, H. C., and Sirica, A. E. (1980): The stages of initiation and promotion in hepatocarcinogenesis. *Biochim. Biophys. Acta,* 605:191–215.
33. Port, R., Stöckle, G., Tennekes, H., and Kunz, W. (1981): Dose-time relations in the induction of enzyme-deficient cell islets and of malignant tumors in rat liver by N-nitrosomorpholine. *(in preparation).*
34. Rabes, H. M., Scholze, P., and Jantsch, B. (1972): Growth kinetics of diethylnitrosamine-induced, enzyme-deficient "preneoplastic" liver cell populations *in vivo* and *in vitro. Cancer Res.,* 32:2,577–2,586.
35. Rajewski, M. M. (1972): Proliferative parameters of mammalian cell systems and their role in tumor growth and carcinogenesis. *Z. Krebsforsch.,* 78:12–30.
36. Rajewski, M. F., Dauber, W., and Frankenberg, H. (1966): Liver carcinogenesis by diethylnitrosamine in the rat. *Science,* 152:83–85.
37. Rossi, L., Ravera, M., Repetti, G., and Santi, L. (1977): Long-term administration of DDT or phenobarbital-Na in Wistar rats. *Int. J. Cancer,* 19:179–185.
38. Scherer, E., and Emmelot, P. (1975): Foci of altered liver cells induced by a single dose of diethylnitrosamine and partial hepatectomy: Their contribution to hepatocarcinogenesis in the rat. *Eur. J. Cancer,* 11:145–154.
39. Scherer, E., Hoffmann, P., Emmelot, P., and Friedrich-Freksa, H. (1972): Quantitative study on foci of altered liver cells induced in the rat by a single dose of diethylnitrosamine and partial hepatectomy. *J. Natl. Cancer Inst.,* 49:93–106.
40. Schauer, H., and Kunze, E. (1968): Enzymhistochemische und autoradiographische Untersuchungen während der Cancerisierung der Rattenleber mit Diäthylnitrosamin. *Z. Krebsforsch.,* 70:252–266.
41. Schieferstein, G., Pirschel, S., Frank, W., and Friedrich-Freksa, H. (1974): Quantitative Untersuchungen über den irreversiblen Verlust zweier Enzymaktivitäten in der Rattenleber nach Verfütterung von Diäthylnitrosamin. *Z. Krebsforsch.,* 82:191–208.
42. Schulte-Hermann, R. (1974): Induction of liver growth by xenobiotic compounds and other stimuli. *Crit. Rev. Toxicol.,* 3:97–158.

43. Schwarz, M., Appel, K. E., Rickart, R., and Kunz, H. W. (1979): Effect of DMN, phenobarbital, and halothane on the sedimentation characteristics of rat liver DNA. In: *Mechanisms of Toxic Action on Some Target Organs. Arch. Toxicol.*, 2:479–482.
44. Solt, D., and Farber, E., (1976): New principle for analysis of chemical carcinogenesis. *Nature*, 263:701–703.
45. Swenberg, J. A., Petzold, G. L., and Harbach, P. R. (1976): *In vitro* DNA damage/alkaline elution assay for predicting carcinogenic potential. *Biophys. Biochem. Res. Commun.*, 72:732–738.
46. Tennekes, H. A., Wright, A. S., Dix, K. M., and Koeman, J. H. (1981): The effects of dieldrin, diet, and bedding on enzyme function and tumour incidence in livers of male CF-1 mice. *Cancer Research (in press).*
47. Thorpe, E., and Walker, A. I. T. (1973): The toxicology of Dieldrin (HEOD). II. Comparative long-term oral toxicity studies in mice with Dieldrin, DDT, Phenobarbitone, β-BHC, and γ-BHC. *Food Cosmet. Toxicol.*, 11:433–442.
48. Tomatis, L., Turosov, V., Day, N., and Charles, R. T. (1972): The effects of long-term exposure to DDT on CF-1 mice. *Int. J. Cancer*, 10:489–506.
49. Walker, A. I. T., Thorpe, E., and Stevenson, D. E. (1973): The toxicology of dieldrin (HEOD). I. Long-term oral toxicity studies in mice. *Food, Cosmet. Toxicol.*, 11:415–432.
50. Weisburger, J. H., Madison, R. M., Ward, J. M., Vignera, C., and Weisburger, E. F. (1975): Modification of diethylnitrosamine liver carcinogenesis with phenobarbital but not with immunosuppression. *J. Natl. Cancer Inst.*, 54:1,185–1,188.
51. Wright, A. S., Akintonwa, D. A. A., and Wooder, M. F. (1977): Studies on the interactions of dieldrin with mammalian liver cells at the subcellular level. *Ecotoxicol. Environ. Safety*, 1:7–16.

Carcinogenesis, Vol. 7, edited by E. Hecker et al.
Raven Press, New York © 1982.

Relevance of Basophilic Foci to Promoting Effect of Sex Hormones on Hepatocarcinogenesis

*S. D. Vesselinovitch, *N. Mihailovich, *K. V. N. Rao, and †S. Goldfarb

Pathology and Radiology Departments, University of Chicago, Chicago, Illinois 60637; and †Pathology Department, University of Wisconsin, Madision, Wisconsin 53706

The advantage of the infant mouse as a highly sensitive model to study hepatocarcinogenesis has been repeatedly demonstrated by our group (3). The integrated studies showed that high macromolecular replication, characteristic during that age period, was of crucial importance for effective initiation of carcinogenesis, and that the sex of the host was responsible for the rate of promotion (2). Dealkylation of diethylnitrosamine (DEN) is apparently an essential step in its biochemical metabolic activation. Infant C57BLxC3H F_1 mice dealkylate DEN with similar rates regardless of sex, and hepatocellular carcinomas develop with the same incidence, although after a longer period of time in females than in males. Thus it is conceivable that a similar number of hepatocytes were initiated in both sexes with DEN treatment but that the rate of neoplastic expression or promotion was dependent on the sex hormonal environment. The present studies were carried out to clarify the mechanism of hormonal modulation of hepatocarcinogenesis by a single administration of a nontoxic dose of DEN. The specific objectives were to (a) identify and characterize early focal hepatocellular changes, (b) correlate these changes with development of hepatocellular carcinoma, and (c) define the effects of the hormonal environment on the onset of kinetics of early focal and nodular lesions in relation to development of carcinoma. The study showed the usefulness of the infant mouse model to analyze quantitatively and qualitatively the initiation and the promotion of hepatocarcinogenesis.

MATERIALS AND METHODS

There were two sets of experiments utilizing C57BLxC3H F_1 mice, 15 days of age, injected i.p. once with DEN. In experiment 1, males received 5.00, 2.50, and 1.25 μg/g body weight (bw) of DEN. In experiment 2, groups of males and females were injected with 2.5 μg/g bw of DEN, and were gonadectomized at 4, 14, and 24 weeks. At autopsy, gross nodular lesions observed on the liver surface were counted and their diameters were measured. Secretions from each liver were made through three main liver lobes: median, at the level of biliary bladder and parallel with dorsal margin, and lateral lobes along maximal, dorso ventral diameters. All lesions were sized and diagnosed microscopically.

RESULTS AND CONCLUSIONS

The first set of studies showed that the early focal lesions induced by DEN were characterized by cells showing increased cytoplasmic basophilia due to elevated ribonucleic acid (RNA), increased ^{3}H-Tdr labeling index, and decrease or absence of glucose-6-phosphatase (1). Dosages of DEN ranging from 5.00 to 1.25 μg/g bw induced hepatocellular carcinomas in time in all animals (Fig. 1). The time and rate at which the carcinomas emerged, however, was dependent on carcinogenic dose. Figure 2 shows that the rate of carcinoma development (percent increment/10-week periods) was positively correlated with the rate of development of the early focal and gross nodular lesions (increase in respective multiplicities/10-week periods). Similar positive correlation was observed between the rates of development of focal and nodular lesions.

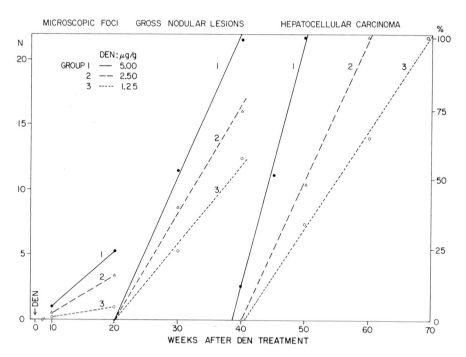

FIG. 1. Dose-dependent development of microscopic foci, gross nodules, and hepatocellular carcinomas following single i.p. injections of DEN to 15-day-old male mice. (*N* = average numbers of foci or nodules per liver cross section or liver surface, respectively; %, incidence of carcinoma-bearing mice).

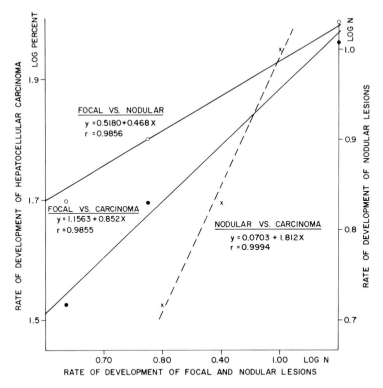

FIG. 2. Relationship between development rates of basophilic foci, nodular lesions, and hepatocellular carcinomas. Multiplicities (focal and nodular average gain in multiplicity/10 weeks) and incidence rates (carcinoma percent increase/10 weeks) were plotted on the logarithmic scale. Note high correlation coefficients.

In the second study, the multiplicities of the nodular lesions in shamgonadectomized animals reached maximal level of 16.0 in males by 40 weeks and 1.9 in females by 60 weeks. Figure 3 shows that orchidectomy prolonged the latent period and slowed the rate at which focal and nodular lesions developed. Figure 4 shows that ovariectomy shortened the latent period and accelerated the rate at which the latter lesions emerged. Nodular multiplicities increased from 2.1 to 4.6 and 8.2 in orchidectomized males, and decreased from 11.9 to 11.8 and 8.1 in ovariectomized females with age at gonadectomy. The serial sacrifice data demonstrated that orchidectomy delayed the onset of the basophilic lesions by an average of 12 weeks. Ovariectomy advanced the onset of the basophilic lesions by 16 weeks and accelerated the rate of their development. The development of carcinomas showed the same trend following gonadectomy. On the average, only 2.2% of all observed lesions in the second study were hepatocellular carcinomas. There were 85.8% basophilic foci, 7.2% hyperplastic nodules, and 4.7 adenomas. The existence of a quantitative relationship between early cellular

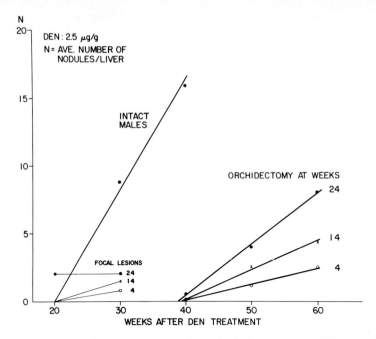

FIG. 3. Delay in the development of focal and nodular lesions due to orchidectomy. Lesions were induced by DEN in 15-day-old mice. Carcinomas were seen at 60 weeks in 100% of intact and in 18.7% of orchidectomized males.

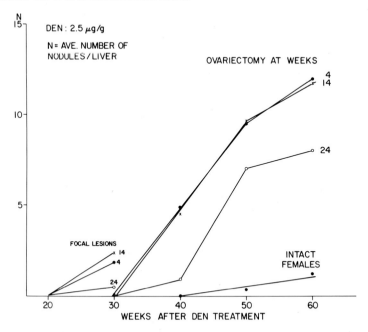

FIG. 4. Acceleration of the emergence of focal and nodular lesions following ovariectomy. Lesions were induced by DEN in 15-day-old females. Carcinomas were seen at 60 weeks in none of the intact and 40.0% of ovariectomized females.

alterations and the rate of appearance of hepatocellular carcinomas (Fig. 2 and the above percent ratio) indicated that certain conclusions could be drawn about development of carcinomas from the kinetics of basophilic foci. It appears that the rate of development of the foci represents the factor limiting the probability at which carcinomas occur. Thus it may be concluded that the mechanism by which sex hormonal environment modified the promoting phase of hepatocarcinogenesis was influencing primarily the time of onset and the rate of development of the basophilic foci. Demonstration that single nontoxic DEN doses were capable of inducing not only early hepatocellular lesions but also carcinomas adds to the practical value of this model system.

ACKNOWLEDGMENTS

Supported in part by FDA 222-76-2004(C) and N. C. I. grants R01 CA-25522 and RO1 CA-25549.

REFERENCES

1. Goldfarb, S., Vesselinovitch, S. D., Pugh, T. D., Mihailovich, N., Koen, H., and He, Y. (1980): Remarkable uniformity of premalignant and malignant hepatocellular foci after single dose injection of diethylnitrosamione (DEN) in infant mice. *Gastroenterology,* 79:1,021.
2. Vesselinovitch, S. D. (1980): Factors modulating response to carcinomutagens: In: *Progress in Environmental Mutagenesis,* edited by M. Alacevic, pp. 281–296. Elsevier Biomedical Press, North Holland.
3. Vesselinovitch, S. D., Rao, K. V. N., and Mihailovich, N. (1979): Neoplastic response of mouse tissues during perinatal age periods and its significance in chemical carcinogenesis. *J. Natl. Cancer Inst.,* 51:239–250.

Carcinogenesis, Vol. 7, edited by E. Hecker et al.
Raven Press, New York © 1982.

Analysis of the Effects of Promoting Agents on Liver and Urinary Bladder Carcinogenesis in Rats

Nobuyuki Ito, Masae Tatematsu, Keisuke Nakanishi,
and Hiroyuki Tsuda

*First Department of Pathology, Nagoya City University Medical School, Mizuho-ku,
Nagoya 467, Japan*

Recent experiments have indicated that promotion is important in the development of several kinds of cancers (1). However, it is difficult to test all possible factors in long-term *in vivo* experiments and no suitable *in vivo* short-term test for promoting agents has yet been established. This work was conducted (a) to test various compounds for their activity to promote preneoplastic liver lesions, (b) to examine the dose-dependent effect of tumor promoters, and (c) to study the organ specific effects of different tumor promoters.

MATERIALS AND METHODS

Chemicals were of the purest grades available. They are listed in Table 1. Male Fischer 344 rats weighing 120 to 150 g were used in all our experiments.

Experimental series I: To test promoting activities of various compounds, rats were injected intraperitoneally with N-nitrosodiethylamine (DEN) [200 mg/kg body weight (bw)] or saline (control) as an initiator and then fed on a basal diet for 2 weeks. Then rats were given one of the test chemicals listed in Table 1 mixed in the basal diet (D) or drinking water (W) for 6 weeks. At the end of week 3, two-thirds partial hepatectomy was performed. The control group was given DEN alone. This experiment was based on our previous results that show the necessity for three components; DEN injection, administration of promoters for 6 weeks, and partial hepatectomy.

Experimental series II: To study of the dose-response of enhancement of N-butyl-N-(4-hydroxybutyl)nitrosamine (BBN)-initiated preneoplastic lesions in rat urinary bladder by treatment with different doses of sodium saccharin as a promoter, rats were divided into six groups. They were initially given drinking water with 0.01% BBN or without BBN for 4 weeks and then a stock diet containing sodium saccharin at a concentration of 5.0%, 1.0%, 0.2%, or 0.04% for 32 weeks.

Experimental series III: For the study of the organ specific effects of two different tumor promoters on the enhancement of neoplastic lesions in rat liver

TABLE 1. Numbers and areas of hyperplastic nodules in the liver promoted by various chemicals in short-term assays in experimental series I

Compound	Dose[b]	Route[c]	Hyperplastic nodules[a]			
			No./cm²		Area (mm²/cm²)	
			Initiator		Initiator	
			DEN[d] (I-1)	0.9% NaCl (I-2)	DEN[d] (I-1)	0.09% NaCl (I-2)
Liver carcinogens						
Ethionine	0.25	D	3.4 ± 1.3^{e} (13)	<0.1 (10)	1.0 ± 0.4^{e}	<0.1
Thioacetamide	0.1	D	10.8 ± 4.2^{e} (12)	0.6 ± 0.4 (9)	6.6 ± 3.0^{e}	0.1 ± 0.1
α-HCH	0.1	D	3.3 ± 1.4^{e} (12)	0 (8)	2.0 ± 0.8^{e}	0
3'-Me-DAB	0.06	D	15.9 ± 4.8^{e} (17)	1.9 ± 1.1 (9)	10.9 ± 5.5^{e}	0.5 ± 0.3
DDT	0.05	D	3.6 ± 1.3^{e} (13)	0 (8)	1.2 ± 0.5^{e}	0
2-AAF	0.02	D	24.3 ± 7.6^{e} (14)	10.0 ± 5.0 (9)	17.1 ± 5.4^{e}	4.3 ± 3.6
Sterigmatocystin	0.012	D	7.8 ± 3.5^{e} (13)	0.1 ± 0.2 (9)	3.7 ± 1.9^{e}	<0.1
DEN	0.01	W	28.7 ± 16.1^{e} (17)	16.7 ± 7.4 (10)	17.2 ± 9.6^{e}	3.6 ± 2.9
Dieldrin	0.01	D•	2.7 ± 0.1^{e} (13)	0 (8)	0.8 ± 0.4^{e}	0
Aldrin	0.005	D	2.5 ± 1.3^{e} (18)	0 (8)	0.5 ± 0.3^{e}	0
Aflatoxin B₁	0.0002	D	31.6 ± 7.4^{e} (12)	3.5 ± 1.0 (9)	10.3 ± 5.5^{e}	1.0 ± 0.3
Nonliver carcinogens						
BBN	0.18	W	2.0 ± 1.4 (14)	0 (10)	0.2 ± 0.2	0
ENU	0.03	W	2.5 ± 1.1^{e} (14)	0 (10)	0.4 ± 0.1^{e}	0
3-MC	0.01	D	1.7 ± 1.0^{e} (14)	0 (10)	0.3 ± 0.2^{e}	0
Miscellaneous compounds						
Saccharin	5.0	D	1.4 ± 1.3 (18)	0 (10)	0.2 ± 0.1	0
Caffeine	0.1	W	1.6 ± 1.0 (20)	0 (10)	0.2 ± 0.1	0
Phenobarbital	0.05	D	3.1 ± 2.3^{e} (15)	0 (10)	1.0 ± 0.7	0
Control(I-3)	—		1.5 ± 1.2 (34)	0 (10)	0	0

[a] Numbers in parentheses: number of animals.
[b] Percentage in the diet or drinking water.
[c] D, in diet; W, in drinking water.
[d] Significantly different from the groups not given DEN (group I-2).
[e] Significantly different from the control (group I-3).

and/or urinary bladder, rats were divided into eight groups. For initiation, rats were fed a stock diet containing 0.02% 2-acetylaminofluorene (2-AAF) for 4 weeks (groups 1, 4, and 7), or given 0.01% BBN in the drinking water for 4 weeks (groups 2, 5, and 8), or neither 2-AAF nor BBN for 4 weeks (groups 3 and 6). Then they were given 0.05% phenobarbital in the diet (groups 1 to 3), or 5.0% sodium saccharin in the diet (groups 4 to 6), or a basal diet (groups 7 and 8) for 32 weeks.

RESULTS AND DISCUSSION

The results in Table 1 show that administration of strong hepatocarcinogens (aflatoxin B_1, DEN, 2-AAF, 3'-methyl-N,N-dimethyl-4-aminoazobenzene (3'-Me-DAB), thioacetamide, sterigmatocystin, and ethionine) resulted in large numbers of hyperplastic liver nodules, whereas, hexachlorobenzene (HCB), dieldrin, 2,2,di(p-chlorophenyl)-1,1,1-trichloroethane (DDT), polychlorinated biphenyls (PCB), and α-hexachlorocyclohexane (α-HCH) had less promoting effects. Nonhepatocarcinogens, such as N-ethylnitrosourea (ENU) and 3-methylcholanthrene (3-MC), also slightly enhanced the induction of hyperplastic nodules. Of the miscellaneous compounds tested, only phenobarbital which is known to have promoting effect in the liver carcinogenesis enhanced the nodule induction (4). Therefore, hepatocarcinogens and chemicals with promoting activity in liver carcinogenesis gave positive results in this system. Thus our system could be used for screening hepatocarcinogens or hepatopromoters.

The results of experimental series II, indicate a clear relationship between the dose of saccharin administered after BBN and the induction of papillary or nodular hyperplasia which are considered to be preneoplastic lesions of bladder cancer (3). If the experimental period had been longer, a dose-response relationship on the induction of papilloma and cancer might have been observed. Similar dose-response relationships for the effect of phenobarbital as a promoter of liver carcinogenesis initiated by 2-AAF have been reported (5).

In experimental series III, after initiation with 2-AAF, phenobarbital greatly enhanced development of neoplastic lesions, and after initiation with BBN, it also induced a significant increase in hyperplastic nodules in the liver (see Table 2). Similarly, after initiation with BBN, saccharin clearly promoted the induction of papillary or nodular hyperplasia, and after initiation with 2-AAF, it slightly promoted the induction of papillary or nodular hyperplasia in the urinary bladder. These results clearly indicate that 2-AAF and BBN act as initiators in both liver and urinary bladder but phenobarbital and saccharin have specific effects on the liver and urinary bladder, respectively.

The present work shows that carcinogens have not only initiating activity but also promoting activity. The promoting effects of promoters were dose-dependent and organ specific. A chemical with strong initiating activity should have strong carcinogenic activity, and a chemical with no initiating activity but strong promoting activity might be a pure promoter. Accordingly, it appears

TABLE 2. Organ specificity of two different tumor promoters in promotion of preneoplastic lesions in the liver and urinary bladder in experimental series III

Group	Initiator	Promotor	No. of animals	Hyperplastic nodules in the liver[a]			Papillary or nodular hyperplasia in the urinary bladder[a]	
				Incidence	No./cm²	Area (mm²/cm²)	Incidence	No./10 cm-BM[b]
1	2-AAF	phenobarbital	24	24 (100)	5.5 ± 3.2[c]	3.5 ± 2.1[c]	0	0
2	BBN	phenobarbital	30	8 (26.7)[d]	<0.04	<0.04	14 (46.7)	0.6 ± 0.7
3	—	phenobarbital	29	0	0	0	0	0
4	2-AAF	saccharin	29	27 (93.1)	3.0 ± 3.6	1.9 ± 2.4	4 (13.8)[e]	0.3 ± 1.1
5	BBN	saccharin	29	0	0	0	24 (82.8)[f]	2.6 ± 2.2[f]
6	—	saccharin	28	0	0	0	0	0
7	2-AAF	—	28	27 (96.4)	3.6 ± 2.6	1.9 ± 1.8	0	0
8	BBN	—	28	0	0	0	11 (39.3)	0.7 ± 1.0

[a] Numbers in parentheses: percentages.
[b] Number of lesions per unit length (10 cm) of basement membrane (BM), mean ± SD
[c] Significantly different from groups 2,3,4,7.
[d] Significantly different from groups 1,3,5,8.
[e] Significantly different from groups 1,5,6,7.
[f] Significantly different from groups 2,4,6,8.

possible to classify chemicals by their potency of initiating and promoting activity. This ability could be helpful in understanding the complicated phenomena involved in chemical carcinogenesis (2).

ACKNOWLEDGMENT

This research was supported in part by Grants-in-Aids for Cancer Research from the Ministry of Education, Science, and Culture of Japan (1979,1980) and the Ministry of Health and Welfare of Japan (1979,1980).

REFERENCES

1. Hicks, R. M., Chowaniec, J., and Wakefield, J. St. J. (1978): Experimental induction of bladder tumors by a two-stage system. In: *Carcinogenesis,* edited by T. J. Slaga, A. Sivak, and R. K. Boutwell, pp. 475–489. Raven Press, New York.
2. Ito, N., Tatematsu, M., Nakanishi, K., Hasegawa, R., Takano, T., Imaida, K., and Ogiso, T. (1980): The effects of various chemicals on the development of hyperplastic liver nodules in hepatectomized rats treated with N-nitrosodiethylamine or N-2-fluorenylacetamide. *Gann,* 71:832–842.
3. Nakanishi, K., Hagiwara, A., Shibata, M., Imaida, K., Tatematsu, M., and Ito, N. (1980): Dose-response of saccharin in the induction of urinary bladder hyperplasias in rats pretreated with N-butyl-N-(4-hydroxybutyl)nitrosamine. *J. Natl. Cancer Inst.,* 65:1,005–1,010.
4. Peraino, C., Fry, R. J. M., Staffeldt, E., and Kisieleski, W. F. (1973): Effects of varying the exposure to phenobarbital on its enhancement on 2-acetylaminofluorene-induced hepatic tumorigenesis in the rat. *Cancer Res.,* 33:2,701–2,705.
5. Takano, T., Tatematsu, M., Hasegawa, R., Imaida, K., and Ito, N. (1980): Dose-response relationship for the promoting effect of phenobarbital on the induction of liver hyperplastic nodules in rats exposed to 2-fluorenylacetamide and carbon tetrachloride. *Gann,* 71:580–581.

Carcinogenesis, Vol. 7, edited by E. Hecker et al.
Raven Press, New York © 1982.

Promotion in Bladder Cancer

R. Marian Hicks

School of Pathology, Middlesex Hospital Medical School, London W 1 P 7LD, England

Evidence that carcinogenesis is a multistage process came from the early work of Berenblum, Rous, Hecker, and Boutwell and their many colleagues working mainly on mouse skin. Up until quite recently, there was a strong consensus that the phenomenon of multistage carcinogenesis, while it applied to mouse skin, had little relevance to any other tissue, despite the accumulating evidence for a multistage process in the lung, liver, and colon. The theory was then expressed in the form of a mathematical model by Armitage and Doll (3) which was subject to epidemiological testing. The assumptions made for this model are that a malignant tumour can arise from a single cell only after that cell has undergone a number of heritable, rare events, each of which must occur in the right sequence over a period of time. Expressed at its simplest, the incidence of tumours, I, is then proportional to time, T, to the power n, where n is the number of events that the cell must experience before it can develop into an autonomous malignant cancer. Epidemiological data for the prevalence of human lung and colon cancer fit this model extremely well, and accumulating evidence suggests that a multistage theory will fit the data for other carcinomas, though not necessarily for leukaemias and sarcomas.

Previously, evidence was presented for a possible two-stage process of carcinogenesis in the urinary bladder based on our work with N-methyl-N-nitrosourea (MNU) given either in small sequential doses or as an initiating dose followed by treatment with other compounds (38). It was suggested that tumour development in the urinary bladder had many points in common with tumour development in skin, and was probably the result of a two-stage or multistage process. Furthermore, it was demonstrated that saccharin and cyclamate were probably not initiators or complete carcinogens when used on their own, but were capable of promoting tumour growth in the bladder. At the time, both these conclusions were novel and the latter was regarded as somewhat controversial, set as it was in the context of a possible ban on the use of saccharin, as well as of cyclamate, in the USA. In this chapter some new evidence will be reviewed that supports the conclusion that carcinogenesis in the urinary bladder is a multistage process. In addition, the probable mode of action of promoters in the bladder will be considered.

INITIATION OF NEOPLASTIC CHANGE IN THE BLADDER

In man, carcinogenesis in the urinary bladder is probably initiated by a small amount only of the activated form of a urine-borne chemical carcinogen that reacts with and produces some alteration of the urothelial cell. In experimental animals the three bladder carcinogens which have been most extensively studied are MNU, the nitrofuran N-[4-(5-nitro-2-furyl)-2-thiazolyl]formamide (FANFT), and the nitrosamine N-butyl-N-(4-hydroxybutyl)nitrosamine (BBN). These initiators of bladder cancer are also complete carcinogens and can bring about all stages in the carcinogenesis process. Because the different stages involve a temporal sequence of events, however, in general even these potent complete carcinogens have to be applied more than once or continually over a period of time in order to complete the process. Thus BBN included as 0.05% in the drinking water has to be administered for 16 weeks or longer, and FANFT incorporated as 0.2% of the diet has to be given for 10 weeks or longer in order to produce bladder cancer in all animals treated (46,48). Repeated exposure over a prolonged period of time is necessary for these carcinogens to bring about all the changes necessary to convert a normal urothelial cell into an autonomous clone of cancer cells. The same is true for MNU where repeated doses have to be given at two-weekly intervals over a period of 6 weeks, in order to produce a 100% incidence of bladder cancer (34,38). In other tissues, tumour incidence is, broadly speaking, proportional to the dose of the initiating carcinogen to which the tissue is exposed (24). Because of the temporal sequence of events involved in a multistage process of carcinogenesis, this cannot readily be demonstrated by measuring the tumour incidence resulting from single doses of different sizes. Instead, each dose has to be fractionated into several small aliquots that are given over a period of time, and the subsequent tumour incidence can then be related to the total cumulative dose. A dose-related response to different cumulative doses of MNU has been demonstrated (34,38). Although there is a good dose-related response for each individual level of split dose, the strict relationship is modified by the toxicity of the carcinogen. Much of the damage produced by reaction of a carcinogen with the cell is lethal rather than mutagenic, and a single high dose may well kill more cells than it leaves alive but initiated. This is illustrated in Fig. 1, which shows the response of the urothelium to multiple doses of MNU of different fraction size. When the tumour incidence is plotted against the total cumulative dose, for any particular dose, the tumour response is greater if it was administered in small fractions than if it was administered in larger fractions. It must be assumed that the lower doses are less cytotoxic and consequently permit more initiated cells to survive and remain available for promotion by subsequent doses. If there is a dose-related toxicity of MNU, although more cells may be initiated by the larger fractions, fewer cells will survive and the surviving population available for subsequent promotion will be progressively reduced. These results suggest that there may well be a greater carcinogenic hazard from the cumulative effect

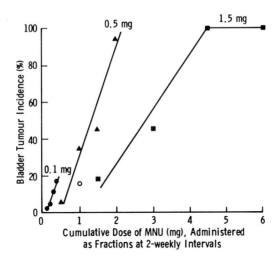

FIG. 1. The effect of fraction size on tumour incidence in response to fractionated doses of MNU. ○, Tumour incidence after single dose of 1.0 mg.

of repeated exposure to very low doses of environmental carcinogens, than there is from a single, episodic exposure to a massive dose. For many toxins, threshold doses can be defined below which there is no detectable biological damage. For carcinogens, by contrast, no theoretical threshold can be defined below which the compound can be regarded as safe, for the initiating effect of the reaction of the carcinogen with the cell is, in effect, permanent, and the effect of repeated exposure to low doses over a period of time is cumulative. This has been confirmed recently in an extensive study using mice, in which the dose-response relationship of the animals to low doses of 2-acetylaminofluorene (2-AAF) was examined (51).

Complete carcinogens, such as MNU, BBN, and FANFT, though they can both initiate and promote tumour growth in the bladder, are not necessarily equally efficient in their action at the different stages of carcinogenesis. There is no *a priori* reason why they should be, for the biochemical events underlying initiation and promotion differ quite fundamentally. For initiation it is generally believed that only a brief, single application of the carcinogen or its ultimate derivative is required to react with the target cell deoxyribonucleic acid (DNA) to produce a permanent mutagenic event (8,61). Initiation thus involves the production of a heritable change in the target cell, whereby it is converted into a latent tumour cell. For promotion, prolonged or repeated treatment with the promoting agent is required and conversion of the initiated cell into a latent tumour cell may involve epigenetic, as opposed to genetic, events. Recently, a further mathematical treatment of multistage carcinogenesis has been made by Day and Brown (23) that enables predictions to be made about the pattern of tumour incidence that will follow a finite exposure of a tissue to an early stage initiating carcinogen, as compared with the pattern of response to be expected after a finite then discontinued exposure to a promoter or late stage carcinogen. According to this model, if exposure is to an initiating, or first stage, carcinogen, tumour incidence continues to rise even after the carcinogen is withdrawn. By contrast, if the exposure is to a promoting agent or to a later stage carcinogen, the excess tumour incidence remains level or may even fall after stopping exposure to the agent. This is illustrated experimentally by the response of the mouse liver and mouse bladder to different periods of exposure to the carcinogen 2-AAF.

This aromatic amine has long been recognised as a bladder carcinogen for the mouse since the work of Bonser and her colleagues in the 1940s (4) and was recently the carcinogen chosen for a study involving over 24,000 mice at the National Center for Toxicological Research in America. In that study, Littlefield et al. (51) confirmed 2-AAF to be a bladder carcinogen and showed a dose-related response of the animals to the carcinogen in terms of bladder cancer prevalence, which might suggest that they were dealing with an initiating carcinogen. There was also a dose-related response in terms of liver cancer, but the liver tumours developed very much later than did the bladder tumours. Indeed, the liver tumours all developed long after the treatment with 2-AAF was discontinued and the shape of the prevalence curves exactly fits the pattern for a first stage, or initiating, carcinogen predicted by Day and Brown's model. These results confirm that 2-AAF is predominantly a first stage, or initiating, carcinogen for the liver. It must also have some promoting activity in the liver since, as a complete carcinogen, it must bring about the subsequent stages in the multistage process. In the bladder, by contrast, the effect of terminating the 2-AAF treatment after 9, 12, or 15 months is completely different from the effect on the liver (52). The tumour incidence did continue to increase very slightly, but at a much slower rate than if the treatment had been continued, so that the tumour prevalence did not increase greatly over that which would have been found if the animals were all killed at the time the treatment was stopped. The prevalence curve was approximately that predicted by Day and Brown's theoretical model for a second stage carcinogen and indicates that in the bladder, 2-AAF is predominantly a second stage, or promoting, carcinogen. The fact that new tumours do continue to arise, albeit very slowly, and that there is a dose-related response to 2-AAF, shows it to be a complete carcinogen for the bladder with weak first stage, or initiating, activity and powerful second stage, or promoting, action. This study with 2-AAF demonstrates that the initiating and promoting capabilities of any compound may vary. It may be predominantly an initiator with little or no promoting activity, for example, urethane; predominantly a promoter with little or no initiating activity, for example, croton oil; or have any balance of activity between these two extremes.

Although initiators are believed to react covalently with the DNA, they do not preferentially react with replicating rather than nonreplicating parts of the genome (69). Since most of the genes are in a repressed state, the areas of the DNA modified by the carcinogen are more likely to be in the unexpressed than in the transcribing areas of the genome, and no difference in phenotypic expression will necessarily be seen after an initiating event. Even if the initiating event is in an unexpressed area of the genome, however, it will be permanent and will leave some cells harbouring misinformation, even though they are phenotypically identical to their unaffected neighbours as judged by their functional proteins, membrane structure, or any other phenotypic marker. Thus, after treating the bladder with a low, initiating dose of MNU, after the initial response of the urothelium to the toxic effect of the drug, differentiation returns to normal and the animal may survive with a normally differentiated urothelium for the rest of its life (68). As long as the altered area remains unexpressed, no change in phenotype will occur, even when the cell divides in the normal course of events. Before a change in phenotype can be seen, a promoting event is required that will allow the altered area of genome to become inducible; the affected area must be morphologically altered into a transcribing rather than a nontranscribing form.

PROMOTION IN THE URINARY BLADDER

Promoters and Later Stage Carcinogens

The action of promoters in skin carcinogenesis has been intensively studied, and we have extended some general observations from skin to promotion in the urinary bladder. Promoters of skin cancer are known to promote hyperplasia by increasing the rate of DNA synthesis and the rate of turnover of the basal cells, so giving any altered transcribable area of the genome a better chance to be expressed and to appear as an altered phenotype. At the same time, this stimulates any altered cells to grow and divide and, in effect, propagates tumour growth. Promoters are also believed to permit expression of the altered information carried by an initiated cell in unexpressed areas of the genome by altering the normal pattern of gene expression (61). Indeed, Cairns (16) suggested that the primary action of promoters is to raise the rate at which the gene regulatory circuits are set, thus increasing the likelihood of expressing hidden or latent damage. Concomitant with disturbing the normal pattern of gene expression, promoters also inhibit the normal differentiation of tissues and tend to produce immature, less well-differentiated, or randomly differentiated cell types, which may be seen as bizarre metaplasias within cancers or as "dedifferentiated" (sic) hyperplasias. This has given rise to the concept of cancer as a disease of maladjusted differentiation, though many of the altered differentiated states may well be epiphenomena and not markers of neoplastic transformation *per se*. At the same time as permitting random differentiation, promoters also inhibit the normal terminal differentiation of the tissue. Many examples are now published in which the phorbol ester series of skin promoters maintain tissues in a relatively undifferentiated state and delay the terminal differentiation of cell lines in culture. They thus increase the time required before a cell will pass into the "differentiate and die" pathway and retain the cells longer in the cell cycle where they can grow and divide. It is a matter of common observation that the aggressive, dividing, malignant cells in solid tumours are not usually those undergoing terminal differentiation, but are the relatively undifferentiated stem cells that remain unspecialised or anaplastic in highly invasive cancers. For example, in the bladder, neoplastic urothelial cells are predominantly small, diploid cells that do not reflect any of the obvious adult differentiation patterns seen in the superficial cells of the normal urothelium (33,37).

Vitamin A Deficiency

A number of compounds that are predominantly promoters or late stage carcinogens for the urinary bladder have now been identified. Vitamin A deficiency clearly acts as a promoting stimulus in the biogenesis of bladder cancer. This was observed nearly 20 years ago by Angrist and his co-workers who used methyl cholanthrene as the initiating carcinogen (17), though at the time it was not interpreted in terms of initiation and promotion. Vitamin A deficiency causes an increase in DNA synthesis and increased mitotic activity in the basal cells of the urothelium leading to hyperplasia. Coincident with this rather nonspecific stimulation of cell division and tumour promotion, vitamin A deficiency also specifically affects the genes controlling the differentiation of the cell, so that bladder tumours in vitamin A-deficient animals are also heavily keratinised. The keratinisation is concomitant with, but not an essential part of, the biogenesis of the neoplasm in initiated tissue, for keratinisation occurs also in vitamin A-deficient urothelia that have not been preinitiated by exposure to a carcinogen (31,32). Keratinisation in this tissue demonstrates a disturbance in the normal control of transcription introduced by vitamin A deficiency, which will automatically increase the chance of transcribing any potentially carcinogenic changes in the genome introduced by previous exposure to an initiator.

Saccharin and Cyclamate

The first unequivocal demonstration of a promoter of bladder cancer came from our work with saccharin and cyclamate following an initiating dose of MNU (36,38,41). If rats are initiated by a single threshold dose of MNU, insufficient to produce tumours on its own, a relatively high concentration of either saccharin or cyclamate subsequently included in the diet of these animals promotes tumour development in 50% of the animals' bladders within 2 years (36,38). The promoting activity of saccharin in the urinary bladder was subsequently confirmed by Friedell's group (22) following an initiating dose of the nitrofuran FANFT. Just as the phorbol ester series of promoters used in isolation induce hyperplasia in skin, we found that saccharin alone causes focal hyperplasia of the urothelium with increased numbers of cells entering into mitosis (20).

Contrary to a previous report (22), this has now been confirmed in another laboratory by Fukushima and Cohen (26), who also observed an increased uptake of tritiated thymidine in focal areas of urothelium in saccharin-treated rats. Tumours promoted by saccharin show a wide variety of differentiation patterns, both within the tumour and in adjacent, nonneoplastic areas of urothelium (35,37). This suggests that saccharin, like skin promoters, in some way disturbs the normal control of differentiation, thus increasing the chance of random transcription of the genome.

In skin carcinogenesis models, it has been demonstrated that the ultimate tumour yield is quantitatively related to the dose of the initiator rather than the dose of the promoter (7,62), and that for unequivocal demonstration of a second promoting stage in carcinogenesis, the initiator must be used at a dose that is not carcinogenic to any marked degree (7,8). The same principles can be shown to apply to initiation and promotion in the urinary bladder. As previously reported, we found that with the same initiating dose of MNU, when animals were maintained on diets containing varying amounts of either saccharin or cyclamate, bladder tumours developed in approximately half of the MNU-treated animals (36,38). Tumour incidence was clearly related to the initiating dose of the MNU and not to the concentration of the sweetener in the diet. The amount of MNU used was apparently sufficient to produce latent tumour cells in about half of the animals that were promoted by the sweeteners in the diet. For these studies the amount of MNU used was insufficient to cause tumour development in the absence of a promoter. In the mouse skin system, Berenblum (7,8) showed that if a high carcinogenic dose of benzo(a)pyrene was used, no increase in tumour incidence could be demonstrated following application of croton oil as a promoter. Similarly, we found when a carcinogenic dose of MNU was used that produced bladder cancer in approximately 30% of the treated animals, no significant increase in tumour incidence resulted from subsequent inclusion of saccharin as a 2% solution in drinking water, even though the number of benign, proliferative lesions in the urothelium did increase (44). Similarly, a carcinogenic dose of MNU producing a 40% incidence of bladder tumours was not increased by ingestion of either saccharin or cyclamate, although in the same experiments, a 28% incidence of urothelial tumours of the renal pelvis was promoted to 57% by saccharin and to 43% by cyclamate (55). These experiments are further evidence that, at high doses, MNU is able to promote all available initiated target cells that survive cytotoxic damage, whereas at lower threshold or subthreshold doses, the cytotoxic damage is less and numerous initiated cells survive and are available for promotion at a later date.

Urinary Calculi

The exact function of urinary calculi in the development of bladder carcinoma has often been debated, and it has even been suggested that the production of urinary calculi is the common aetiological denominator in many experimental investigations of chemical carcinogenesis in rodents (21). We have long disputed this view and have published evidence that calculi, though commonly found in association with tumours, are also found in tumour-free bladders and, conversely, that tumours develop in carcinogen-treated rats that have no urinary lithiasis (34,37). The possible association between artificial sweeteners, urolithiasis, and the induction of bladder cancer has also been debated in some depth, but we could demonstrate no positive correlation between calcification and tumour formation either in our own laboratories (20,37) or in the work done elsewhere (44), and this has now been confirmed by other investigators (28). Undoubtedly, however, where a calculus is present in a bladder in which the urothelium has already been exposed to initiating and promoting stimuli, it will accelerate tumour growth by increasing the rate of urothelial cell turnover in response to the diffuse irritation and abrasion that it causes. The effect of urinary calculi is thus comparable to the effect of irritant chemicals such as turpentine (9) on initiated and promoted skin, or the effect of wounding previously tarred rabbit ears (53). Chapman et al. (18) demonstrated tumour incidence in surgically constructed rat bladder pouches to be increased in the presence of urine from 27% to 66% by insertion of a stone into the pouch. If contact with urine was prevented, no tumours developed. In these experiments a urine-borne carcinogen, probably of dietary origin, must have been present in sufficient concentration to both initiate and promote a few cells in the urothelium, from which tumour growth was accelerated by the local trauma of the surgery involved in constructing the pouch. This would be comparable to the effect of wounding previously tarred rabbit ears. The additional diffuse hyperplasia produced by including a stone in the pouch would then act like turpentine on initiated and promoted skin, to further accelerate and propagate tumour growth from microscopic tumour foci in the urothelium.

Bilharziasis

In patients with bilharziasis, there is an elevated prevalence of bladder cancer in some, but not all, areas of endemic S. haematobium infection (13,43,45). This may be explained if exposure to low doses of environmental carcinogens, which may well vary from area to area, is required in order to bring about the early stages of carcinogenesis and produce microscopic foci of tumour cells in the urothelium. Such foci, if small enough, could remain undetectable until further growth is stimulated by a second or later stage carcinogen or by irritation and hyperplasia caused by the erupting live and/or calcified dead schistosoma ova in the bladder wall (39,40,42). The effect of schistosomiasis is thus to accelerate, but not to initiate, bladder cancer development.

Tryptophan

For many years tryptophan and its metabolites have been implicated in the biogenesis of bladder cancer, but the results have been very difficult to interpret.

Abnormalities of tryptophan metabolism have been reported frequently in patients with bladder cancer (12,14,59), but in experimental animals, dietary tryptophan alone is not carcinogenic. As demonstrated by Boyland and his colleagues (1,11) and subsequently confirmed by Bryan et al. (15), however, a number of tryptophan metabolites were found to be carcinogenic for the urinary bladder by the mouse bladder inplantation test. Furthermore, addition of either tryptophan or the related compound indole to the diet of 2-AAF-treated rats markedly increased the incidence of bladder cancer (25). Tryptophan has now been demonstrated to promote the initiating effect of low doses of FANFT, although its effect is much less marked than that of saccharin (22). It is also a promoter of bladder cancer in mice following initiation by FANFT (54) and in dogs after treatment with aromatic amines (60). Collectively, these observations show that although tryptophan and/or its metabolites may be unable to initiate bladder cancer, they will act as weak promoters of carcinogens if the urothelium has previously been exposed to some other initiating compound.

Cyclophosphamide

Another compound about which there has been much controversy in recent years is cyclophosphamide, or cytoxan. There are regular, though infrequent, reports of carcinoma in the bladder developing in patients with no history of urinary tract disease, who have been treated with cyclophosphamide as part of a multiple cytotoxic therapy programme for malignant disease elsewhere in the body. On the other hand, bladder cancer is an infrequent complication for renal transplant patients who have been immunosuppressed with cyclophosphamide (47). Most (2,38,49) but not all (30) investigators who have tested the effect of repeated doses of cyclophosphamide have found it to be noncarcinogenic for the rat urinary bladder. However, it has now been reported to be cocarcinogenic for the mouse bladder (58), and doses of cyclophosphamide, which *per se* are not carcinogenic for the rat bladder, will nevertheless promote tumour growth in animals previously initiated with FANFT (2). If cyclophosphamide proves to be a promoter of bladder carcinogenesis in man as well as in rodents, its use in combined cytotoxic therapy could be potentially dangerous if other compounds with known mutagenic or carcinogenic potential are also being administered. This is a particularly important consideration when treating patients in younger age groups with a relatively long life expectancy.

REQUIREMENT FOR PROLONGED PERIOD OF PROMOTION

Clinical Consequences

Although the process of carcinogenesis can be initiated by only a brief exposure of the tissues to a threshold or subcarcinogenic dose of a complete carcinogen, all available evidence indicates that prolonged exposure to promoters is required before converted tumour cells develop the property of autonomous growth that, more than any other single factor, characterises malignant neoplasms. In skin, the preneoplastic hyperplasias seen in the early stages of promotion will be arrested or regress if the promoters are withdrawn soon enough (8). This demonstrates that the early stages of tumour development in skin are partially reversible and that, for a time, the newly converted tumour cells can be repaired or else revert to the dormant, but still initiated, state in which they will remain until promoted once again. If, however, promotion is prolonged, the biochemical events that underlie promotion persist and, at some stage, the cell will develop autonomy, and its new, neoplastic phenotype will then continue to be fully expressed even in the absence of further doses of promoter. As previously reported (38,41), in the urinary bladder a single dose of cyclophosphamide fails to promote tumour growth following a subthreshold initiating dose of MNU, even though it temporarily causes marked urothelial hyperplasia (19,38,49); but repeated doses of cyclophosphamide over 40 weeks will promote the initiating effect of a threshold dose of FANFT (2). Even though the early hyperplasia produced in the initial stages of promotion may regress, the production of persistent low-grade hyperplasia by a promoting agent may be diagnostic for subsequent development of carcinomas. This was demonstrated in the mouse study with 2-AAF, where it was observed that the tumour incidence could have been predicted 9 months in advance from the state of persistent hyperplasia in the urothelium (27,51,52). The speed at which a tumour develops from fully committed cells in an area of persistent hyperplasia depends partly on the inherent proliferative capacity of the tissue and partly on the presence or absence of cofactors such as a calculus that can accelerate cell division, as discussed above. This has an important bearing on the treatment of bladder cancer patients. It is evident that tumour growth is accelerated significantly by any agent or procedure that stimulates an increased rate of cell turnover in an initiated and promoted urothelium. By analogy with the proven stimulus to tumour growth given by wounding tumour-free but previously initiated skin, there is a strong argument for restricting to an absolute minimum the number of urothelial biopsies taken from patients with a history of neoplastic disease. Any programme involving serial biopsies of areas of either of carcinoma *in situ* or of atypical hyperplasia should be meticulously avoided, or the rate at which the next neoplasm develops may well be accelerated by the surgical trauma. On the other hand, the facts that prolonged exposure to promoters is required for autonomous tumour growth and that, in the early stages of promotion, the effects are reversible, offer new hopes for treatment of the cancer patient. In people, it may require many years for the necessary number of cellular events to be experienced in the right order to produce a malignant growth from an initiated cell. Potentially, this long promotion phase of tumour development offers the most hopeful period for the eventual control of bladder cancer. Interest is now centering upon antipromoters such as retinoids (65), antiinflammatory steroids (6,63), and protease inhibitors (66) which specifically antagonise different stages of carcinogenesis (64). The retinoids and antiinflammatory steroids reinforce the normal differentiation of the cell and reduce the opportunity for atypical expression of normally suppressed areas of the genome. Consequently they reduce the opportunity for expression of any malignant change that has been introduced into nontranscribing areas of the normal DNA by previous exposure to an initiator. It has been demonstrated in animal models that retinoids can delay the onset of tumour growth in animals previously exposed to carcinogens (5,29). We have investigated the efficacy of two retinoids, namely 13-*cis*-retinoic acid and N-ethylretinamide, to prevent the development of bladder cancer in rats treated with BBN. We find that these compounds delay the onset of tumour growth but do not reduce the rate of development of fully promoted cancers already growing autonomously (37a). This is just what would be predicted if they delay the rate of conversion of an initiated cell to a promoted cell, but have no effect on the rate of cell turnover or propagation of a committed clone of tumour cells.

CONCLUSIONS

No reports are available of any biochemical events that accompany promotion in the bladder, comparable to the extensive literature on the biochemistry of promoters in skin systems reviewed by Boutwell (10), Scribner and Suss (61), and extended in the last few years by many other investigators (57, and see T. J. Slaga, *this volume*). When tested in parallel with other compounds in the same animal model, saccharin appears to be the most effective promoter of bladder carcinogenesis discovered so far. It is more effective than tryptophan or cyclophosphamide and equally effective as cyclamate. It produces at least some of the same effects as the phorbol ester series of promoters produce in skin, including mild hyperplasia, by accelerating the rate of mitosis, thus also helping to accelerate tumour growth. In addition, it encourages the appearance of abnormal phenotypes in the urothelium, presumably by disturbing the control of gene expression and permitting random readout. Saccharin also behaves as a promoter in other tissues in *in vitro* assay systems. Thus it acts as a promoter in a mouse embryo fibroblast test system (56) and, like other promoters of the phorbol-ester type, blocks metabolic cooperation, a form of cell-to-cell communication, in Chinese hamster V79 cells *in vitro* (67). Very recently it has been reported that saccharin and cyclamate, like TPA and other related diterpenes, inhibit the binding of labelled mouse epidermal growth factor (EGF) to HeLa cells (50). There are thus good grounds for believing that saccharin may prove to be as useful a tool for the investigation of multistage carcinogenesis in the bladder as the phorbol esters have been for multistage carcinogenesis in skin.

Until now, the multistage nature of carcinogenesis in the bladder has been established on a purely biological basis using whole animal experimental models. Such studies have provided a valuable base line for further research now urgently needed to supply a biochemical explanation for the phenomenon of promotion in the urinary bladder, comparable to the data that already exist for promotion in skin.

ACKNOWLEDGMENTS

Work on multistage models and the biogenesis of bladder cancer in the School of Pathology, Middlesex Hospital Medical School, has been supported over a number of years by generous grants from the Cancer Research Campaign. I am indebted to all my colleagues, past and present, who have worked with me on these problems, and in particular to J. St. J. Wakefield, J. Chowaniec, and N. Severs.

REFERENCES

1. Allen, M. J., Boyland, E., Dukes, C. E., Horning, E. S., and Watson, J. G. (1957): Cancer of the urinary bladder induced in mice with metabolites of aromatic amines and tryptophan. *Br. J. Cancer,* 17:212–228.
2. Arai, M., Cohen, S. M., and Friedell, G. H. (1977): Promoting effect of cyclophosphamide (CP) on rat urinary bladder carcinogenesis following initiation by N-[4-(5-nitro-2-furyl)-2-thiazolyl]formamide (FANFT). Proceedings of the Japanese Cancer Association: 36th Annual Meeting, October 1977, Tokyo, p. 39. Published as a supplement to Gann., Japanese Cancer Association, Tokyo.
3. Armitage, P., and Doll, R. (1961): Stochastic models for carcinogenesis. In: *Proceedings of the Fourth Berkeley Symposium on Mathematical Statistics and Probability, Vol. 4,* edited by J. Neyman, pp. 19–38. University of California Press, Berkeley.
4. Armstrong, E. C., and Bonser, G. M. (1944): Epithelial tumours of the urinary bladder in mice induced by 2-AAF. *J. Pathol. Bacteriol.,* 56:507–511.
5. Becci, P. J., Thompson, H. J., Grubbs, C. J., Brown, C. C., and Moon, R. C. (1979): Effect of delay in administration of 13-*cis*-retinoic acid on the inhibition of urinary bladder carcinogenesis in the rat. *Cancer Res.,* 39:3,141–3,144.
6. Belman, S., and Troll, W. (1978): Hormones, cyclic nucleotides, and prostaglandins. In *Carcinogenesis, Vol. 2: Mechanisms of Tumor Promotion and Carcinogenesis,* edited by T. J. Slaga, A. Sivak, and R. K. Boutwell, pp. 117–134. Raven Press, New York.
7. Berenblum, I. (1941): The mechanism of carcinogenesis: A study of the significance of cocarcinogenic action and related phenomena. *Cancer Res.,* 1:807–814.
8. Berenblum, I., (1974): *Carcinogenesis as a Biological Problem.* North Holland, Amsterdam.
9. Boutwell, R. K. (1964): Some biological aspects of skin carcinogenesis. *Prog. Exp. Tumor Res.,* 4:207–250.
10. Boutwell, R. K. (1978): Biochemical mechanism of tumour promotion. In: *Carcinogenesis, Vol. 2: Mechanisms of Tumor Promotion and Cocarcinogenesis,* edited by T. J. Slaga, A. Sivak, and R. K. Boutwell, pp. 49–58. Raven Press, New York.
11. Boyland, E., Busby, E. R., Dukes, C. E., Grover, P. L., and Manson, D. (1964): Further experiments on implantation of materials into the urinary bladder of mice. *Br. J. Cancer,* 18:575–581.
12. Boyland, E., and Williams, D. C. (1956): Metabolism of tryptophan: Metabolism of tryptophan in patients suffering from cancer of the bladder. *Biochem. J.,* 64:578–582.
13. Brand, K. G. (1979): Schistosomiasis—cancer: Aetiological considerations. *Acta Trop.,* 36:203–214.
14. Brown, R. R., Price, J. M., Friedell, G. H., and Burney, S. W. (1969): Tryptophan metabolism in patients with bladder cancer: Geographical differences. *J. Natl. Cancer Inst.,* 43:295–301.
15. Bryan, G. T., Brown, R. R., and Price, J. M. (1964): Incidence of mouse bladder tumours following implantation of paraffin pellets containing certain tryptophan metabolites. *Cancer Res.,* 24:582–585.
16. Cairns, J. (1977): Some thoughts about cancer research in lieu of a summary. In: *Origins of*

Human Cancer. Book C. Human Risk Assessment, edited by H. H. Hiatt, J. D. Watson, and J. A. Winsten, pp. 1,813–1,820. Cold Spring Harbor Laboratory, Cold Spring Harbor, New York.

17. Capurro, P., Angrist, A., Black, J., and Moumgis, B. (1960): Studies in squamous metaplasia in rat bladder. 1. Effects of hypovitaminosis A, foreign bodies, and methylcholanthrene. *Cancer Res.,* 20:563–567.

18. Chapman, W. H., Kirchheim, D., and McRoberts, J. W. (1973): Effect of the urine and calculus formation on the incidence of bladder tumors in rats implanted with paraffin wax pellets. *Cancer Res.,* 33:1,225–1,229.

19. Chaves, E. (1968): Induction of bladder hyperplasia in rats after a single dose of cyclophosphamide. *Rev. Fr. Chem. Biol.,* 13:56–61.

20. Chowaniec, J., and Hicks, R. M. (1979): Response of the rat to saccharin with particular reference to the urinary bladder. *Br. J. Cancer,* 39:355–375.

21. Clayson, D. B. (1974): Bladder carcinogenesis in rats and mice: Possibility of artifacts. *J. Natl. Cancer Inst.,* 52:1,685–1,689.

22. Cohen, S. M., Arai, M., Jacobs, J. B., and Friedell, G. H. (1979): Promoting effect of saccharin and *DL*-tryptophan in urinary bladder carcinogenesis. *Cancer Res.,* 39:1,207–1,217.

23. Day, N. E., and Brown, C. C. (1980): Multistage models and primary prevention of cancer. *J. Natl. Cancer Inst.,* 64:977–989.

24. Druckrey, H. (1967): Quantitative aspects in chemical carcinogenesis. In: *Potential Carcinogenic Hazards from Drugs, UICC Monograph Series, Vol. 7,* edited by R. Truhaut, pp. 60–78. Springer-Verlag, Berlin.

25. Dunning, W. F., Curtis, M. R., and Maun, M. E. (1950): Effect of added dietary tryptophan on occurrence of 2-acetylaminofluorene-induced liver and bladder cancer in rats. *Cancer Res.,* 10:454–459.

26. Fukushima, S., and Cohen, S. M. (1980): Saccharin-induced hyperplasia of the rat urinary bladder. *Cancer Res.,* 40:734–736.

27. Gaylor, D. W. (1980): The ED_{01} study: Summary and conclusions. *J. Environ. Pathol. Toxicol.,* 3:179–183.

28. Green, U., and Rippel, W. (1979): Bladder calculi in rats treated with nitrosomethylurea and fed artificial sweeteners. *Exp. Pathol. (Jena),* 17:561–564.

29. Grubbs, C. J., Moon, R. C., Squire, R. A., Farrow, G. M., Stinson, S. F., Goodman, D. G., Brown, C. C., and Sporn, M. B. (1977): *β-cis*-Retinoic acid: Inhibition of bladder carcinogenesis induced in rats by N-butyl-N-(4-hydroxybutyl)nitrosamine. *Science,* 198:743–744.

30. Habs, M., and Schmähl, D. (1978): Carcinogenic action of low-dose cyclophosphamide (CP) in rats. *Proc. Am. Assoc. Cancer Res.,* 19:14.

31. Hicks, R. M. (1968): Hyperplasia and cornification of the transitional epithelium in the vitamin A-deficient rat. *J. Ultrastruct. Res.,* 22:206–230.

32. Hicks, R. M. (1969): Nature of the keratohyalin-like granules in hyperplastic and cornified areas of transitional epithelium in the vitamin A-deficient rat. *J. Anat.,* 104:327–339.

33. Hicks, R. M. (1976): Changes in differentiation of the urinary bladder during benign and neoplastic hyperplasia. In: *Progress in Differentiation Research,* edited by N. Müller-Berat, pp. 339–353. North Holland, Amsterdam.

34. Hicks, R. M. (1980a): Multistage carcinogenesis in the urinary bladder. *Br. Med. Bull.,* 36:39–46.

35. Hicks, R. M. (1980b): Early carcinogenesis differentiation and promotion. *Br. J. Cancer,* 41:661–663.

36. Hicks, R. M., and Chowaniec, J. (1977): The importance of synergy between weak carcinogens in the induction of bladder cancer in experimental animals. *Cancer Res.,* 37:2,943–2,949.

37. Hicks, R. M., and Chowaniec, J. (1978): Experimental induction, histology, and ultrastructure of hyperplasia and neoplasia in the urinary bladder epithelium. *Int. Rev. Exp. Pathol.,* 18:199–280.

37a. Hicks, R. M., Chowaniec, J., Twiton, J. A., Massey, E. D., and Harvey, A. (1981): The effects of dietary retinoids on experimentally induced carcinogenesis in the rat bladder. In: *Molecular Interrelations of Nutrition and Cancer, 34th Annual Symposium on Fundamental Cancer Research, University of Texas System Cancer Center and M. D. Anderson Hospital and Tumor Institute.* Raven Press, New York (in press).

38. Hicks, R. M., Chowaniec, J., and Wakefield, J. St. J. (1978): Experimental induction of bladder

tumors by a two-stage system. In: *Carcinogenesis, Vol. 2: Mechanisms of Tumor Promotion and Cocarcinogenesis,* edited by T. J. Slaga, A. Sivak, and R. K. Boutwell, pp. 475–489. Raven Press, New York.

39. Hicks, R. M., Gough, T. A., and Walters, C. L. (1978): Demonstration of the presence of nitrosamines in human urine: Preliminary observations on a possible aetiology for bladder cancer. In: *Environmental Aspects of N-nitroso Compounds,* edited by E. Walker, L. Griciute, M. Castegnaro, and R. E. Lyle, pp. 465–475. IARC Scientific Publications, No. 19, IARC, Lyon.

40. Hicks, R. M., James, C., and Webbe, G. (1980): The effect of Schistosoma haematobium and N-butyl-N-(4-hydroxybutyl) nitrosamine on the development of urothelial neoplasia in the baboon. *Br. J. Cancer,* 42:730–755.

41. Hicks, R. M., Wakefield, J. St. J., and Chowaniec, J. (1975): Evaluation of a new model to detect bladder carcinogens or cocarcinogens: Results obtained from saccharin, cyclamate, and cyclophosphamide. *Chem. Biol. Interact.,* 11:225–233.

42. Hicks, R. M., Walters, C. L., Elsebai, I., El-Aasser, A. B., El-Merzabani, M., and Gough, T. (1977): Demonstration of N-nitrosamines in human urine. Preliminary observations on a possible aetiology for bladder cancer in association with chronic urinary tract infections. *Proc. R. Soc. Med.,* 70:413–417.

43. Higginson, J., and Oettlé, A. G. (1962): Cancer of the bladder in the South African Bantu. *Acta. Univ. Int. Contra Cancrum,* 18:579–584.

44. Hooson, J., Hicks, R. M., Grasso, P., and Chowaniec, J. (1980): o-Toluene sulphonamide and saccharin in the promotion of bladder cancer in the mouse. *Br. J. Cancer,* 42:129–147.

45. Houston, W. (1964): Carcinoma of the bladder in Southern Rhodesia. *Br. J. Urol.,* 36:71–76.

46. Ito, N., Hiasa, Y., Tamai, A., Okajima, E., and Kitamura, H. (1969): Histogenesis of urinary bladder tumors induced by N-butyl-N-(4-hydroxybutyl)nitrosamine in rats. *Gann,* 60:401–410.

47. Ito, T. Y., and Martin, D. C. (1977): Tumours of the bladder in renal transplant patients: Report of a case of adenocarcinoma and review of known cases. *J. Urol.,* 117:52–53.

48. Jacobs, J. B., Arai, M., Cohen, S. M., and Friedell, G. H. (1977): A long-term study of reversible and progressive urinary bladder cancer lesions in rats fed N-[4-(5-nitro-2-furyl)-2-thiazolyl] formamide. *Cancer Res.,* 37:2,817–2,821.

49. Koss, L. G. (1967): A light and electron microscope study of the effects of cyclophosphamide on various organs in the rat. 1. The urinary bladder. *Lab Invest.,* 16:44–65.

50. Lee, L. S. (1980): Inhibition of epidermal growth factor by phorbol esters, saccharins, and cyclamate. In: *Cancer Detection and Prevention.* 3 (1), Abstract no. 014.

51. Littlefield, N. A., Farmer, J. H., Gaylor, D. W., and Sheldon, W. G. (1980): Effects of dose and time in a long-term, low-dose carcinogenic study. *J. Environ. Pathol. Toxicol.,* 3:17–34.

52. Littlefield, N. A., Greenman, D. L., Farmer, J. H., and Sheldon, W. G. (1980): Effects of continuous and discontinued exposure to 2-AAF on urinary bladder hyperplasia and neoplasia. *J. Environ. Pathol. Toxicol.,* 3:35–53.

53. MacKenzie, I., and Rous, P. (1941): Experimental disclosure of latent neoplastic changes in tarred skin. *J. Exp. Med.,* 73:391–416.

54. Matsushima, M. (1977): The role of the promoter L-tryptophan on tumorigenesis in the urinary bladder. 2. Urinary bladder carcinogenity of FANFT (initiating factor) and L-tryptophan (promoting factor) in mice. *Jap. J. Urol.,* 68:731–736.

55. Mohr, U., Green, U., Althoff, J., and Schneider, P. (1979): Syncarcinogenic action of saccharin and sodium-cyclamate in the induction of bladder tumours in MNU-pretreated rats. In: *Health and Sugar Substitutes,* edited by B. Guggenheim, pp. 64–69. Karger, Basel.

56. Mondal, S., Brankow, D. W., and Heidelberger, C. (1978): Enhancement of oncogenesis in C3H/10T½ mouse embryo cell cultures of saccharin. *Science,* 201:1,141–1,142.

57. Mufson, R. A., Fischer, S. M., Verma, A. K., Gleason, G. L., Slaga, T. J., and Boutwell, R. K. (1980): Effects of 12-0-tetradecanoylphorbol-13-acetate and mezerein on epidermal orthithine decarboxylase activity, isoproterenol-stimulated levels of cyclic adenosine 3′:5′ -monophosphate, and induction of mouse skin tumors *in vivo. Cancer Res.,* 39:4,791–4,795.

58. Otsuka, H., Akagi, A., and Akagi, G. (1974): Effects of Endoxan on experimental bladder carcinogenesis. *Proc. Jap. Cancer Assoc.,* 33:58.

59. Quagliariello, E., Tancredi, F., Fedele, L., and Saccone, C. (1961): Tryptophan-nicotinic acid metabolism in patients with tumours of the bladder. Changes in the excretory products after treatment with nicotinamide and vitamin B6. *Br. J. Cancer,* 15:367–372.

60. Radomski, J. L., Radomski, T., and MacDonald, W. E. (1977): Carcinogenic interaction between DL-tryptophan and 4-aminobiphenyl or 2-napthylamine in dogs. J. Natl. Cancer Inst., 58:1,831–1,834.
61. Scribner, J. D., and Suss, R. (1978): Tumor initiation and promotion. Int. Rev. Exp. Pathol., 18:137–198.
62. Slaga, T. J., Bowden, G. T., Scribner, J. D., and Boutwell, R. K. (1974): Dose-response studies on the ability of 7,12-dimethylbenz(a)anthracene and benz(a)anthracene to initiate skin tumours. J. Natl. Cancer Inst., 53:1,337–1,340.
63. Slaga, T. J., Fischer, S. M., Viaje, A., Berry, D. L., Bracken, W. M., LeClerc, S., and Miller, D. R. (1978): Inhibition of tumour promotion by antiinflammatory agents: An approach to the biochemical mechanisms of promotion. In: Carcinogenesis, Vol. 2: Mechanisms of Tumor Promotion and Cocarcinogenesis, edited by T. J. Slaga, A. Sivak, and R. K. Boutwell, pp. 173–196. Raven Press, New York.
64. Slaga, T. J., Klein-Szanto, J. P., Fischer, S. M., Weeks, C. E., Nelson, K., and Major S. (1980): Studies on mechanism of action of antitumor-promoting agents: Their specificity in two-stage promotion. Proc. Natl. Acad. Sci. USA, 77:2,251–2,254.
65. Sporn, M. B. (1978): Pharmacological prevention of carcinogenesis by retinoids. In: Carcinogenesis, Vol. 2: Mechanisms of Tumor Promotion and Cocarcinogenesis, edited by T. J. Slaga, A. Sivak, and R. K. Boutwell, pp. 545–551. Raven Press, New York.
66. Troll, W., Meyn, M. S., and Rossman, T. G. (1978): Mechanisms of protease action in carcinogenesis. In: Carcinogenesis, Vol. 2: Mechanisms of Tumor Promotion and Cocarcinogenesis, edited by T. J. Slaga, A. Sivak, and R. K. Boutwell, pp. 301–312. Raven Press, New York.
67. Trosko, J. E., Dawson, B., Yotti, L. P., and Chang, C. C. (1980): Saccharin may act as a tumour promoter by inhibiting metabolic co-operation between cells. Nature (Lond.), 285:109–110.
68. Wakefield, J. St. J., and Hicks, R. M. (1973): Bladder cancer and N-methyl-N-nitrosourea, 2. Sub-cellular changes associated with a single non-carcinogenic dose of MNU. Chem. Biol. Interact., 7:165–179.
69. Yuspa, S. H., DelSol, A. E., Morgan, D. L., and Bates, R. R. (1969): The binding of 7,12-dimethylbenz(a)anthracene to replicating and non-replicating DNA in cell cultures. Chem. Biol. Interact., 1:223–233.

Carcinogenesis, Vol. 7, edited by E. Hecker et al.
Raven Press, New York © 1982.

Studies on the Multistage Nature of Radiation Carcinogenesis

R. J. M. Fry, *R. D. Ley, †D. Grube, and †E. Staffeldt

Biology Division, Oak Ridge National Laboratory, Oak Ridge, Tennessee 37830; and †Division of Biological and Medical Research, Argonne National Laboratory, Argonne, Illinois 60439

The radiations to which man is exposed vary in wavelength by many orders of magnitude. It is not surprising that the type of molecular lesions that are induced and the subsequent biological effects also vary (Table 1). The range of wavelengths of radiations that have been shown to be carcinogenic is much less than for cell killing. In fact, although carcinogenic studies with longer wavelengths have been far from extensive, wavelengths above 320 nm are usually considered noncarcinogenic. Despite the fact that the radiation dose-response curves for cell killing, mutagenesis, and carcinogenesis are similar in form, it seems reasonable to believe that the molecular lesions and their expression may differ in these biological effects. It has been difficult to demonstrate unequivocally such differences. Recently, Elkind et al. (11) have shown that mutation and *in vitro* cell transformation can be induced by ultraviolet radiation (UVR) of a particular emission spectrum without measurable cell killing. Conversely, Harisiadis et al. (19) have shown that hyperthermia, induced by much longer wavelengths than UVR, causes cell killing without any measurable *in vitro* cell transformation. These results suggest that there may be qualitative as well as

TABLE 1. *Adverse biological effects of several types of radiation*

Type of radiation	Wavelength (nm)	Adverse biological effects
Gamma	1×10^{-7}–$\sim 5 \times 10^{-3}$	Cell killing Mutagenesis Teratogenesis
X-rays	$\sim 5 \times 10^{-3}$–~ 2	Carcinogenesis
Ultraviolet	40–390	Cell killing Carcinogenesis
Wavelengths greater than 320 nm are not considered carcinogenic		
Visible	390–780	
Infrared	780–4×10^5	Cell killing
Radio waves	10^5–3×10^{13}	Cell killing

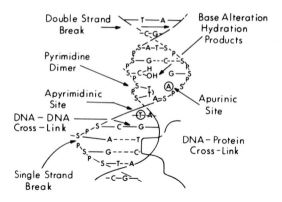

FIG. 1. Schematic of DNA- and radiation-induced lesions.

quantitative differences in the molecular lesions, or their repair, that induce malignant changes from those that induce cell killing.

Studies in radiation cocarcinogenesis (17, see refs. in 32) suggest that the expression of radiation-induced lesions involves processes that are different from those that induce initiation. A myriad of molecular lesions induced by various radiation qualities has been identified (Fig. 1). The quantitative differences are much greater than the qualitative differences in the types of specific lesions induced by the different radiations. In the case of high linear energy transfer radiations, such as neutrons, the number of two track events, such as double strand breaks, will be greater than with more sparsely ionizing radiations, such as gamma radiation. The more densely ionizing radiations are also more effective than the sparsely ionizing for the induction of various biological endpoints, including carcinogenesis. In the case of UVR, many workers believe that there is a correlation between the wavelengths that interact with deoxyribonucleic acid (DNA) and those that cause cancer. But there is no evidence that a DNA lesion common to the different radiation qualities is involved in tumorigenesis. The apparent lack of specificity of the molecular lesions suggests that either the appropriate lesion(s) has not been identified or that an essential event in the tumorigenic process is subsequent to the initially radiation-induced lesion.

Although interpretations of animal experiments are difficult, the spatial and temporal characteristics of the deposition of energy of radiation, together with the range of macromolecular lesions that can be both identified and quantified, make radiations of different qualities useful probes for investigating the mechanisms of carcinogenesis and cocarcinogenesis.

IONIZING RADIATION CARCINOGENESIS

Most of the studies carried out with ionizing radiation have been designed on the premise that radiation is a complete carcinogen. Whereas a number of experiments have investigated the cocarcinogenic effects of radiation, especially in combination with chemical carcinogens, there are very few experiments that have been designed to test the initiating and promoting effects of radiation separately. Both Berenblum and Shubik, who had carried out much of the early work on cocarcinogenesis and the promotion properties of croton oil, did establish, to their satisfaction, that ionizing radiation was an effective initiator. Shubik et al. (31) found that exposures of the skin to β-rays which alone produced no tumors in the period of the experiment did so if they were followed by treatments with croton oil. Berenblum and Trainin (3) found that doses of X-rays that they considered nonleukemogenic resulted in an appreciable incidence of leukemia if followed by treatment with urethan. They interpreted these results to indicate that radiation at dose levels insufficient for complete carcinogenesis was an effective initiator.

This is not the only example of the use of carcinogenic agents in small dose levels to increase the expression of radiation-induced initiation; McGregor (26) used tar from cigarettes to enhance skin tumorigenesis initiated by β-rays. More recently Hoshino and Tanooka (21) found that latent carcinogenic events induced by β-irradiation in the skin were expressed after treatment with 4-nitroquinoline-1-oxide even if the treatment was carried out as much as 400 days after irradiation. These results and others indicate clearly that irradiation initiates events that are retained in viable cells for long periods without any evidence that the lesions undergo further change or expression until a subsequent event is induced.

Cocarcinogenic effects on tumor induction, especially in skin, have been found in both experimental animals and man by a number of workers when carcinogenic levels of various chemical carcinogens and irradiation were combined (1,6,7,9,24,25,26,30).

Unless it is assumed or established that there is a threshold dose for a carcinogen, the use of such terms as subcarcinogenic in describing the protocol for a classical initiation-promotion experiment is purely operational (20). In the case of ionizing radiation, both known biophysical factors and experimental data suggest that in the case of most tissues there is no threshold, and, therefore, most experiments are strictly studies of cocarcinogenesis. Skin has been a popular tissue for cocarcinogenic studies with radiation as well as with chemical carcinogens, but it is now established that other epithelial tissues, such as the mammary and Harderian glands, can be used for experiments designed to study separately initiation and expression or promotion. Yokoro et al. (33) have shown that the initiation can be induced by irradiation in the rat mammary gland and promoted by subsequent increases in the prolactin levels. The hormonal promotion was effective as long as 7 months after initiation. We have also used increased prolactin secretion from pituitary isografts for investigating the expression of radiation-induced Harderian gland tumors in mice (15).

It can be seen from Fig. 2 that the hormonal effect on the naturally occurring tumors of Harderian glands is to advance the time of appearance rather than increase the incidence. In the case of radiation-induced tumors the increased

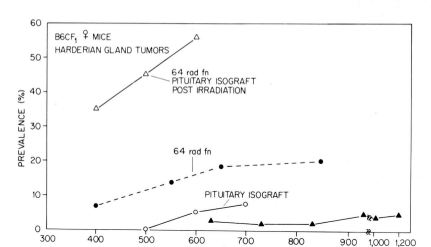

FIG. 2. The prevalence of Harderian gland tumors in female B6CF₁/Anl after pituitary isograft only (▲——▲); after a single exposure to 64 rad fn only (●---●); and to 64 rad fn followed by pituitary isograft on the same day (△——△).

levels of pituitary hormones not only decrease the time to appearance but also increase the incidence.

Figure 3 illustrates the quantitative difference in tumor incidence when the expression of latent initiated cells is enhanced by hormonal stimulation. These

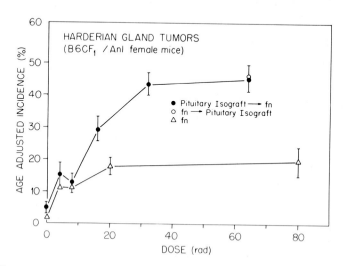

FIG. 3. The age-adjusted incidence of Harderian gland tumors as a function of dose of JANUS reactor fission neutrons in B6CF₁ mice with (●——●), and without (△——△), pituitary isografts. The incidence of tumors in mice exposed to 64 rads fn before receiving pituitary isografts: (○).

results show that the initiation of cells is a more common event than would be predicted by the cumulative tumor incidence when radiation is given alone. Similarly, these results illustrate the competence of the intact animal to suppress expression of initiated cells.

In humans there is a similar indication that ionizing irradiation may induce latent tumor cells that can be "promoted" to express their carcinogenic potential. Psoriasis patients who had received X-ray treatment and were treated subsequently with 8-methoxypsoralen plus UVA radiation (PUVA) had a significantly higher skin tumor incidence than patients who received only X-ray or PUVA treatment (R. S. Stern and J. A. Parrish, *personal communication*).

STUDIES OF UVR CARCINOGENESIS

We have studied a very particular form of cocarcinogenesis involving two agents, neither of which alone is carcinogenic (16,18). The agents are 8-methoxypsoralen (8-MOP) and long-wavelength UVR (320 to 400 nm), often called UVA. Certain photobiologically active furocoumarins, commonly called psoralens, photoreact with DNA during exposure to UVR and extend the action spectrum of UVA for lethal, mutagenic, and carcinogenic effects (10,14,28,29). Since exposure to 8-MOP and UVA (PUVA) results in specific photoproducts that can be assayed, it is possible to carry out carcinogenesis experiments with dosimetry based on the quantity of specific DNA photoproducts. In our experiments we have used two stocks of mice with a mutation at the hr locus: SKH:hairless-1 and HRS/J/Anl mice. Topical applications of 8-MOP followed by irradiation with UVA from a Magnaflux mercury vapor lamp (365 nm), or a Westinghouse F40BLB fluorescent lamp filtered through 3-mm window glass to give a 320 to 400 nm emission spectrum, induced skin cancer in both stocks of mice.

Figure 4 shows that the incidence of skin carcinomas was dependent on dose (number of treatments) and that the tumor response was significantly different in the two stocks of mice. This experiment had been designed so that the same number of psoralen-DNA crosslinks were induced in the basal cells of the epidermis of both stocks of mice. On the assumption that initiation was similar in the two stocks, we chose to investigate whether or not the difference in susceptibility was due to differences in expression of the initial events.

It was necessary to establish whether or not a promoter such as 12-O-tetradecanoylphorbol-13-acetate (TPA) could be used to modulate the incidence of tumors induced by 8-MOP plus UVA. It can be seen from Fig. 5 that 18 exposures to 8-MOP plus UVA (320 to 400 nm) over a 6-week period resulted in no carcinomas. If TPA was applied three times a week after the completion of the 8-MOP plus UVA treatment, however, the cumulative incidence reached almost 60%. Treatment with TPA alone resulted in no carcinomas. These results are consistent with those reported for results for promotion of UVR-induced lesions (13,22,27). It should be noted that multiple applications of TPA alone

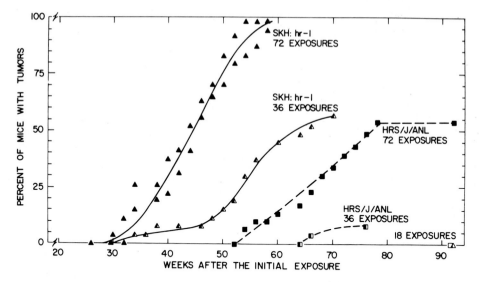

FIG. 4. The incidence of epidermal carcinomas after 18 exposures: HRS/J/Anl (□); SKH:hairless-1 (△); 36 exposures: HRS/J/Anl (■); SKH:hairless-1 (▲); and 72 exposures: HRS/J/Anl (■); SKH:hairless-1 (▲); to 250 μg 8-MOP plus 5.5 J/m² 365 nm.

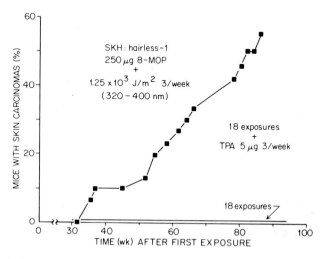

FIG. 5. The incidence of carcinomas in the skin of SKH:hairless-1 mice exposed to: (a) 18 exposures of 250 μg 8-MOP applied topically followed 45 min later by 1.25 × 10³ J/m² (320–400 nm) given three times per week (——); and (b) the same regimen plus subsequent applications of 5 μg TPA three times per week for 50 weeks (■——■).

have been reported as carcinogenic in other strains of hairless mice (2,8,23).

Groups of both stocks of mice were given 36 exposures to 8-MOP plus UVA with and without subsequent promotion with TPA. It was found that most of the difference in the tumor responses between the two stocks disappeared when the irradiation regimen was followed by TPA treatment (Fig. 6). These results suggested that the major factors in the difference in susceptibility were associated with differences in expression of the initial events in the two stocks of mice. We have established that these results were not dependent on the initiating agent, as similar findings were obtained with benzo(a)pyrene.

In order to determine whether or not the difference in susceptibility for carcinomas between the two stocks of mice was due to a systemic difference that affected other tissues, we investigated sarcomagenesis by implanting silastic discs under the skin. It was found that sarcomas arising in the subcutaneous tissue appeared earlier and at a higher incidence in HRS/J/Anl than in SKH:hairless-1 mice, whereas, as has been noted, the SKH:hairless-1 mice were more susceptible to epidermal carcinomas than the HRS/J/Anl mice.

If we assume that TPA acts as a promoter of initiation by 8-MOP plus UVA, as appears to be the case (Fig. 5), it becomes possible to investigate dose-response relationships for initial events and tumor incidence separately. Dose-response curves were constructed from data obtained in experiments in which the cumulative incidence of carcinomas had been determined as a function of total dose by varying the dose per fraction or the total number of fractions. It can be seen in Fig. 7 that exposure regimens that were not followed with applications of TPA resulted in a sigmoid dose-response curve. In contrast, if

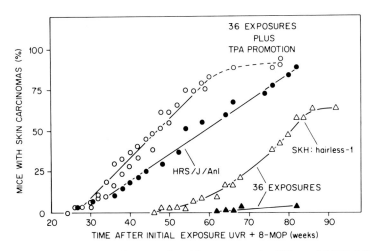

FIG. 6. The incidence of carcinomas after 36 exposures to 250 μg 8-MOP followed by 1.25 $\times$ 10^3 J/m^2 (320–400 nm) with and without subsequent promotion with 5 μg of TPA three times per week in HRS/J/Anl mice: without promotion (▲——▲), and with promotion (●——●); SKH:hairless-1 mice: without promotion (△——△), and with promotion (○——○).

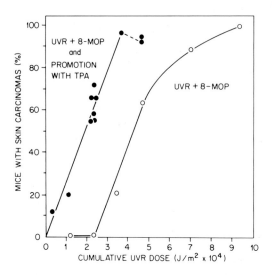

FIG. 7. The percent of mice with squamous cell carcinomas as a function to total dose of 320–400 nm UVR given in various numbers of fractions plus 8-MOP (○———○); and similar exposures but followed at the end of the fractionation regimen by treatment with 5 μg of TPA three times per week (●———●). (Reproduced from Fry et al. (17), with permission from Elsevier/North-Holland Biomedical Press.)

similar regimens, but with lower total doses, were followed by TPA treatments, the relationship of the response to dose was not a threshold-linear response.

It has long been recognized that a considerable number of exposures to UVR are required for cancer production (5). This has also been shown to be the case with 8-MOP plus UVA (Figs. 5 and 7). The relationship of the number of fractions to the incidence of tumors suggests that many of the later fractions are necessary for the expression of the tumors. It was therefore of interest to determine if there was a wavelength dependency for the effect of UVR on expression. Groups of mice were exposed to 36 combined treatments of 8-MOP and UVA and were then given either (a) no further treatment, or (b) a series of exposures to one of the following: 365 nm, 320 to 400 nm, 280 to 400 nm, or TPA. The results, seen in Fig. 8, show that the longer wavelength spectra had little or no effect, but that exposures to 280 to 400 nm (Westinghouse FS40 sunlamp), which includes the tumorigenic 280 to 320 nm spectrum (UVB), enhanced the tumor incidence induced by the 8-MOP plus UVA treatment even more than TPA. The dose level of the 280 to 400 nm spectrum is sufficient to initiate cells, so it is not yet possible to determine if the mechanisms of initiation and promotion involve different molecular lesions.

There have been a number of studies of UVR cocarcinogenesis (see refs. in 32). Unfortunately, interpretation of the results has been complicated, because many of the chemical carcinogens that have been used show photodynamic activity. Also, exposure of the skin to either UVR or chemical carcinogens

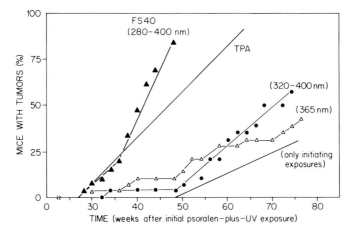

FIG. 8. The incidence of epidermal carcinomas as a function of time after 36 exposures to 8-MOP plus 1.25×10^3 J/m². 320–400 nm (———); a similar regimen followed by 72 exposures of 5.5×10^3 J/m² 365 nm ($\triangle$———$\triangle$); or 1.25×10^3 J/m² 320–400 nm ($\circ$———$\circ$); or 500 J/m² 280–400 nm ($\blacktriangle$———$\blacktriangle$); or 5 μg TPA three times/week for 24 weeks (———).

may alter the distribution of cells in the cell cycle which, in turn, may alter the susceptibility to subsequent treatments. Changes in proliferation, in particular hyperplasia, must be taken into account when designing cocarcinogenesis studies involving UVR.

Some experiments, such as those of Epstein (12), suggest that UVR does enhance or promote chemical carcinogenesis of the skin. An unusual example of UVR-cocarcinogenesis has been reported by Bingham and Nord (4). They found that skin tumors were produced in C3H/HeJ mice by topical treatment with *n*-decane or *n*-dodecane followed by exposures to UVR (> 350nm), neither of which treatment independently is carcinogenic. It is apparent that cocarcinogenesis involving UVR is poorly understood.

CONCLUSIONS

It is clear that with low-dose levels of ionizing or UVR, the number of initiation events exceeds the numbers of tumors that grow to a detectable size. Ionizing radiation, which is a complete carcinogen, appears to be a more effective initiator than an enhancer or promoter. However, the initiation and promotion aspects of ionizing radiation have been studied in very few organ systems. In the case of UVR, with or without photosensitizers such as psoralens, the requirement of a relatively large number of exposures for carcinogenesis suggests that the expression of the initiated cells as frank tumors requires a number of events spread out over the time of the development of the tumor. Both ionizing and UVR are, perhaps, underutilized as tools for probing the mechanism of both initiation and promotion.

ACKNOWLEDGMENTS

Research sponsored by the Office of Health and Environmental Research, U.S. Department of Energy, under contract W-7405-eng-26 with the Union Carbide Corporation and Argonne National Laboratory, Illinois, under contract W-31-109-eng-38.

REFERENCES

1. Arseneau, J. C., Fowler, E., and Bakemeier, R. F. (1977): Synergistic tumorigenic effect of procabazine and ionizing radiation in (BALB/c x DBA/2)F$_1$ mice. *J. Natl. Cancer Inst.,* 59:423–425.
2. Astrup, E. G., Iverson, O. H., and Elgjo, K. (1980): The tumorigenic and carcinogenic effect of TPA (12-O-tetradecanoylphorbol-13-acetate) when applied to the skin of BALB/c A mice. *Virchows Arch. (B Cell Path.),* 33:303–304.
* 3. Berenblum, I., and Trainin, N. (1960): Possible two-stage mechanism in experimental leukemogenesis. *Science,* 132:40–41.
4. Bingham, E., and Nord, P. J. (1977): Cocarcinogenic effects of *n*-alkanes and ultraviolet light on mice. *J. Natl. Cancer Inst.,* 58:1,099–1,101.
5. Blum, H. F. (1959): *Carcinogenesis by ultraviolet light.* Princeton University Press, Princeton.
* 6. Burns, F. J., Strickland, P., and Albert, R. E. (1977): The combined carcinogenic action of ionizing radiation and DMBA on rat skin. *Radiat. Res.,* 70:607.
7. Canellos, G. P., Arseneau, J. C., DeVita, V. T., Wlang-Peng, J., and Johnson, R. E. C. (1975): Second malignancies complicating Hodgkin's disease in remission. *Lancet,* 1:947–949.
8. Chouroulinkov, I., and Lazar, P. (1974): Actions cancérogène et cocancérogène du 12-O-tetradecanoylphorbol-13-acetate (TPA) sur la peau de souris. *C. R. Acad. Sci. Paris, Ser. D.,* 278:3,027–3,030.
9. Cloudman, A. M., Hamilton, K. A., Clayton, R. S., and Brues, A. M. (1955): Effects of combined local treatment with radioactive and chemical carcinogens. *J. Natl. Cancer Inst.,* 15:1,077–1,083.
10. Cole, R. S. (1971): Inactivation of *Escherichia coli* F' episomes at transfer and bacteriophage lambda by psoralen plus 360 nm light: Significance of deoxyribonucleic acid cross-links. *J. Bacteriol.,* 107:846–852.
11. Elkind, M. M., Han, A., and Lankas, G. R. (1980): "Sunlight"-induced cell killing, mutation, and neoplastic transformation: Relevance to the ozone depletion problem. *Proc. Am. Assoc. Cancer Res.,* 21:95.
* 12. Epstein, J. H. (1965): Comparison of the carcinogenic and cocarcinogenic effects of ultraviolet light on hairless mice. *J. Natl. Cancer Inst.,* 34:741–745.
* 13. Epstein, J. H., and Roth, H. L. (1968): Experimental ultraviolet light carcinogenesis. *J. Invest. Dermatol.,* 50:387–389.
14. Fowlks, W. L., Griffith, D. G., and Oginsky, E. L. (1958): Photosensitization of bacteria by furocoumarins and related compounds. *Nature,* 181:571–572.
15. Fry, R. J. M., Garcia, A. G., Allen, K. H., Sallese, A., Staffeldt, E., Tahmisian, T. H., Devine, R. L., Lombard, L. S., and Ainsworth, E. J. (1976): The effect of pituitary isografts on radiation carcinogenesis in the mammary and Harderian glands of mice. In: *Biological Effects of Low-Level Radiation Pertinent to Protection of Man and His Environment,* pp. 213–227. IAEA, Vienna.
16. Fry, R. J. M., Ley, R. D., and Grube, D. D. (1978): Photosensitized reactions and carcinogenesis. In: *Ultraviolet Radiation Carcinogenesis. Natl. Cancer Inst. Monogr.,* 50:39–43.
17. Fry, R. J. M., Storer, J. B., and Ullrich, R. L. (1980): Radiation toxicology: Carcinogenesis. In: *The Scientific Basis of Toxicity Assessment,* edited by H. P. Witschi, pp. 291–304. Elsevier/North-Holland Biomedical Press, New York.
18. Grube, D. D., Ley, R. D., and Fry, R. J. M. (1977): Photosensitizing effects of 8-methoxypsoralen on the skin of hairless mice. II. Strain and spectral differences for tumorigenesis. *Photochem. Photobiol.,* 25:269–276.

19. Harisiadis, L., Miller, R. C., Harisiadis, S., and Hall, E. I. (1980): Oncogenic transformation and hyperthermia. *Br. J. Radiol.,* 53:479–482.
20. Hecker, E. (1975): Cocarcinogens and cocarcinogenesis. In: *Handbüch der allgemeinem pathologie, Vol. 6,* pp. 651–676. Springer-Verlag, Berlin-Heidelberg.
21. Hoshino, H., and Tanooka, H. (1975): Interval effect of β-irradiation and subsequent 4-nitro-quinoline-1-oxide painting on skin tumor induction in mice. *Cancer Res.,* 35:3,663–3,666.
22. Hsu, T., Forbes, P. D., Harber, L. C., and Lakow, E. (1975): Induction of skin tumors in hairless mice following single exposure to ultraviolet radiation. *Photochem. Photobiol.,* 21:185–188.
23. Iversen, U. M., and Iversen, O. H. (1979): The carcinogenic effect of TPA (12-O-tetradecanoyl-phorbol-13-acetate) when applied to the skin of hairless mice. *Virchows Arch. (B Cell Path.),* 30:33–42.
• 24. Lurie, A. G. (1977): Enhancement of DMBA tumorigenesis in hamster cheek pouch epithelium by repeated exposures to low level X-radiation. *Radiat. Res.,* 72:499–511.
25. McGandy, R. B., Kennedy, A. R., Terzaghi, M., and Little, J. B. (1974): Experimental respiratory carcinogenesis: Interaction between alpha radiation and benzo(a)pyrene in the hamster. In: *Experimental Lung Cancer: Carcinogenesis and Bioassays,* edited by E. Karbe and T. F. Park, pp. 485–491. Springer-Verlag, New York.
26. McGregor, J. F. (1976): Tumor-promoting activity of cigarette tar in rat skin exposed to radiation. *J. Natl. Cancer Inst.,* 56:429–430.
• 27. Mondal, S., and Heidelberger, C. (1976): Transformation of C3H/10T½ CL8 mouse embryo fibroblasts by ultraviolet irradiation and a phorbol ester. *Nature,* 260:710–711.
28. Musajo, L., and Rodighiero, G. (1972): Mode of photosensitizing action of furocoumarins. In: *Photophysiology, Vol. IV,* edited by A. C. Giese, pp. 115–147. Academic Press, New York.
29. O'Neal, M. A., and Griffin, A. C. (1954): The effect of oxypsoralen upon ultraviolet carcinogenesis in albino mice. *Cancer Res.,* 17:911–916.
• 30. Shellabarger, C. J. (1967): Effect of 3-methylcholanthrene and X-irradiation given singly or combined on rat mammary carcinogenesis. *J. Natl. Cancer Inst.,* 38:73–77.
31. Shubik, P., Goldfarb, A. R., and Ritchie, A. C. (1953): Latent carcinogenic action of Beta-irradiation on mouse epidermis. *Nature,* 171:934–935.
32. Ullrich, R. L. (1980): Interaction of radiation and chemical carcinogens. In: *Carcinogenesis, Vol. 5: Modifiers of Chemical Carcinogenesis,* edited by T. J. Slaga, pp. 169–184. Raven Press, New York.
33. Yokoro, K. Nakano, M., Ito, A., Nagao, K., Kodama, Y., and Hamada, K. (1977): Role of prolactin in rat mammary carcinogenesis: Detection of carcinogenicity of low-dose carcinogens and of persisting dormant cancer cells. *J. Natl. Cancer Inst.,* 58:1,777–1,783.

Carcinogenesis, Vol. 7, edited by E. Hecker et al.
Raven Press, New York © 1982.

Esophageal Cancer in Linxian County, China: A Possible Etiology and Mechanism (Initiation and Promotion)

†S. J. Cheng, *M. Sala, †M. H. Li, and *I. Chouroulinkov

*Institut de Recherches Scientifiques sur le Cancer, 94800-Villejuif, France; and †Cancer Institute, Chinese Academy of Medical Sciences, Peking, China

The esophageal cancer (EC) is one of the most common varieties of cancer in China. It ranks second to that of gastric carcinoma as a cause of death. Between 1973 and 1975, the adjusted death rate was 14.59/100,000 for the entire country, and 21.8% of deaths from all malignant tumors. But epidemiological studies carried out among 50 million people from 181 countries and cities showed that the mortality rate in the province of Henan is 32.22/100,000 and 40.55% of all malignant tumors. Moreover, Linxian county has the highest adjusted mortality rate for EC, with 161.33 for males and 102.88 for females (3,5,7,9).

The epidemiological and experimental data allow us to define EC as a multistep and multicausal environmental cancer.

EPIDEMIOLOGICAL DATA

The geographical distribution of EC in China is well defined (for review, see ref. 7). The Linxian county of Henan province has the highest rate of mortality adjusted for age and sex (3). In the same zone the incidence of EC in chickens is significantly higher (10 times that in other counties) (7). These two observations indicate the exogenous causes common to man and to chickens and exclude the use of tobacco. Such suspected exogenous factors can only be chemicals. In effect, the mortality rate for EC as a function of age is practically nil below 30 years and has its highest level between 60 and 69 years (7).

Present knowledge indicates that the latency of chemically provoked tumors in man varies from 20 to 40 years. Epidemiological studies have also established a direct relationship between the mortality rate due to EC and the consumption of pickled vegetables (PV). This is a food that has been widely used in the concerned area for many years; and the adjusted mortality rate was constant for 30 years (from 1941 to 1970): 130.3/100,000. This high incidence of EC was also observed among migrants who still keep the old alimentary habits. Moreover, it was established that PV were permanently contaminated with fungi, which indicates the possible presence of chemical carcinogens. In fact, nitrosamines were identified in corn bread contaminated with fungi found in food stuffs from Linxian county (8,10).

Finally, epidemiological and clinical studies have shown that the frequency of esophageal hyperplasia is higher in north Linxian than in south Linxian and that this hyperplasia frequency is related to the level of EC (Table 1). Advanced hyperplasia frequently evolves into the cancer (Table 2) but may also regress to normal. These observations indicate that the hyperplasia precedes the development of the cancer and suggest the intervention of a promoter(s) that has the property to induce a reversible epidermal hyperplasia in mice.

EXPERIMENTAL DATA

The epidemiological results have suggested a number of experimental studies that confirm the hypothesis that carcinogens and/or cocarcinogens play an important role in the development of EC in China.

It must be remembered that nitrosamines were identified in corn bread contaminated with fungi from foodstuffs in Linxian county and to which small amounts of $NaNO_2$ were added (8,10). A raised level of nitrates and nitrites in the soil and in the vegetables has been found and their accumulation was explained by a molibdenum deficiency in the soil. Molibdenum is a necessary component of some enzymes, such as nitrate reductase (4).

The role of the fungi was demonstrated experimentally. The culture medium of *Geotrichum candidum,* the most common PV contaminant, enhances the carcinogenic action of methylbenzylnitrosamine in the mouse forestomach. It is therefore conceivable that PV contaminated with *Geotrichum candidum* contains chemical carcinogens.

The oral administration in mice of a liquid concentrate of PV induces hyperplasia in the esophagus and in the forestomach and papillomas in the forestomach (M. H. Li and S. J. Cheng, *in preparation).* The extract of PV has been shown to be mutagenic in bacteria (12) and has induced sister chromatid exchanges (SCE) and HGPRT⁻ mutants in V79 cells (2). This extract has also shown a

TABLE 1. *The incidences between dysplasia and carcinoma in different areas*

Areas	Total persons examined	No. of cases			Rate (per 1,000)		
		Mild dysplasia	Marked dysplasia	Cancer	Mild dysplasia	Marked dysplasia	Cancer
Northern Linhsien	4,377	1,117	98	57	255	22	13
Southern Linhsien	2,835	518	21	20	183	7	7

From: The Coordinating Group for the Research of Esophageal Carcinoma, Chinese Academy of Medical Sciences and Honan Province (1975): Studies on the relationship between epithelial dysplasia and carcinoma of the esophagus. *Chin. Med. J.* I:110–116.

TABLE 2. *Results of follow-up on 79 cases with marked dysplasia*

Time intervals of follow-up (yr)	No. of cases					%				
	Progressing to carcinoma	Remaining marked dysplasia	Recurring marked dysplasia	Regressing to normal or to mild dysplasia	Total	Progressing to carcinoma	Remaining marked dysplasia	Recurring marked dysplasia	Regressing to normal or to mild dysplasia	Total
2	14	10	10	24	58	24.12	17.24	17.24	41.40	100.0
3	4	—	1	5	10	40.00	—	10.00	50.00	100.0
4	3	2	3	3	11	27.27	18.19	27.27	27.27	100.0
Total	21	12	14	32	79	26.60	15.20	17.70	40.50	100.0

From: The Coordinating Group for the Research of Esophageal Carcinoma, Chinese Academy of Medical Sciences and Honan Province (1975): Studies on the relationship between epithelial dysplasia and carcinoma of the esophagus. *Chin. Med. J.* l:110–116.

direct transforming effect on Syrian Hamster Embryo (SHE) cells (2). These results suggest the probable presence in PV of mutagen(s) and of carcinogen(s). Moreover, the results obtained with PV extract in C3H/10T1/2 cells previously initiated with 3-methylcholanthrene (MCA) (Table 3) showed the presence of a compound, or compounds, with the properties of a promoter such as 12-O-tetradecanoylphorbol-13-acetate (TPA).

Preliminary chemical analyses demonstrate the presence in PV of benzo(a)pyrene, of quercetine, and of nitroso-compounds among which the dimethylthiotetranitrosodiiron, or Roussin's red, has been identified (7,13). The biological assays with this compound have shown that it is neither mutagenic nor transforming in SHE cells. However, Roussin's red induced foci type 3 (Fig. 1) in C3H/10T1/2 cells previously initiated with MCA (Table 4) and has shown a positive action in short-term skin tests in mice (Fig. 2): a significant decrease of the sebaceous gland number and a significant increase of the epidermal thickness, like the effect of TPA (1,6). These results indicate Roussin's red as one of the possible natural promoters present in PV.

POSSIBLE PATHOGENESIS OF EC

The high level of nitrates, nitrites, and secondary amines in the environment, and the fungal contamination of the food favor the formation of nitrosamines and other carcinogens. The mutagenic activity of the PV extract, the promoting

TABLE 3. *Transforming and promoting effects of PV extract in C3H/10T1/2 cells[a]*

| Experimental schedule | | | | |
Treatment[b] for 24 hr (μg/ml)	Treatment at each medium change[c] (μg/ml)	Plating efficiency	No. of dishes with foci[d]/ Total no. of dishes	Dishes with foci (%)
Acetone (0.5%)	—	32	0/43	0
MCA (1.0)	—	30	12/38	31.5
MCA (0.1)	—	31	0/32	0
MCA (0.1)	TPA (0.1)	34	7/41	17.1
—	TPA (0.1)	22	0/18	0
MCA (0.1)	PV extract (1.0)	30	1/15	6.7
MCA (0.1)	PV extract (5.0)	33	7/33	21.2
MCA (0.1)	PV extract (10.0)	33	6/31	19.4
PV extract (20.0)	—	34	0/9	0
PV extract (60.0)	—	30	0/20	0
PV extract (20.0)	TPA (0.1)	33	0/20	0
PV extract (60.0)	TPA (0.1)	23	0/18	0
—	PV extract (20.0)	24	0/18	0

[a] The transformation assays using C3H/10T1/2 cells were carried out according to the method of Mondal et al., ref. 11.
[b] 24 hr after plating.
[c] 3 days after the first 24-hr treatment.
[d] The numbers of dishes containing type-3 foci were scored 40 days after plating.

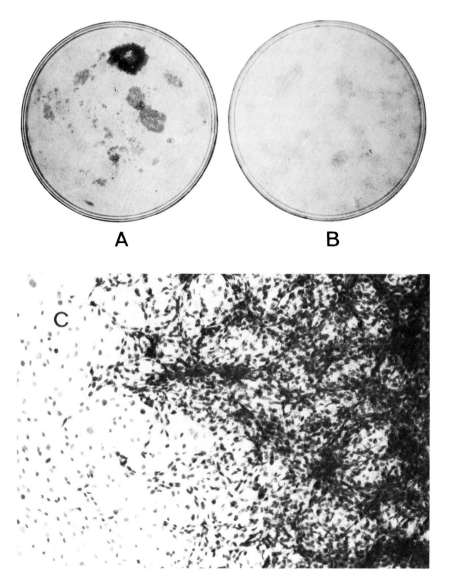

FIG. 1. Culture of C3H/10T1/2 cells fixed and stained 40 days after plating. **A:** Transformed focus (type 3) from cells initiated with MCA (0.1 μg/ml) and then treated with Roussin's red (2 μg/ml) at each medium change. **B:** Acetone control. **C:** Photomicrograph of the type-3 focus **(A)** (×42).

effect of the same extract and of the Roussin's red, and the relationship of the PV consumption to the EC rate in Linxian county indicate that EC is a complex problem; many factors may be interacting. Nevertheless, the pathogenesis can be schematized, as shown in Fig. 3.

TABLE 4. *Transforming and promoting effects of Roussin's red in C3H/10T1/2 cells*[a]

Experimental schedule		Plating efficiency	No. of dishes with foci[d]/ total no. of dishes	Dishes with foci (%)
Treatment for 24 hr (μg/ml)[b]	Treatment at each medium change[c] (μg/ml)			
Acetone (0.5%)	—	32	0/37	0
MCA (1.0)	—	30	13/60	21.7
MCA (0.1)	—	30	0/55	0
MCA (0.1)	TPA (0.1)	33	9/38	23.7
—	TPA (0.1)	22	0/18	0
MCA (0.1)	Roussin's red (0.5)	28	1/20	5.0
MCA (0.1)	Roussin's red (1.0)	29	2/53	3.8
MCA (0.1)	Roussin's red (2.0)	34	12/40	30.0
Roussin's red (3.0)	—	17	0/24	0
Roussin's red (2.0)	TPA (0.1)	30	0/20	0
—	Roussin's red (2.0)	31	0/19	0

[a] The transformation assays using C3H/10T1/2 cells were carried out according to the method of Mondal et al., ref. 11.
[b] 24 hr after plating.
[c] 3 days after the first 24-hr treatment.
[d] The numbers of dishes containing type-3 foci were scored 40 days after plating.

The esophageal epithelium is first initiated by the carcinogens (nitrosamines or others) formed in the food or even *in vivo*. This phase may occur at an early age. Later, the intervention of promoters or cocarcinogens present in PV, such as Roussin's red, produce epithelial hyperplasia. This hyperplasia may

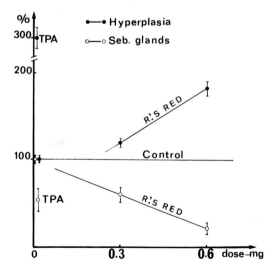

FIG. 2. Suppression of sebaceous glands and induction of hyperplasia in mouse skin treated with Roussin's red or TPA.

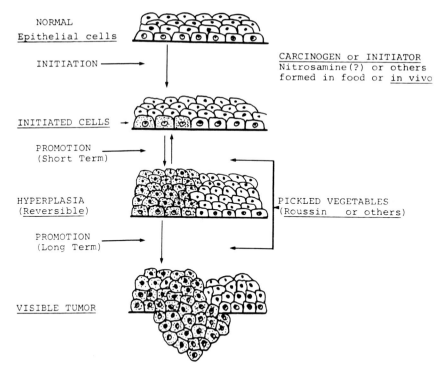

FIG. 3. Pathogenesis of esophageal cancer.

be reversible if the promoting effect is of short duration. If, however, the promotion continues, the hyperplasia may evolve into a visible tumor. This pattern was observed in pathological studies in man that showed the formation of mild hyperplasia, marked hyperplasia, carcinoma *in situ,* and infiltrating cancer (7).

It would appear, therefore, that the concept of two or multistage chemical carcinogenesis is applicable to man in at least one case: EC in China.

REFERENCES

1. Cheng, S. J., Sala, M., Li, M. H., Courtois, I., and Chouroulinkov, I. (1981): Promoting effect of Roussin's red identified in pickled vegetables from Linxian China. *Carcinogenesis,* 2:313–319.
2. Cheng, S. J., Sala, M., Li, M. H., Wang, M. Y., Pot- Deprun, J., and Chouroulinkov, I. (1980): Mutagenic, transforming, and promoting effect of pickled vegetables from Linxian county, China. *Carcinogenesis,* 1:685–692.
3. The coordinating group for research on etiology of esophageal cancer in North China (1975): The epidemiology and etiology of esophageal cancer in North China: A preliminary report. *Chin. Med. J.,* 3:167–183.
4. Department of chemical etiology, Cancer Instituts, Chinese Academy of Medical Science (1978): Further studies on the etiology of esophageal cancer. *Chin. Med. J.,* 58:593–597.
5. Department of epidemiology, Cancer Institute, Department of Statistics, Institute of Medical

Information, Chinese Academy of Medical Science, and Institute of Microbiology, Acad. Sinica. (1977): A preliminary survey on epidemiological factors of esophageal cancer in China, Research on Cancer Treatment and Control, 2:1–8.

6. Lazar, P., Liberman, C., Chouroulinkov, I., and Guérin, M. (1963): Test sur la peau de souris pour la détermination des activités carcinogènes: Mise au point méthodologique. *Bull. Cancer*, 50:567–577.

7. Li, M., (Li Min-Hsin), Li, P., and Li, B. (Li Pao-Jung) (1980): Recent progress in research on esophageal cancer in China. *Adv. Cancer Res.*, (33):123–249.

8. Li, M. X., Lu, S. X., Ji, C., Wang, M. Y., Cheng, S. J., and Jin, C. L. (1979): Formation of carcinogenic N-nitroso compounds in corn bread inoculated with fungi. *Scientia Sinica,* 22:471–477.

9. Li, P., and Li, J. Y. (1980): National survey of cancer mortality in China. *Chin. J. Oncol.,* 2:1–10.

10. Lu, S. X., Li, L. X., Ji, C., Wang, M. T., Wang, Y. L., and Huang, L. (1979): A new N-nitroso compound, N-3-methylbutyl-N-1-methylacetonylnitrosamine, in corn bread inoculated with fungi. *Scientia Sinica,* 22:601–607.

11. Mondal, S., Brankow, W. D., and Heidelberger, C. (1976): Two-stage chemical oncogenesis in cultures of C3H/10T1/2 cells. *Cancer Res.,* 36:2,254–2,260.

12. Takahashi, Y., Nagao, M., Fugino, T., Yamaizumi, Z., and Sugimura, T. (1979): Mutagens in japanese pickle identified as flavonoids. *Mutat. Res.,* 68:11–123.

13. Wang, G. H., Zhang, W. X., and Chai, W. G. (1980): The identification of natural Roussin red methyl ester. *Acta Chim. Sinica* (Chinese), 3:95–102.

Carcinogenesis, Vol. 7, edited by E. Hecker et al.
Raven Press, New York © 1982.

Mechanisms of Promotion in Nutritional Carcinogenesis

John H. Weisburger, Bandaru S. Reddy, Leonard A. Cohen, Peter Hill, and Ernst L. Wynder

American Health Foundation, Valhalla, New York 10595

Most cancers, although environmentally caused, have nonoccupational origins that have been obscure until recently. Major advances have resulted from considering each cancer separately, such as cancer of the lung and cancer of the large bowel, and seeking answers in relation to the causative and modifying factors for each one. Current concepts of cancer etiology stem from multidisciplinary research efforts based on three major approaches, namely: (a) the variation in incidence of a specific type of cancer as a function of area of residence, with particular regard to migrant populations; (b) the changes in incidence as a function of time, and (c) detailed laboratory studies in man, in animal models, or through *in vitro* systems (4).

Colon cancer has exhibited a slight upward trend in incidence over the last 40 years in the United States (14). Likewise, cancers of the breast and prostate have also only slightly increased in rate in the United States. This suggests that industrial pollution, intentional food additives, and inadvertent food contaminants, the levels of which have altered dramatically, are not associated with the development of these three important types of human cancers in the Western world. In Japan, a highly industrialized country comparable to the Western world, these three cancer types have a low incidence. Recently, an increasing trend has appeared there, that may be associated with the progressive Westernization of the Japanese diet since 1945 (7,16). Thus, this is evidence that the dietary pattern rather than industrial activity is most important in relation to causative mechanisms for these human cancers.

Epidemiologic data from migrant studies with respect to colon and breast cancer have provided further leads on mechanisms of carcinogenesis for these two organs. Colon cancer risk increases in the first generation of migrants from low-risk Japan to higher-risk US. In contrast, the incidence of breast cancer in Japanese migrants rises only in the second generation. The difference in increase of colon and breast cancers as a function of migrant generation has been discussed in terms of exposure to genotoxic carcinogens during periods of high tissue and cell proliferation (15). Epidemiologic data demonstrate a clear association between a high intake level of dietary fat and colon, breast, and prostate cancers. The underlying mechanism appears to stem from promotion. Results obtained in human and animal studies provide the evidence supporting this view (see recent reviews 5 and 12).

A dietary intake of total fat levels typical of the Western diet, accounting for about 40% of calories, together with a relatively low fiber consumption, results in considerable amounts, as well as high concentrations, of bile acids in the gut. Animal experimentation shows that rats given several types of colon carcinogens had a high incidence of large bowel cancer when fed fat at 20% in the diet (corresponding to 40% of calories). In contrast, intake of diets containing 5% fat (equivalent to 10% of calories, which mimics a low-risk Japanese population) shows a lower incidence of colon cancer. Western people, and animals on a high fat diet not only excrete more total bile acids in their stools, but also have higher levels of specific secondary bile acids, compared to low-risk Japanese or African people or rats on a 5% fat diet. Thus, data from humans and animals drew attention to the levels of bile acids in the gut. Indeed, tests in germ-free and conventional rats show that they have an appreciable promoting action in large bowel carcinogenesis (but not on mouse skin). Cholesterol and neutral sterols, however, are not promoters.

Specific fibers, such as wheat bran and pectin, have an inhibiting effect in large bowel carcinogenesis in animals. The mechanism may be simple dilution of intestinal bile acids, but the phenomenon may be more complex; more research is necessary. Adequate intake of fiber in man results in larger stool bulk and a lower incidence of large bowel cancer. For example, in Finland or areas like Utah, even though there is a high dietary fat intake, a high fiber intake is customary. Thus, such people have a dietary fat intake similar to that of high-risk New Yorkers, accounting for their equal risk for coronary heart disease. Because of the high fiber intake in Finland, however, and perhaps in Utah, the concentration of bile acids in the intestinal tract and in the stools is similar to that of low-risk Japanese people. Thus, it is well documented that in animal models and in man, dietary fat and fiber exert an opposite controlling influence in the development of large bowel cancer by affecting the concentration of promotional stimuli (Figs. 1 and 2).

Similarly, data on the incidence of cancers of the breast and prostate show the same relationship to total dietary fat intake as found with colon cancer. The question is not yet resolved as to the mechanisms whereby dietary fat translates to cancer risk for these diseases. On the basis of a number of lines of evidence, it is noted that development of these two types of cancer can be modulated by endocrine factors.

A number of investigators have examined the urinary hormone excretion pattern in women at diverse risk for breast cancer. Thus, Bulbrook (2) thought that the ratio of androgens to estrogens was relevant. At the present time, this British group has a large-scale prospective study underway in which these factors are monitored and in which other endocrine parameters are tested at the same time. Eventually, this should present useful parallel information. Mac-

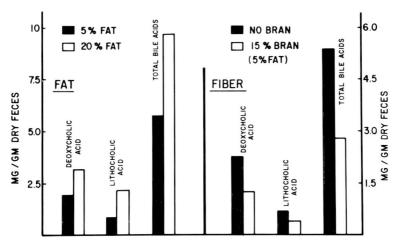

FIG. 1. Fecal secondary bile acids in rats fed high fat or high wheat bran diets. **Left:** Male Fischer strain rats fed a high fat diet show more total bile acids, as well as deoxycholic and lithocholic acids, in their stools than rats fed a low fat diet. **Right:** Addition of 15% bran to a low fat diet reduces the concentration of total bile acids and also of deoxycholic and lithocholic acids. (Note different scales for right and left sides of chart. See Reddy et al., ref. 12, for detailed comments.)

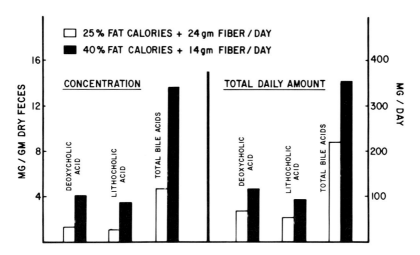

FIG. 2. Human volunteers were fed either a low fat, high fiber diet or a high fat, low fiber diet. **Right:** The total dietary amount of total bile acids and deoxycholic and lithocholic acid is related to the dietary fat content. **Left:** The concentration of bile acids in the feces is modulated by fat and fiber content. Thus, the concentration of total bile acids and also of specific acids is considerably lower on a low fat, high fiber diet.

Mahon and colleagues (10) noted that the ratio of estradiol metabolites in urine, specificially estriol/estradiol ratios, might be relevant.

In more recent years, however, studies have concentrated more on blood plasma levels of hormones, inasmuch as the tissues are continuously bathed in hormones. Moreover, research has yielded specific cell surface and intracellular molecular receptors for specific hormones that may bear on the modulation of growth of a given normal or neoplastic cell. This laboratory, on the basis of various lines of evidence has introduced consideration of the pituitary hormone prolactin as part of the total endocrine balance requiring consideration. Indeed, in animal models, Furth (3) demonstrated many years ago that the growth of experimental mammary tumors was highly prolactin dependent. Prolactin exhibits considerable diurnal as well as seasonal variation. Its daily rhythm includes a peak during the phases of deep sleep. We have noted a higher peak in women on a high fat standard Western diet compared to the peak seen in the same individuals on a low fat regimen (12 and Fig. 3).

More recently Petrakis (11) and we (12) have concerned ourselves with the question of effector systems within the breast as observed in the small amounts of breast fluid obtained from many women by gentle application of a vacuum.

Supporting the human evidence is a considerable amount of information obtained from animal models over the last 25 years. These uniformly show that female rats or mice on a high fat diet, when given a carcinogen (or, in the presence of mammary tumor virus in mice), have a higher incidence of breast cancer earlier than when the comparable groups are placed on a low fat diet (Fig. 4). Varying protein content shows little effect in this system. In man also, protein intake is relatively constant, at 10 to 15% of the diet. With an identical fat intake, animals on high sucrose diets have a higher breast cancer incidence than when the carbohydrate component was starch (8).

The situation for prostate cancer is somewhat unclear at the present time. The international comparisons basically parallel the findings for colon cancer; thus a suggested relationship of dietary fat seems warranted. There are curious exceptions, however, such as a higher prevalence of prostate cancer in US black males compared to white males. Also, Mormon men have a higher incidence of prostate cancer, whereas Mormon women tend to have a lower incidence of breast cancer. An additional problem is that, thus far, there are no really good models for chemically or virally induced prostate cancer (9,13). In this institute, we are endeavoring to develop such models for the purpose of gaining more information as to whether nutrition and dietary fat actually do play a role in prostate cancer and to have additional tools with which to study the relevant mechanisms.

The metabolic epidemiology of prostate cancer attempting to account for mechanisms whereby diet affects endocrine status in diverse population groups requires more research. Akazaki (1) described the high incidence of latent prostate carcinoma in Japanese men, but the risk of invasive clinical cancer is low.

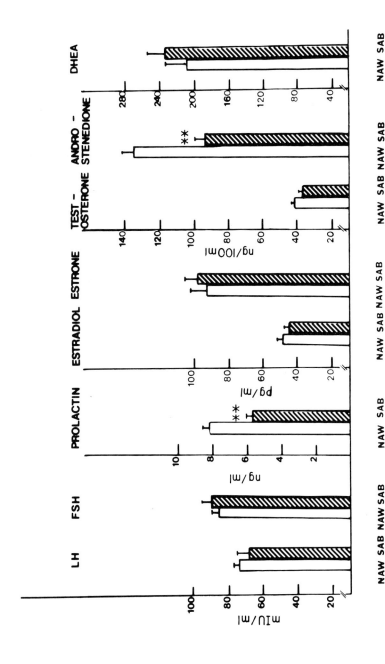

FIG. 3. Serum hormones: North American white women (NAW) and rural South African Bantu blacks (SAB) representing a Western high fat, low fiber, meat-eating population compared to a largely vegetarian, low fat, high fiber-eating population, respectively. Note the differences in adrenal and pituitary hormones. (See Reddy et al., ref. 12, for detailed comments.)

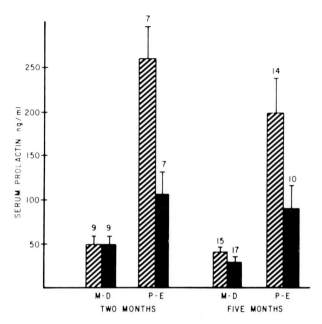

FIG. 4. Serum prolactin levels in female Sprague-Dawley rats fed a high fat (20%, *solid bars*) and a low fat (5%, *stippled bars*) diet are similar in metestrus and diestrus stages, but there are significant differences at proestrus and estrus after 2 or 5 months on the diets. Animals on a high fat diet develop breast cancer to a greater extent and with a greater multiplicity than animals on a low fat diet. (See Reddy et al., ref. 12, for detailed comments.)

Thus, initiation may have taken place, but promotion is weak. The key element, then, is to assess the nature of the promoting stimuli in Western man.

Recently, it was noted that a Western diet yielded distinct urinary estrogens and androgens as well as higher levels of circulating estrogens, androgens, follicle-stimulating hormone (FSH), and luteinizing hormone (LH) compared to the same individuals fed lower fat vegetarian diets. In black South Africa men, black North American men, and white North American men, hormone levels were also different in older men, age 60 to 73, compared with middle-aged men, ages 40 to 55 (6). This situation is quite complex, and no clear endocrine balances reflecting nutritionally related risk for prostate cancer can be described at this time.

CONCLUSIONS

For these important human cancers at high risk in the Western world, namely, colon, breast, and prostate cancers, the key nutritional element appears to be the level of total dietary fat consumed. Dietary fat accounts for 40% of calories in a high-risk country, whereas in a low-risk country, such as Japan, the intake is only 10 to 15% of calories. In recent years, with a progressive Westernization of the Japanese diet, the amount of fat consumed has increased, as has the incidence of the fat-sensitive cancers. Indeed, this change in nutrition, with a concomitant change in incidence, provides more evidence. The mechanism whereby fat translates to risk has been sketched out rather satisfactorily for colon cancer, where there is a relationship between the amount of fat consumed and the quantity of cholesterol biosynthesized in the liver. In turn, there is a relationship between cholesterol and bile acids derived metabolically from cholesterol. Bile acids are transferred to the gut via the bile. In independent studies in germ-free and conventional animals, bile acids were shown to be promoters in colon cancer. The role of fibers, such as wheat bran, is to control the concentration of bile acids in the gut, thereby playing a role in colon cancer development in man and animal models.

With the endocrine-related cancers, namely, breast and prostate, it is quite reasonable to assume that certain endocrine imbalances can act as promoters. It is not yet known exactly what kind of endocrine balances would favor the growth of neoplastic cells, or indeed would inhibit such growth. It is also unclear as yet precisely through what steps dietary fat affects endocrine balances. It seems most probable, however, that these factors are related and deserve further investigation. It is known that steroids alone do not exert a primary controlling effect, but that the entire complex pituitary-gonad-adrenal relationship is involved and even thyroid hormones may play a role.

Thus, for cancers of the colon, breast, or prostate, and possibly other nutrition-linked cancers such as those in the ovaries, endometrium, pancreas, or kidney, undetermined endogenously produced promoting factors, in turn related to nutritional elements, play a key role.

REFERENCES

1. Akazaki, K. (1973): Comparative histological studies on the latent carcinoma of the prostate under different environmental circumstances. In: *Host Environment Interactions in the Etiology of Cancer in Man,* edited by R. Doll and I. Vodopija, pp. 89–98. International Agency for Research on Cancer, Lyon, France.
2. Bulbrook, R. D. (1972): Urinary androgen excretion and the etiology of breast cancer. *J. Natl. Cancer Inst.,* 48:1,039–1,042.
3. Furth, J. (1975): Hormones as etiological agents in neoplasia. In: *Cancer: A Comprehensive Treatise, Vol. I,* edited by F. F. Becker, pp. 75–120. Plenum Publishing Corp., New York.
4. Hiatt, H. H., Watson, J. D., and Winsten, J. A. (1977): *Origins of Human Cancer,* Cold Spring Harbor Laboratory, Cold Spring Harbor, New York.
5. Higginson, J. (1979): Environmental carcinogenesis: A global perspective. In: *Environmental Carcinogenesis: Occurrence, Risk Evaluation, and Mechanisms,* edited by P. Emmelot and E. Kriek, pp. 1–8. Elsevier/North Holland, Amsterdam.
6. Hill, P., Wynder, E. L., Garnes, H., and Walker, A. R. P. (1980): Environmental factors, hormone status, and prostatic cancer. *Prev. Med.,* 9:657–666.
7. Hirayama, T. (1979): Diet and cancer. *Nutr. Cancer,* 1:67–81.
8. Hoehn, S. K., and Carroll, K. K. (1979): Effects of dietary carbohydrate on the incidence of mammary tumors induced in rats by 7,12-dimethylbenz(a)anthracene. *Nutr. Cancer,* 1(3):27–30.

9. Isaacs, J. T., and Coffey, D. S. (1979): Animal models in the study on prostatic cancer. *Cancer Detect. Prev.,* 2:587–600.
10. MacMahon, B., Cole, P., and Brown, J. (1973): Etiology of human breast cancer: A review. *J. Natl. Cancer Inst.,* 50:21–42.
11. Petrakis, N. L. (1977): Breast secretory activity in nonlactating women, postpartum breast involution, and the epidemiology of breast cancer. *Natl. Cancer Inst. Monogr.,* 47:161–164.
12. Reddy, B. S., McCoy, G. D., Cohen, L. A., Hill, P., Weisburger, J. H., and Wynder, E. L. (1980): Nutrition and its relationship to cancer. *Adv. Cancer Res.,* 32:237–345.
13. Rivenson, A., and Silverman, J. (1979): The prostatic carcinoma in laboratory animals. *Invest. Urol.,* 16:468–472.
14. Schottenfeld, D. (1975): *Cancer Epidemiology and Prevention,* Charles Thomas Publishing Co., Springfield, Illinois.
15. Weisburger, J. H. (1979): Mechanism of action of diet as a carcinogen. *Cancer,* 43:1,987–1,995.
16. Wynder, E. L., and Hirayama, T. (1977): Comparative epidemiology of cancers of the United States and Japan. *Prev. Med.,* 6:567–594.

Carcinogenesis, Vol. 7, edited by E. Hecker et al.
Raven Press, New York © 1982.

Epidemiological Evidence of Promoting Effects—
The Example of Breast Cancer

Nicholas E. Day

*Biostatistics Programme, Division of Epidemiology and Biostatistics, International Agency
for Research on Cancer, 69732 Lyon Cedex 2, France*

Epidemiological data, being observational by nature, are inherently less well structured than experimental results. The type of experimental design that enables one to demonstrate directly the phenomenon of promotion, even the simplest, is more complex than one would hope to observe. On the few occasions where the joint action of two or more agents has been studied, there has usually been too little information on the variations in the times of exposures to the different agents to be able to infer clearly an initiating or promoting action. So to examine the extent to which promoting action may be an important determinant of risk for human cancers requires a less direct approach. One approach is to examine the response to a single exposure, rather than the joint action of several exposures, and to explore ways in which one might determine the mode of action. In particular, if the agent is assumed to be capable of producing tumors on its own, to determine whether its main mode of action is at an early or at a late stage in the carcinogenic process. In this chapter we shall examine the consequences of assuming that carcinogenesis is a multistage process, investigate the differences in response that might be used to distinguish between early and late stage carcinogens, show that these distinctions are observed in practice both epidemiologically and experimentally, and then outline how this approach might be helpful in describing the general epidemiological features of female breast cancer.

If exposure is continuous since birth to an agent capable on its own of producing tumors, then for the majority of epithelial tumors, incidence increases as the power of age (7,9). These tumors have been referred to as log-log tumors (20). If exposure is continuous from some time after birth, then incidence will rise as the power of duration of exposure, if no other exposures are in operation. This behavior has been observed both experimentally and epidemiologically (14,21). Suppose, now, that other factors are in operation, or that there is a certain background incidence of the disease, and that the exposure of interest is of limited duration. The uniformity of behavior seen in the continuous exposure situation no longer holds, and a wide variety of patterns of evolving incidence may be seen (8). One can contrast, for example, the appearance many years later of an excess number of epithelial tumors following short exposure to irradiation with the rapid increase in risk for endometrial cancer (admittedly not a log-log cancer) associated with continuous exposure to exogenous estrogens, an increase in risk that disappears rapidly following cessation of exposure.

One way of describing the variety of behavior observed is in terms of simple models of the carcinogenic process, models that are really no more than mathematical descriptions of experimental situations. We shall assume that a tumor arises from a single cell by means of a process consisting of several stages, which we shall characterize in no greater detail than by saying that some of the stages (at least one) occur early, and are then analogous to initiation in the mouse skin model, and some of the stages (again at least one) occur late, and are thus analogous to promotion in the mouse skin model. The population dynamics of cells that have passed through the early stages may differ from the population dynamics of normal cells of the relevant tissue, although direct observation of this difference may not be possible.

LATE STAGE ACTION AND THE EFFECT OF REMOVING EXPOSURE

Now, in these terms, an agent that produces tumors can be assumed to increase the rate at which either early or late stages occur, or to increase the proliferative advantage of intermediate cells. Most agents would probably increase the rate of all stages, but for many, the effect might well be predominantly early or late. In the following figures, we compare the differences in behavior the model would predict for early as opposed to late stage carcinogens, under a variety of circumstances where the exposure is of limited duration (8). Figure 1A com-

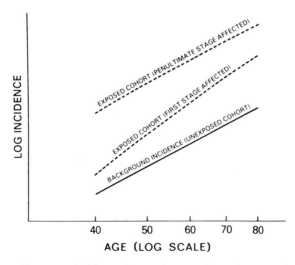

FIG. 1A. Age-specific cancer incidence for a cohort continuously exposed to a carcinogen from 20 years of age. (From Day and Brown, ref. 8.)

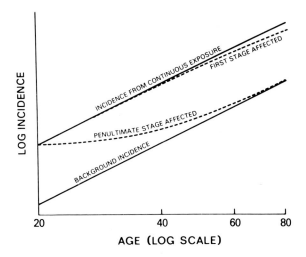

FIG. 1B. Effect of stopping exposure at 20 years of age when carcinogenic exposure started at birth. Age-specific incidence. (From Day and Brown, ref. 8.)

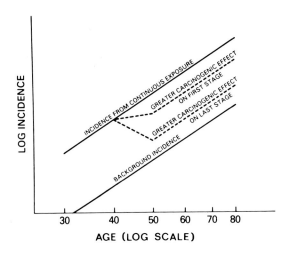

FIG. 1C. Age-specific incidence after exposure stopped: first and last stages affected. Exposure started at birth and stopped at 40 years of age. (From Day and Brown, ref. 8.)

pares the difference between early and late stage carcinogens when exposure starts in adult life; Figs. 1B and 1C compare the differences when exposure starts early, but is of limited duration in the situation where a carcinogen is either completely or only predominantly early or late stage. The differences between the two types of behavior predicted by the model are marked. We shall concentrate mainly on the differences shown in Figs. 1B and 1C, consequent to stopping exposure.

Mouse skin-painting experiments have been reported (P. N. Lee, *personal communication*) in which a limited exposure to benzo[a]pyrene (BP) and an extract of a tobacco smoke condensate (GT57) were compared. The full results are reported elsewhere; a summary representation is shown in Fig. 2. BP behaves as if it were a predominantly early stage carcinogen; the tobacco smoke extract behaves more like a late stage carcinogen.

A large series of experiments (Littlefield, *unpublished data*) has been reported on the effect of 2-acetylaminofluorene (2-AAF) on BALB/c mice, both with continuous lifetime and with short-term exposure. Two types of tumor are induced, those of the bladder and those of the liver. The difference in behavior between the tumors at the two sites is striking (Figs. 3A and 3B). For the liver, discontinuing the treatment has little effect on the subsequent evolution of incidence. By contrast, for the bladder, stopping the treatment freezes the incidence (in fact, the effect may be even greater, since in the report there is no clear distinction between incidence and prevalence). In this situation, 2-AAF or its metabolites appear to have predominantly an early stage effect on the liver but a late stage effect on the bladder.

As a final experimental example, we shall consider some stopping experiments done with 2,2-di(*p*-chlorophenyl)-1,1,1-trichlorethane (DDT), using CF-1 mice (26,27,30). The results, shown in Table 1, would indicate that DDT has a predominantly late stage effect, the change in incidence at stopping exposure being

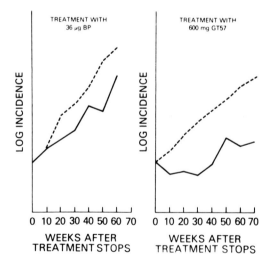

FIG. 2. Effect of discontinued treatment on incidence of skin tumours induced by BP and GT57. *Dotted line* shows average incidence if treatment continued; *continuous line* shows average observed incidence after treatment stopped. (From Day and Brown, ref. 8.)

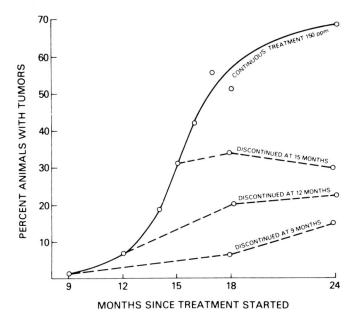

FIG. 3A. Effect of discontinued treatment on incidence of 2-AAF-induced bladder tumors in mice. (From Day and Brown, ref. 8.)

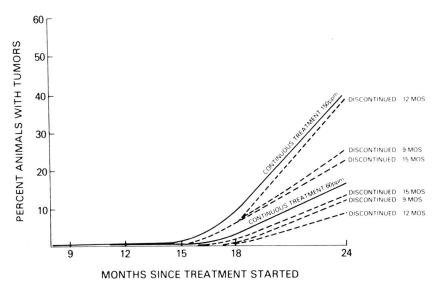

FIG. 3B. Effect of discontinued treatment on incidence of 2-AAF-induced liver tumors in mice. (From Day and Brown, ref. 8.)

TABLE 1. *Induction of liver tumors by DDT (250 ppm) in CF1 mice[a]*

Wk of treatment	Killed at week:								
	65			95			120		
	0	0–15	0–30	0	0–15	0–30	0	0–15	0–30
Males[b]	70(12)	60(13)	60(38)	83(24)	60(25)	60(41)	98(33)	69(25)	60(37)
Females[b]	69(0)	69(3)	54(4)	72(0)	60(11)	55(11)	90(1)	60(5)	54(11)

[a] From Tomatis et al. (26). Treatment groups considered in present series are shown.
[b] No. of animals killed or that died in the interval; no. of mice with hepatomas at or before death are in parentheses.

probably more marked than would appear due to the same confusion between incidence and prevalence noted for the 2-AAF experiment.

Thus, in summary, it would appear from stopping experiments that the two distinct types of behavior predicted are those that occur; one, interpretable as the action of early stage carcinogens, the other, as the action of late stage carcinogens.

We shall now consider some epidemiological examples, to see if a similar distinction can be observed. Two exposures apparently acting mainly on the early stages are radiation and asbestos: radiation for sites other than leukemia, and asbestos for both lung cancer and mesothelioma. A brief summary of the data appears in Tables 2, 3, and 4 (2,4,12,17,19,22,23,24,25). For asbestos, some doubt must be cast on this interpretation, since exposure to the tissue cannot be assumed to have stopped simply because external exposure has been removed. Asbestos bodies will remain in the lung, and a recent paper claims a promoting action for asbestos. For mesothelioma, however, an early-stage action would seem necessary, given the very long latent periods.

The effect of stopping cigarette smoking is equivalent to that of removing exposure to a late stage carcinogen (11) (Table 5). The fact that the rate in continuing smokers is similar to that for early stage carcinogens in Fig. 1A would indicate that both early and late stage action are important with cigarette smoke. After stopping smoking, however, the late stage effect is the one that determines the evolution of incidence.

The effect of nickel exposure (or some compound of nickel) on the nasal sinuses is rather similar (10). After exposure stops, the incidence rate freezes (Table 6), which one can interpret as indicating that nickel has a strong late stage effect.

Exogenous estrogens have an effect on the incidence of endometrial cancer that is overwhelmingly late stage. Excess tumors arise soon after exposure starts (cf. Fig. 1A), and the excess decreases rapidly following withdrawal of the drug. The effect of exogenous estrogens on breast cancer incidence is discussed later.

These results, experimental and epidemiological, indicate that the carcinogenic action of a compound for a particular site, in a particular species, may be classified as strongly early stage, or late stage, or both.

A MODEL FOR THE EPIDEMIOLOGY OF BREAST CANCER

We shall now attempt to show how this approach, considering action at different stages in the carcinogenic process, can be useful in attempting to understand the complex epidemiological behavior of female breast cancer, and how it leads to specific hypotheses testable by further epidemiological studies.

First, a general description of some of the ways in which breast cancer risk varies between and within populations.

TABLE 2. *Evolution of relative risk following limited exposure to radiation*[a]

	Time since exposure (yr)	Relative risk
A. Atomic bomb survivors with cancers other than leukemia[b]	5–9	1.4(29)
	10–13	1.0(18)
	14–17	1.4(33)
	18–21	1.1(34)
	22–25	1.3(40)
	26–29	1.5(45)
B. Atomic bomb survivors with breast cancer[c]	5–9	4.0(5)
	10–14	2.4(6)
	15–19	2.4(11)
	20–24	4.9(12)
C. Breast cancer after repeated fluoroscopies[d]	0–4	1.1(1)
	5–9	0.8(2)
	10–14	0.9(2)
	15–19	1.4(5)
	20–24	2.4(11)
	25–29	1.8(8)
	30–34	1.7(6)
	35+	2.7(6)
D. Breast cancer after irradiation for postpartum mastitis[e]	0–9	1.0(1)
	10–19	1.5(14)
	20–34	3.4(22)
E. Irradiation for ankylosing spondylitis: heavily exposed sites other than leukemia[f]	0–2	1.4
	3–5	1.3(27)
	6–8	1.2(21)
	9–11	1.9(45)
	12–14	1.7(46)
	15–17	1.6(43)
	18–20	1.5(26)
	21–23	1.3(11)
	24–26	0.9(4)
F. Irradiation for metropathia hemorraghica: heavily irradiated sites[g]	0–4	0.3(2)
	5–9	1.6(15)
	10–14	1.6(17)
	15–19	1.4(14)
	20–24	1.3(9)
	25–29	1.4(4)

[a] No. of cases are in parentheses.
[b] Mortality: relative risk of those exposed to 100+ rads to those exposed to 0–9 rads. From Beebe et al. (2).
[c] Morbidity: Relative risk of those exposed to 100+ rads to those exposed to 0–9 rads. From McGregor et al. (17).
[d] From Boice and Monson (4).
[e] From Shore et al. (23).
[f] From Smith and Doll (25).
[g] From Smith and Doll (24).

TABLE 3. *Percentage increment in the excess cumulative probability of lung cancer[a]*

Length of exposure (mo)	Yr since first exposure				
	5–9	10–14	15–19	20–24	25–30
<1	−0.15	−0.24	−0.35	1.09	2.67
1	−0.21	0.74	2.74	−0.51	0.47
2	−0.27	−0.38	0.69	1.89	4.20
3–5	−0.24	−0.34	0.91	1.51	0.11
6–11	−0.19	0.47	1.83	2.43	0.20
12–23	−0.15	2.24	1.33	1.21	2.80
Average increment	−0.215	0.415	1.192	1.270	1.742

[a] Difference between observed and expected cumulative probabilities. From Seidman et al. (22).

TABLE 4. *Mesothelioma mortality rates following exposure to asbestos[a]*

Time since first exposure (yr)	Rate per 10^5 person-years[b]
10–14	6(1)
15–19	45(6)
20–24	152(15)
25–29	171(11)
30+	318(12)

[a] From Newhouse and Berry (19).
[b] No. of cases are in parentheses.

TABLE 5. *Evolution of mortality from lung cancer among ex-cigarette smokers[a]*

Measurement	Years since smoking stopped				
	0	<5	5–9	10–14	≥15
No. of deaths among ex-smokers[b]		10	12	8	7
No. of deaths as percent of no. expected among continuing smokers	100	68	35	25	11
No. of deaths divided by no. expected among lifelong nonsmokers	15.8	10.7	5.9	4.7	2.0

[a] From Doll and Peto (11).
[b] Excluding those who stopped smoking after developing lung cancer.

TABLE 6. *Number of men developing nasal sinus cancer by calendar year of observation and number expected after standardization for year and age at first employment[a]*

Calendar year of observation	No. of nasal sinus cancers		No. observed/ No. expected
	Observed	Expected[b]	
1939–41	7	3.63	1.93
1942–46	8	7.28	1.10
1947–51	9	9.66	0.93
1952–56	5	9.34	0.54
1957–61	6	6.28	0.96
1962–66	5	3.82	1.31
All years	40	40.01	

χ^2 for trend = 0.95; df = 1; $p > 0.30$

[a] From Doll et al. (10).
[b] The expected numbers are not based on population incidence data but were obtained from the observed cases by assuming that the incidence was proportional to the man-year at risk after standardizing for calendar year and age at first employment. The uniformity of the observed to expected ratio thus reflects a constancy over follow-up time of the absolute rather than relative excess risk.

Age

The earlier distinction that used to be made between the change of incidence with age in high- and low-risk countries (US and Japan, say) has been shown to be a misconception of how to look at age-incidence curves. If one constructs such curves for women born in a particular time period, irrespective of the country, then every cohort of women gives rise to a curve of similar shape (18). Data from Iceland (3) are shown as an example in Figs. 4A and 4B, and mortality data from China in Fig. 4C (6). These latter data are interesting as they represent a low-risk country where change, if any has occurred, has occurred only recently, and where the cross-sectional age curve should be similar to the cohort age curves, and show the typical shape of Fig. 4B. This typical cohort age curve for breast cancer incidence bears considerable resemblance to the shape an age-incidence curve for lung cancer would have for a group who smoked regularly from age 15 to age 45.

Age at First Birth and Parity

A large number of studies have shown an increasing risk with increasing age at first full-term pregnancy (16). Some studies have shown, in addition, that further full-term pregnancies (28) after the first confer additional protection.

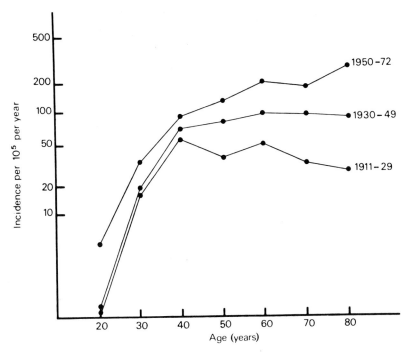

FIG. 4A. Age-specific incidence of breast cancer in Iceland for the three time periods 1911–29, 1930–49, and 1950–72. (From Bjarnason et al., ref. 3.)

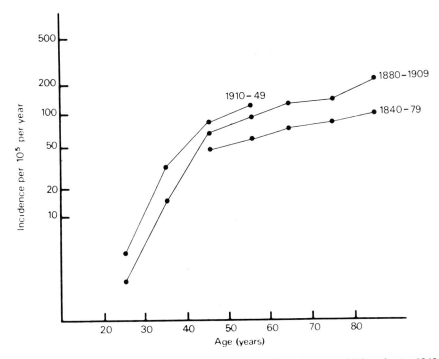

FIG. 4B. Age-specific incidence of breast cancer in Iceland for three birth cohorts, 1840–1879, 1880–1909, and 1910–1949. (Adapted from Bjarnason et al., ref. 3.)

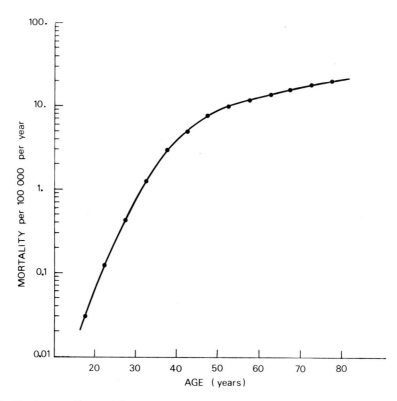

FIG. 4C. Age-specific mortality rates for breast cancer in the Peoples Republic of China. (From ref. 6.)

Age at Menarche and Age at Menopause

A consistent, if not very large, increase in risk with early menarche has been regularly demonstrated (28). Of perhaps greater interest is the indication of a strong correlation between average age at menarche in a cohort of women and their overall risk for breast cancer. Late age at menopause increases risk to some degree, but early oopharectomy has a strong protective effect (15).

Radiation

The increase in risk for breast cancer following irradiation is more pronounced for women irradiated in the 10 to 20 age group; earlier irradiation appears to have little effect, and later irradiation is associated with lower increase in risk. Of particular interest is the indication that the risk is greatest for nulliparous women, and for women irradiated around the time of menarche (5).

Exogenous Estrogens

The effect on breast cancer risk of replacement estrogens at the menopause is much less marked than the effect on risk of endometrial cancer, and several early studies showed no increase in risk. Recent, more rigorous cohort studies have shown that risk is increased, but only 10 to 15 years after beginning administration, and at most by a factor of two (13).

Predisposing Factors

A family history of breast cancer has been recognized for many years as a risk factor, two- or threefold risks being observed for women whose mothers or sisters have had the disease (29). The risks are higher for premenopausal and for bilateral breast cancer (1).

A previous history of benign breast disease also predisposes to breast cancer, and it is of interest that the principal characteristics of the benign lesions leading to highest risk are those with evidence of epithelial hyperplasia. The role of obesity or height is not clear. Several studies report an increased risk among obese women, particularly after the menopause, whereas other observations suggest that height may be of greater importance. The effect, anyway, is small.

A MODEL FOR BREAST CANCER DEVELOPMENT

We have proposed as a model for breast cancer development (23), into which these epidemiological findings fit comfortably, a process similar to the one discussed earlier in this chapter, which was shown for other types of tumor to be capable of describing many experimental and epidemiological results. This model consists of early stages in which normal cells undergo some alteration, a period of proliferation of these altered cells, and then late stages in the process that lead to the formation of malignant cells, which progress into a clinical malignancy. The process is shown graphically in Fig. 5. For breast cancer, we

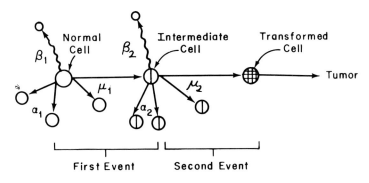

FIG. 5. A two-stage model for carcinogenesis. (From Moolgavkar et al., ref. 18.)

have to impose the following restrictions to take account of the physiology of mammary tissue.

(a) The number of normal cells at risk is not constant, but increases with the development of breast tissue, i.e., very low until the year or two before menarche, then increasing rapidly to reach a stable, adult level.

(b) The proliferation of intermediate cells is hormone dependent. The term $(\alpha_2\text{-}\beta_2)$ (see Fig. 5) in the rate of growth of the intermediate cell population falls in the years before the menopause, and may even become negative.

(c) A full-term pregnancy reduces the number of normal cells available for initiation. The effect of this reduction is clearly most marked for the first birth, but later full-term pregnancies deplete further the pool of susceptible cells. This reduction is probably a reflection of the increase in differentiation of mammary cells in the last trimester of pregnancy, thus depleting the reservoir of stem cells.

With these modifications to the basic process, which generates the log–log behavior for most other epithelial tumors, we can explore the type of epidemiological behavior that would be predicted. By elementary fitting techniques as described elsewhere, one obtains a close approximation to the standard age-incidence curve (Fig. 6A), to the change of risk with age at first birth (Fig. 6B), the effect of age at menarche and of age at menopause. The effect of replacement estrogens is exactly what one would predict if the effect were simply to replace for a limited period the action of ovarian estrogens. The excess risk resulting from mammary hyperplasia is also what one would expect. The role of hormones appears to be to increase the rate of late stage events. There is no need to invoke early stage effects mediated by hormones, in keeping with their apparent lack of mutagenic activity.

Many aspects of the epidemiology of the disease are thus what one would predict if the pathogenesis of the disease followed roughly along the lines of the proposed model. Beyond being an alternative description of the same phenomenon, however, one has to ask whether testable hypotheses arise from the model that may advance one's understanding of the etiology of the disease, or whether steps for primary prevention might be suggested by the model. One could argue as follows. The risk for breast cancer seems to be set in the first few years after menarche, if not earlier, and the evolving risk as a woman ages is then determined. The major differences in risk between different populations thus arise from early life exposures. The results of migrant studies support this conclusion (15). In terms of the proposed model, these differences in risk must relate to the rate at which cells are initiated, a rate that depends both on the concentration of whatever agent it may be that causes initiation and on the number of susceptible cells. Since age at menarche and breast cancer risk are strongly inversely correlated among different populations, it would seem that breast tissue at the time of menarche in high-risk populations may be subject to greater proliferative stimulation than in low-risk populations. (The factors that determine the differences of age at menarche between women within a given population are probably many. A factor that decreases the average age at menarche by a year may have a much greater influence on breast cancer risk than would be predicted from the within-population relative risks, since out of the many factors affecting menarche, it may be the one specifically related to breast cancer risk.) Thus one would predict that histological studies of breast

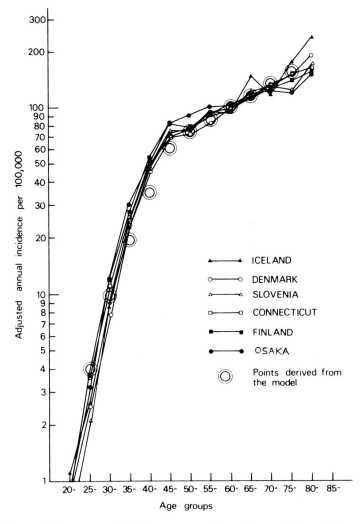

FIG. 6A. Shapes of the age-specific incidence curves of breast cancer in females from different populations after adjustment for temporal trends, and the shape of the incidence curve generated by the model (parameters obtained from fit to Connecticut data). All curves have been normalized so that the sum of the rates over all age groups is the same. Note that incidence is on a logarithmic scale. (From Moolgavkar et al., ref. 18.)

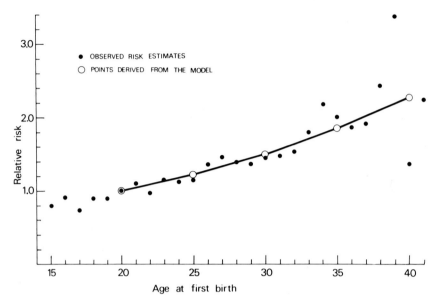

FIG. 6B. Risk for different ages at first full-term pregnancy relative to first full-term pregnancy at age 20 compared with predictions from the model.

cancer in the first few years after menarche in populations at high and low risk for breast cancer should demonstrate tissue differences consistent with a greater population of cells at risk. Such a result would be of biological interest but singularly useless as far as disease prevention is concerned. It is not plausible to consider intervention studies at premenarche ages aimed at reducing future breast cancer risk. The only way to achieve primary prevention of the disease is by manipulation of the late-stage processes of the disease. Hormonal regulation of the population dynamics of mammary cells might be conceivable, if one could guarantee the preservation of a woman's life-style. Perhaps, as an alternative, direct intervention in the promotion mechanism could be considered.

REFERENCES

1. Anderson, D. E. (1977): Breast cancer in families. *Cancer,* 40:1,855–1,860.
2. Beebe, G. W., Kato, H., and Land, C. E. (1977): Mortality experience of atomic bomb survivors 1950–74. Life Span Study Report 8. *Radiation Effects Research Foundation Technical Report TR 1–77.24.*
3. Bjarnason, O., Day, N. E., Snaedal, G., and Tulinius, H. (1974): The effect of year of birth on the breast cancer age-incidence curve in Iceland. *Int. J. Cancer,* 13:689–696.14.
4. Boice, J. D., and Monson, R. R. (1977): Breast cancer in women after repeated fluoroscopic examinations of the chest. *J. Natl. Cancer Inst.,* 59:823–832.29.
5. Boice, J. D., and Stone, B. J. (1978): Interaction between radiation and other breast cancer risk factors. In: *Late Biological Effects of Ionizing Radiation,* pp. 231–249. International Atomic Energy Agency, Vienna.
6. Cancer Control Office, Ministry of Health, Peking (1980): Atlas of Cancer Mortality for the People's Republic of China, *(in press).*

7. Cook, P. J., Doll, R., and Fellingham, S. A. (1969): A mathematical model for the age distribution of cancer in man. *Int. J. Cancer,* 4:93–112.
8. Day, N. E., and Brown, C. C. (1980): Multistage models and primary prevention of cancer. *J. Natl. Cancer Inst.,* 64:977–989.
9. Doll, R. (1971): The age distribution of cancer. Implications for models of carcinogenesis. *J. R. Statist. Soc. A,* 134:133–155.22.
10. Doll, R., Morgan, L. G., and Speizer, F. E. (1970): Cancers of the lung and nasal sinuses in nickel workers. *Br. J. Cancer,* 24:623–632.
11. Doll, R., and Peto, R. (1976): Mortality in relation to smoking: 20 years' observations on male British doctors. *Br. Med. J.,* 2:1,525–1,526.
12. Hempelmann, L. H., Hall, W. J., Phillips, M., Cooper, R. A., and Ames, W. R. (1975): Neoplasms in persons treated with X-rays in infancy. *J. Natl. Cancer Inst.,* 50:519–530.
13. Hoover, R., Gray, L. A., Cole, P., and MacMahon, B. (1976): Menopausal estrogens and breast cancer. *N. Engl. J. Med.,* 295:401–405.
14. Lee, P. N., and O'Neill, J. A. (1971): The effect of both time and dose applied on tumour incidence rates in benzopyrene skin-painting experiments. *Br. J. Cancer,* 23:582–586.
15. MacMahon, B., Cole, P., and Brown, J. (1973): Etiology of human breast cancer: A review. *J. Natl. Cancer Inst.,* 50:21–42.
16. MacMahon, B., Cole, P., Lin, T. M., Lowe, C. R., Mirra, A. P., Ravnihar, B., Salber, E. J., Valaoras, V. G., and Yuasa, S. (1970): Age at first birth and breast cancer risk. *Bull. WHO,* 43:209–221.
17. McGregor, D. H., Land, C. E., Choi, K., Tokuoka, S., Liu, P. I., Wakabayashi, T., and Beebe, G. W. (1977): Breast cancer incidence among atomic bomb survivors, Hiroshima and Nagasaki 1950–69. *J. Natl. Cancer Inst.,* 59:799–811.
18. Moolgavkar, S. H., Day, N. E., and Stevens, R. G. (1980): Two-stage model for carcinogenesis: Epidemiology of breast cancer in females. *J. Natl. Cancer Inst.,* 65:559–569.
19. Newhouse, M. L., and Berry, G. (1976): Predictions of morality from mesothelial tumours in asbestos factory workers. *Br. J. Ind. Med.,* 33:147–151.
20. Peto, R. (1977): Epidemiology, multistage models, and short-term mutagenicity tests. In: *Origins of Human Cancer,* edited by H. H. Hiatt, J. D. Watson, and J. A. Winsten, pp. 1,403–1,428. Cold Spring Harbor Press, New York.
21. Peto, R., Roe, F. J., Lee, P. N., Levy, L., and Clack, J. (1975): Cancer and aging in mice and men. *Br. J. Cancer,* 32:422–426.
22. Seidman, H., Lilis, R., and Selikoff, I. J. (1977): Short-term asbestos exposure and delayed cancer risk. In: *Prevention and Detection of Cancer, Part 1: Prevention,* edited by H. E. Mieburgs, pp. 943–960. Marcel Dekker, New York.
23. Shore, R. E., Hempelmann, L. H., Kowaluk, E., Mansur, P. S., Pasternack, B. S., Albert, R. E., and Haughie, G. E. (1977): Breast neoplasms in women treated with X-rays for acute postpartum mastitits. *J. Natl. Cancer Inst.,* 59:813–822.
24. Smith, P. G., and Doll, R. (1976): Late effects of X-irradiation in patients treated for metropathia haemorrhagica. *Br. J. Radiol.,* 49:224–232.
25. Smith, P. G., and Doll, R. (1978): Age- and time-dependent changes in the rates of radiation-induced cancers in patients with ankylosing spondylitis following a single course of X-ray treatment. In: *Late Biological Effects of Ionizing Radiation,* pp. 205–214. International Atomic Energy Agency, Vienna.
26. Tomatis, L., Turusov, V., Charles, R. T., Boicchoi, M., and Gati, E. (1974): Liver tumors in CF-1 mice exposed for limited periods to technical DDT. *Z. Krebsforsch.,* 82:25–35.
27. Tomatis, L., Turusov, V., Day, N., and Charles R. T. (1972): The effect of long-term exposure to DDT on CF-1 mice. *Int. J. Cancer,* 10:489–506.
28. Tulinius, H., Day, N. E., Johannesson, G., Bjarnason, O., and Gonzalez, M. (1978): Reproductive factors and risk for breast cancer in Iceland. *Int. J. Cancer,* 21:724–730.
29. Tulinius, H., Day, N. E., Sigvaldason, H., Bjarnason, O., Johannesson, G., Liceaga de Gonzalez, M., Grimsdottir, K., and Bjarnadottir, G. (1980): A population-based study on familial aggregation of breast cancer in Iceland, taking some other risk factors into account. In: *Genetic and Environmental Factors in Experimental and Human Cancer,* edited by H. V. Gelboin, B. MacMahon, T. Matsushima, T. Sugimura, S. Takayama, and H. Takebe, pp. 303–312. Japan Scientific Societies Press, Tokyo.
30. Turusov, V. S., Day, N. E., Tomatis, L., Gati, E., and Charles, R. T. (1973): Tumors in CF-1 mice exposed for six consecutive generations to DDT. *J. Natl. Cancer Inst.,* 51:983–987.

Carcinogenesis, Vol. 7, edited by E. Hecker et al.
Raven Press, New York © 1982.

Phenotypic and Chromosomal Alterations in Cell Cultures as Indicators of Tumor-Promoting Activity

Norbert E. Fusenig and Rule T. Dzarlieva

German Cancer Research Center, Institute of Biochemistry, 6900 Heidelberg, Federal Republic of Germany

RELEVANCE OF *IN VITRO* SYSTEMS FOR PROMOTION STUDIES

Cell cultures are important tools with which to study normal and aberrant growth behavior. They offer a spectrum of experimental possibilities to analyze effects of carcinogens and promoters at the *cellular level* which are difficult or impossible to perform *in vivo.* The pleiotropic effects of phorbol esters on a variety of cell types in culture provide important clues to the process of tumor promotion. One has to consider, however, that many manifestations of cultured cells may result solely from the *in vitro* conditions. Separated from their tissue architecture and from their normal intercellular communications, cells *in vitro* are studied under rather artificial conditions. In population densities up to 10^5-fold lower than *in vivo,* they are restricted to growth in two dimensions, on an artificial substrate, in a partly synthetic medium enriched with heterologous serum.

An appreciation of the discrepancies between the conditions *in vivo* and *in vitro* compels one to critically examine the relevance of data obtained in cell culture systems. It is important to compare observations gathered from one particular *in vitro* system, under special conditions, with observations from other culture systems or cell types and, of course, with the *in vivo* system.

Another point concerns the question of whether a normal (i.e., untreated) cell system—either *in vivo* or *in vitro*—is appropriate to study promotion effects at all, since these occur, per definition, on initiated cells. Since most biochemical *in vivo* data have also been obtained from noninitiated skin and correlate to promotion by analogy, it is generally assumed that changes effected by promoters in normal cells or tissues are similar or identical to those induced in initiated cells.

Since promoter effects are studied *in vitro* in primary or early passage cultures, as well as in cell lines from different tissues, these studies might also give an answer as to whether or not this assumption is correct. The so-called "normal" *permanent lines* often used for transformation or promotion experiments, such as 3T3 or 10T1/2, are *nontransformed* by morphologic criteria, but can grow to tumors when transplanted under appropriate conditions (2). They are also called "conditionally neoplastic" and may well represent one type of *initiated cells,* similar to the genetically altered human fibroblasts used by Kopelovich et al. (19) or the nontumorigenic epithelial lines studied by Colburn et al. (5). Transformation of these cells *in vitro* by tumor promoters may thus reflect some further steps of the multistep process of tumor formation, steps that are *in vivo* only observed during promotion of initiated cells. On the other hand, it may well be that promoters do not act primarily on initiated cells but on their surrounding normal cells in reducing or blocking potential intercellular control mechanisms, thus rendering the environment permissive for the expression of the transformed phenotype and the expansion of the initiated cells.

TUMOR PROMOTION BY PHORBOL ESTERS IN CULTURED CELLS

Phorbol esters induce a whole variety of pleiotropic effects on cells in culture, including changes in morphology and growth characteristics, alteration of membrane properties, induction of enzyme activities, and modification of various cell functions. The effects can occur within seconds or are expressed only after days, and they may vary qualitatively and quantitatively depending on the cell or tissue type and the test condition used. Many of the biological effects of promoters in mesenchymal cells, particularly the early and short-term effects, can be associated with the well-known mitogenic effect of phorbol esters. The biochemical changes noted in 12-0-tetradecanoylphorbol-13-acetate (TPA)-treated cellular or subcellular test systems may thus relate merely to differences between growing and nongrowing cells and may not be relevant to the transformed state of a cell. However, since several of the TPA-induced changes mimic a reversibly altered phenotype that eventually may develop into a permanently altered or transformed state, they are related to the *in vitro cocarcinogenic* activity of tumor promoters (4).

There is good reason for this correlation, since the two-stage phenomenon has been demonstrated in several *in vitro* systems designed to measure transformation and mutagenesis. Rat, hamster, and mouse fibroblasts could be promoted to transformed phenotypes by TPA following initiation with chemicals, ultraviolet radiation (UV), or X-rays (21,27,32). Enhancement of Epstein-Barr virus-induced lymphocyte transformation by TPA (49) was reported, as well as TPA-induced phenotypic expression of malignancy in genetically predisposed human fibroblasts (19).

It should be emphasized, however, that clear-cut two-stage carcinogenesis has not yet been achieved in epithelial cell cultures, with the probable exception of a recent report of a two-stage transformation experiment in a pancreatic organ culture system (30). It has been shown that phorbol esters active in stimulating proliferation in primary and permanent epidermal cultures (13,52) enhance the establishment of permanent lines in rat tracheal epithelial cultures (39) and stimulate the incidence of altered foci in 7,12-dimethylbenz(a)anthracene (DMBA)-initiated mouse salivary gland cultures (18). Using nontumorigenic cell lines derived from primary mouse epidermal cultures, Colburn et al. (5) identified several lines that could be "promoted" by TPA to irreversibly acquire the capacity to grow in soft agar.

IN VITRO CRITERIA FOR TRANSFORMED CELLS

A whole variety of phenotypic changes associated with tumor cells in vivo have been described which, to a certain extent, are also expressed in vitro (for review, see ref. 7). There is, however, so far no specific function or its loss that can be directly correlated to the onset of malignancy.

In vitro transformed cells differ from their normal counterparts by changes in growth behavior or social behavior. These include alterations in cell-to-cell, cell-to-substrate, and cell-to-medium interactions, which phenotypically lead to an altered growth pattern referred to as "morphological transformation." There exist characteristic changes indicative for the transformed state of mesenchymal cells, but only some are also applicable to epithelial cells (for review, see ref. 3). Many of the alterations in the social behavior of transformed cells only become manifest when cells grow in contact with each other, and are thus probably secondary and due to membrane effects. Those membrane changes, including functional and structural alterations, have been demonstrated in many cell systems after chemical or viral transformation.

TRANSFORMATION CRITERIA FOR EPITHELIAL AND MESENCHYMAL CELLS

The so-called early transformation features, such as morphologic transformation, membrane changes, alteration in density inhibition, nutrient requirement, etc., used as indicators in mesenchymal cultures are often not applicable to "carcinoma" cells (3,45). This does not invalidate the criteria when used in mesenchymal systems, but it leaves some doubt as to their general applicability and probably also to their causal relationship to neoplastic transformation.

In contrast to mesenchymal cells, morphology and growth patterns in epithelial cultures are generally not drastically changed during transformation, whether cells are grown in confluent cultures or at clonal densities. Transformed epithelial cells also may pile up, but this is not an early and general phenomenon; multilayering is often a normal feature of epithelial cultures (for review, see ref. 11). There are several other phenotypic changes of cultured cells following phorbol ester treatment that may only be called transformation associated in mesenchymal systems.

As demonstrated earlier, mesenchymal cells transformed by various agents showed increased plasminogen activator (PA) production (42). It could also be demonstrated that active phorbol esters also induce PA in normal chick and hamster fibroblasts, macrophages, and other cells, thus mimicking one aspect of the transformed phenotype (46). As far as carcinomas or epithelial cultures are concerned, PA activity is not strictly correlated to the transformed state (26,28,31,50). These observations indicate that PA activation may not be a valid criterion for cell transformation or promotion when epithelial cells are concerned.

The loss of LETS-protein or fibronectin from the surface of cells, another putative marker for transformation (43), appears to occur only with mesenchymal cells too. This protein is not present, or is present only in minute amounts, on transformed *and* normal epithelial cells (26,47,50).

Another phorbol ester-mediated effect is the induction of ornithine decarboxylase (ODC). Whether the induction of ODC observed *in vivo* and *in vitro* in mesenchymal and epithelial systems is causally related to promotion or merely linked to stimulated cell proliferation is not unequivocally answered. Stimulated cell proliferation appears to be a general phenomenon induced by tumor promoters, but its significance for the promotion process even *in vivo* remains questionable (23,25,37). Nevertheless, induction of ODC is considered a useful and early marker of tumor-promoting activity, although it may not be considered a specific marker for cell transformation.

TUMOR PROMOTION AND ALTERED DIFFERENTIATION *IN VITRO*

By 1954 Berenblum (1) had already postulated that tumor promotion involves a nonspecific proliferative stimulus and a specific inhibition of differentiation.

TABLE 1. *Effect of TPA and related phorbol esters on morphologic differentiation of mouse keratinocytes in culture (line HEL-30)[a]*

Phorbol ester	Dose (M)	PE[b] (%)	DC[c] (%)
TPA	10^{-9}	89	58
	10^{-8}	75	51
	10^{-7}	67	27
4-O-ME-TPA	10^{-9}	105	118
	10^{-8}	106	97
	10^{-7}	100	94
PDD[d]	10^{-9}	86	108
	10^{-8}	69	91
	10^{-7}	65	55
4-α-PDD	10^{-9}	81	110
	10^{-8}	81	108
	10^{-7}	77	105

[a] HEL cells were grown at clonal density with 3T3 feeder cells and treated three times per week (total four times) starting 1 day after plating. Colonies were stained with hematoxylin and rhodamin B.
[b] PE, Plating efficiency/% of control.
[c] DC, Differentiated (rhodamin-stained) colonies/% of control.
[d] PDD, Phorbol-12,13-didecanoate.

TABLE 2. *Effect of TPA and RA on morphologic differentiation of mouse keratinocytes in culture (line HEL-30)[a]*

	PE[b] (%)	DC[c] (%)
Medium control	100	100
DMSO[d], 0.05%	89	105
TPA, 10^{-6} M	88	11
RA, 0.1 μg/ml	80	0

[a]HEL cells were grown at clonal density with 3T3 feeder cells and treated three times per week (total four times) starting 5 days after plating when colonies had already formed. Colonies were stained with hematoxylin and rhodamin-B.
[b]PE, Plating efficiency/% of control.
[c]DC, Differentiated (rhodamin-stained) colonies/% of control.
[d]DMSO, Dimethylsulfoxide.

Raick (34) reported that phorbol esters induced changes in the ultrastructure of mouse epidermis, which he interpreted as inhibition of differentiation, or "dedifferentiation." Effects of phorbol ester on the chalon control mechanism were interpreted in the same direction (20). Inhibition of terminal differentiation by phorbol esters has recently been demonstrated *in vitro* with cells of varying origins, but promoters can also stimulate differentiation in other cells (for review, see refs. 7, 44).

We could demonstrate that phorbol esters inhibit terminal differentiation of mouse epidermal cells in primary culture (13). Keratinization is also inhibited in an epidermal cell line (HEL-30) with highly preserved differentiation capacity. The effect can be analyzed morphologically by the stainability of keratinized colonies with rhodamin-B when cells are cultivated at clonal density with or without 3T3 feeder cells (11) (Table 1). Although nonpromoting phorbol esters do not inhibit differentiation, the effect is by no means promoter specific, since other factors such as retinoic acid (RA) have similar or even more dramatic effects on keratinization. The inhibition is equally observed with either TPA or RA treatment started immediately after plating, or when colonies with beginning differentiation had formed (Table 2). The effect is reversible for both substances.

ALTERED MULTICELLULAR ORGANIZATION WITH TRANSFORMED CELLS

Tumor cells are also characterized by another alteration in tissue-specific functions, namely the strictly organized architecture of cells within a tissue, e.g. in proliferating and differentiating compartments, as it is particularly well expressed in the epidermis. The alteration of this cell function—also called loss of "positional control (38)"—is typically induced by promoters in the skin during the development of hyperplasia, papillomas, and invasive carcinomas. The loss of positional control is a typical criterion of tumor cells, but has been difficult to test in cultured cells. Our laboratory developed a cell culture system in which epidermal cells can grow in their "organotypical" pattern and form a regularly organized multicellular architecture—quite similar to that of the epidermis *in vivo* (10,11). While normal keratinocytes organize to a typical stratified multicellular structure with proliferating basal and superimposed differentiating cell layers, this organizational behavior is lost in transformed epidermal cells (Fig. 1a). Early passages of transformed cell lines may still express a nearly normal arrangement of proliferating and differentiating cell layers (Fig. 1b). Tumorigenic cells only form amorphous nodules with randomly distributed proliferating cells and occasional centrally positioned horn-pearl-like keratinization areas (Figs. 1c and d). Further experiments have to test whether phorbol esters and other promoters interfere with the organizational behavior of normal or early passage (presumably initiated) cells in that the positional control is reversibly or permanently affected.

Recent reports by Trosko and co-workers (41,51) and Murray and Fitzgerald (29) on the phorbol ester-induced inhibition of cellular communication or metabolic cooperation led to other speculations concerning a more indirect mechanism of promotion. Metabolic cooperation is a form of intercellular communication in which the mutant phenotype, for example, is corrected by normal cells by direct cell-to-cell transfer of substances. Following these lines it might be an attractive hypothesis that phorbol esters are effective promoters in that they interfere with the intercellular growth control mechanisms. Earlier *in vitro* data about the TPA-enhanced expression of transformed 3T3 colonies when cocultivated with normal 3T3 cells (36) can be similarly interpreted as the TPA-mediated loss in sensitivity to chalone in the epidermis *in vivo* (20). The well-known phenomenon of the so-called spontaneous transformation of rodent cells in culture and the inverse relationship between cell density and transformation frequency indicate that cell cooperation *in vitro* is similarly important for growth control as *in vivo* (15). Such considerations raise the question of whether the isolated cell is a proper unit of expression of the regulated behavior of animal cells and its alterations in transformed cells.

PROMOTER-INDUCED CHROMOSOMAL ALTERATIONS

Although modulating effects on differentiation, growth regulation, and structural organization may not be specific for promoters, they suggest a relationship between the type of epigenetic control involved in development and the loss of control in malignancy. Phorbol esters do not appear to be mutagenic, but are able to induce inheritable changes. Kinsella and Radman (17) reported

FIG. 1. Structural organization of mouse keratinocytes from primary cultures **(a)**, early passages **(b)**, and late passages **(c)** of a spontaneously transformed line (HEL) and from a DMBA-transformed cell line (PDV) **(d)**. Cells were grown for 2 weeks on a lifted collagen gel in organotypical cultures (Hematoxylin and eosin, × 250).

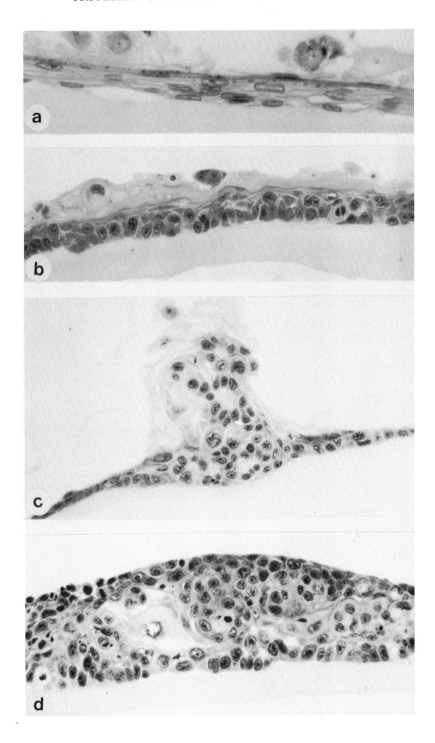

that phorbol esters increase the rate of sister chromatid exchange (SCE) in chinese hamster V-79 cells. Based on this observation, they proposed a challenging hypothesis on phorbol ester-induced genetic recombination as the result of epigenetic changes. Attempts to repeat these results have been mostly unsuccessful (e.g., ref. 40). In mouse epidermal cell cultures that respond to the growth stimulatory and differentiation inhibitory effects of TPA (11,13), we could demonstrate distinct cytogenetic alterations after short-term TPA treatment. Primary epidermal cell cultures (PEC) with a high rate of spontaneous chromosomal aberrations (8) and spontaneously transformed heteroploid mouse epidermal cell lines (HEL) with stable marker chromosomes were treated with TPA (10^{-6} and 10^{-8}M) for two cell cycles, either with or without bromodeoxyuridine (BrdU)(10^{-5}M). While SCEs were only slightly induced in all cell types by TPA, a significant increase in numerical and structural chromosomal aberrations was observed.

In PEC, TPA induced only a 20 to 70% induction of SCEs depending on dose when calculated per metaphase or per chromosome (Table 3). The percentage of tetraploid cells (already 16% in normal cultures 3 to 4 days after plating) was essentially unchanged by TPA, but the fraction of hypodiploid cells was clearly increased. Structurally, the changes included elevated levels of metacentric chromosomes and particularly chromatid and chromosome breaks and exchanges with the formation of tri- and quadriradials (Fig. 2). The increase in numerical and structural aberrations was similar whether TPA was administered alone or simultaneously with BrdU (data not shown).

Two sublines from a spontaneously transformed mouse epidermal cell line (HEL-30 and HEL-37), which express different levels of keratinization but are of monoclonal origin as indicated by a common marker chromosome (12), were analyzed at high and low passage levels, yielding very similar results. TPA

TABLE 3. *Spontaneous and TPA-induced numerical and structural chromosome aberrations and SCEs in PECs[a]*

	Hypodiploidy/ hyperdiploidy (%)	Metacentrics (%)	Structural chromo- somal aberrations[b] (%)	SCEs[c] per metaphase/ per chromosome
Control	2.0/0	2.0	2.0	6.4/0.15
	2.0/0	2.0	8.0	6.7/0.16
TPA 10^{-8} M	10.0/ 0	5.0	24.0	10.4/0.20
54 hr	7.5/3.0	9.0	30.0	8.0/0.18
TPA 10^{-6} M	10.0/2.0	8.0	31.0	10.8/0.23
54 hr	14.0/6.0	12.0	52.0	9.5/0.22

[a] 50–100 metaphases were examined 4 days after plating at 37°C. Modal chromosome number 40, tetraploidy 14–18%. Data from two different experiments.
[b] Chromatid and chromosome breaks and exchanges (triradials, quadriradials, rings); no BrdU.
[c] BrdU 10^{-5} M.

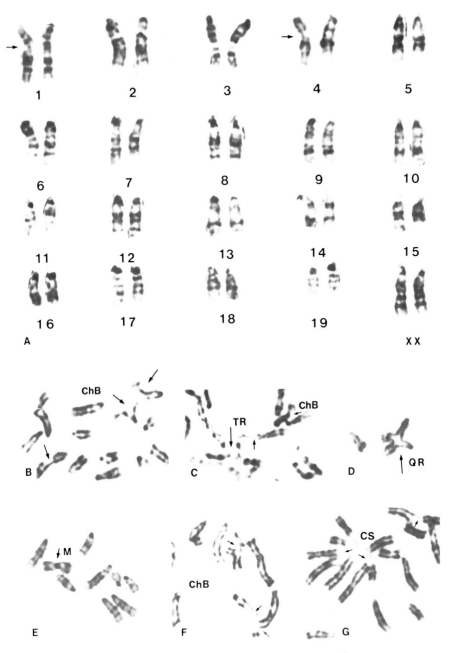

FIG. 2. Structural chromosome aberrations in PECs 4 days after plating and after 54 hr TPA (10^{-8} or 10^{-6} M) treatment without *Brd*U addition (Giemsa banding). **A:** Karyotype with large chromosome and chromatid breaks on chromosome No. 1 and 4 (*arrows*) after 10^{-8} M TPA. **B:** TPA 10^{-6} M; chromatid and isochromatid breaks (ChB). **C:** TPA 10^{-8} M; triradial configuration (TR) and ChB. **D:** TPA 10^{-6} M; quadriradial configuration (QR). **E:** TPA 10^{-6} M; metacentric chromosome (M). **F:** TPA 10^{-8} M; ChB. **G:** TPA 10^{-8} M; centrometric splitting (CS) with associations between chromosomes.

TABLE 4. Spontaneous and TPA-induced numerical and structural chromosome aberrations in permanent mouse epidermal cell lines (HEL-30 and HEL-37)[a]

Cell Line	HEL-30/9				HEL-37/38			
Treatment (M)	None	$BrdU$ 10^{-5}	TPA 10^{-8} $+ BrdU$	TPA 10^{-6} $+ BrdU$	None	$BrdU$ 10^{-5}	TPA 10^{-8} $+ BrdU$	TPA 10^{-6} $+ BrdU$
Polyploidy ($\geq$ octaploidy)[b]	2.0	1.0	7.0	9.0	2.0	3.0	8.0	7.0
Structural chromosome aberrations[b,c]	4.0	5.0	16.0	21.0	2.0	9.0	26.0	27.0
SCEs per metaphase		20.7	25.0	28.5		12.3	14.2	14.1
per chromosome		0.25	0.29	0.35		0.17	0.18	0.18

[a] $\geq$ 50 metaphases examined.
[b] Percent of metaphases.
[c] Chromatid and chromosome breaks and exchanges (rings, dicentrics, triradials, quadriradials). Minutes and double minutes are not included.

induced SCEs by only 20 to 40% (HEL-30) and 5% (HEL-37) as calculated per chromosome. The same treatment (for two cell cycles) increased the polyploidization rate in both lines by a factor of four to five, particularly ploidy steps of more than octaploidy (Table 4). Structural aberrations were similarly induced by TPA in HEL as in PEC cells, whether or not *Brd*U was included in the culture medium. Predominantly, a significant increase in chromatid and chromsome breaks and exchanges was noted and the formation of rings, dicentrics, and tri- or quadriradials (Fig. 3).

Thus, TPA, a putative nonmutagenic substance, caused distinct numerical and structural chromosomal aberrations in mouse epidermal cell cultures after short-term treatment with low doses (10^{-8} M). The cells used in this study, both the normal PEC and the permanent line HEL, are genetically very labile mouse cells with a high rate of spontaneous chromosomal aberrations in culture. Nevertheless, the alterations induced by TPA are so clearly distinct from the background level and reproducibly produced that the effect of TPA on the genetic material is beyond doubt. Moreover, recent results from another laboratory using primary phytohemagglutinine (PHA)-stimulated human lymphocytes demonstrated very similar structural chromosomal aberrations by nmole concentrations of TPA (I. Emerit and P. Cerutti, *personal communication*). In addition, the nonpromoting phorbol ester derivative 4-O-methyl-TPA (2×10^{-6} M) induced neither SCEs nor significant structural chromosomal aberrations in HEL cells.

ANCHORAGE-INDEPENDENT AND TUMORIGENIC GROWTH

Growth in suspension or semisolid media is the most valid criterion for transformed cells *in vitro* (35). Evidence is accumulating that this anchorage independence reflects a certain degree of nutritional autonomy, since its manifestation depends on various culture conditions such as medium type, serum concentration, and cell number (e.g., see refs. 6,22). The ability of a cell line to produce colonies in agar increases or is often only acquired with higher passage numbers and may be characteristic for late stages of transformation (24). Its frequency can thus be enhanced or "promoted" by continued growth *in vitro*. In a mouse keratinocyte cell line (HEL), the plating efficiency on plastic and in agar rises with increasing passage numbers, while the morphologic differentiation decreases (Table 5). The plating efficiency of early passage HEL cells in agar could not be increased by long-term treatment with TPA. It has been demonstrated by others that TPA can enhance the growth of nontumorigenic cells in agar and irreversibly "promote" these cells to the anchorage-independent state (5,6). Thus, anchorage independence may be considered a criterion for testing promotion *in vitro*, although this ability is acquired rather late and may represent a late stage in the transformation process. In most transformed cells, the capacity for growth in soft agar corresponds to their tumorigenic potential, but exceptions have been reported (26).

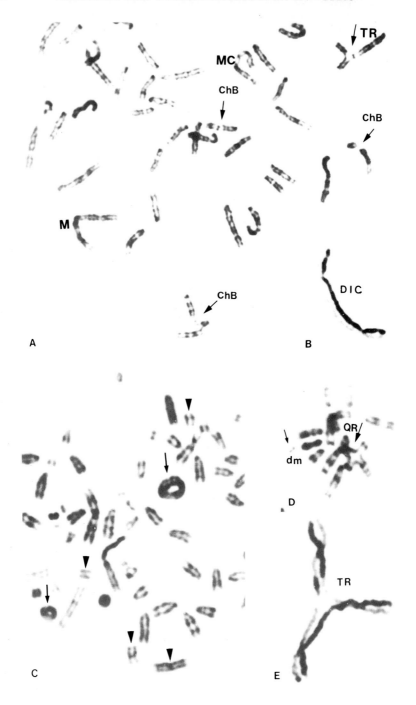

TABLE 5. *Clonal growth capacity of HEL-30 and HEL-37 cells in soft agar and on plastic, depending on passage number*

| Strain | Passage No. | Mean colony no./dish plated cell no. on agar | | | On plastic | |
		10^3	10^4	10^5	PE[b]	DC[c]
HEL-30	20	5	53	580	4	37
HEL-30	44	3	63	672	(−)	(−)
HEL-30	97	135	652	TMC[a]	25	10
HEL-37	68	11	58	345	42	7
HEL-37	262	81	351	TMC	49	0

[a] TMC, Too many to count.
[b] PE, Plating efficiency (%).
[c] DC, Differentiated colonies (% of total).

TUMORIGENICITY OF TRANSFORMED CELLS

Although cells may grow in agar and possess severe chromosomal changes, they often do not grow to tumors when injected into newborn or adult syngeneic animals or even nude mice, possibly due to problems with histocompatibility of the host, antigenicity of tumor cells, or volume and cell number of the inoculum (e.g., see refs. 16,33). It may be questioned whether the methods by which tumorigenicity is usually tested, i.e., by subcutaneous, intraperitoneal, or intramuscular injection, are appropriate and sensitive enough to detect early transformation changes, such as those occurring in early invading carcinomas. In order to improve the *in vivo* tumorigenicity test, we developed a transplantation assay to analyze early oncogenic capacities of cultured cells, such as the invasive growth behavior after retransplantation (10,11,14,48).

Cells are transplanted as suspensions or intact cultures on a well-vascularized granulation tissue induced under the back skin of mice. Transplanted cancer cells grow rapidly and infiltrate the granulation tissue within a few days, whether the tested cells are of syngeneic or allogeneic origin. With appropriate conditioning (thymectomy and X-irradiation), even cells from a human skin squamous cell carcinoma can grow invasively for up to three weeks in C3H mice (Boukamp et al., *in preparation*). Thus, a rapid and sensitive tumorigenicity test is now available to analyze promoted cells for their tumorigenic potentials at an early stage of their development.

FIG. 3. Structural chromosome aberrations in permanent mouse epidermal cell lines (HEL-37 passage 38 and HEL-30 clone 1 passage 42) after TPA (10^{-8} or 10^{-6} M) treatment for two cell cycles with or without addition of *BrdU*. A: HEL-37/38 and TPA 10^{-8} M; ChB, TR, M, and multicentric (MC). B: HEL-37/38, TPA 10^{-8} M and *BrdU* 10^{-5} M; dicentric chromosome (DIC). C: HEL-37/38, TPA 10^{-8} M; metaphase plate with ring chromosomes (*arrows*), chromosome breaks, minutes, double minutes, and acentric chromosome (*arrow heads*). D: HEL-37/38, TPA 10^{-8} M; QR and double minute (dm). E: HEL-30C1/42, TPA 10^{-6} M and *BrdU* 10^{-5} M; TR between three Ms.

CONCLUSION

In conclusion, there is so far no unique promotion test *in vitro* that could substitute for the *in vivo* experiment. The analysis of promotion *in vitro* requires multiple test assays which should be chosen depending on the target cells involved. Evidences are accumulating that the promotion processes understood as occurring *in vivo* can be imitated in culture and studied under *in vitro* conditions. This is at least true for mesenchymal cell systems, while the conditions for two-stage carcinogenesis with defined epithelial cell cultures still have to be developed. The lack of clear-cut promotion results may be related to the problems with malignant transformation *in vitro* of epithelial cells in general. Whether this discrepancy between the transformability of cultured mesenchymal and epithelial cells is due to endogenous regulatory differences or to inadequate culture conditions for epithelia has still to be determined. There are, however, several sensitive test assays available now that allow an investigation of these questions in epithelial cultures from tissues of various origin.

ACKNOWLEDGMENTS

The technical assistance of Charlotte Rausch, Birgit Kahl, and Sabine Stuhlert, and the preparation of the manuscript by Monika Matejka are gratefully acknowledged.

REFERENCES

1. Berenblum, I. (1954): A speculative review: The probable nature of promoting action and its significance in the understanding of the mechanism of carcinogenesis. *Cancer Res.,* 14:471–477.
2. Boone, Ch. W., and Jacobs, J. B. (1976): Sarcomas routinely produced from putatively nontumorigenic balb/3T3 and C3H/10T1/2 cells by subcutaneous inoculation attached to plastic platelets. *J. Supramol. Struct.,* 5:131–137.
3. Borek, C. (1979): Malignant transformation *in vitro:* Criteria, biological markers, and application in environmental screening of carcinogens. *Radiat. Res.,* 79:209–232.
4. Chang, Ch.-Ch., Trosko, J. E., and Warren, S. T. (1978): *In vitro* assay for tumor promoters and antipromoters. *J. Environ. Pathol. Toxicol.,* 2:43–64.
5. Colburn, N. H., Former, B. F., Nelson, K. A., and Yuspa, S. H. (1979): Tumour promoter induces anchorage independence irreversibly. *Nature,* 282:589–591.
6. Colburn, N. H., Vorger Bruegge, W. F., Bates, J. R., Gray, R. H., Rossen, J. D., Kelsey, W. H., and Shimada, T. (1978): Correlation of anchorage-independent growth with tumorigenicity of chemically transformed mouse epidermal cells. *Cancer Res.,* 38:624–634.
7. Diamond, L., O'Brien, T. G., and Baird, W. M. (1980): Tumor promoters and the mechanism of tumor promotion. *Adv. Cancer Res.,* 32:1–75.
8. Dzarlieva, R. T., Schütz, S., and Fusenig, N. E. (1981): Spontaneous and cocarcinogen-induced chromosome aberrations in primary and permanent mouse epidermal cells. *J. Cancer Res. Clin. Oncol.,* 99:A61.
9. Fisher, P. B., Dorsch-Häsler, K., Weinstein, I. B., and Ginsberg, H. S. (1979): Tumour promoters enhance anchorage-independent growth of adenovirus-transformed cells without altering the integration pattern of viral sequences. *Nature,* 281:281–594.
10. Fusenig, N. E., Amer, S. M., Boukamp, P., and Worst, P. K. M. (1978): Characteristics of chemically transformed mouse epidermal cells *in vitro* and *in vivo. Bull. Cancer,* 65:271–280.
11. Fusenig, N. E., Breitkreutz, D., Boukamp, P., Lueder, M., Irmscher, G., and Worst, P. K. M.

(1979): Chemical carcinogenesis in mouse epidermal cell cultures: Altered expression of tissue-specific functions accompanying cell transformation. In: *Neoplastic Transformation in Differentiated Epithelial Cell Systems in vitro,* edited by L. M. Franks and C. B. Wigley, pp. 37–98. Academic Press, New York.

12. Fusenig, N. E., Breitkreutz, D., Lueder, M., and Dzarlieva, R. T. (1980): Correlation between differentiation, proliferation, karyotype, and transformed phenotype of a mouse epidermal cell line. *Proc. Am. Assoc. Cancer Res.,* 21:40.

13. Fusenig, N. E., and Samsel, W. (1978): Growth-promoting activity of phorbol ester TPA on cultured mouse skin keratinocytes, fibroblasts, and carcinoma cells. In: *Carcinogenesis, Vol. 2: Mechanisms of Tumor Promotion and Cocarcinogenesis,* edited by T. J. Slaga, A. Sivak, and R. K. Boutwell, pp. 203–220. Raven Press, New York.

14. Fusenig, N. E., Valentine, E. A., and Worst, P. K. M. (1980): Growth behaviour of normal and transformed mouse epidermal cells after reimplantation *in vivo.* In: *Tissue Culture in Medical Research (I),* edited by R. J. Richards and K. T. Rajan, pp. 87–95. Pergamon Press, Oxford.

15. Haber, D. A., Fox, D. A., Dynan, W. S., and Thilly, W. G. (1977): Cell density dependence of focus formation in the C3H/10T1/2 transformation assay. *Cancer Res.,* 37:1,663–1,648.

16. Jamasbi, R. J., and Nettesheim, P. (1977): Increase in immunogenicity of a pulmonary squamous cell carcinoma, propagated *in vitro. Int. J. Cancer,* 20:817–823.

17. Kinsella, A. R., and Radman, M. (1978): Tumor promoter induces sister chromatid exchanges: Relevance to mechanisms of carcinogenesis. *Proc. Natl. Acad. Sci. USA,* 75:6,149–6,153.

18. Knowles, M. A. (1979): Effects of the tumor-promoting agent 12-O-tetradecanoylphorbol-13-acetate on normal and "preneoplastic" mouse submandibular gland epithelial cells *in vitro. J. Natl. Cancer Inst.,* 62:349–352.

19. Kopelovich, L., Bias, N. E., and Helson, L. (1979): Tumour promoter alone induces neoplastic transformation of fibroblasts from humans genetically predisposed to cancer. *Nature,* 282:619–621.

20. Krieg, L., Kühlmann, I., and Marks, F. (1974): Effect of tumor-promoting phorbol esters and of acetic acid on mechanisms controlling DNA synthesis and mitosis (chalones) and on the biosynthesis of histidine-rich protein in mouse epidermis. *Cancer Res.,* 34:3,135–3,146.

● 21. Lasne, C., Gentil, A., and Chouroulinkov, I. (1974): 2-stage malignant transformation of rat fibroblasts in tissue culture. *Nature,* 247:490–491.

22. Leavitt, J. C., Crawford, B. D., Barrett, J. C., and Ts'o, P. O. (1977): Regulation of requirements for anchorage independent growth of Syrian hamster fibroblasts by somatic mutation. *Nature,* 268:63–65.

23. Lichti, U., Slaga, T. J., Ben, Th., Patterson, E., Hennings, H., and Yuspa, S. H. (1977): Dissociation of tumor promoter-stimulated ornithine decarboxylase activity and DNA synthesis in mouse epidermis *in vivo* and *in vitro* by fluocinolone acetonite, a tumor-promotion inhibitor. *Proc. Natl. Acad. Sci.,* 74:3,908–3,912.

24. Marchock, A. C., Rhoton, J. C., and Nettesheim, P. (1978): *In vitro* development of oncogenicity in cell lines established from tracheal epithelium preexposed *in vivo* to 7,12-dimethylbenz(a)anthracene. *Cancer Res.,* 38:2,030–2,037.

25. Marks, F., Bertsch, S., and Fürstenberger, G. (1979): Ornithine decarboxylase activity, cell proliferation, and tumor promotion in mouse epidermis *in vivo. Cancer Res.,* 39:4,183–4,188.

26. Marshall, C. J., Franks, L. M., and Carbonell, A. W. (1977): Markers of neoplastic transformation in epithelial cell lines derived from human carcinomas. *J. Natl. Cancer Inst.,* 58:1,743–1,747.

● 27. Mondal, S., Brankow, D. W., and Heidelberger, Ch. (1976): Two-stage chemical oncogenesis in cultures of C3H/10T1/2 cells. *Cancer Res.,* 36:2,254–2,260.

28. Montesano, R., Drevon, C., Kuroki, T., Saint Vincent, L., Handleman, S., Sanford, K. K., DeFeo, D., and Weinstein, I. B. (1977): Test for malignant transformation of rat liver cells in culture: Cytology, growth in soft agar, and production of plasminogen activator. *J. Natl. Cancer Inst.,* 59:1,651–1,658.

29. Murray, A. W., and Fitzgerald, D. J. (1979): Tumor promoters inhibit metabolic cooperation in cocultures of epidermal and 3T3 cells. *Biochem. Biophys. Res. Commun.,* 91:395–401.

30. Parsa, I., Marsh, W. H., and Sutton, A. L. (1980): An *in vitro* model of pancreas carcinogenesis. Two-stage MNU-TPA effect. *Am. J. Pathol.,* 98:649–662.

31. Pearlstein, E., Hynes, R. O., Franks, L. M., and Hennings, V. J. (1976): Surface proteins and fibrinolytic activity of cultured mammalian cells. *Cancer Res.,* 36:1,475–1,480.

• 32. Poiley, J. A., Raineri, R., and Pienta, R. J. (1979): Two-stage malignant transformation in hamster embryo cells. *Br. J. Cancer,* 39:8–14.

33. Ponten, J. (1976): The relationship between *in vitro* transformation and tumor formation *in vivo. Biochim Biophys. Acta,* 458:397–422.

34. Raick, A. N. (1973): Ultrastructural, histological, and biochemical alterations produced by TPA in mouse epidermis and their relevance to skin tumor promotion. *Cancer Res.,* 33:269–286.

35. San, R. H. C., Laspia, M. F., Soiefer, A. I., Maslansky, C. J., Rice, J. M., and Williams, G. M. (1979): A survey of growth in soft agar and cell surface properties as markers for transformation in adult rat liver epithelial-like cell cultures. *Cancer Res.,* 39:1,026–1,034.

36. Sivak, A., and van Duuren, B. L. (1967): Phenotypic expression of transformation: Induction in cell culture by a phorbol ester. *Science,* 157:1,443–1,444.

37. Slaga, T. J., Scribner, J. D., Thompson, S., and Viaje, A. (1976): Epidermal cell proliferation and promoting ability of phorbol esters. *J. Natl. Cancer Inst.,* 57:1,145–1,149.

38. Smets, L. A. (1979): Neoplastic transformation: The relevance of *in vitro* studies for the understanding of tumor pathogenesis and neoplastic growth. In: *Chromatin Structure and Function, Part B,* edited by C. A. Nicolini, pp. 683–703. Plenum Publishing Corporation, New York.

39. Steele, V. E., Marchock, A. C., and Nettesheim, P. (1978): Establishment of epithelial cell lines following exposure of cultured tracheal epithelium to 12-O-tetradecanoylphorbol-13-acetate. *Cancer Res.,* 38:3,563–3,565.

40. Thompson, L. H., Baker, R. M., Carrano, A. V., and Brookman, K. W. (1980): Failure of the phorbol ester 12-O-tetradecanoylphorbol-13-acetate to enhance sister chromatid exchange, mitotic segregation, or expression of mutations in chinese hamster cells. *Cancer Res.,* 40:3,245–3,251.

41. Trosko, J. E., Chang, C.-C., Yotti, L. P., and Chu, E. H. Y. (1977): Effect of phorbol myristate acetate on the recovery of spontaneous and ultraviolet light-induced 6-thioguanine and ouabain-resistant chinese hamster cells. *Cancer Res.,* 37:188–193.

42. Unkeless, J., Dano, K., Kellermann, G. M., and Reich, E. (1974): Fibrinolysis associated with oncogenic transformation. Partial purification and characterization of the cell factor, a plasminogen activator. *J. Biol. Chem.,* 249:4,295–4,305.

43. Vaheri, A., and Mosher, D. F. (1978): High molecular weight, cell surface-associated glycoprotein (fibronectin) lost in malignant transformation. *Biochim. Biophys. Acta,* 516:1–25.

44. Weinstein, I. B., Mufson, R. A., Lee, L. S., and Fisher, P. B. (1980): Membrane and other biochemical effects of the phorbol esters and their relevance to tumor promotion. In: *Carcinogenesis: Fundamental Mechanisms and Environmental Effects,* edited by B. Pullman, P. O. P. Ts'o, and H. Gelboin, pp. 543–563, D. Reidel Publishing Company.

45. Weinstein, I. B., Orenstein, J. M., Gebert, R., Kaighn, M. E., and Stadtler, U. C. (1975): Growth and structural properties of epithelial cell cultures established from normal rat liver and chemically induced hepatomas. *Cancer Res.,* 35:253–263.

46. Wigler, M., and Weinstein, I. B. (1976): Tumor promoter induces plasminogen activator. *Nature,* 259:232–233.

47. Wigley, C. B., and Summerhayes, I. C. (1979): Loss of LETS protein is not a marker for salivary gland or bladder epithelial cell transformation. *Exp. Cell Res.,* 118:394–398.

48. Worst, P. K. M., and Fusenig, N. E. (1976): Rücktransplantation epidermaler Mäusezellkulturen mit Ausbildung einer neuen Epidermis in syngenen und allogenen Empfängern. *Z. Immun. Forsch.,* 152:273–342.

49. Yamamoto, N., and zur Hausen, H. (1979): Tumour promoter TPA enhances transformation of human leukocytes by Epstein-Barr virus. *Nature,* 20:244–245.

50. Yang, N.-S., Kirkland, W., Jorgensen, T., and Furmanski, P. (1980): Absence of fibronectin and presence of plasminogen activator in both normal and malignant human mammary epithelial cells in culture. *J. Cell Biol.,* 84:120–130.

51. Yotti, L. P., Chang, C. C., and Trosko, J. E. (1979): Elimination of metabolic cooperation in Chinese hamster cells by a tumor promoter. *Science,* 206:1,089–1,091.

52. Yuspa, S. H., Ben, Th., Patterson, E., Michael, D., Elgjo, K., and Hennings, H. (1976): Stimulated DNA synthesis in mouse epidermal cell cultures treated with 12-O-tetradecanoylphorbol-13-acetate. *Cancer Res.,* 36:4,062–4,068.

Carcinogenesis, Vol. 7, edited by E. Hecker et al.
Raven Press, New York © 1982.

The Study of Tumor Promotion in a Cell Culture Model for Mouse Skin—A Tissue That Exhibits Multistage Carcinogenesis *In Vivo*

Stuart H. Yuspa, Henry Hennings, Molly Kulesz-Martin, and Ulrike Lichti

In Vitro *Pathogenesis Section, Laboratory of Experimental Pathology, National Cancer Institute, Bethesda, Maryland 20205*

If one studies a list of model systems where promotion or cocarcinogenesis has been demonstrated (19), it is clear that the phenomenon occurs in the epithelium of complex tissues. Most commonly, target epithelial cells are organized in a stratified or maturing arrangement, usually in a terminally differentiating lining epithelium. Is this by chance, is it due to inadequate studies in other tissues, or is it a fundamental requirement for a multistage mechanism? In mouse skin, basic biological observations have indicated that tissue complexity contributes to the multistage nature of the process of carcinogenesis. Table 1 outlines some biological observations derived from two-stage skin carcinogenesis experiments. It should be particularly noted that two-stage protocols with phorbol esters are most efficient at producing benign tumors and very inefficient at producing malignant tumors, although carcinomas ultimately arise from some papillomas even when promotion has long since been terminated (3,18,22). This is in contrast to repeated application of initiating agents that produce more carcinomas, often without an obvious precursor lesion (18). These facts are often overlooked in mechanistic studies relating to phorbol esters. A further finding not widely recognized is that multiple exposures to 12-O-tetradecanoyl-phorbol-13-acetate (TPA) in mouse skin result in increased sensitivity for certain responses such as ornithine decarboxylase (ODC) induction (14,15) and stimulation of deoxyribonucleic acid (DNA) synthesis (17). This observation suggests that selection of responsive cells may be occurring with multiple exposures.

Our laboratory has been using cultured mouse epidermal cells for a variety of studies relating to multistage carcinogenesis (25). For this chapter and that of Hennings et al. (*this volume*), we have focused on three specific questions of primary importance in understanding the process of tumor promotion. First, which cells in the complex structure of the epidermis are most responsive to tumor promoters? Second, do all responsive cells respond in the same way? And finally, what is the nature of the initiated cell? Clarification of this latter

TABLE 1. *Biology of skin tumor promotion*

(a) Requires initiated cells
(b) Primarily produces benign tumors
(c) Probably involves more than one mechanism
(d) Repeated exposures appear to select for cells with increased sensi-
    tivity for some responses
(e) Stable intermediate stages probably occur prior to tumor formation

point would seem to be a prerequisite to understanding the mechanism of tumor
promotion.

RESULTS AND DISCUSSION

The Epidermal Target Cell for Phorbol Esters

The versatility of our *in vitro* model has been enhanced recently by the finding
that growth of cell isolates from mouse epidermis in medium with reduced
ionic calcium concentration (0.02 to 0.09 mM) selects for the basal cell population
(8,9). The supporting data are summarized in Table 2 and are based on morphological, cell kinetic, and specific marker protein information. When the medium
calcium concentration of basal cell cultures is subsequently elevated to levels
found in most culture media (1.4 mM), proliferation ceases and terminal differentiation rapidly ensues with squamous differentiation and sloughing of cells occurring by 72 to 96 hr. This simple, physiological manipulation has been useful
in determining the identity of the target cell for phorbol esters.

The induction of the enzyme ODC has been a useful marker for responsiveness
to TPA in epidermis *in vivo* and *in vitro* (15,26). Induction of ODC was compared
in basal cells cultured under low calcium conditions and in cells plated under
standard calcium conditions that we know to be a mixture of basal and differentiating cells. The experimental details are presented in the chapter by Hennings
et al. (this volume). TPA causes a 2- to 10-fold greater induction of ODC in
basal cells than in cells plated under standard calcium conditions that are a
mixture of basal and differentiating cells. By various techniques we have ruled

TABLE 2. *Basal cell properties of keratinocytes cultured in*
0.02–0.09 mM calcium

(a) Basal cell morphology by light and electron microscopy
(b) High proliferation rate
(c) Growth fraction approaches 100%
(d) Synthesizes pemphigoid antigen but not pemphigus anti-
    gen
(e) Basal cell protein pattern by gel electrophoresis
 (f) Can be induced to terminally differentiate into squames
    by 1.4 mM calcium

out a direct effect of medium calcium concentration on inducibility of ODC (12) so that the most plausible explanation for these findings is the presence of a greater proportion of responsive cells under low calcium conditions. Cells grown under low calcium conditions maintain their responsiveness to TPA during prolonged culture time (12) whereas cells grown under standard calcium conditions that differentiate extensively during the first 6 days in culture rapidly lose the ability to respond (14). When cells grown under low calcium conditions are induced to differentiate by increasing the calcium concentration to 1.2 mM, responsiveness to TPA is rapidly lost, so that by 6 hr cells are only marginally responsive (Hennings et al., *this volume*). Even when the treatment with TPA is simultaneous with the switch to high calcium medium, there is already a substantial reduction in ODC inducibility (Hennings et al., this volume). The enhanced responsiveness to ODC induction in basal cell cultures coupled with the rapid decline in responsiveness following induced differentiation indicate that only basal cells are responsive to this aspect of TPA exposure. The mechanisms controlling responsiveness of basal cells and the loss of responsiveness with terminal differentiation remain to be elucidated. Since we know that differentiating cells are capable of an ODC response by other stimuli (12), an obvious site of regulation for TPA insensitivity would be at the level of the phorbol ester receptor. Studies to define receptor differences are currently in progress.

Heterogeneity of Response Among Basal Cells

Early in our studies on the induction of ODC in keratinocytes under standard culture conditions, we had reported that exposure to weak promoters induced ODC activity with a peak at 3 hr whereas peak activity after exposure to strong promoters was at 9 hr (14). We had suggested that this was due to subpopulations of keratinocytes with different sensitivities to phorbol esters. A similar conclusion was made concerning the stimulation of DNA synthesis induced by phorbol esters in keratinocytes (27). This question was reexplored with basal cell populations. Figure 1 indicates the time of peak ODC activity for basal cells treated with different concentrations of TPA. TPA exposure at 1 ng/ml produces a maximum ODC induction at 3 hr after the start of treatment, and higher doses actualy inhibit this peak. Treatment with 100 ng or more gives maximum induction at 9 hr. These results are consistent with the presence of at least two populations of cells, a particularly sensitive population with peak ODC activity at 3 hr after exposure that seems to be inhibited at higher doses and a less sensitive population with later peak activity.

Other data support the idea of divergence of responses among basal cell subpopulations. Basal cell cultures are composed of a monolayer of relatively uniform polygonal cells with a few round, floating cells that we know have undergone a form of terminal differentiation that occurs in low calcium medium (8,9). When such cultures are exposed to TPA, morphological changes result in a more or less equal mixture of rounded cells, or cells in the process of

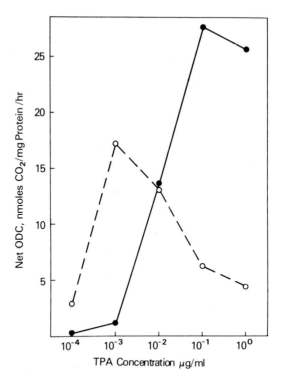

FIG. 1. Kinetics of ODC response in epidermal basal cells exposed to TPA. Cells grown in medium containing 0.09 mM calcium were treated with the indicated concentrations of TPA, and ODC activity was determined at 3 hr and 9 hr after the start of TPA treatment. Each point represents the average of duplicate determinations on duplicate dishes that varied by $< \pm 10\%$. (○----○): 3 hr after TPA; (●----●): 9 hr after TPA.

rounding that eventually detach from the monolayer, and attached polygonal cells that look relatively unaffected by TPA. Thus, within the same population, morphological variability is easily documented. This result was reminiscent of a paradox we had reported in our earlier work. Epidermal keratins studied by polyacrylamide gel electrophoresis shifted from a basal cell to a stratum corneum pattern within 12 to 24 hr of exposure to TPA (21). A late effect of TPA in these same cell cultures, however, was to inhibit the natural process of terminal differentiation that occurred during the first week *in vitro* (27). Thus it appeared from earlier studies that TPA had both accelerating and inhibitory effects on keratinocyte differentiation.

In order to clarify these observations, the effect of TPA on basal cell differentiation was studied through the enzyme epidermal transglutaminase. This cross-linking enzyme plays an integral part in epidermal differentiation by catalyzing the formation of the cornified envelope (4). High enzyme activity is characteristic of differentiated cells whereas basal cells have very low activity. In basal cell cultures (0.02 to 0.09 mM Ca^{2+}), transglutaminase activity can be increased by inducing differentiation through elevation of the calcium concentration in culture medium to 1.2 to 1.4 mM. Figure 2 indicates that transglutaminase activity increases in basal cell cultures exposed to TPA after a lag of 6 to 8 hr. Peak activity increases of three- to fivefold occur generally 12 to 14 hr after TPA exposure commences and returns toward basal levels by 24 to 72 hr. This activity increase is inhibited by either actinomycin D or cycloheximide at doses that inhibit ribonucleic acid (RNA) or protein synthesis by more than 95% (23). TPA does not directly activate the enzyme when added to cell lysates, and other promoting phorbol esters and mezerine are also active in inducing transglutaminase, whereas nonpromoting analogues are ineffective (23). Combined with the morphological data, these observations suggested that at least a portion of the epidermal basal cell population, presumably that represented by the rounding cells, could be induced to differentiate by TPA. But what about the other population that was morphologically unaffected? These cells

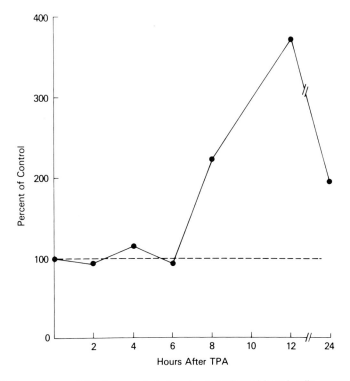

FIG. 2. Epidermal transglutaminase activity in mouse epidermal basal cells exposed to TPA. Epidermal cells were grown for 6 days in 0.02 mM Ca^{2+} medium and exposed to TPA (0.01 μg/ml) or dimethylsulfoxide solvent (0.1% DMSO). Samples were removed at intervals for transglutaminase assay (23). Control samples varied little during the 24-hr period and values were approximately 1–1.5 cpm/mg protein/10 min ($\times 10^{-3}$) whereas peak TPA-induced activity (●----●) was 4.5 cpm/mg protein/10 min ($\times 10^{-3}$).

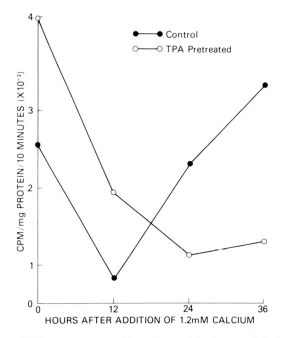

FIG. 3. The effect of TPA exposure on epidermal transglutaminase activity induced by calcium. Epidermal cells were grown in 0.02 mM calcium medium for 6 days and exposed to 0.01 μg/ml TPA or 0.1% DMSO for 72 hr. Cultures were then switched to medium with 1.2 mM calcium and transglutaminase activity was monitored for an additional 36 hr. Each point represents duplicate samples that varied by $< \pm 10\%$.

appeared to be resistant to TPA-induced differentiation. It was possible, in fact, that TPA exposure made these cells resistant to differentiation. To test this idea, basal cells previously treated with TPA for 72 hr and thus representing the morphologically unchanged population were stimulated to differentiate by increasing their extracellular calcium levels, a treatment that would normally increase transglutaminase activity. As seen in Fig. 3, transglutaminase activity did not increase in this population when induced by elevating calcium in culture medium. In untreated controls, transglutaminase activity increased as expected. Taken together, these results indicate that TPA can induce subpopulations of epidermal basal cells to differentiate or can prevent some basal cells from undergoing differentiation by physiological stimuli. This heterogeneity in response within the same tissue could form the basis for the promoting activity of phorbol esters and other agents. The realization that within the same tissue, subsets of target cells can respond differently, might serve to clarify seemingly disparate reports when cell lines are exposed to phorbol esters.

The Biological Nature of Initiation

In order to extrapolate experimental results in phorbol ester research to a mechanism of tumor promotion, we must first begin to understand the nature of the initiated cell. Our laboratory has developed a model system which we believe may help in resolving this problem (11,29). In carcinogenesis in a terminally differentiating tissue, an alteration in terminal differentiation must accompany tumorigenesis. Thus it seemed reasonable that if basal cells were treated with a carcinogen, clones of cells resistant to terminal differentiation could be induced. Such cells would be expected to represent an early obligatory stage in transformation, perhaps initiation. Furthermore, we would expect that if differentiation were induced in the entire basal cell population, normal cells would cease to proliferate and would die while carcinogen-altered cells might continue to proliferate and form countable foci. Thus a protocol evolved in which basal cells grown in 0.02 mM Ca^{2+} medium were exposed briefly to carcinogen and maintained under low calcium conditions for sufficient time to allow clonal expansion of altered colonies. Colonies, however, would not be distinguished under these culture conditions. Differentiation was then induced by 1.2 mM calcium medium, leading to sloughing of normal cells from the culture dish; the colonies that continued to proliferate under these conditions were selected.

Culture dishes were ultimately fixed and the colonies were counted after staining with rhodamine to identify their epidermal origin (11,29). Figure 4 shows characteristic results from such experiments. In control dishes, no or very few small countable foci survive an induced differentiation. The number of surviving control colonies increases with longer times under low calcium growth prior to selection, indicating that a finite level of spontaneous changes can occur within the basal cell population *in vitro*. Carcinogen treatment causes a substantial increase in the number (and size) of altered foci. In numerous experiments this increase has ranged between 4- and 30-fold. The increase in colony number is dependent on the dose of carcinogen, as can be seen in Table 3, for the two carcinogens N-methyl-N'-nitro-N-nitrosoguanidine (MNNG) and 7,12-dimethylbenz[a]anthracene (DMBA). The colonies that evolve are epidermal in morphology and undergo a vertical stratification process similar to normal cells. What is distinctive about these colonies is that they continue to proliferate under conditions favoring terminal differentiation and form a new population balance in which cell renewal exceeds cell death. We have isolated cell lines from a number of such colonies and found none to be tumorigenic; nor do any grow in soft agar. All lines can be subpassaged. Studies in progress suggest that prolonged subculture ($\geq$ 10 additional passages) leads to progression of some lines to a tumorigenic cell type producing squamous cell carcinomas upon reinjection to nude mice.

To test the validity of the selection procedure for neoplasia, we have used epidermal cell lines, termed Pam lines, that are tumorigenic but that have retained epidermal specific functions and appear morphologically similar to cells derived from altered colonies in the differentiation assay (24). We wondered if these cells could be selected in experiments using a protocol similar to the differentiation assay. Pam cells were mixed with normal basal cells in 0.02 mM Ca^{2+} medium at a ratio of $100 : 2 \times 10^6$. Controls were plated at 2×10^6 without

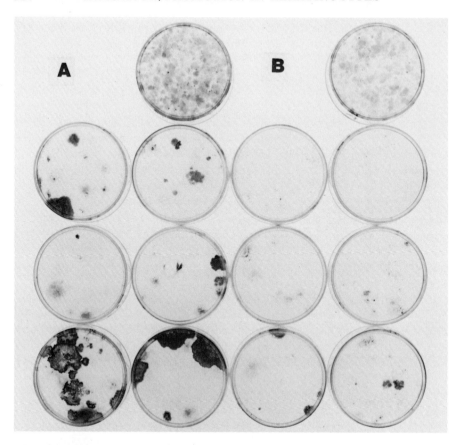

FIG. 4. Rhodamine-positive colonies resistant to differentiation after selection by high calcium medium. Epidermal cells were plated in 0.02 mM calcium medium and treated on day 3 with **(A)** 1.5 μg/ml MNNG × 1 hr or **(B)** 0.1% ethanol × 1 hr. After 5 additional weeks in low calcium medium, differentiation was induced by growth in 1.4 mM calcium for 4 weeks. Cultures were fixed in 10% formalin and stained with 1% rhodamine B. Carcinogen treatment results in many more surviving epidermal colonies (11). Single dish at top of **A** or **B** shows cell density by Giemsa staining at time just prior to selection with 1.4 mM calcium.

Pam cells. Two weeks later, cells were switched to a high calcium medium, and were stained with rhodamine after several more weeks. In these experiments, only cultures containing Pam cells demonstrated colonies. Thus a selection for differentiation variants seems a valid technique for recognizing transformants in a mixed population of normal and malignant epidermal cells.

Is this alteration in differentiation characteristic of initiation? This is a difficult but appropriate question. We have initiated mouse dorsal skin *in vivo* with a single application of DMBA (25 μg) and 6 weeks later placed the epidermal cells in low calcium culture in parallel with epidermal cells of control mice. After 11 weeks without further treatment, differentiation was induced by increasing calcium; 4 weeks later cultures were fixed and stained with rhodamine. In

TABLE 3. *Quantitation of epidermal colonies stained with rhodamine after switch from low to high calcium culture*

Experiment[a]		Treatment	Plates (+)/ total plates (%)		Corrected[b] colonies/ plate
6 weeks low Ca^{2+}	Control	(0.2% acetone × 24 hr)	8/18	(44%)	0.9
8 × 10^5 cells/35-mm dish	DMBA	(0.04 ng/ml × 24 hr)	5/12	(42%)	0.9
	DMBA	(0.4 ng/ml × 24 hr)	8/12	(67%)	1.3
	DMBA	(4 ng/ml × 24 hr)	13/15	(87%)	3.8
	DMBA	(20 ng/ml × 24 hr)	8/12	(67%)	3.0
	DMBA	(100 ng/ml × 24 hr)	5/12	(42%)	1.4
6 weeks low Ca^{2+}	Control	(0.2% acetone × 1 hr)	2/14	(14%)	0.3
8 × 10^5 cells/35-mm dish	MNNG	(0.1 μg/ml × 1 hr)	7/16	(44%)	1.4
	MNNG	(0.2 μg/ml × 1 hr)	9/17	(53%)	2.2
	MNNG	(0.5 μg/ml × 1 hr)	10/15	(67%)	4.5
5 weeks low Ca^{2+}	Control	(0.2% ethanol × 1 hr)	1/8	(13%)	0.3
4 × 10^6 cells/60-mm dish	MNNG	(1.5 μg/ml × 1 hr)	6/8	(75%)	5.4

[a] Balb/c newborn epidermal cells were plated at the indicated density in medium containing 0.02 mM calcium. Three days after plating, cultures were exposed to carcinogen or solvent as described in column 2. After an additional 7–10 days, several dishes in each group were used for cell counts to determine carcinogen-induced cytotoxicity and establish a survival index relative to controls. The remaining dishes were maintained for an additional 4–5 weeks in 0.02 mM calcium and then switched to a medium containing 1.4 mM calcium for 4 weeks. Plates were fixed in 10% formalin, stained with 1% rhodamine B, and the number of surviving colonies counted. For more details see Kulesz-Martin et al. (11).

[b] Corrected colonies/plate = total colonies/plate × 1/survival index.

cultures derived from control mice, very few colonies (2 colonies in 99 dishes) were present, whereas in most dishes from treated mice, multiple colonies persisted and were expanding (30). All colonies had the identical morphological characteristics as those selected in the *in vitro* assay, but biological properties have not yet been documented. Nevertheless these results are consistent with the idea that initiation is characterized by a fundamental alteration in the program of differentiation that allows initiated cells to continue to proliferate under conditions where normal cells are obligated to differentiate.

SUMMARY AND SPECULATION

Can we now attempt to consolidate all of this data derived from *in vitro* and *in vivo* studies on the epidermis into a scheme that might reflect the biological events in multistage carcinogenesis? Since two-stage skin carcinogenesis results primarily in benign tumors, the proposal should be restricted to the formation of papillomas. In reviewing *in vivo* data, we would predict that additional, probably different, and perhaps randomly determined (that is promoter-independent) events are required for subsequent malignant change.

In order to establish a working hypothesis, we must first consider the dynamics of normal epidermis, as shown in Fig. 5. Several assumptions, more or less based on experimental data, must be accepted. Normal epidermis is composed of three keratinocyte categories: (a) stem cells mainly located in the neck of the hair follicle that differentiate into basal cells; (b) interfollicular basal cells that become committed to mature; and (c) maturing cells. Once a basal cell leaves the basement membrane area, either actively or passively, it is committed to mature and to die. In normal skin, agents that produce chemical hyperplasia, such as promoters, induce terminal differentiation in some of the basal cells, indicated as the induced committed cell in Fig. 5. Other basal cells and stem

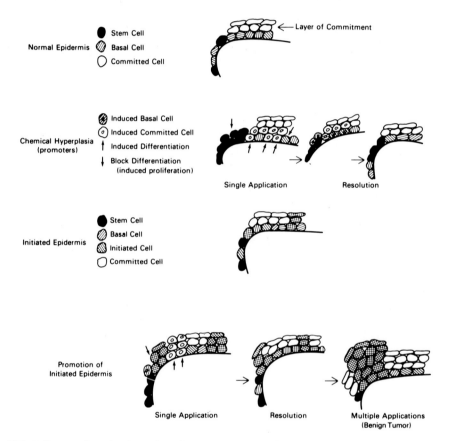

FIG. 5. Proposed mechanism of papilloma induction by promoters. In normal skin, maturation of basal and stem cells is strongly regulated by location on the basement membrane, and commitment to differentiate is inescapable in the upper layers. In initiated skin, cells with an altered commitment to differentiate (the initiated cells) reside within the basal or stem cell populations. Promoters induce a regenerative hyperplasia because they can both stimulate and inhibit basal cell differentiation in separate target cells. This allows a repopulation of vacated basal cell sites by initiated cells. Since such cells can continue to proliferate in the layers of commitment, their clone size increases until they are recognized as a benign tumor. Subsequent malignant change may be independent of promoter action.

cells are stimulated to proliferate by the same promoter treatment. Stem cell progeny that leave the basement membrane area as a result of promoter stimulation become committed as basal cells (induced basal cell in Fig. 5) and repopulate the basal area in conjunction with other proliferating basal cells. TPA is particularly good at producing this heterogenous response, whereas other hyperplastic agents that are not promoting, or are only weakly so, are effective at producing only proliferation (without differentiation) or producing differentiation (or cytotoxicity) indiscriminately (including initiated cells). The induction of both differentiation and proliferation results in a process similar to regeneration, in that repopulation of the basal cell area is required because of loss of basal cells through induced terminal differentiation. Regeneration is accomplished both by migration of induced (from stem cells) basal cells and by proliferation of subpopulations of basal cells stimulated by the promoter (Fig. 5). Although maturation is transiently blocked in cells stimulated to proliferate, integrity of commitment to differentiate in the upper layers is intact and balance is ultimately restored.

In initiated skin, a new cell type is introduced—the initiated cell that has an inherent alteration in its program of commitment and is derived from a basal or stem cell. Initiated cells continue to express differentiative functions including terminal differentiation but have the potential to bypass normal regulatory processes in the layer of commitment (Fig. 5). The phenotypic alteration is not expressed under normal circumstances, since the population dynamics are such that surrounding normal cells maintain control over their own domains thereby limiting space for expansion in the upper layers. When such epidermis is promoted, initiated cells, along with other stem and basal cells, assume the repopulation function and fill areas left vacant by induced committed cells. At resolution, a new balance is achieved in which initiated cells occupy several domains in the basal and committed levels. Repetition of these exposures results first in a miniclone of initiated cells in which proliferative functions are maintained in the layers of commitment (16). Ultimately a benign tumor, with multiple proliferative layers, can result. Continued promoter exposure is required to maintain most tumors, particularly when they are small, since these clones of initiated cells maintain partial differentiative capacity (11) and might regress without the proliferative and antidifferentiative stimuli provided by promoters. In the case where regression occurs, one might expect a balance to be achieved above the layer of commitment where small clones of initiated cells would continue to proliferate. Such "microtumors" have been reported in skin previously containing papillomas that were allowed to regress (2).

While this working hypothesis requires several assumptions, it is consistent with the biological observations in skin carcinogenesis *in vivo* and *in vitro* and addresses the known biological activity of phorbol esters in skin. Such a scheme provides rational approaches to more molecular studies on promoter action and allows certain predictions relating to skin carcinogenesis. Since benign tumors would be clonal expansions of initiated cells, such tumors must be monoclonal. Studies on chimeric mice have shown this to be true (10). Stimulation of growth and migration of specific epidermal cell types should be apparent after promoter exposure. Dark cells may represent one such cell type, perhaps the stem cell (16). The phenotype of the initiated cells, of early benign growths (miniclones), and of the final papillomas should be the same. Although this is not known for skin, studies in liver carcinogenesis have indicated that the distribution of preneoplastic phenotypes does not change during prolonged promotion with phenobarbital (Pitot et al., *this volume*). This model suggests that population redistribution is essential to promotion and predicts that other techniques to produce such a change will act as promoting stimuli. In this regard, wounding (7) and skin abrasion (1) are promoting influences in skin. In contrast, a purely hyperplastic stimulus that does not involve regeneration, such as skin massage, is not a promoting influence (6). This model also predicts that agents that interfere with either the differentiative or proliferative effects of phorbol esters will inhibit promotion. Antipromoting steroids are potent inhibitors of TPA-induced proliferation (13) and retinoids are known to alter epidermal differentiation (28). One might also expect that a critical element in promotion would be the early escape of initiated cells from the confines of neighboring normal cells to form a miniclone less subject to the negative regulation of its surroundings. TPA may be particularly effective in this regard, whereas other agents such as mezerine are less effective or are particularly damaging to initiated cells. Once a miniclone is established, other agents can complete the clonal expansion. This would explain the apparent multistage nature of promotion (20).

In summary, this scheme suggests that the primary effect of initiators is to alter the normal differentiative commitment of the epidermal basal or stem cells. Promoters then act on both initiated and surrounding normal cells to redistribute subpopulations as in regenerative hyperplasia. This results in benign tumors. Individual cells in a papilloma then may undergo a subsequent change, perhaps a random genetic event (recombination, amplification, or mutation), that results in a malignant cell. The high proportion of proliferating cells, concentrated in the papilloma, makes this latter event more likely to occur in that lesion (5). That last step is likely to be independent of promoter action in mouse skin.

REFERENCES

1. Argyris, T. S. (1980): Tumor promotion by abrasion-induced epidermal hyperplasia in the skin of mice. *J. Invest. Dermatol.,* 75:360–362.
2. Burns, F. J., Vanderlaan, M., Sivak, A., and Albert, R. A. (1976): Regression kinetics of mouse skin papillomas. *Cancer Res.,* 36:1,422–1,427.
3. Burns, F. J., Vanderlaan, M., Snyder, E., and Albert, R. E. (1978): Induction and progression kinetics of mouse skin papillomas. In: *Mechanisms of Tumor Promotion and Cocarcinogenesis,* edited by T. J. Slaga, A. Sivak, and R. K. Boutwell, pp. 81–96. Raven Press, New York.
4. Buxman, M. M., and Weupper, K. D. (1975): Keratin cross-linking and epidermal transglutaminase. *J. Invest. Dermatol.,* 65:107–112.

5. Cairns, J. (1975): Mutation selection and the natural history of cancer. *Nature,* 255:197–200.
6. Clark-Lewis, I., and Murray, A. W. (1978): Tumor promotion and the induction of epidermal ornithine decarboxylase activity in mechanically stimulated mouse skin. *Cancer Res.,* 38:494–497.
7. Hennings, H., and Boutwell, R. K. (1970): Studies on the mechanism of skin tumor promotion. *Cancer Res.,* 30:312–320.
8. Hennings, H., Holbrook, K., Steinert, P., and Yuspa, S. H. (1980): Growth and differentiation of mouse epidermal cells in culture: Effects of extracellular calcium. In: *Biochemistry of Normal and Abnormal Epidermal Differentiation,* edited by I. A. Bernstein and M. Seiji, pp. 3–22. University of Tokyo Press, Tokyo.
9. Hennings, H., Michael, D., Cheng, C., Steinert, P., Holbrook, K., and Yuspa, S. H. (1980): Calcium regulation of growth and differentiation of mouse epidermal cells in culture. *Cell,* 19:245–254.
10. Iannaccone, P. M., Gardner, R. L., and Harris, H. (1978): The cellular origin of chemically induced tumors. *J. Cell Sci.,* 29:249–269.
11. Kulesz-Martin, M., Koehler, B., Hennings, H., and Yuspa, S. H. (1980): Quantitative assay for carcinogen-altered differentiation in mouse epidermal cells. *Carcinogenesis,* 1:995–1,006.
12. Lichti, U., Patterson, E., Hennings, H., and Yuspa, S. H. (1981): The tumor promoter 12-O-tetradecanoylphorbol-13-acetate induces ornithine decarboxylase in proliferating basal cells but not in differentiating cells from mouse epidermis. *J. Cell Physiol.,* 107:261–270.
13. Lichti, U., Slaga, T. J., Ben, T., Patterson, E., Hennings, H., and Yuspa, S. H. (1977): Dissociation of tumor promoter stimulated ornithine decarboxylase activity and DNA synthesis in mouse epidermis *in vivo* and *in vitro* by fluocinolone acetonide, a tumor-promotion inhibitor. *Proc. Natl. Acad. Sci. USA,* 74:3,908–3,912.
14. Lichti, U., Yuspa, S. H., and Hennings, H. (1978): Ornithine and s-adenosylmethionine decarboxylases in mouse epidermal cell cultures treated with tumor promoters. In: *Mechanisms of Tumor Promotion and Cocarcinogenesis,* edited by T. J. Slaga, A. Sivak, and R. K. Boutwell, pp. 221–232. Raven Press, New York.
15. O'Brien, T. G. (1976): The induction of ornithine decarboxylase as an early, possibly obligatory, event in mouse skin carcinogenesis. *Cancer Res.,* 36:2,644–2,653.
16. Raick, A. N. (1974): Cell differentiation and tumor-promoting action in skin carcinogenesis. *Cancer Res.,* 34:2,915–2,925.
17. Raick, A. N., Thumm, K., and Chivers, B. R. (1972): Early effects of 12-O-tetradecanoylphorbol-13-acetate on the incorporation of tritiated precursor into DNA, and the thickness of the interfollicular epidermis, and their relation to tumor promotion in mouse skin. *Cancer Res.,* 32:1,562–1,568.
18. Saffiotti, U., and Shubik, P. (1956): The effects of low concentrations of carcinogen in epidermal carcinogenesis. A comparison with promoting agents. *J. Natl. Cancer Inst.,* 16:961–969.
19. Sivak, A. (1978): Mechanisms of tumor promotion and cocarcinogenesis: A summary from one point of view. In: *Mechanisms of Tumor Promotion and Cocarcinogenesis,* edited by T. J. Slaga, A. Sivak, and R. K. Boutwell, pp. 553–564. Raven Press, New York.
20. Slaga, T. J., Fisher, S. M., Nelson, K., and Gleason, G. L. (1980): Studies on the mechanism of skin tumor promotion: Evidence for several stages in promotion. *Proc. Natl. Acad. Sci. USA,* 77:3,659–3,663.
21. Steinert, P., and Yuspa, S. H. (1978): Biochemical evidence for keratinization by mouse epidermal cells in culture. *Science,* 200:1,491–1,493.
22. Verma, A. K., and Boutwell, R. K. (1980): Effects of dose and duration of treatment with the tumor promoting agent, 12-O-tetradecanoylphorbol-13-acetate on mouse skin carcinogenesis. *Carcinogenesis,* 1:271–276.
23. Yuspa, S. H., Ben, T. B., Hennings, H., and Lichti, U. (1980): Phorbol ester tumor promoters induce epidermal transglutaminase activity. *Biochem. Biophys. Res. Commun.,* 97:700–708.
24. Yuspa, S. H., Hawley-Nelson, P., Koehler, B., and Stanley, J. R. (1980): A survey of transformation markers in differentiating epidermal cell lines in culture. *Cancer Res.,* 40:4,694–4,703.
25. Yuspa, S. H., Hawley-Nelson, P., Stanley, J. R., and Hennings, H. (1980): Epidermal cell culture. *Transplant. Proc.,* 12:114–122.
26. Yuspa, S. H., Lichti, U., Ben, T., Patterson, E., Hennings, H., Slaga, T. J., Colburn, N., and Kelsey, W. (1976): Phorbol esters stimulate DNA synthesis and ornithine decarboxylase activity in mouse epidermal cell cultures. *Nature,* 262:402–404.

27. Yuspa, S. H., Lichti, U., Ben, T., Patterson, E., Michael, D., Elgjo, K., and Hennings, H. (1976): Stimulated DNA synthesis in mouse epidermal cell cultures treated with 12-O-tetradeca-noylphorbol-13-acetate. *Cancer Res.,* 36:4,062–4,068.
28. Yuspa, S. H., Lichti, U., and Hennings, H. (1981): Modulation of terminal differentiation and tumor promotion by retinoids in mouse epidermal cell cultures. *Ann. N.Y. Acad. Sci.,* 359:260–273.
29. Yuspa, S. H., Lichti, U., Morgan, D., and Hennings, H. (1980): Chemical carcinogenesis studies in mouse epidermal cell cultures. In: *Biochemistry of Normal and Abnormal Epidermal Differenti-ation,* edited by I. A. Bernstein and M. Seiji, pp. 173–190. University of Tokyo Press, Tokyo.
30. Yupsa, S. H., and Morgan, D. L. (1981): Mouse skin cells resistant to terminal differentiation associated with initiation of carcinogenesis. *Nature,* 293:72–74.

Carcinogenesis, Vol. 7, edited by E. Hecker et al.
Raven Press, New York © 1982.

The Role of Mitogenic Stimulation and Specific Glycoprotein Changes in the Mechanism of Late-Stage Promotion in JB-6 Epidermal Cell Lines

Nancy H. Colburn, L. David Dion, and Edmund J. Wendel

Laboratory of Viral Carcinogenesis, National Cancer Institute, Frederick Cancer Research Center, Frederick, Maryland 21701

We have recently described the JB-6 epidermal cell (3,6) model which is being used for studying the mechanism of late-stage promotion. The JB-6 cells respond to phorbol (3) and nonphorbol (4) tumor promoters with a shift to anchorage independence and tumorigenicity (2,3). This promotion of tumor cell phenotype occurs irreversibly (3) by a mechanism that appears to involve induction of a new phenotype rather than selection of preexisting variants (2). Whether late-stage promotion requires promoter-dependent mitogenic stimulation, specific enzyme induction, gene rearrangements, or specific changes in cellular glycoconjugate synthesis is the subject of current studies in our laboratory. The studies reported here suggest that promotion of anchorage independence in JB-6 cells does not involve a "release from growth restraint" type of mitogenesis, but may involve specific changes in glycoprotein synthesis.

LACK OF REQUIREMENT FOR MITOGENIC STIMULATION

Although promoters as a class are mitogenic, the issue of whether any or all stages of tumor promotion require promoter-dependent mitogenesis has been unresolved. Recent findings in our laboratory (Colburn and Ozanne, *unpublished data*) have indicated that promotion of anchorage independence during monolayer exposure to 12-O-tetradecanoylphorbol-13-acetate (TPA) occurs without "release-from-stationary-phase" mitogenesis by TPA. In order to further verify these findings, promotable JB-6 clonal derivatives were selected for resistance to resting phase mitogenic stimulation by TPA. A mitogenic stimulation requirement for late-stage promotion would predict that such mitogen-resistant variants should also become nonpromotable.

The selection for mitogen resistance (7) was carried out by a procedure similar to that described by Pruss and Herschman (9) which involves treating JB-6 C141 cells (4) at plateau density with colchicine (0.12 μg/ml) and TPA (10 ng/ml) in medium containing 5% fetal bovine serum. These cells undergo a twofold increase in plateau density in response to TPA alone, but in the

TABLE 1. *Resistance of epidermal cell variants to mitogenic stimulation by TPA[a]*

	Plateau cell density (number cells/25-cm² flask × 10⁻⁶)				
		TPA			10% Serum
Cell line	DMSO	1 ng/ml	10 ng/ml	100 ng/ml	control
R24	1.3	ND[b]	1.3	ND	2.8
R219	2.8	2.4	2.3	2.6	3.3
R6101	5.2	4.8	5.2	5.0	7.0

[a] Cells were allowed to reach plateau density in minimal essential medium (MEM) containing 5% fetal bovine serum. At plateau, the same medium without or with TPA (in 0.1% dimethylsulfoxide, DMSO) at indicated concentrations or medium containing 10% serum was added and changed daily.
[b] ND, Not determined.

presence of colchicine the responders are killed. The nonresponders were recovered and the colchicine selection was repeated for a total of six cycles. At the end of six selections, the cells showed 25% of the original mitogenic response to TPA (data not shown). The selected cells were cloned in order to seek lines showing zero mitogenic response. Several nonresponders were obtained. Three such mitogen-resistant cell lines are shown in Table 1. All three failed to show a plateau density mitogenic stimulation response to TPA at concentrations from

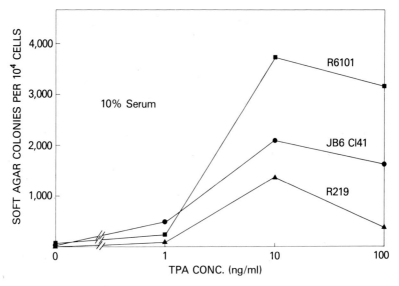

FIG. 1. Promotability of mitogen-resistant variants. Cells were suspended in 0.33% agar medium containing 10% serum and TPA or solvent alone and scored for colony formation as described (3,6).

1 to 100 ng/ml, the concentration range effective in promotion of anchorage independence. That the failure to respond was due to a specific lack of response to TPA and not to a general inability to reach a higher density was demonstrated by the capacity of these three cell lines to reach a higher plateau density after a shift to 10% serum.

These mitogen-resistant cell lines were then tested for "promotability" in 0.33% agar. R24 turned out to be anchorage independent, a not unexpected result in view of the prolonged exposure to TPA experienced by these promotable cells during the selection. As shown in Fig. 1, lines R219 and R6101 were promotable to anchorage independence by 1 to 100 ng/ml TPA, with R219 showing a lower promotion response and R6101 a higher promotion response than the parent line JB-6 C141. These results therefore suggest a lack of requirement for a "release from growth arrest" type of promoter-dependent mitogenesis in late-stage promotion.

POSSIBLE INVOLVEMENT OF A DECREASE IN A 180,000 MW GLYCOPROTEIN

In order to further investigate the possibility of an inducible or repressible molecular event that might be required for late-stage promotion, and since various changes in fibronectin and other glycoprotein synthesis have been found to occur in response to tumor promoters (1), the effect of TPA on glycoprotein synthesis in promotable JB-6 cells was studied. As shown in Fig. 2, cellular glycoprotein synthesis was followed by incorporation of labeled sugars, in this case, 2-^{3}H-mannose, followed by sodium dodecyl sulfate-polyacrylamide gel electrophoresis (SDS-PAGE), and radioautography of the gels. Lanes 3 and 6 indicate that 80 hr of exposure to TPA produced a relatively specific decrease in terminal 8-hr ^{3}H-mannose or ^{3}H-leucine incorporation into a 180,000 MW glycoprotein. This decrease was apparent from 4 to 80 hr post-TPA exposure and occurred in response to 1 to 100 ng/ml concentrations of TPA, the effective promoting range (8). As one approach to investigating the relevance of this change to promotion of tumor cell phenotype, we made use of the previously published observation (4,5) that promotion of anchorage independence can be inhibited by simultaneous exposure to the antipromoter retinoic acid. As shown in Fig. 2, lanes 2 and 5, retinoic acid produced an increased synthesis of the glycoprotein-180 in JB-6 cells and, in combination with TPA, antagonized the promoter effect (lanes 4 and 8). This glycoprotein-180 has been identified as procollagen (8). Decreased procollagen synthesis may therefore play a role in late-stage promotion and may be a target of antipromoting retinoids.

CONCLUSION AND SUMMARY

Studies with the JB-6 model system for late-stage promotion of tumor cell phenotype indicate that the mechanism occurs by induction of events that do

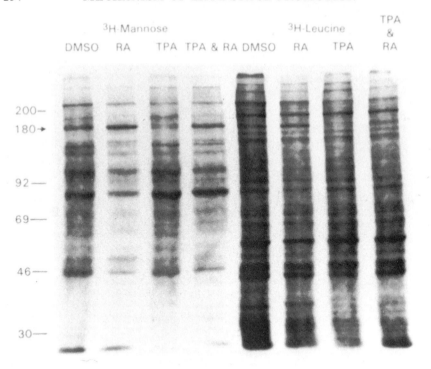

FIG. 2. Antagonistic effects of promoter and antipromoter on the synthesis of a 180,000 MW glycoprotein. JB-6 cells in logarithmic phase were exposed to TPA (10 ng/ml), retinoic acid (10^{-6} M), or both for 80 hr. During the terminal 8 hr, cells were incubated with 2-^{3}H-mannose. SDS-PAGE was carried out on 7.5% gels.

not require promoter-dependent mitogenic stimulation, since some of the mitogen-resistant variants derived from a promotable clone of JB-6 cells were still promotable to anchorage independence. Whether earlier stages of promotion require mitogenesis by the promoter is unanswered by these experiments. However, studies of Peraino et al. on liver promotion, Marks et al. on skin promotion, and Little et al. on $10T_{1/2}$ cell promotion *(this volume)* suggest a lack of requirement for hyperplasia in promotion.

One of the events required for late-stage promotion may be a "switching off" of a 180,000 MW glycoprotein identified as procollagen. The sensitivity of this change to the antipromoter retinoic acid suggests its possible significance.

REFERENCES

1. Colburn, N. H. (1980a): Tumor promotion and preneoplastic progression. In: *Carcinogenesis, Vol. 5: Modifiers of Carcinogenesis,* edited by T. J. Slaga, pp. 33–56. Raven Press, New York.
2. Colburn, N. H. (1980b): Tumor promoter produces anchorage independence in mouse epidermal cells by an induction mechanism. *Carcinogenesis,* 1:951–954.

3. Colburn, N. H., Former, B. F., Nelson, K. A., and Yuspa, S. H. (1979): Tumor promoter induces anchorage independence irreversibly. *Nature,* 281:589–591.
4. Colburn, N. H., Koehler, B., and Nelson, K. A. (1980): A cell culture assay for tumor promoter-dependent progression toward neoplastic phenotype: Detection of tumor promoters and promotion inhibitors. *Teratogenesis, Carcinogenesis, Mutagenesis,* 1:87–96.
5. Colburn, N. H., Ozanne, S., Licht, U., Ben, T., Yuspa, S. H., Wendel, E., Jardini, E., and Abruzzo, G. (1981): Retinoids inhibit promoter-dependent preneoplastic progression in mouse epidermal cell lines. *Ann. N. Y. Acad. Sci.,* 359:251–259.
6. Colburn, N. H., Vorderbruegge, W. F., Bates, J. R., Gray, R. H., Rossen, J. D., Kelsey, W. H., and Shimada, T. (1978): Correlation of anchorage-independent growth with tumorigenicity of chemically transformed mouse epidermal cells. *Cancer Res.,* 38:624–634.
7. Colburn, N. H., Wendel, E. J., Abruzzo, G. (1981): Dissociation of mitogenesis and late stage promotion of tumor cell phenotype by phorbol esters: Mitogen resistant variants are sensitive to promotion. *Proc. Natl. Acad. Sci. USA,* 78(11).
8. Dion, L. D., DeLuca, L. M., and Colburn, N. H. (1981): Phorbol ester-induced anchorage independence and its antagonism by retinoic acid correlates with altered expression of specific glycoproteins. *Carcinogenesis* 2(10).
9. Pruss, R. M., and Herschman, H. R. (1977): Variants of 3T3 cells lacking mitogenic response to epidermal growth factor. *Proc. Natl. Acad. Sci. USA,* 74:3,918–3,921.

Carcinogenesis, Vol. 7, edited by E. Hecker et al.
Raven Press, New York © 1982.

Dynamics of Phorbol Diester Promoters in Epidermal Cells in Culture

*David L. Berry, †Thomas J. Slaga, ‡Gerhard Fürstenberger, and
‡Friedrich Marks

*Toxicology Unit, U.S.D.A. Western Regional Research Center, Berkeley, California 94710;
†Biology Division, Oak Ridge National Laboratory, Oak Ridge, Tennessee 37830; and
‡Institute for Biochemistry, German Cancer Research Center,
D-6900 Heidelberg 1, West Germany*

In the phorbol diester series, 12-O-tetradecanoylphorbol-13-acetate (TPA) is the most potent tumor promoter in mouse skin (7). TPA elicits several biochemical responses both *in vivo* and *in vitro* at nanomolar doses (6,7) and many of the responses occur within 5 min after TPA exposure (4,7,8). Most of the biochemical responses occur with a dose-dependent relationship, and other phorbol diesters or the parent alcohol phorbol are much less active than TPA (4,7,8).

The increased use of phorbol diesters *in vitro* to study the biochemical events involved in cell proliferation, cell differentiation, and processes associated with tumor promotion is further evidence that these compounds are extremely potent probes in experimental cell research. The dynamics of the phorbol diesters in culture is not well defined and such factors as rapid metabolism, possible metabolic activation, and conjugation can markedly affect the experimental results. The stability of the phorbol diester in culture medium, serum, solvents, and the prolonged exposure to CO_2 and 37°C temperatures should be considered. In view of the above considerations, a detailed study of the dynamics of ^{3}H-TPA and ^{3}H-phorbol-12,13-didecanoate (PDD) was undertaken in primary mouse epidermal cells in culture.

METHODS

Newborn or adult mouse epidermal cells from BALB/c, SENCAR, or Swiss Webster were isolated via the trypsin floatation technique developed by Yuspa et al. (8). Cells were plated at a density of 2.5×10^4 cells per cm^2 in plastic dishes in medium M199 or a modified Waymouths MB752/1 supplemented with 10% fetal bovine serum. Cells were treated with labeled phorbol diesters for selected times, washed once with phosphate-buffered saline, and the cells and/or media were extracted with a mixture of ethylacetate/acetone (2.5:1). Samples of media alone, serum, and serum plus media were also treated with labeled phorbol diester and extracted as above. The organic phase was concentrated and prepared for high pressure liquid chromatography (HPLC) as previously described (2). Water soluble metabolites were acidified, treated with β-glucuronidase, and extracted with chloroform/methanol (2:1) and the organic phase prepared for HPLC.

TPA, 12-O-tetradecanoylphorbol (T12P), phorbol-13-acetate (P13A), PDD, phorbol, and ^{3}H-TPA (5.0 mCi/mmole) were purchased from Dr. Peter Borchert, Minneapolis, Minnesota. Phorbol-12,13-dibutyrate (PDBu), phorbol-12,13-diacetate (PDA), and 4-O-methyl-12-O-tetradecanoylphorbol-13-acetate (4-O-Me-TPA) were kindly provided by Prof. E. Hecker, Heidelberg, West Germany. Phorbol-13-decanoate (P13D), phorbol-12-decanoate (P12D), and ^{3}H-PDD (1.6 mCi/mmole) were synthesized by the method of Baird and Boutwell (1).

RESULTS

Newborn BALB/c, SENCAR, and Swiss Webster epidermal cells rapidly assimilate ^{3}H-TPA and ^{3}H-PDD from the culture medium. Cell-associated phorbol diester reached a plateau level by 3 to 6 hr after treatment, and the levels of phorbol diester remained about the same for up to 96 hr of continuous treatment. Both ^{3}H-TPA and ^{3}H-PDD were stable to the extraction conditions. As shown in Table 1, the major compound associated with the epidermal cell is the diester; the monoesters accumulate in the media. The epidermal cell converts TPA into T12P, P13A, and phorbol, whereas PDD was converted primarily into P13D. The cell-associated phorbol diester ranged from 0.11 to 0.21 pmole/μg cellular deoxyribonucleic acid (DNA) and it was not possible to differentiate

TABLE 1. *Phorbol diester associated with primary mouse epidermal cells and media at selected times after treatment[a]*

Time	^{3}H-TPA				^{3}H-PDD			
	TPA	T12P	P13A	Phorbol	PDD	P12D	P13D	Phorbol
3 hr								
Cells	0.62	0.07	0.18	0.04	0.72	—	—	—
Media	5.11	0.43	0.26	0.14	5.7	—	0.12	—
12 hr								
Cells	0.58	0.20	0.12	0.14	0.70	—	0.05	—
Media	3.17	1.76	0.81	0.68	5.2	—	0.18	0.10
24 hr								
Cells	0.60	0.32	0.08	0.26	0.65	—	0.15	0.05
Media	2.25	1.08	1.73	1.04	5.2	0.10	0.34	0.15
96 hr								
Cells	0.62	0.16	0.10	0.08	0.65	0.10	0.10	0.05
Media	1.28	1.04	1.27	2.78	3.6	0.25	0.95	0.58

[a] Values expressed as pmole/10 μl sample injected onto HPLC column. TPA metabolism was measured in SENCAR and BALB/c cells, and PDD metabolism in Swiss Webster cells.

between membrane-associated and intercellular diesters. The epidermal cells were able to make glucuronides of P13A and P13D and, by 96 hr, the levels of these glucuronides ranged from 1 to 3% of the total media metabolites.

Both ^{3}H-TPA and ^{3}H-PDD were stable in cell-free culture medium containing 10% fetal bovine serum at 37°C for up to 96 hr. Autooxidation at either the C6, C7, or C20 position was not detected. The appearance of monoesters or phorbol was cell dependent and was most probably esterase mediated.

Media in the presence of cells contained the majority of the label from either ^{3}H-TPA or ^{3}H-PDD. The levels of ^{3}H-TPA decreased rapidly with time as shown in Fig. 1. Newborn SENCAR cells metabolized ^{3}H-TPA more rapidly than adult SENCAR cells ($T_{1/2}$ = 8.2 versus 10.5 hr) as shown in Fig. 1. On

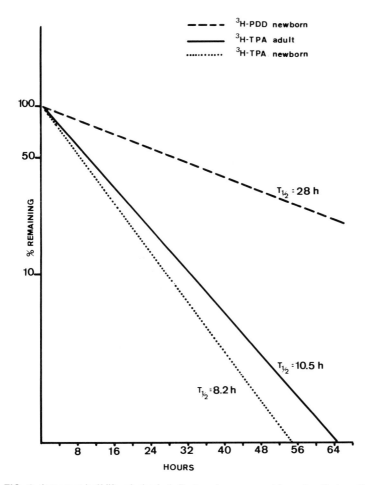

FIG. 1. Apparent half-life of phorbol diesters in mouse epidermal cells in culture.

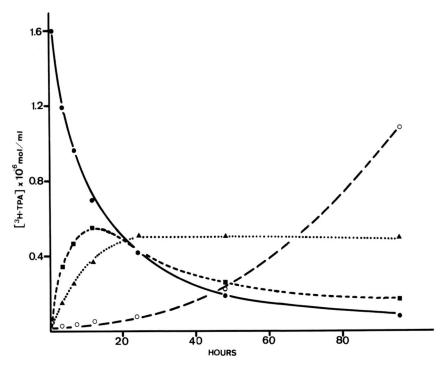

FIG. 2. Dynamics of ³H-TPA in the media of mouse epidermal cells in culture. (●—●) TPA, (■---■) T12P, (▲· · · ·▲) P13A, and (○---○) phorbol.

the other hand, ³H-PDD had an apparent half-life of 28 hr in Swiss Webster epidermal cells.

In newborn SENCAR cells, levels of ³H-TPA in the media decreased rapidly and at a nonlinear rate (Fig. 2). The two monoesters were produced rapidly but at a nonlinear rate. Phorbol increased at a slow, almost linear rate up to 96 hr. The cells appeared to metabolize the monoesters to phorbol. Media levels

TABLE 2. *Tumor-promoting activity of phorbol diesters in NMRI mice at 12 and 24 weeks of promotion*[a]

	Papillomas/mouse		Potency relative to TPA
Compound, dose, treatment	12 weeks	24 weeks	
TPA, 10 nM, 2 ×	1.9	5.9	1.0
PDD, 20 nM, 2 ×	0.64	2.4	0.20
PDBu, 40 nM, 2 ×	0.0	0.01	0.0004
PDA, 40 nM, 2 ×	0.0	0.0	—
4-O-Me-TPA, 400 nM, 2 ×	0.0	0.04	0.0002

[a] Animals were initiated with 100 nM 7,12-dimethylbenz(a,c)anthracene in 0.1 ml acetone 1 week prior to phorbol diester tumor promotion.

of ^{3}H-PDD and its metabolites indicate that PDD has a lower turnover rate than TPA and that the 13-monoester is the predominate ester formed from PDD (Table 1).

TPA and PDD stimulate DNA synthesis in newborn epidermal cells in a dose-dependent relationship. On a molar basis, TPA is more effective than PDD by a factor of two, whereas PDBu, PDA, and 4-O-Me-TPA are not mitogenic agents at up to 1,000 times the molar concentration of TPA. These data correlate with the tumor-promoting data on the phorbol esters *in vivo* shown in Table 2.

DISCUSSION

The increased application of phorbol diesters for *in vitro* transformation studies and experimental cell research makes it important to understand the bioavailability of the phorbol diesters in culture. From the early investigations of Kreibich et al. (3) and, more recently, O'Brien and Saladik (5), it is apparent that TPA is metabolized by a wide variety of fibroblasts. Results presented here indicate that primary mouse epidermal cells rapidly metabolize TPA to monoesters and phorbol. The less potent tumor promoter PDD is more slowly metabolized by primaries. In both cases, however, the major cell-associated diester was either TPA or PDD (> 95%) and the monoesters and phorbol accumulated in the media. No evidence was observed for metabolic activation of TPA or PDD; it must be assumed that metabolism leads to inactivation of the phorbol diester.

The ability of the phorbol diesters to stimulate DNA synthesis *in vitro* correlates with their promoting efficacy (8). TPA is twofold more potent in stimulating DNA synthesis than PDD, whereas *in vivo,* TPA is fivefold more potent in promoting activity. At 1,000-fold greater concentrations *in vitro,* PDA, 4-O-Me-TPA, and PDBu were ineffective mitogens, and *in vivo* these compounds were very weak or nonpromoting diesters (Table 2). As pointed out by Marks et al. (4), the stimulation of DNA synthesis is a necessary but not sufficient condition for tumor promotion *in vivo,* and, although promotion has not been adequately defined *in vitro,* it would seem prudent to suspect that DNA synthesis and cell proliferation are necessary components for promotion. Hence, effective promoters *in vitro* should stimulate DNA synthesis and cell proliferation.

Clearly, TPA and PDD are effective promoters *in vivo* and stimulate DNA synthesis *in vitro.* If one suspects that a particular cell rapidly metabolizes TPA so that an effective dose cannot be assured, one might consider the use of a diester with a longer biological half-life. In so doing, however, it should be recognized that there are major differences in potencies and that these differences may have important biological implications.

REFERENCES

1. Baird, W. M., and Boutwell, R. K. (1971): Tumor-promoting activities of phorbol and four diesters of phorbol in mouse skin. *Cancer Res.,* 31:1,074–1,079.

2. Berry, D. L., Bracken, W. M., Fischer, S. M., Viaje, A., and Slaga, T. J. (1978): Metabolic conversion of 12-O-tetradecanoylphorbol-13-acetate in adult and newborn mouse skin and mouse liver microsomes. *Cancer Res.*, 39:2,301–2,306.
3. Kreibich, G., Süss, R., and Kinzel, V. (1974): On the biochemical mechanism of tumorigenesis in mouse skin. V. Studies on the metabolism of tumor-promoting and nonpromoting phorbol derivatives *in vivo* and *in vitro*. *Z. Krebsforsch.*, 81:135–149.
4. Marks, F., Bertsch, S., and Fürstenberger, G. (1979): Ornithine decarboxylase activity, cell proliferation, and tumor promotion in mouse epidermis *in vivo*. *Cancer Res.*, 39:4,183–4,188.
5. O'Brien, T. G., and Saladik, D. (1980): Differences in the metabolism of [3]H-12-O-tetradecanoylphorbol-13-acetate and ^{3}H-phorbol-12,13-didecanoate by cells in culture. *Cancer Res.*, 40:4,433–4,437.
6. Scribner, J. D., and Suss, R. (1978): Tumor initiation and promotion. *Int. Rev. Exp. Pathol.* 18:138–198.
7. Slaga, T. J., Sivak, A., and Boutwell, R. K., editors (1978): *Carcinogenesis, Vol. 2: Mechanisms of Tumor Promotion and Cocarcinogenesis.* Raven Press, New York.
8. Yuspa, S. H., Lichti, U., Ben, T., Patterson, E., Hennings, H., and Slaga, T. J. (1976): Phorbol esters stimulate DNA synthesis and ornithine decarboxylase activity in mouse epidermal cell cultures. *Nature (Lond)*, 262:402–404.

Carcinogenesis, Vol. 7, edited by E. Hecker et al.
Raven Press, New York © 1982.

Promotion of X-Ray Transformation *In Vitro*

John B. Little and Ann R. Kennedy

*Laboratory of Radiobiology, Harvard University School of Public Health,
Boston, Massachusetts 02115*

Berenblum (1), Rous and Kidd (23), and others demonstrated that skin tumors could be induced in experimental animals exposed to subcarcinogenic doses of polycyclic hydrocarbons if treatment was followed by repeated applications of a noncarcinogenic irritant agent. These early observations led to the interest in carcinogenesis as a multistage process. Research efforts were focused on the study of croton oil as the "promoting" agent in mouse skin carcinogenesis. More recently, Hecker (4) and Van Duuren (29) isolated and characterized the phorbol esters as the active components of croton oil; one of the most active of these is 12-O-tetradecanoylphorbol-13-acetate (TPA). For many years, however, a clear-cut demonstration of this phenomenon of tumor promotion by phorbol esters was restricted to the induction of skin papillomas.

That promotion was a more general phenomenon in carcinogenesis was given impetus by the *in vitro* observations of Lasne et al. (11) and Mondal et al. (14) that phorbol esters could accelerate or enhance transformation of cultured cells exposed to polycyclic hydrocarbons. In this chapter, we will review our findings on promotion of X-ray transformation in mouse C3H 10T½ cells, and discuss these results in the light of those for chemical carcinogen-induced transformation in established cell lines.

MATERIALS AND METHODS

Mouse C3H 10T½ cells were orginally isolated and characterized by Reznikoff et al. (21,22) and adapted by us for studies of radiation transformation (12,28). They were grown and maintained in Eagle's basal medium supplemented with 10% heat-inactivated fetal calf serum as described in detail elsewhere (12,28). Cells were passaged every 7 days at a 1:20 dilution; they were used between passages 7 and 15, and subsequently discarded. They were irradiated with either a Philips MG-100 X-ray generator operating at 100 kV and 9.6 mA, or a G.E. Maximar Unit operating at 220 kV and 15 mA. Both generators yielded a dose-rate to the cells of approximately 80 rads/min. TPA was obtained either from Consolidated Midland Co., Brewster, New York (lot numbers 007 and 016) or Chemical Carcinogenesis, Eden Prairie, Minnesota, and used at a concentration of 100 ng/ml of complete medium. TPA solutions were prepared and used as previously described (8,9). Other agents were obtained from the Sigma Chemical Co. Antipain was kindly provided by the U.S.-Japan Cooperative Cancer Research Program.

The protocol for the usual transformation experiment is shown in the upper line of Fig. 1. Cells are seeded at low density in 100-mm Petri dishes, allowed to attach, and irradiated 24 hr later. The cells are initially seeded at a density such that approximately 300 viable cells will result when the cloning efficiency and the toxicity of the particular radiation exposure or other treatment are accounted for. The cultures are then returned to the incubator, the medium changed at twice weekly intervals, and the cells allowed to proliferate until they become confluent. This takes about 10 to 14 days; the cells will on the average undergo approximately 13 rounds of cell division during this interval. Subsequently, the cultures are maintained in the incubator for an additional 4 to 5 weeks with weekly medium changes until transformed foci develop (12); Types II and III foci were scored, as previously described (21,28).

The results of our earlier experiments are presented in terms of the transforma-

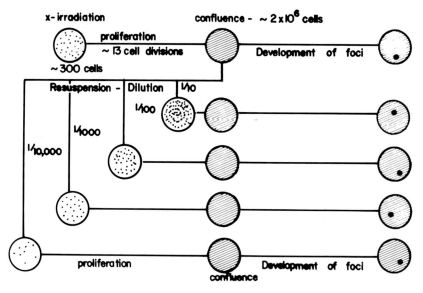

FIG. 1. Protocol for transformation experiments. The usual experiment is shown on the top line. Cells are seeded in 100-mm Petri dishes in sufficient numbers such as to yield approximately 300 viable cells when the cloning efficiency and toxicity of the particular treatment are accounted for. The dishes are irradiated 24 hr later, then returned to the incubator for 6–7 weeks to allow for the expression of transformation. The cells will undergo on the average about 13 rounds of division before confluence is reached 10–14 days after seeding. In some experiments, varying numbers of cells from 1 to approximately 400 were initially seeded. In others, dishes seeded with 300 cells were harvested as soon as they reached confluence, resuspended, and reseeded at various dilutions as shown in the lower part of the figure. These reseeded dishes were allowed the full 6–7-week expression period before scoring for transformed foci.

tion frequency per initial viable cell (12,28). As will be described later, however, the ultimate yield of transformed foci appears to be independent of the initial number of cells seeded. Thus, the parameter transformation frequency per viable cell has no meaning in absolute terms. When the initial number of viable cells seeded is held constant (around 300 cells), however, this parameter may be used to compare the effects of different treatments, doses, etc. In our recent experiments, the results are expressed in terms of the average number of foci that developed per dish.

In some experiments, the cultures were initially seeded with varying numbers of viable cells, ranging from 1 to 400. In others, the cultures were trypsinized just when they reached confluence, and the cells were resuspended and reseeded in new dishes at various dilutions, as shown in the lower portion of Fig. 1. These dishes were again allowed to reach confluence, and then held for 4 to 5 weeks until transformed foci developed. Reseeding at 1:1,000 dilution yielded approximately the same number of viable (colony-forming) cells as were initially seeded (300 to 400). The results of these experiments are presented in terms of the average number of transformed foci per dish, as calculated by the Poisson method (5).

RESULTS

The effect of exposure to TPA on the frequency of X-ray-induced transformation of 10T½ cells is shown in the dose-response curves in Fig. 2. The lower curve was obtained following exposure to X-rays alone, whereas the upper curve resulted when the cells were in addition incubated with TPA for the full 6 to 7 week expression period following irradiation. TPA induced no transformation by itself. As can be seen in Fig. 2, however, TPA enhanced the X-ray-induced transformation frequency at all radiation dose levels, though the relative effect was much greater following low X-ray doses (25 to 100 rads) than following a high dose (400 rads). This finding is consistent with the observations of Mondal et al. (14,16) who found that TPA was most effective in enhancing transformation induced by ultraviolet light (16) or polycyclic hydrocarbons (14) when the cells were treated with very low or subcarcinogenic doses of these initiating agents.

The results of experiments designed to examine the time-dependence of this effect are shown in Fig. 3. Cultures exposed to 100 rads were continuously incubated with TPA for various time intervals ranging from 48 hr to 6 weeks after X-irradiation. Clearly, TPA had its greatest effect in enhancing transformation during the earlier period when the cells were actively proliferating. This conclusion was confirmed in separate experiments in which TPA was added to cultures irradiated with 100 rads after confluence was reached and then maintained for either 2 weeks or until the end of the experiment (9). A maximum enhancement of 1.5- to 2.0-fold occurred in these groups. A similar finding was reported by Mondal et al. (14) for transformation induced by polycyclic hydrocarbons. Transformation was not enhanced in benzo(a)pyrene (BP)-treated

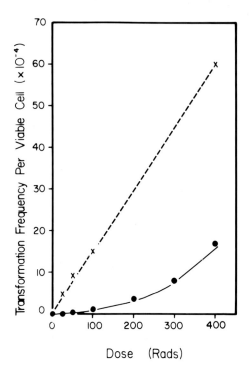

FIG. 2. Effect of TPA on X-ray transformation *in vitro*. The lower curve represents dose-response data for the induction of transformation in 10T½ cells by X-rays alone (28). The upper curve is the dose-response relationship obtained when the cells were incubated with 0.1 µg/ml TPA following irradiation for the full expression period (8).

cultures, and only minimally enhanced in cultures treated with 0.1 µg/ml of 7,12-dimethylbenz(a)anthracene (DMBA) or 3-methylcholanthrene (MCA) when TPA was added 10 days after carcinogen treatment when the cultures had reached confluence.

One of the characteristics of promotion of mouse skin tumors by phorbol esters is that the promoting agent is effective even when applied many months after exposure to the initiating carcinogen. In order to examine this phenomenon *in vitro*, cells seeded at low density were irradiated with 400 rads, returned to the incubator, and allowed to proliferate until the cultures reached confluence. The cells were then harvested, diluted, and reseeded in new dishes at the initial cell density (250 to 300 viable cells per dish). TPA was added to one group of cultures (another group received no TPA treatment), and they were maintained an additional 6 to 7 weeks until transformed foci developed. The results of these experiments are summarized in Table 1. There was no significant difference in the ultimate yield of transformants between the group subcultured at confluence (group 2) and that maintained without subculture (group 1). When TPA was added after subcultivation (group 3), however, the transformation frequency

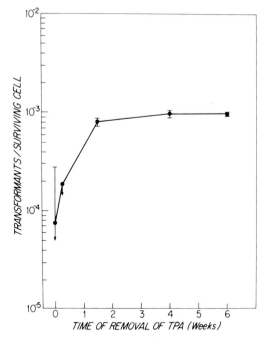

FIG. 3. Effect of duration of exposure to TPA on X-ray transformation. TPA was added after irradiation with 100 rads, and subsequently removed at the indicated times. Each data point represents the mean results ± 1 SE of three separate experiments. Complete data are tabulated in Kennedy et al. (9).

increased by a factor of three—an enhancement similar to that previously observed when the cells were incubated with TPA immediately after irradiation (Fig. 2).

This finding indicates that X-irradiated cells do retain the capacity to respond

TABLE 1. *Effect on transformation of exposure to TPA at late times after X-irradiation*[a]

Group	Treatment	Total no. of dishes	Total no. of cells	No. transformed foci observed	Average no. foci per dish
1	400 rads	77	18,292	39	0.51
2	400 rads + subcultivation[b]	74	18,195	22	0.30
3	400 rads + subcultivation[b] + TPA[c]	60	19,980	90	1.50

[a] Data are pooled from five separate experiments. Data for individual experiments are tabulated in Kennedy et al. (9).
[b] Cells irradiated at low density were harvested when they reached confluence, diluted, reseeded at low cell density (~250–300 cells/dish), and allowed full expression period.
[c] TPA added after subcultivation only.

to TPA even when many generations of cell division have elapsed since the radiation exposure. Furthermore, they suggest that the effect of TPA does not result from a simple stimulation of cell proliferation, as the transformation frequency was not significantly elevated in the cultures allowed an additional 13 rounds of cell division with no TPA (group 2, Table 1). A similar conclusion was reached by Mondal et al. (14) and Peterson et al. (20) for TPA enhancement of polycyclic hydrocarbon transformation.

Another related hypothesis concerning the mechanism of action of TPA is that TPA confers to cells transformed in its presence a selective growth advantage over normal cells. In order to test this hypothesis, the growth rates of normal 10T½ cells, an established line of X-ray-transformed 10T½ cells (F-17) (28), and cells transformed by X-rays in the presence of TPA were compared. As can be seen in Fig. 4, there were no significant differences among these cell lines in their growth rates to confluence either in the presence or absence of TPA in the medium. The small increase in the saturation density at confluence of normal cells incubated with TPA has been observed by several investigators (9,13,30).

In preliminary experiments, we have examined several other classes of agents for possible inhibiting or promoting effects on X-ray transformation. These include epidermal growth factor (EGF), the bee venom toxin melittin (a stimulator

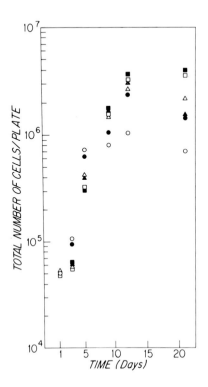

FIG. 4. Effect of incubation with TPA on the growth rate and saturation density of normal and transformed 10T½ cells. *Open symbols* are for cultures without TPA: (○), normal cells; (△), radiation-transformed cells (F-17 strain); (□), cells transformed in the presence of TPA. *Closed symbols* are for the same cell lines grown in the presence of 0.1 μg/ml TPA. Data and figure from Kennedy *et al.* (9).

of prostaglandin synthesis), the steroid antiinflammatory agents cortisone and dexamethasone, the nonsteroid antiinflammatory agent indomethacin, and certain protease inhibitors. Antiinflammatory agents have been reported to inhibit promotion *in vivo.* The cells were incubated with nontoxic or minimally toxic concentrations of these agents for the entire 6- to 7-week postirradiation expression period. The results of some of these experiments are presented in Tables 2 and 3.

The effects of several antiinflammatory agents on X-ray transformation are shown in Table 2. Cortisone and indomethacin both induce a fairly high yield of transformants by themselves; the yield of transformants in cultures treated with 400 rads and cortisone was consistently higher than that expected by a simple additive effect. In cultures treated with X-rays and indomethacin, on the other hand, the yield was less than that expected. Also included in Table 2 are results for the protease inhibitor antipain. Antipain induced no transformation by itself (6), but markedly suppressed transformation induced by X-rays. It also completely inhibited the promotion of X-ray transformation by TPA (6,7). Indomethacin also inhibited the TPA enhancement of X-ray information (data not shown). Similar experiments with the antiinflammatory steroid hormones are currently underway in our laboratory, but Mondal and Heidelberger (17) have reported that these hormones inhibit TPA-induced promotion of transformation in 10T½ cells initiated by MCA or 5-azacytidine. Thus, both the steroidal and nonsteroidal antiinflammatory agents suppressed TPA promotion *in vitro,* but had no systematic effect on the expression of transformation induced by X-rays alone.

Among potential tumor promoters, EGF did not transform by itself, but consistently enhanced the yield of transformants induced by either X-rays (Table 3) or ultraviolet light (UV) exposures (data not shown). The enhancement was similar in magnitude to that induced by TPA in the same experiments but, unlike in the case of TPA, it was not significantly inhibited by indomethacin (data not shown). Melittin, on the other hand, appeared to suppress both X-ray and UV-induced transformation.

As is also shown in Table 3, no promoting effect was observed when X-irradiated cells were incubated during the entire expression period in the presence of low concentrations of mitomycin-C. Some investigators have found that TPA induces a low level of sister chromatid exchanges (SCE) in mammalian cells (3,10,19), and it has been hypothesized that this phenomenon may reflect mitotic recombinational activity that leads to promotion by facilitating the segregation of specific recessive mutations in daughter cell populations (10). Mitomycin-C is a potent inducer of SCE; at the concentration employed it enhanced the spontaneous SCE frequency by a factor of about 1.5, a similar enhancement to that produced in 10T½ cells by TPA (19).

In a separate series of experiments, cultures were irradiated with 400 to 600 rads after they were initially seeded at varying cell densities, ranging from 1 to approximately 300 viable cells. In other experiments, the cultures were initially

TABLE 2. *Effect of antiinflammatory agents on X-ray transformation*

Treatment[a] 1	2	Total no. of dishes	Total no. of cells	No. transformed foci observed	Average no. foci per dish
—	—	93	31,750	0	0
—	Cortisone (10^{-7}M)	40	14,600	16	0.40
—	Dexamethasone (10^{-7}M)	40	21,170	2	0.05
—	Indomethacin (0.1 µg/ml)	33	11,645	37	1.12
100 rads	—	73	26,335	17	0.23
400 rads	—	37	15,040	34	0.65
400 rads	Cortisone	38	13,300	58	1.53
400 rads	Dexamethasone	36	16,520	41	1.14
100 rads	Indomethacin	11	5,885	2	0.18
600 rads	Antipain (50 µg/ml)	26	9,625	1	0.04

[a] Second treatment begun 24 hr after seeding (immediately after irradiation) and maintained for full 6–7-week expression period. Data pooled from several experiments.

TABLE 3. *Effect of potential promoting agents on X-ray transformation*

Treatment[a]		Total no. of dishes	Total no. of cells	No. transformed foci observed	Average no. foci per dish
1	2				
—	—	120	28,640	1	0.01
—	EGF (50 ng/ml)	28	9,575	0	0
—	Mitomycin-C (10^{-9}M)	17	6,075	1	0.06
100 rads	—	105	34,335	21	0.20
100 rads	EGF	29	11,010	26	0.90
100 rads	Mellitin (2 µg/ml)	18	6,210	0	0
100 rads	TPA (0.1 µg/ml)	32	12,400	36	1.12
100 rads	Mitomycin-C	30	10,530	4	0.13

[a] Second treatment begun 72 hr after seeding (48 hr after irradiation) and maintained for entire 6–7-week expression period.

seeded and irradiated at a density of about 300 cells; when the cells reached
confluence they were harvested and reseeded at 10-fold dilutions as shown in
Fig. 1. The unexpected finding in these experiments was that the average number
of transformed foci that developed per confluent dish was roughly constant
over a wide range of initial and reseeded cell densities; that is, it was independent
of the number of cells actually exposed to the radiation or the number of progeny
of irradiated cells reseeded after confluence. These results have been presented
and discussed in detail elsewhere (5).

Similar experiments were designed to examine the effects of TPA on transformation when the irradiated progeny were subcultured at confluence. Results
of these experiments are summarized in Fig. 5. As can be seen in Fig. 5, the
number of transformed foci that developed per subcultivated dish (open circles
and crosses) remained roughly constant, even though the total number of cells
reseeded ranged over three orders of magnitude, and was similar to that observed
in the nonsubcultivated dishes (open triangle and square). The ultimate yield
of transformants did not differ significantly whether TPA was present for the
entire experiment (circles in Fig. 5) or whether it was removed at the first
confluence (crosses) and thus present only during the initial proliferative phase
of expression. No transformation was seen in nonirradiated cultures with or
without TPA exposure.

The results of experiments in which cultures treated with 100 rads and incu-

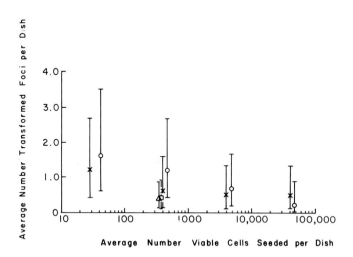

FIG. 5. Effect of subcultivation at confluence and reseeding at various cell densities on the
yield of transformants. Protocol as shown in Fig. 1: All cultures irradiated with 100 rads: (×),
radiation only; (○), radiation plus incubation with TPA for entire experiment. Other symbols
(□,△) are initial cell densities for similarly treated cultures that were not subcultivated, but
left undisturbed and allowed the usual expression time for transformation (*upper line*, Fig.
1). Vertical bars are 95% confidence limits. Average number of transformed foci per dish
calculated by Poisson method (5).

bated with TPA were not reseeded but the initial cell density was varied are summarized in Fig. 6. The yield of transformants was very low in cultures exposed to either 100 rads or TPA alone. When cultures exposed to 100 rads were subsequently incubated with TPA, however, a large increase in the yield of transformants occurred. As can be seen in Fig. 6, the effect of TPA appeared to be further enhanced when the initial cell density was decreased from 370 to less than 100 cells per dish. It should be noted in Fig. 6 that the average number of foci per dish in cultures initially seeded with a single viable cell was 2.1; that is, one or more transformed foci ultimately developed overlying the normal monolayer in nearly every confluent dish.

The finding that under appropriate conditions transformation will occur among one or more of the progeny of most cells irradiated with 100 rads and subsequently incubated with TPA suggests that the initial alteration produced by radiation is a common event involving most or all of the irradiated cells. We hypothesize that it may be epigenetic in nature, such as an alteration in gene expression (2). This change is transmitted to the progeny of surviving cells, and is sensitive to the effects of TPA. We hypothesize further that this initial change enhances the probability of the occurrence of a second event. This second event is the transformation of one or more of the progeny of the irradiated cell when they are maintained under conditions of confluence. This second event is not altered by incubation with TPA. That transformation occurs

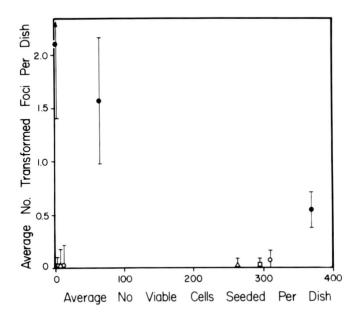

FIG. 6. Effect of varying the initial cell density on the yield of transformants: (□), nontreated controls; (○), 100 rads only; (△), TPA only; (●), 100 rads plus TPA. Vertical bars are 95% confidence limits. Average number of foci per dish calculated by Poisson method (5).

after confluence is reached is indicated by the results of the subculture experiments in Fig. 5. Had transformation occurred earlier, clones of transformed cells would be present at confluence, and the number of foci in reseeded dishes should have increased markedly with increasing numbers of cells reseeded.

CONCLUSIONS AND DISCUSSION

These results from studies on promotion of transformation in established cell lines suggest several conclusions concerning the promoting effect of TPA *in vitro.* These include: (a) it is not due to a simple conversion of premutational deoxyribonucleic acid (DNA) lesions to mutations; (b) it is not due to an effect on DNA repair processes; (c) it is not due to a simple stimulation of cell proliferation, though TPA is effective primarily in proliferating cells; and (d) it does not result primarily from stimulating quiescent cells to proliferate or from releasing cells from contact inhibition. Finally, our recent results with X-ray transformation suggest that TPA may be acting to enhance some sort of a reversible epigenetic change, such as an alteration in gene expression induced by the radiation exposure that increases the probability that the actual transforming event will occur at some later time.

The first two of these conclusions can be drawn largely from the results of Table 1; that is, TPA was equally as effective in enhancing transformation when treatment began many rounds of cell division following exposure to the primary carcinogen as it was when applied immediately thereafter. Generally, the conversion of a premutational lesion in DNA (usually assumed to be some sort of base damage) to a mutation is thought to occur either during DNA replication or as the result of the action of DNA repair processes. Most DNA repair appears to be complete within 24 hr of exposure to radiation or chemical agents. It is true that some DNA base damage may be bypassed at replication and passed on to daughter cells; depending on the nature and degree of this damage, these cells may be viable. Even on the assumption that, owing to bypass mechanisms, some persistent nonlethal base damage remained unrepaired at subsequent divisions, this should be so diluted out by 12 to 13 consecutive rounds of DNA replication as to be inconsequential. Furthermore, there is no experimental evidence for the existence of such persistent radiation-induced DNA base damage or DNA-carcinogen adducts, nor is there evidence for persistent DNA repair activity at long times after exposure to DNA-damaging agents.

The data in Table 1 also speak against the hypothesis that promotion by TPA results primarily from a stimulation of cell proliferation. When previously irradiated cells were subcultivated at confluence and allowed to undergo another 12 to 13 rounds of cell division, no increase in the yield of transformants occurred. Such an increase would have been expected if promotion resulted from additional proliferative activity. This conclusion is further supported by the results in Fig. 4 which show that TPA had no measurable effect on the growth rate of either normal or transformed cells. On the other hand, TPA appeared to be effective in enhancing transformation when it was applied while the cells were actively proliferating (Fig. 3). This may explain why its enhancing effect in mouse skin has usually been associated with increased proliferation; the irritant effect of croton oil may have led to the proliferative response necessary for the phorbol ester to be effective as a promoter.

The results in Fig. 3 indicate in addition that the promoting effect of TPA does not result primarily from an effect on quiescent cells, such as by releasing them from contact inhibition. This latter result is in contradistinction to the earlier findings of Sivak and Van Duuren (25,26) who studied the enhancing effect of phorbol esters on the clonal growth of either virally or chemically transformed cells in a mixed culture system containing a large excess of contact-inhibited normal cells. In a preliminary communication, Sivak et al. (24) also reported that a phorbol ester tumor promoter was effective during the postconfluence interval of the transformation assay in 3T3 cells.

The results of the experiments we have described, however, cannot exclude the possibility that the promoting effect of TPA might result from its conferring a subtle growth advantage to potentially transformed cells. If the initial cellular alteration induced by radiation indeed involves a relatively large fraction of the irradiated cells, as is suggested by the evidence presented earlier (Figs. 5 and 6), the proportion of altered cells at confluence could be considerably enhanced if they possessed a relative small growth advantage during the proliferative phase. The probability of a transformational event occurring after confluence would thus be enhanced proportionally. Unfortunately, we have at present no way of identifying such potentially transformed progeny prior to confluence and focus formation.

Several agents other than TPA have now been shown to have promotional activity *in vitro* in established cell lines. These include EGF (Table 3), saccharin (15), anthralin, and mezereine (18). It is not known whether the mechanism of action of these agents may be similar to that of TPA or not. The lack of a promoting effect of melittin suggests that promotion *in vitro* is not mediated by prostaglandins (27). The lack of an effect of mitomycin-C, however, does not necessarily argue against the hypothesis that a terminal event in promotion may involve aberrant mitotic segregation. At least some SCE appear to be derived from the presence of long-lived base lesions in DNA (31) such as may be induced by mitomycin-C. This mechanism is likely very different from that involved in SCE production by TPA; SCE resulting from such base damage would thus bear no relation to promotion.

Finally, the results shown in Figs. 5 and 6 suggest, as was discussed earlier, that the initial alteration produced by radiation in cells is a common event involving most or all of the irradiated cells. This would imply that this alteration was epigenetic in nature. Evidence has recently been presented (2) that chemical carcinogens are effective in the induction of altered gene expression; more effective, perhaps, than in inducing mutations. It is attractive to hypothesize that the effects of tumor promoters and certain inhibitors of carcinogenesis are on an initial, presumably reversible, epigenetic change involving an alteration in gene expression. It is this initial change that would determine the probability with which the ultimate transformational event would eventually occur.

ACKNOWLEDGMENTS

This research was supported by grants CA-11751, CA-22704, and ES-00002 from the National Institutes of Health.

REFERENCES

1. Berenblum, I. (1941): The cocarcinogenic action of croton resin. *Cancer Res.,* 1:44–48.
2. Fahmy, M. J., and Fahmy, O. G. (1980): Intervening DNA insertions and the alteration of gene expression by carcinogens. *Cancer Res.,* 40:3,374–3,382.
3. Gentil, A., Renault, G., and Margot, A. (1980): The effect of the tumor promoter 12-O-tetradecanoylphorbol-13-acetate (TPA) on UV- and MNNG-induced sister chromatid exchanges in mammalian cells. *Int. J. Cancer,* 26:517–521.
4. Hecker. (1968): Cocarcinogenic principles from the seed oil of croton tigluim and from other euphorbraceae. *Cancer Res.,* 28:2,332–2,349.
5. Kennedy, A. R., Fox, M., Murphy, G., and Little, J. B. (1980): On the relationship between X-ray exposure and malignant transformation in C3H 10T½ cells. *Proc. Natl. Acad. Sci. USA,* 77:7,262–7,266.
6. Kennedy, A. R., and Little, J. B. (1978): Protease inhibitors suppress radiation-induced malignant transformation *in vitro. Nature,* 276:825–826.
7. Kennedy, A. R., and Little, J. B. (1980): Radiation transformation *in vitro:* Modification by exposure to tumor promoters and protease inhibitors. In: *Radiation Biology and Cancer Research,* edited by R. E. Meyn and H. R. Withers, pp. 295–307. Raven Press, New York.
8. Kennedy, A. R., Mondal, S., Heidelberger, C., and Little, J. B. (1978): Enhancement of X-ray transformation by 12-O-tetradecanoylphorbol-13-acetate in a cloned line of C3H mouse embryo cells. *Cancer Res.,* 38:439–443.
9. Kennedy, A. R., Murphy, G., and Little, J. B. (1980): The effect of time and duration of exposure to 12-O-tetradecanoylphorbol-13-acetate (TPA) on x-ray transformation of C3H 10T½ cells. *Cancer Res.,* 40:1,915–1,920.
10. Kinsella, A. R., and Radman, M. (1978): Tumor promoter induces sister chromatid exchanges: Relevance to mechanisms of carcinogenesis. *Proc. Natl. Acad. Sci. USA,* 75:6,149–6,153.
11. Lasne, C., Gentil, A., and Chouroulinkov, I. (1974): Two-stage malignant transformation of rat fibroblasts in tissue culture. *Nature,* 274:490–491.
12. Little, J. B. (1977): Radiation carcinogenesis *in vitro:* Implications for mechanisms. In: *Origins of Human Cancer, Vol. IV,* edited by H. H. Hiatt, J. D. Watson, and J. A. Winston, pp. 923–939. Cold Spring Harbor Conferences on Cell Proliferation, Cold Spring Harbor, New York.
13. Mondal, S. (1980): C3H/10T½ cl 8 mouse embryo cell line: Its use for the study of carcinogenesis and tumor promotion in cell culture. In: *Mammalian Cell Transformation by Chemical Carcinogens,* edited by N. K. Mishra, V. Dunkle, and M. Mehlman, pp. 181–211. Senate Press, Princeton Junction, N.J.
14. Mondal, S., Brankow, D. W., and Heidelberger, C. (1976): Two-stage chemical oncogenesis in cultures of C3H/10T½ cells. *Cancer Res.* 36:2,254–2,260.
15. Mondal, S., Brankow, D. W., and Heidelberger, C. (1978): Enhancement of oncogenesis in cultures of C3H/10T½ mouse embryo cell cultures by saccharin. *Science,* 201:1,141–1,142.
16. Mondal, S., and Heidelberger, C. (1976): Transformation of C3H/10T½ cl 8 mouse embryo fibroblasts by ultraviolet irradiation and a phorbol ester. *Nature,* 260:710–711.
17. Mondal, S., and Heidelberger, C. (1980a): Cell differentiation and tumor promotion (abstract). *Proc. Am. Assoc. Cancer Res.,* 21:96.

18. Mondal, S., and Heidelberger, C. (1980*b*): Inhibition of induced differentiation of C3H/10T½ clone 8 mouse embryo cells by tumor promoters. *Cancer Res.,* 40:334–338.
19. Nagasawa, H., and Little, J. B. (1979): Effect of tumor promoters, protease inhibitors, and repair processes on X-ray-induced sister chromatid exchanges in mouse cells. *Proc. Natl. Acad. Sci. USA,* 76:1,943–1,947.
20. Peterson, A. R., Mondal, S., Brankow, D. W., Thon, W., and Heidelberger, C. (1977): Effects of promoters on DNA synthesis in C3H/10T½ mouse fibroblasts. *Cancer Res.,* 37:3,223–3,227.
21. Reznikoff, C. A., Bertram, J. S., Brankow, D. W., and Heidelberger, C. (1973): Qualitative and quantitative studies of chemical transformation of cloned C3H mouse embryo cells sensitive to postconfluence inhibition of cell division. *Cancer Res.,* 33:3,239–3,249.
22. Reznikoff, C. A., Brankow, D. W., and Heidelberger, C. (1973): Establishment and characterization of a cloned line of C3H mouse embryo cells sensitive to postconfluence inhibition of cell division. *Cancer Res.,* 33:3,231–3,238.
23. Rous, P., and Kidd, J. G. (1941): Conditional neoplasms and subthreshold neoplastic states. A study of the tar tumors of rabbits. *J. Exp. Med.,* 73:365–390.
24. Sivak, A., Rudenko, L., and Simons, I. (1978): Carcinogen-induced neoplastic transformation in BALB/C 3T3 cells. (Abstract). *Proc. Am. Assoc. Cancer Res.,* 19:36.
25. Sivak, A., and Van Duuren, B. L. (1970): A cell culture system for the assessment of tumor-promoting activity. *J. Natl. Cancer Inst.,* 44:1,091–1,097.
26. Sivak, A., and Van Duuren, B. L. (1976): Phenotypic expression of transformation: Induction in cell culture by a phorbol ester. *Science,* 157:1,443–1,444.
27. Tashjian, A. H., Ivey, J. L., Delclos, B., and Levine, L. (1978): Stimulation of prostaglandin production in bone by phorbol diesters and melittin. *Prostaglandins,* 16:221–232.
28. Terzaghi, M., and Little, J. B. (1976): X-radiation-induced transformation in a C3H mouse embryo-derived cell line. *Cancer Res.,* 36:1,367–1,374.
29. Van Duuren, B. L. (1969): Tumor-promoting agents in two-stage carcinogenesis. *Prog. Exp. Tumor Res.,* 11:31–68.
30. Weinstein, I. B., Wigler, M., Fisher, P. B., Sisskin, E., and Pietropaolo, C. (1978): Cell culture studies on the biological effects of tumor promoters. In: *Carcinogenesis, Vol. 2: Mechanisms of Tumor Promotion and Cocarcinogenesis,* edited by T. J. Slaga, A. Sivak, and R. K. Boutwell, pp. 313–333. Raven Press, New York.
31. Wolff, S. (1978): Relation between DNA repair, chromosome aberrations, and sister chromatid exchanges. In: *DNA Repair Mechanisms,* edited by P. C. Hanawalt, E. C. Friedberg, and C. F. Fox, pp. 751–760. Academic Press, New York.

Carcinogenesis, Vol. 7, edited by E. Hecker et al.
Raven Press, New York © 1982.

Genetic Forms of Neoplasia in Man: A Model for the Study of Tumor Promotion *In Vitro*

L. Kopelovich

Memorial Sloan-Kettering Cancer Center and Cornell University Graduate School of Medical Sciences, New York, New York, 10021

It is generally believed that all forms of cancer are due to heritable and permanent changes in the cell genome (3,18,40). A view that considers tumor cells as an expression of a particular state of differentiation rather than as a genetic variant has also been stated (42). Presumably, genetic and epigenetic mechanisms are associated with both the initiation and maintenance of the malignant state (40).

Malignant transformation is a multiphase process apparently caused by carcinogens and subject to the influence of promoters (5,6,13,17,51). A potent class of tumor-promoting agents are the naturally occurring phorbol esters (17,51,58), such as 12-O-tetradecanoylphorbol-13-acetate (TPA). Through the use of TPA, a two-stage process of malignant transformation has been demonstrated in the mouse skin model (5,51) as well as in various organs of other rodents (16; also *this volume*), and, more recently, in cell culture systems (20, 32,38,41,43). The role of TPA is presumably to increase the probability of expression of the malignant phenotype (51,59). Nonetheless, studies *in vitro* suggest that it reversibly affects terminal differentiation and differentiated cell functions (51,59).

This chapter summarizes experiments on the effects of TPA on skin fibroblasts obtained from individuals with hereditary adenomatosis of the colon and rectum. The growth properties *in vitro* and the growth *in vivo* of human mutant cells exposed to TPA alone are described.

THE MODEL SYSTEM

Our approach toward the elucidation of mechanisms associated with initiation and promotion in human cancer has been to study in detail an inherited form of cancer. Adenomatosis of the colon and rectum (ACR) is a disease in which numerous adenomatous polyps develop from the mucosa of the large intestine, and in which frank tumors presumably arise from these polyps. The trait is expressed through an autosomal dominant gene (2,15,44), but it seems probable that additional genes may pleiotropically modify its expression (2,15,44). The

Gardner syndrome has been considered a special variant of ACR in which, in addition to colon cancer, a tendency to develop both benign and malignant growths from extracolonic tissues is indicated (15). To date, no sharp distinction between these two disease entities has been made (44).

As part of a study of human mutant cells *in vitro,* we have found that whereas cutaneous biopsies of ACR patients and their progeny are apparently normal, the cultured skin fibroblasts (SF) were abnormal in several aspects of *in vitro* growth control, increased proteolytic activity, cell architecture, susceptibility to further transformation by viral probes, and, more recently, a spontaneous loss of anchorage sensitivity (Table 1). These findings suggested a *systemic disorder* of stromal cells in ACR patients that might provide insight about cancer initiation and cancer promotion in man (28,29,32). Based on these results, we have assumed that the ACR cell exists in an *initiated state* due to a dominant

TABLE 1. *A phenotypic profile of an initiated ACR cell*[a]

A. Growth Parameters
    (1) Growth in nutrient-deprived environment (27,36,46).
    (2) Loss of contact inhibition (27,36,46).
    (3) Formation of cell aggregates (36).
    (4) Increased cloning efficiency (36).

B. Cytoskeletal Structures
    (1) Defective actin-containing cables (α-actin) (35).
    (2) Defective myosin-associated cables (α-meromyosin) *(unpublished data).*
    (3) Normal organization of microtubules (α-tubulin) *(unpublished data).*
    (4) Normal organization of intermediate filaments (α-vinmentin) *(unpublished data).*

C. Membrane-Associated Parameters
    (1) Increased Con A agglutination (in suspension and onto derivatized matrices) (8, and A. Braun and L. Kopelovich, *unpublished data).*
    (2) Increased intra- and extracellular levels of plasminogen activator (27).
    (3) Normal expression of LETS (S. Renard and L. Kopelovich, *in preparation).*
    (4) Defective polymerization of collagen (E. M./hydroxy and cishydroxyproline)? (R. Scott and E. Gardner, *personal communication;* L. Kopelovich, *unpublished data).*
    (5) Proteoglycans (not done).
    (6) A partial loss of anchorage sensitivity (32).

D. Increased Sensitivity to Further Transformation by Oncongenic Viruses
    (1) KiMSV (associated with an expression of a human fetal-like antigen) (45).
    (2) SV40 (associated with an expression of a human placenta-like antigen) (37).

E. Increased Sensitivity to Further Transformation by Chemical Agents
    (1) TPA (associated, presumably, with induced alteration followed by selection, and characterized by a decreased toxicity of ACR cells, and the occurrence of a human fetal-like antigen) (32,33,34).
    (2) MNNG (associated, presumably, with selection toward more resistant variants) (48).

F. Miscellaneous
    (1) Normal cholesterol feedback regulation (HMG CoA reductase) (27).
    (2) Apparently normal radiosensitivity (X-ray, U.V.) (32).

---

[a] Numbers in parenthesis provide the appropriate references for each finding.

mutation and that expression of the malignant phenotype might presumably only require treatment with a tumor-promoting agent (32).

We believe that *autosomal dominant traits* that predispose individuals to cancer (24,32) truly reflect genetic information directly related to this disease. In this connection, an association of the transformed state with a dominant mutation has been previously suggested (11,54). An autosomal dominant pattern has also been recently recognized in familial aggregates predisposed to cancer, comprising a large segment of all cancers reported (14,39,55). In our opinion, the ACR system provides a unique and a relatively uncomplicated approach for the study of cancer promotion in human cells *in vitro*.

RESULTS

Dose-Response Relationship to TPA and Human-Derived Bile Acid Analogues

We have shown that treatment of high density ACR cell cultures (5×10^4 cells/cm²) with TPA resulted in a dose-dependent stimulation of cell proliferation (Fig. 1, top; T. Gansler and L. Kopelovich, *in preparation*). In contrast, addition of TPA to sparse cultures (0.25×10^2 to 4×10^3 cells/cm²) produced a biphasic (concaved upward) dose-response curve with maximum inhibition in the range of 2 to 10 ng/ml of TPA (Fig. 1, bottom, and Fig. 2). These experiments did not require a continuous exposure to TPA. For example, the presence of TPA for approximately 48 hr and its subsequent removal from the cell culture medium yielded maximum values at the time of scoring, i.e., about 10 days later. Normal SF were considerably more sensitive to the toxic effects of TPA. At a TPA concentration of 2 to 10 ng/ml, the inhibition of proliferation of normal cells was essentially complete. We have used this differential toxicity to TPA to

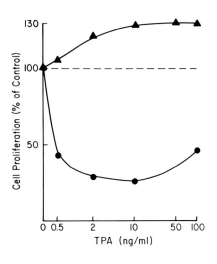

FIG. 1. The effects of TPA on cell proliferation. Cells were plated at a density of 4×10^3 cells/cm² (sparse cultures) and at a density of 5×10^4 cells/cm² (near confluence) and were exposed the following day to various concentrations of TPA. Cell counts were taken 4 days later. *Closed triangles* represent high density cultures, and *closed circles* represent sparse cultures.

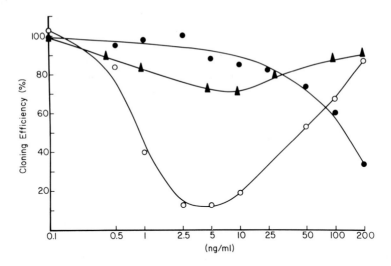

FIG. 2. The effects of TPA and 4-O-methyl TPA on cloning efficiency (CE). The SF were plated a density of 500 cells/60-mm Petri dish and allowed to attach overnight. At day 1 postplating, the medium was changed to a growth medium containing the appropriate concentration of the test compound. The results represent the CE in the presence of the test compound as percent of the CE in their absence (set up to 100%), in five dishes of five different experiments. *Open circles* represent the effects of TPA following acute exposure; *closed triangles* represent the effects of TPA on cells rescued from agar-growing colonies (AgI); and *closed circles* represent the effects of 4-O-methyl TPA following an acute exposure.

distinguish between normal persons and colorectal-prone individuals (31). It is of interest to note that a biphasic dose-response to TPA was not seen in sparse cultures of established normal fibroblastic cell lines (C3H/3T3, C3H/-10T 1/2).

The bimodal dose-response pattern to TPA in sparse cultures suggests the occurrence of two types of receptors: a high affinity receptor which, upon binding to the ligand, confers inhibition of cell growth, but can be saturated at a TPA concentration below 10 ng/ml, and another receptor of lower affinity (> 10 ng/ml) which, upon binding, causes stimulation of cell proliferation (Fig. 2). The apparent discrepancy in the dose-response pattern to TPA between sparse and near confluent human cell cultures (Figs. 1 and 2) may suggest that the "high affinity receptor" has been rendered inactive in the latter condition. This high affinity receptor is apparently absent from normal rodent SF lines (see above), indicating perhaps that these cells, unlike the human cell strains, are further along the transformation process. Whether these results suggest the existence of at least two cell populations, each of which displays a distinct type of receptor for TPA, or a single cell population with at least two types of receptors to TPA remains to be established. We believe that the latter condition is more likely, since the occurrence of two distinct cell types would conceivably permit a selection at high TPA concentration (> 10 ng/ml) and/or upon chronic exposure, to a cell population distinctly different from the mock-treated parent culture. The chronic exposure of ACR cells to TPA (about 10 population doublings), however, produced no significant differences in either the sensitivity or the pattern of response observed upon acute exposure to this promoter.

The nontumor promoter analogues of TPA, phorbol, and 4-O-methyl-12-O-tetradecanoylphorbol-13-acetate, showed a usual dose-response pattern characteristic of a drug with a single mode of action. In addition, human-derived bile acid analogues, such as lithocholate, chenocholate, cholate, and deoxycholate, believed to act as cancer promoters in man (19,47), effected little or no change in cell proliferation and were essentially nontoxic to either normal or ACR SF cultures both at low and high cell densities (slight stimulation).

Thymidine Uptake and Deoxyribonucleic Acid Distributions in TPA-Treated Cells

Experiments on the thymidine uptake and the thymidine-labeling indices in sparse cultures suggest that whereas the fraction of cells undergoing mitosis in exponentially growing SF (e.g., Fig. 1, bottom, and Fig. 2) is not appreciably affected by TPA, the absolute number of cells and possibly the rate at which deoxyribonucleic acid (DNA) synthesis proceeds might be primarily responsible for the effect seen with this compound. In confluent ACR cultures, however, TPA appears to induce an increase of both the thymidine uptake and the thymidine-labeling index in a manner consistent with the pattern shown in Fig. 1 (top). *In the context of these studies it is of interest that we have not been able to show any effects by TPA on ornithine decarboxylase in this cell system* (T. O'Brien and L. Kopelovich, *unpublished data*). Flow-cytometry analysis of DNA distributions showed that acute exposure of asynchronous ACR cells to TPA (100 ng/ml) caused the SF to accumulate primarily in G_1 and early S phase with few cells in late S or G_2. On the other hand, asynchronous agar I cell isolates (see below) growing in the absence of TPA showed a normal DNA distribution pattern, whereas in the presence of TPA there was an immediate and considerable accumulation of cells in G_2/M at the expense of G_1 (J. Fried and L. Kopelovich, *unpublished data*). A variety of similarly transient changes that were induced by TPA at different phases of the cell cycle of HeLa cells have been reported (23). These changes resembled the effects seen in cell cultures following X-ray irradiation (49).

Loss of Anchorage Sensitivity and Growth *In Vivo* of TPA-Treated Cells

The chronic application of TPA (100 ng/ml) to ACR cell cultures (Fig. 3) effected a change in cell morphology from the smooth fibroblastic-like to a dendritic-like cell. This effect was most pronounced at the early periods of exposure to TPA (first passage), and largely disappeared in later passages. This amount of TPA has also effected an increase in growth rate, saturation density,

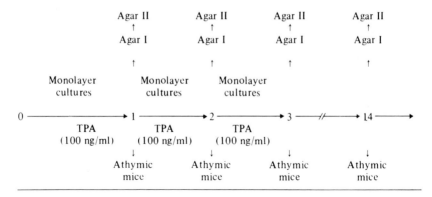

FIG. 3. The protocol for TPA-treated cells. Nutrient agar (Difco), 1.84% (wt/vol), was melted in boiling water and equilibrated at 45°C. It was then mixed with 2 × EMEM-40% FCS containing 200 ng ml^{-1} TPA/0.02% dimethylsulfoxide (DMSO)1:1 (vol/vol) at 45°C; 4 ml were plated onto each of 3–5 60-mm dishes as an underlayer and allowed to firm for 15 min at room temperature. Another portion of this solution was mixed with a cell suspension of 5 × 10^4 cells ml^{-1} in 1 × EMEM, 1:1 (vol/vol) containing 100 ng ml^{-1} of TPA in 0.01% of DMSO or DMSO alone. This preparation (4 ml), representing 1 × 10^5 cells per dish, was plated over the base layer and allowed to firm for 1 hr at room temperature in a chamber irrigated with 5% CO_2. Agar colonies were scored microscopically after about 4 weeks of incubation at 37°C in a humidified 5% CO_2 incubator. Inoculation of the nude mice (CD-1) was carried out with cells that were trypsinized, counted, and washed twice with physiological buffered saline (PBS) to give a final cell concentration of 1 × 10^6 per 0.02 ml of PBS. A volume of 0.02 ml was injected under a magnifying glass bilaterally into the anterior chamber of the eye. The mice were checked every week for the appearance of tumors. These usually became apparent at 2 weeks postinjection and were removed 1–2 weeks later. Each number represents a consecutive passage.

plasminogen-dependent activity occurring in very dense foci, and anchorage-insensitive colonies (30,32,33). These effects by TPA did not necessarily occur concurrently, however; they were transient during consecutive passages, and they were variable for a given human cell strain during different periods of TPA application (32). Furthermore, as already noted, TPA sensitivity following chronic exposure was both qualitatively and quantitatively similar to that observed in cells acutely exposed to this compound.[1]

We have previously demonstrated the induction by TPA of anchorage-insensitive ACR colonies (30). Since our initial report, the conditions for growing cells in agar have been optimized and we now find that ACR cells grow spontaneously in agar, albeit at low frequency (Table 1). Under these conditions, TPA has been shown at times to induce an increase of about 50- to 100-fold in anchorage-insensitive colonies. Other reports with cells that are probably further along the transformation process than are ACR cells also showed an increase in anchorage-insensitive colonies due to TPA (10,12). The effects seen in these

---

[1] The appearance of new genetic variants in a small member of cells during a chronic exposure to TPA should not be excluded (see below). The relationship of these variants to the TPA-induced phenotypic changes is not clear at present.

later studies, however, were both more uniform and permanent than those reported by us (30,32,33,34). The agar-growing cells showed a tighter clonal morphology, and about a threefold increase in proliferation in monolayer cultures, and in Ag II (33). The AgI cells (Fig. 3) also showed a dose-response to TPA considerably less concaved than that shown by nonagar-growing cells (Fig. 2), indicating perhaps a transient selection toward cells in which a portion of the "high affinity" receptors are apparently functionally inactive. Whether these results suggest that the "low-affinity" receptors are primarily responsible for some of the promoting activity of TPA (e.g., stimulation of cell proliferation; Figs. 1 and 2) remains to be seen. The agar-growing cells could not, however, be sustained beyond two passages in agar (Fig. 3; Ag II), and they eventually senesced (33,34). Our results, put together from a large number of experiments, suggest a high degree of heterogeneity, possibly coupled with an adaptive response and/or reversibility during selection of human cells in the continuous presence of TPA.

Previous attempts in our laboratory to inoculate TPA-treated ACR cells s.c. in the nude mouse have failed to yield any tumors (Fig. 3). Recently, however, the inoculation of these cells from 2 different individuals into the anterior chamber of the eye of a nude mouse gave rise to a moderately differentiated fibrosarcoma which is characterized by uniformly appearing, highly basophilic, fibroblast-like cells (34). These cells did not necessarily grow in agar, nor did they acquire an infinite life-span *in vitro* (32,34). Indeed, not all cells obtained from spontaneously occurring human tumors appear to grow indefinitely in culture (52). At present, we are studying a larger number of different individuals to provide a reliable measure about the probability of such an event occurring upon repeated exposures of cells from the same individuals and those taken from different gene carriers.

We have recently demonstrated that TPA-treated ACR cells that grew in athymic mice showed about 33% increase in cell aneuploidy (L. Kopelovich and R. Moon, *unpublished data*). The same proportion of cells has also been shown to be positive with respect to a first trimester human fetal antigen in the perinuclear region. An antigen with a similar specificity was also seen in KiMSV transformed ACR cells (32). These cells, however, were negative for ribonucleic acid (RNA)-associated viral expressions using antibodies directed against disrupted whole viruses of Gibbon ape leukemia, endogenous baboon virus, and endogenous cat RD-114. In addition, we found no correlation in the cellular levels of the sarc gene of Avian sarcoma virus in mock-treated normal and ACR cells, or TPA-treated cells (A. Goldberg and L. Kopelovich, *unpublished data*).

DISCUSSION

It has been suggested that cellular aging of fibroblasts is a differentiation process leading either to cellular degeneration or to neoplastic transformation (4,26). TPA may occupy a pivotal role in cell differentiation, capable of both the inhibition and stimulation of this process in a number of model systems (59). These observations could possibly be explained through the bimodal effect of TPA, which is characteristic of a drug with two modes of action. Although we do not yet fully understand the nature of this effect, these results may also suggest an interaction by TPA with a constitutive promoter-like factor (polypeptide?) that exists in both normal and ACR cells and is preferentially expressed through TPA in ACR cells. Incidentally, the parallel between this system and the concentration-dependent agonist-antagonist action of the opiates and their naturally occurring endorphins (53) is mechanistically intriguing. If, as has been suggested, the dominant cancer trait occurs in a class of tissue-differentiation genes (25), the elucidation of their mechanism of action in response to tumor promoters *vis-à-vis* differentiation would be important not only for the problem of cancer but also for the understanding of normal development. It would be of interest to extend these findings to study the effects of TPA on metabolic cooperation (60) and differentiation (59) of human fibroblasts.

TPA has been shown to enhance the stable transformation of murine and, more recently, of human foreskin fibroblasts previously exposed to a carcinogen (20,38,41,43). Thus, our results may indicate that the ACR mutation is a complete one for malignancy, representing an initiated state (32,34), and that the chronic application of TPA, in support of the two-stage "Berenblum hypothesis (5,6)," can precipitate the final oncogenic event. Alternatively, the enhancement of agar-insensitive colonies and the growth of cells *in vivo* may represent an intermediary state, similar perhaps to the TPA-induced papillomas in the mouse skin model (5,6,51) or to the clinical appearance of polyps in the colon; these may or may not regress spontaneously upon withdrawal of the stimulating factor. The latter would suggest that an additional mutation(s) is necessary for the malignant transformation of ACR cells with certain promoters acting during all phases of oncogenesis to increase the probability of expression of the malignant phenotype. Our ability to understand reversibility and adaptation (acquired resistance) in relation to inflammation, hyperplasia (transient and sustained), and promotion in TPA-sensitive animals (16,51) would provide insight about the effects of TPA in human cells *in vitro*.

Various hypotheses have been advanced to explain the promoting action of TPA. Thus, mechanisms involving membrane-induced sequential alterations in the response of the same cell type to TPA, presumably leading to increased probability for the expression of the malignant phenotype, have been indicated (21,59). Genomic effects due to TPA have also been proposed. For example: (a) aberrant mitotic segregation event(s) facilitated by a TPA-induced sister chromatid exchange (SCE), which might lead to the cosegregation of recessive chromosomal lesions (22); (b) a TPA-mediated enhancement in the frequency of specific locus mutations following insult with a carcinogen(s) (57); and (c) a TPA-induced aneuploidy (this chapter). Partial evidence that promotion by TPA does not proceed through mechanisms involving either genetic recombination or the altered suppression of newly mutated alleles has also been presented (56).

We speculate, nevertheless, that both initiators and promoters, in that order (51,59), can be mutagenic. Carcinogens are mutagenic due perhaps to their direct interaction with DNA, whereas TPA is mutagenic because it might cause chromosomal aberrations and an increase in cell ploidy. Aneuploidy, associated with aberrant chromosomal segregation, if stable, may conceivably be consistent with the expression of a recessive mutation(s) (32,34). Along similar lines we have recently, for example, noted that TPA inhibited the expression (about 99%) of SV40-induced T antigen display in ACR cells. Virus adsorption was not affected by this treatment. TPA has also been shown to induce the expression of persisting viral genomes (61). In addition, TPA effected the reexpression of malignancy in (human × mouse) hybrids whose tumorigenic phenotype was stably suppressed (7,8,9). The complex nature of changes occurring in eukaryotic chromosomes (e.g., transposable genes) has been recently documented (1). Clearly, the proper monitoring of subtle mutations and mutation frequencies in human cells due to TPA will be of great significance.

SUMMARY

In the studies described here, we demonstrated a unique dose-response (concaved upward) to TPA in sparse human cell cultures and a dose-dependent stimulation of cell proliferation in confluent cultures, suggesting a functional difference in putative TPA receptors between these two conditions. This bimodal dose-response to TPA was not seen in sparse cultures of established normal rodent cell lines.

The phenotypic profile of ACR cells chronically exposed to TPA, although effecting a change toward a more transformed phenotype (e.g., growth in agar), was in large measure neither stable nor uniform during consecutive passages or for a given cell strain during different periods of TPA application.

ACR cells when exposed to TPA alone appear to grow in the anterior chamber of the eye of a nude mouse. We speculated that TPA-induced aneuploidy in these cells, coupled with DNA instability and aberrant chromosomal segregation, may conceivably be consistent with neoplasia in initiated ACR cells.

Finally, the apparent susceptibility of ACR cells to further transformation by TPA and N-methyl-N^1-nitro-N-nitrosoguanidine (MNNG) (34,48) and by ocongenic viruses (37,45) indicates that *genetic information* residing within these cells, probably in the form of an ACR mutation, renders them more sensitive to these *two distinct classes* of carcinogens.

ADDENDUM

A bimodal dose reponse to TPA has recently been observed in cloned ACR skin fibroblasts (Kopelovich, L., *in preparation*). This further supports our contention that a single cell population of the same lineage possesses at least two receptor sites to TPA *(this review)*. Following our observation, Dr. M. Eisinger of this Institute found a bimodal dose response to TPA in human keratinocytes, but only the stimulatory portion of the curve for melanocytes *(personal communication)*. If our assumption about the potential role of these two types of receptors is correct *(this review),* the expected incidence of melanoma should be relatively high under conditions of sufficient exposure to potential promoters and/or carcinogens. Indeed, the incidence of melanotic foci increases considerably with age.

We have recently found that the following TPA analogues, in diminishing order of toxicity, showed a bimodal dose-response: PDD, PDBu, PDB, and PDA. They were all considerably less toxic than TPA. However, mezerine exhibited the usual dose response, characteristic of a drug with a single mode of action. Its toxicity greatly exceeded that shown for 4-0 Me-TPA and phorbol *(this review).*

At present, we have extended our observations about the growth of TPA-treated ACR cells *in vivo* to 10 individuals. Attempts are currently underway to retrieve these cells from the eye and to establish their human origin by karyotyping.

ACKNOWLEDGMENTS

I thank Dr. S. Rasheed for the determination of RNA-associated viral expressions in TPA-treated cells.

I thank Ms. R. Vuolo, Ms. T. Shapiro, and M. P. Monoghan for excellent technical assistance. This work was supported, in part, by grants CA-19259 and CA-21623 from the National Large Bowel Cancer Project and an institute grant CA-08748 from the National Cancer Institute.

REFERENCES

1. Abelson, J., and Butz, E. (editors) (1980): Recombinant DNA. *Science,* 209:1,317–1,438.
2. Almy, T., and Licznerski, G. (1973): The intestinal polyposes. *Clin. Gastroentrol.,* 2:577–601.
3. Ames, B. N., McCann, J., and Yamasaki, B. (1975): Methods for detecting carcinogens and mutagens with the salmonella/mammalian-microsome mutagenicity test. *Mutat. Res.,* 31:347–364.
4. Bell, E., Marek, L. F., Levinstone, D. S., Merrill, L., Sher, S., Young, T. I., and Eden, M. (1978): Loss of division potential *in vitro:* Aging or differentiation? *Science,* 202:1,158–1,163.
5. Berenblum, I. (1975): Sequential aspects of chemical carcinogenesis, skin. In: *Etiology: Chemical and Physical Carcinogenesis, Vol. 1: Cancer, A Comprehensive Treatise,* edited by F. F. Becker, pp. 323–344. Plenum Publishing Corp., New York.
6. Berenblum, I. (1978): Established principles and unresolved problems in carcinogenesis. *J. Natl. Cancer Inst.,* 60:723–726.
7. Chopan, M., and Kopelovich, L. (1981): The suppression of tumorigenicity in human X mouse cell hybrids. I. Derivation of hybrid clones, chromosome analysis, and tumorigenicity studies. *Exp. Cell Biol.,* 79:78–90.
8. Chopan, M., and Kopelovich, L. (1981): The suppression of tumorigenicity in cell hybrids. II. The relationship between tumorigenicity and transformation-related parameters *in vitro. Exp. Cell Biol.,* 49:132–140.
9. Chopan, M., and Kopelovich, L. (1981): A nontumorigenic (mouse × human) cell hybrid inhibits tumorigenicity of its malignant mouse parent cell and unrelated human tumor cells *in vivo. Oncology,* 38:240–242.

10. Colburn, N. H., Former, B. F., Nelson, K. A., and Yuspa, S. H. (1979): Tumor promoter induces anchorage independence irreversibly. *Nature,* 281:589–591.
11. Comings, D. E. (1973): A general theory of carcinogenesis. *Proc. Natl. Acad. Sci. (U.S.A.),* 70:3,324–3,328.
12. Fisher, P. B., Dorsch-Hasler, K., Weinstein, B. I., and Ginsburg, H. S. (1979): Tumor promoters enhance anchorage-independent growth of adenovirus-transformed cells without altering the integration pattern of viral sequences. *Nature,* 281:591–594.
13. Foulds, L. (1969): Current Concepts of Neoplastic Transformation *in vivo.* Neoplastic Transformation. Academic Press, New York.
14. Fraumeni, J. F., Jr. (1977): Clinical patterns of familial cancer. In: *Genetics of Human Cancer,* edited by J. J. Mulvihill, R. W. Miller, and J. F. Fraumeni, Jr., pp. 223–235. Raven Press, New York.
15. Gardner, E., and Richards, R. (1953): Multiple cutaneous and subcutaneous lesions occurring simultaneously with hereditary polyposis and osteomatosis. *Am. J. Hum. Genet.,* 5:139–148.
16. Goerttler, K., Loehrke, H., Schweizer, J., and Hesse, B. (1980): Two-stage tumorigenesis of dermal melanocytes in the back skin of the Syrian golden hamsters using systemic initiation with 7,12-dimethylbenz(a) anthracene and topical promotion with 12-O-tetradecanoylphorbol-13-acetate. *Cancer Res.,* 40:155–161. *(Also, this volume).*
17. Hecker, E. (1971): Isolation and characterization of the cocarcinogenic principle from croton oil. *Methods Cancer Res.,* 6:439–484.
18. Heidelberger, C. (1975): Chemical carcinogenesis. *Ann. Rev. Biochem.,* 44:79–121.
19. Kelsey, M. I., Molina, J. E., and Hwang, K. K. (1979): A comparison of litocholic acid metabolism by intestinal microflora in subjects of high- and low-risk colon cancer populations. *Front. Gastorintest. Res.,* 4:38–50.
20. Kennedy, A. R., Mondal, S., Heidelberger, C., and Little. J. B. (1978): Enhancement of X-ray transformation by 12-O-tetradeconoylphorbol-13-acetate in a cloned line of C3H mouse embryo cells. *Cancer Res.,* 38:439–443.
21. Kennedy, A. R., Murphy, G., and Little, J. B. (1980: The effect of time and duration of exposure to 12-O-tetradecanoylphorbol-13-acetate (TPA) on X-ray transformation of C3H 10T½ cells. *Cancer Res.,* 40:1,915–1,920.
22. Kinsella, A. K., and Radman, M. (1978): Tumor promoter induces sister chromatid exchanges: Relevance to mechanisms of carcinogenesis. *Proc. Natl. Acad. Sci. USA,* 75:6,149–6,153.
23. Kinzel, V., Richards, J., and Stohr, M. (1980): Tumor promoter TPA mimics irradiation effects on the cell cycle of HeLa cells. *Science,* 210:429–431.
24. Knudson, A. G. (1977): Genetics and etiology of human cancer. In: *Advances in Human Genetics,* edited by H. Harris and K. Hirshhorn, pp. 1–66. Raven Press, New York.
25. Knudson, A. G. (1979): Hereditary Cancer. *JAMA,* 241:279.
26. Kontermann, K., and Bayreuther, K. (1979): The cellular aging of rat fibroblasts *in vitro* is a differentiation process. *Gerontology,* 25:261–274.
27. Kopelovich, L. (1977*a*): Phenotypic markers in human skin fibroblasts as possible diagnostic indices of hereditary adenomatosis of the colon and rectum. *Cancer,* 40:2,534–2,541.
28. Kopelovich, L. (1977*b*): Familial polyposis: A model of tumor progression. In: *Workshop on Cancer Invasion and Metastasis Biologic Mechanisms and Therapy,* edited by S. Day, pp. 375–387. Raven Press, New York.
29. Kopelovich, L. (1978*a*): Cutaneous manifestations occurring systemically in heritable forms of cancer. Proceedings 1st Int. Symposium on Inborn of Metabolism in Man. *Monogr. Hum. Genet.,* 10:156–169.
30. Kopelovich, L. (1978*b*): TPA-induced agar-insensitive colonies in human mutant cells. *Cold Spring Harbor Symp.,* p. 11.
31. Kopelovich, L. (1981): The use of a tumor promoter as a single parameter approach for the detection of individuals genetically predisposed to colorectal cancer. *Cancer Letters,* 12:67–74.
32. Kopelovich, L. (1980*b*): Hereditary adenomatosis of the colon and rectum. Recent studies on the nature of cancer promotion and cancer prognosis *in vitro.* In: *Colorectal Cancer: Prevention, Epidemiology, and Screening,* edited by S. Winawer, D. Schottenfield, and P. Sherlock, pp. 91–108. Raven Press, New York.
33. Kopelovich, L., and Bias, N. (1979): Tumor promoter induces loss of anchorage dependence in human skin fibroblasts from individuals genetically predisposed to cancer. *Exp. Cell Biol.,* 48:207–217.

34. Kopelovich, L., Bias, N., and Helson, L. (1979): Tumor promoter alone induces malignant transformation of human skin fibroblasts from individuals genetically predisposed to cancer. *Nature,* 282:619–621.
35. Kopelovich, L., Conlon, S., and Pollack, R. (1977): Defective organization of actin in cultured skin fibroblasts. *Proc. Natl. Acad. Sci. USA,* 74:3019–3022.
36. Kopelovich, L., Pfeffer, L., and Bias, N. (1979): Growth characteristics of human skin fibroblasts *in vitro.* A simple experimentation approach for the identification of hereditary adenomatosis of the colon and rectum. *Cancer,* 43:218–223.
37. Kopelovich, L., and Sirlin, S. (1980): Human skin fibroblasts from individuals genetically predisposed to cancer are sensitive to an SV40-induced T antigen display and transformation. *Cancer,* 45:1,108–1,111.
38. Lasne, C., Gentil, A., and Chouroulinkov, I. (1974): Two-stage malignant transformation of rat fibroblasts in tissue culture. *Nature,* 247:490–491.
39. Lynch, H. T., Harris, R. E., Lynch, P. M., Guirgis, H. A., Lynch, J. P., and Bardawil, W. A. (1977): Role of heredity in multiple primary cancers. *Cancer,* 40:1,845–1,849.
40. Miller, E. C. (1978): Some current perspectives on chemical carcinogenesis in humans and experimental animals. *Cancer Res.,* 38:1,479–1,496.
41. Milo, G. F., and Dipaolo, J. A. (1978): Neoplastic transformation of human diploid cells *in vitro* after chemical carcinogen treatment. *Nature,* 275:130–132.
42. Mintz, B., and Illmensee, K. (1975): Normal genetically mosaic mice produced from malignant teratocarcinoma cells. *Proc. Natl. Acad. Sci. USA,* 72:3,585–3,589.
43. Mondal, S., Barnkow, D. W., and Heidelberger, C. (1976): Two-stage oncogenesis in cultures of C3H 10T½ cells. *Cancer Res.,* 36:2,254–2,260.
44. Morson, B., and Bussey, H. (1970): Predisposing causes of intestinal Cancer. *Curr. Probl. Surg.,* 1–50.
45. Pfeffer, L., and Kopelovich, L. (1977): Differential genetic susceptibility of cultured human skin fibroblasts to transformation by Kirsten murine sarcoma virus. *Cell,* 10:313–320.
46. Pfeffer, L., Lipkin, M., Stutman, O., and Kopelovich, L. (1976): Growth abnormalities of cultured human skin fibroblasts derived from individual with hereditary adenomatosis of the colon and rectum. *J. Cell. Physiol.,* 80:29–38.
47. Reddy, B. S., and Watanable, K. (1979): Effect of cholesterol metabolites and promoting effects of litocholic acid in colon carcinogenesis in germ-free and conventional F344 rats. *Cancer Res.,* 39:1,521–1,527.
48. Rhim, J. S., Huebner, R. J., Arnstein, P., and Kopelovich, L. (1980): Chemical transformation of cultured human skin fibroblasts derived from individuals with hereditary adenonatosis of the colon and rectum. *Int. J. Cancer,* 26:565–569.
49. Sinclair, W. K. (1968): Cylic X-ray responses in mammalian cells *in vitro. Radiat. Res.,* 33:620–643.
50. Sivak, A., and Van Duuren, B. L. (1967): Phenotypic expression of transformation: Induction in cell culture by a phorbol ester. *Science,* 157:1,443–1,444.
51. Slaga, T. J., Sivak, A., and Boutwell, R. K. (editors) (1978): *Mechanism of tumor promotion and cocarcinogenesis, Vol. 2,* pp 1–715. Raven Press, New York.
52. Smets, L. A. (1980): Cell transformation as a model for tumor induction and neoplastic growth. *Biochem. Biophys. Acta,* 605:93–111.
53. Snyder, H. (1977): Opiate receptors and internal opiates. *Sci. Am.,* 236:44–66.
54. Stanbridge, E. J., and Wilkinson, J. (1978): Analysis of malignancy in human cells: Malignant and transformed phenotypes are under separate genetic control. *Proc. Natl. Acad. Sci. USA,* 75:1,466–1,469.
55. Swift, M. (1976): Malignant disease in heterozygote carriers. Cancer and genetics. *Birth Defects,* 12:133–144.
56. Thompson, L. H., Baker, R. M., Carrano, A. V., and Brookman, K. W. (1980): Failure of the phorbol ester 12-O-tetradecanoylphorbol-13-acetate to enhance sister chromatid exchange, mitotic segregation, or expression of mutations in Chinese hamster cells. *Cancer Res.,* 40:3,245–3,251.
57. Trosko, J. E., Cheng, C. C., Yotti, L. P., and Chu, E. H. Y. (1977): Effect of phorbol myristate acetate on the recovery of spontaneous and ultraviolet light-induced 6-thioguanine and ouabain-resistant Chinese hamster cells. *Cancer Res.,* 37:188–193.
58. Van Duuren, B. N. (1976): Tumor-promoting and cocarcinogenic agents in chemical carcinogen-

esis. In: *Chemical Carcinogens, Monograph 173,* edited by C. E. Searle, pp. 24–51. American Chemical Society, Washington, D.C.

59. Weinstein, I. B., Mufson, A., Lee, L. S., Fisher, P. B., Laskin, J., Horowitz, A. D., and Ivanovic, V. (1980): Membrane and other biochemical effects of the phorbol esters and their relevance to tumor promotion. 13th Jerusalem Symposium, Carcinogenesis. Fundamental Mechanisms and Environmental Effects, edited by B. Pullman, P. O. P. Tso, and H. Gelboin. R. Eidel Publishing Co., Amsterdam *(in press).*

60. Yotti, L. P., Chang, C. C., and Troski, J. (1979): Elimination of metabolic cooperation in Chinese hamster cells by a tumor promoter. *Science,* 206:1,089–1,091.

61. Zur Hausen, H., Bornkamm, G. W., Schmidt, R., and Hecker, E. (1979): Tumor initiators and promoters in the induction of Epstein-Barr virus. *Proc. Natl. Acad. Sci. USA,* 76:782–785.

Carcinogenesis, Vol. 7, edited by E. Hecker et al.
Raven Press, New York © 1982.

Regulation of Mammalian Cell Transformation

J. A. DiPaolo, C. H. Evans, N. C. Popescu, and J. N. Doniger

Laboratory of Biology, National Cancer Institute, Bethesda, Maryland 20205

Transformation *in vitro* of mammalian cells by carcinogens to the neoplastic state has been extensively proven (2). Furthermore, neoplastic markers are identical for both *in vitro* results and *in vivo* experimental data. With Syrian hamster embryo cells (HEC), it is possible to demonstrate morphologic transformation after only 7 days of culture. A statistical analysis of the transformation dose-response phenomenon indicates that the transformation is inductive and due to a one-hit-type of event. In addition, failure to find evidence of C-type particles or of viruses known to transform mammalian cells indicates that transformation of HEC is due to the direct effect of the agent used. The transformation frequency can be inhibited or enhanced by biological modifiers or chemical treatment. Thus, studies utilizing these cells are relevant to the study of the mechanism(s) of carcinogenesis and for the investigation of cocarcinogenic and anticarcinogenic effects of a variety of agents.

The transformation frequency associated with a chemical carcinogen can be increased by sequential use of other chemicals or physical agents. For example, enhancement of transformation occurs when X-irradiation or methyl-methane-sulfonate precedes chemical carcinogen or ultraviolet (UV) irradiation (3,4,5). Since the enhancement is time dependent, the increased transformation is considered due to a transitory change in specific cells; however, no changes were noted in cell cycle, in progression of cells from G_1 to S, nor was any difference noted in the frequency of aberration or ploidy compared to time intervals when the transformation was no longer elevated.

X-ray alone causes no transformation whereas UV induces a frequency of 10^{-3}/erg/mm² which is 10^2- to 10^4-fold greater than reported mutation frequencies with mammalian cells. Excision and postreplication deoxyribonucleic acid (DNA) repair of UV-induced damage were studied to determine whether enhanced transformation frequencies were associated with either of these repair mechanisms (5). Independent of pretreatment, approximately 25% of the pyrimidine dimers are excised within 24 hr in cells irradiated with UV (3 J/m²). During this period, more than 70% of the cell's genome has been replicated. Regardless of X-ray pretreatment, 1 and 3 hr are required for pulse-labeled DNA in control and in irradiated cells to reach parental size. Therefore, no correlation exists between changes in the rate of excision or postreplication repair and enhancement of transformation. Cells UV-irradiated have a 70% survival rate and multiply with more than 10^5 pyrimidine dimers per genome in the DNA. Therefore, other repair mechanisms must be responsible for cell survival as well as enhanced transformation. Caffeine has a cocarcinogenic effect if added after UV or chemical carcinogen. We asked whether the modulation by caffeine of post-UV DNA replication might be responsible for the enhanced frequency of transformed colonies (6). After cells are irradiated with UV, two modes of DNA replication occur. During the early mode that operates for the first 3 to 4 hr post-UV, nascent DNA strands were smaller than those in nonirradiated cells. During the late mode, the nascent strands were of normal size. Incubating the cells with caffeine post-UV irradiation (10 J/m²) inhibited the conversion of the early mode to the late mode. The change from early mode to late mode replication occurs at about 4 hr post-UV and with the time interval for caffeine's greatest effect on transformation. The observed caffeine-induced changes in the post-UV DNA replication can account for the potentiation of UV-induced lethality by caffeine and may be partially responsible for the enhancement of transformation.

An important aspect of our *in vitro* transformation studies is shown to elucidate the role of chromosomal changes in carcinogenesis. Therefore, a coordinated transformation and cytogenic study was designed to determine the relationship of the tumor promoter 12-O-tetradecanoylphorbol-13-acetate (TPA) to chromosomal changes during the process of transformation (8). Whereas TPA was ineffective in influencing transformation frequency by itself, it did enhance transformation obtained with N-methyl-N'-nitro-N-nitrosoguanidine (MNNG) and a series of hydrocarbons that are known to be weak or noncarcinogens. The enhanced transformation frequency indicates that the number of cells initiated by a low dose of carcinogen is greater than those cells transformed by a carcinogen alone. TPA alone was ineffective in inducing SCE, or in altering SCE frequency in MNNG cells that were growing logarithmically or had been treated with TPA and released from confluency. Nor did TPA post-MNNG alter the percent of cells with aberrations or the total number of aberrations per 100 metaphases. A lack of effect by TPA is consistent with the evidence that TPA does not covalently bind with DNA.

Interference with transformation can be demonstrated in cell cultures. Lymphokines, biologically active hormone-like substances produced by stimulated lymphocytes, are an effective growth inhibitor of a variety of tumor cells and have very little effect on nontumorigenic cells. With carcinogen-treated guinea pig cells, lymphotoxin susceptibility generally develops when the cells acquire the ability to produce tumors *in vivo*. The frequency of benzo[a]pyrene-, MNNG-, N-acetoxyacetylaminofluorene-, or 254-nm UV irradiation-induced transformation is reduced in direct proportion to the concentration of lymphotoxin from mitogen-stimulated Syrian hamster leukocytes (7). Transformation is prevented when lymphotoxin is added either simultaneously or 1 to 4 days after carcinogen. Furthermore, refeeding with medium lacking lymphotoxin results in no increase in transformation frequency. Thus, the anticarcinogenic activity of lymphotoxin is irreversible.

Postcarcinogen treatment, but not pretreatment, with varying concentrations of antipain also inhibits transformation (1). DNA replication is not affected by MNNG, antipain, or the combination of the two, and no synergistic lethality occurs. MNNG causes a variety of chromosomal aberrations primarily of the chromatid type including exchanges. No specificity in terms of chromosome involvement or chromosome segments was noted. Because chromosomal abnormalities are often associated with neoplasia, a relationship has been assumed between changes in chromatid function and cancer. On the basis of the average number of SCE per metaphase or chromosome, antipain did not alter the 5-bromodeoxyuridine (BrdUrd)-induced rate of untreated controls or the frequency of MNNG-induced rate when added 10 min post- or 24 hr pre-MNNG. Our results with HEC that undergo transformation, however, demonstrate an increased frequency of chromosomal aberrations (per metaphase) when treated with MNNG followed by antipain, the same procedure used for the transformation studies. The increase in the number of aberrations per metaphase with MNNG and antipain compared to MNNG alone was statistically significant at 10, 26, and 40 hr after treatment. Although the mode of action of antipain is unknown, it is unlikely that the mechanism of gene conversion leading to transformation involves a proteolytic sensitive step that controls the formation of chromatid exchanges. A possibility may be that the reduction in transformation frequency simply reflects cell death due to the increase in chromosome aberrations and thus is responsible for eliminating a subpopulation that was destined to be transformed.

It has been intellectually more satisfying and consistent with the irreversibility of the initiating event to presume that a mutation-like process occurs very rapidly and that the long latent period of carcinogenesis involves the promoting phase. The time dependence for enhanced transformation with X-ray and alkylating agents followed by a potent carcinogen or UV suggested that mechanisms other than point mutations are responsible for HEC survival and for the radiation-type enhanced transformation. Since the damage persists and cells survive with that damage, DNA alteration is probably responsible for the transformation. What is unresolved is whether DNA leads to mutation(s) that are involved in the conversion of nonmalignant cells to malignancy.

REFERENCES

1. DiPaolo, J. A., Amsbaugh, S. C., and Popescu, N. C. (1980): Antipain inhibits N-methyl-N'-nitro-N-nitrosoguanidine-induced transformation and increases chromosomal aberrations. *Proc. Natl. Acad. Sci. USA,* 77:6,649–6,653.
2. DiPaolo, J. A., and Casto, B. C. (1978): *In vitro* carcinogenesis with cells in early passages. *Natl. Cancer Inst. Monogr.,* 48:245–257.
3. DiPaolo, J. A., and Donovan, P. J. (1976): *In vitro* morphologic transformation of Syrian hamster cells by UV-irradiation is enhanced by X-irradiation and unaffected by chemical carcinogens. *Int. J. Radiat. Biol.,* 30:41–53.

4. DiPaolo, J. A., Donovan, P. J., and Popescu, N. C. (1976): Kinetics of Syrian hamster cells during X-irradiation enhancement of transformation *in vitro* by chemical carcinogen. *Radiat. Res.,* 66:310–325.
5. Doniger, J., and DiPaolo, J. A. (1980): Excision and postreplication DNA repair capacities, enhanced transformation, and survival of Syrian hamster embryo cells irradiated by ultraviolet light. *Cancer Res.,* 40:582–587.
6. Doniger, J., and DiPaolo, J. A. (1981): Modulation of *in vitro* transformation and the early and late modes of DNA replication of UV-irradiated Syrian hamster cells by caffeine. *Radiat. Res.,* 87:565–575.
7. Evans, C. H., and DiPaolo, J. A. (1981): Lymphotoxin: An anticarcinogenic lymphokine as measured by inhibition of chemical carcinogen or ultraviolet irradiation-induced transformation of Syrian hamster cells. *Int. J. Cancer,* 27:45–49.
8. Popescu, N. C., Amsbaugh, S. C., and DiPaolo, J. A. (1980): Enhancement of N-methyl-N'-nitro-N-nitrosoguanidine transformation of Syrian hamster cells by a phorbol diester is independent of sister chromatid exchanges and chromosome aberrations. *Proc. Natl. Acad. Sci. USA,* 77:7282–7286.

Carcinogenesis, Vol. 7, edited by E. Hecker et al.
Raven Press, New York © 1982.

In Vitro Modulation of Oncogenesis and Differentiation by Retinoids and Tumor Promoters

Carmia Borek, R. C. Miller, C. R. Geard, D. L. Guernsey, and
J. E. Smith

*Departments of Radiology, Pathology, Biochemistry, and Medicine, Cancer Center/Institute
of Cancer Research, Columbia University College of Physicians & Surgeons,
New York, New York 10032*

Retinoids, the family of vitamin A and its analogues, have multiple functions. They control growth and differentiation and they are effective inhibitors of neoplastic development *in vivo* and *in vitro* (for review, see ref. 9). Conversely, promoters, in particular 12-O-tetradecanoylphorbol-13-acetate (TPA) (8), have been shown to inhibit differentiation in many systems and serve as enhancers of carcinogenesis (12).

In recent years it has become increasingly evident that there exists an antagonism between retinoids and tumor promoters in their effect on differentiation and in their influence on normal and neoplastic cells (for review, see ref. 9). In this chapter we show this antagonism in two systems: (a) The ability of retinoids to inhibit, in rodent fibroblasts, radiation-induced transformation and its promotion by TPA; and (b) The effectiveness of retinoids in antagonizing the inhibitory effect of TPA on differentiation in rat liver epithelial cells. TPA inhibits the production of Vitamin A (retinol) binding proteins (RBP) and Vitamin A can overcome this inhibitory effect (5).

RETINOIDS AS INHIBITORS OF RADIATION TRANSFORMATION AND ITS PROMOTION BY TPA

In earlier work we described the inhibition of radiation transformation by a Vitamin A analogue in C3H/10T½ cells (7). In the present work we used two cell systems, the C3H 10T½ mouse heteroploid line (10) and freshly explanted diploid hamster embryo cells (1). We asked the following questions: (a) Will TPA promote radiation transformation in both cell systems? (b) Will the retinoids inhibit the promotional effect of TPA? (c) If they do, is the inhibition reflected in patterns of deoxyribonucleic acid (DNA) damage using sister chromatid exchange (SCE) analysis? (d) Are the effects of retinoids and TPA on transformation reflected in the level of membrane-associated ion transport enzymes Na$^+$/K$^+$ ATPase, Mg$^+$ ATPase, and 5'nucleotidase, since both TPA and retinoids have been reported to modify cell membranes?

Materials and Methods

Detailed experimental procedures have been described elsewhere (3). TPA (Consolidated Midland Corp., N.Y.) was dissolved in dimethylsulfoxide (DMSO) and added to the cells at 0.16 μM in a final DMSO concentration of 0.01%. Retinoids included β all-transretinoic acid (RA) and trimethylmethoxyphenyl analogue of N-ethyl retinamide (TMMP-ERA). In the SCE studies colcemide was used at 5 μM and BrdU at 3 μM (3).

Cells were X-irradiated with 300 or 400 rad as described (3,4).

Analysis of the membrane-ion transport enzymes was carried out using a modification of established method, as described elsewhere (2).

Cells were exposed to radiation 24 hr after seeding, in the presence of retinoids. The retinoids were removed 4 days later. TPA was added immediately after irradiation and left on throughout the experiments (2 weeks for the hamster cells and 6 weeks for the 10T½). Hamster cells were fed twice weekly whereas C3H 10T½ cells were fed every 6 days. All cells were maintained at 37°C in a humidified incubator in 5% CO_2 in air for the duration of the experiment, after which the plates were fixed and stained with Giemsa. Transformed colonies in the hamster cultures (1) and transformed foci type II and III in the 10T½ cultures (10) were identified morphologically and scored as described (3,4). The distinct, dense, multilayered growth pattern with irregular cell-cell orientation distinguished the transformed cells from the untransformed counterparts.

SCE analysis was carried out on the C3H 10T½ cells. Cells were incubated with 3 μM BrdU for 24 or 26 hr prior to irradiation, TPA, and/or retinoid treatment. Cells were fixed at various times after irradiation with mitoses being accumulated with colcemide for the final 6 hr and stained with Giemsa (3).

For the determination of membrane-associated enzymes Na$^+$/K$^+$ ATPase, Mg$^+$ ATPase, and 5'nucleotidase, cells were incubated with TPA and/or all transretinoic acid for 4 days, along with untreated controls.

Results

Modification of Transformation in C3H/10T½ and Syrian Hamster Embryo Cells

Exposure of cells to TPA alone, retinoid alone, or the combination of the two compounds produced no transformation (Table 1). Addition of TPA immediately followed by continuous exposure of cells to TPA, however, resulted in enhanced transformation frequency. In contrast, exposing cells to X-rays and retinoid reduced the transformation frequency by half. The combination of X-

TABLE 1. *TPA and retinoid modulating X-ray induced transformation in hamster embryo and C$_3$H-10T½ cells*[a]

Treatment	Hamster embryo		C$_3$H-10T½	
	Surviving fraction[b]	Mean rate of transformation (10^{-3}) ± standard error	Surviving fraction	Mean rate of transformation (10^{-4}) ± standard error
Control	1.00	0	1.00	0
TPA (0.16μM)	0.70	0	0.93	0
Retinoid (7.1 μM)	0.62	0	0.75	0
Retinoid, TPA	0.89	0	0.67	0
X-rays	0.42	6.99 ± 1.65	0.32	8.78 ± 1.29
X-rays, TPA	0.53	12.52 ± 1.81	0.52	16.15 ± 1.59
X-rays, retinoid	0.38	2.94 ± 0.79	0.30	4.37 ± 0.93
X-rays, retinoid, TPA	0.41	2.41 ± 0.85	0.36	2.46 ± 0.54

[a] In experiments where cells were exposed to X-rays, hamster cells were irradiated with 300 rad while C$_3$H 10T½ were treated with 400 rad.

rays, continuous exposure to TPA, and a 4-day exposure of cells to retinoid resulted in a transformation frequency similar to exposure of cells to X-rays and retinoid. Retinoid for only 4 days completely inhibited the promoting effects of a continuous exposure to TPA and much of the inducing effects of X-rays.

SCE

Results from five replicate experiments with the retinoid TMMP-ERA are described in detail elsewhere (3) and are illustrated in Fig. 1. Retinoids and TPA had little influence on SCE frequencies, though both show small increases over the control. Radiation, at 300 rad of X-rays, increased SCE frequencies by 50%, and both TPA and retinoid alone or in combination increased this level slightly. Figure 1 displays the striking contrast between the findings for SCE and for transformation. The overall mean incidences of SCE per chromosome are presented as a histogram for each treatment alongside the overall frequencies for transformation. While retinoid and TPA slightly increased SCE, they produced no transformation. Radiation produced both transformation and increased SCEs. Furthermore, while the added retinoid completely eliminated

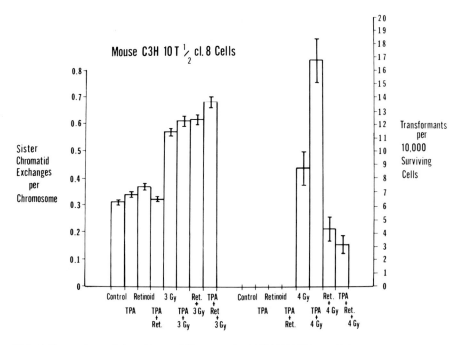

FIG. 1. Comparison of the effects of X-rays, retinoid TMMP-ERA, and TPA on transformation induction (*right side*) and SCEs (*left side*) in C3H/10T½ cells. Standard errors of the mean (transformation) and 2 × SE x̄ (SCEs) are indicated. For the SCE studies, cells were scored up to 20 hr after irradiation, while transformation incidence was assessed at 5 weeks after irradiation with TPA in continuous cell contact and retinoid present for 4 days only.

TABLE 2. *The effect of RA and TPA on membrane enzyme activities in hamster embryo and C$_3$H-10T½ cells^a*

Treatment	Na$^+$/K$^+$ ATPase	Mg$^+$ ATPase	5'-Nucleotidase
Hamster embryo			
Control	1.21 ± 0.21	1.35 ± 0.17	1.73 ± 0.28
TPA (0.16 μM)	1.53 ± 0.43	1.44 ± 0.45	1.89 ± 0.31
Retinoid (7.1 μM)	0.78 ± 0.19	1.32 ± 0.36	1.75 ± 0.21
Retinoid, TPA	1.13 ± 0.27	1.19 ± 0.41	1.91 ± 0.32
C$_3$H-10T½			
Control	1.79 ± 0.32	1.26 ± 0.31	0.56 ± 0.08
TPA (0.16 μM)	2.18 ± 0.31	1.26 ± 0.26	0.60 ± 0.12
Retinoid (7.1 μM)	1.13 ± 0.20	1.32 ± 0.26	0.68 ± 0.05
Retinoid, TPA	1.73 ± 0.23	1.23 ± 0.28	0.64 ± 0.10
Transformed Hamster embryo			
Control	2.46 ± 0.27	1.54 ± 0.31	5.75 ± 1.21
TPA (0.16 μM)	2.31 ± 0.21	1.38 ± 0.21	5.90 ± 1.38
Retinoid (7.1 μM)	2.50 ± 0.29	1.42 ± 0.21	5.83 ± 1.10
Retinoid, TPA	2.34 ± 0.31	1.50 ± 0.32	5.92 ± 1.23
Transformed C$_3$H-10T½			
Control	0.97 ± 0.09	0.87 ± 0.08	0.40 ± 0.07
TPA (0.16 μM)	1.21 ± 0.12	1.38 ± 0.22	0.46 ± 0.06
Retinoid (7.1 μM)	0.82 ± 0.21	8.99 ± 0.06	0.59 ± 0.02
Retinoid, TPA	1.04 ± 0.18	1.05 ± 0.10	0.47 ± 0.16

^{a} All values are mean ± standard error in moles Pi/hr/mg protein.

the promotional effect of TPA on radiation-induced transformation, SCEs are slightly increased.

The results on the effect of the retinoids and TPA on membrane enzymes are presented in Table 2. The level of Na$^+$/K$^+$ ATPase is enhanced by TPA and decreased by all-transretinoic acid. When cells were exposed to both retinoid and TPA, the enzyme returned to control level. The effect is specific to the Na$^+$/K$^+$ ATPase system since Mg$^+$ ATPase and 5'nucleotidase were unaffected by the two compounds. When neoplastic C3H 10T½ and hamster embryo cells were exposed to TPA and retinoid alone or in combination, there was no significant effect on the membrane enzymes.

REGULATION OF RBP BY RETINOIDS AND TPA

Retinol, a water soluble lipid alcohol, is the major form of Vitamin A normally found in the plasma. Retinol circulates in the plasma bound to RBP (6,11) which has been purified from a variety of species including humans and rats. RBP is a small protein with a MW of about 20,000 daltons, which has a single binding site for one molecule of retinol.

In our earlier studies we have shown that the differentiated hepatoma cell line H$_4$II EC$_3$ (H$_4$) produced RBP as well as albumin, and that the production

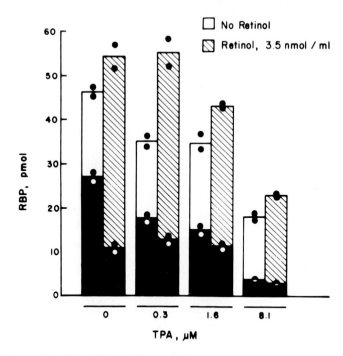

FIG. 2. Histogram describing TPA inhibition on RBP production in H₄ cells and the effect of retinol in suppressing the TPA effect. *Dark black areas* represent cellular content of RBP. *White and notched areas* represent RBP measured in the medium. Details of RBP measurements using radioimmunoassay are in ref. 11.

of RBP is enhanced by retinol (6,11). The current experiments were undertaken to evaluate the effect of TPA on both RBP and albumin. Nongrowing high density cultures of H₄ (5) were treated with a range of doses of TPA (0.2 μg/ml to 5.0 μg/ml) for 3 days. RBP, determined by radioimmunoassay (6), was found to decrease proportionally to the increasing TPA dose, e.g., from 500 ng/cell homogenate in control cultures to 100 ng per cell homogenate (6 × 10⁶ cells) in the cultures treated with 5.0 μg/ml TPA. When 1 μg/ml Vitamin A was added concomitantly with TPA we found, as illustrated in Fig. 2, a total inhibition of TPA effect at low dose levels 0.2 μg/ml and partial inhibition at intermediate and high doses. The inhibitory effect of TPA was specific to RBP since no effect was seen on albumin synthesis by the cells.

DISCUSSION

The studies described above address two areas in which the antagonistic interaction between retinoid and TPA is observed; an effect on transformation and on differentiation, on initiation of events and on gene expression. Our results on transformation show that radiation-induced transformation in both hamster and mouse cells is enhanced by TPA and inhibited by retinoid. Furthermore, the retinoid, present for 4 days, completely eliminates the promotional effects of TPA to which the cells are chronically exposed for 2 to 6 weeks.

In our study on the site of action of the antagonistic effect, we found that whereas initiation of transformation by radiation is reflected at a chromosomal level in increased SCE frequency, the modulation of this transformation by retinoid or TPA is not reflected in DNA damage. It is reflected rather at the membrane level, in alteration of Na^+/K^+ transport enzymes. These enzymes may be involved in the progression of expression of the neoplastic state. Once this neoplastic is fully expressed as in transformed neoplastic cells, these enzymes are no longer responsive to the modulating factors, in the manner of their normal counterparts.

The effectiveness and specificity of the interaction between TPA and retinoids on gene expression is further observed in our results on differentiation. Here, TPA inhibited liver RBP synthesis and secretion whereas albumin production in the same cells remained unaltered. Retinol was effective in eliminating the inhibitory effect of TPA on RBP in a dose-response manner, but did not modify albumin. The mechanisms of these effects are currently being pursued.

ACKNOWLEDGMENTS

This investigation was supported by Contract DE-AC02-78EV0 4733 from the Department of Energy and by Grant No. CA 12536 to the Radiological Research Laboratory/Department of Radiology, and Grant No. CA 13696 to the Cancer Center/Institute of Cancer Research, awarded by the National Cancer Institute, DHEW.

REFERENCES

1. Borek, C. (1979): Malignant transformation *in vitro:* Criteria, biological markers, and application in environmental screening of carcinogens. *Radiat. Res.,* 79:209–232.
2. Borek, C., and Guernsey D. (1981): Membrane-associated ion transport enzymes in normal and oncogenically transformed fibroblasts and epithelial cells. *Studia Biophys.,* 84:53–55.
3. Borek, C., Miller, R. C., Geard, C. R., Guernsey, D., Osmak, R. S., Rutledge-Freeman, M., Ong, A., and Mason, H. (1981): The modulating effect of retinoids and a tumor promoter on malignant transformation, sister chromatid exchanges, and Na/K ATPase. *Ann. N.Y. Acad. Sci. (in press).*
4. Borek, C., Miller, R. C., Pain, C., and Troll, W. (1979): Conditions for inhibiting and enhancing effects of the protease inhibitor antipain on X-ray-induced neoplastic transformation in hamster and mouse cells. *Proc. Natl. Acad. Sci. USA,* 76:1,800–1,803.
5. Borek, C., and Smith, J. E. (1978): Tumor promotor inhibits production of liver retinol binding protein. *J. Cell Biol.,* 79:78a.
6. Borek, C., Smith, J. E., and Goodman, D. W. (1980): Liver cells in culture: A model for investigating the regulation of retinol binding protein metabolism. In: *Differentiation and Carcinogenesis in Liver Cells,* edited by C. Borek and G. M. Williams. *Ann. N.Y. Acad. Sci.,* 349:221–227.
7. Harisiadis, L., Miller, R. C., Hall, E. J., and Borek, C. (1978): A vitamin A analogue inhibits radiation-induced oncogenic transformation. *Nature,* 274:486–487.

8. Hecker, E. (1971): Isolation and characterization of the cocarcinogenic principles from croton oil. *Methods Cancer Res.,* 6:439–489.
9. Lotan, R. (1980): Effects of vitamin A and its analogs (retinoids) on normal and neoplastic cells. *Biochem. Biophys. Acta. Rev. Cancer,* 3,605:33–91.
10. Reznikoff, C. A., Bertram, J. S., Brankow, D. W., and Heildelberger, C. (1973): Quantitative and qualitative studies of chemical transformation of cloned C3H mouse embryo cells sensitive to postconfluence inhibition of cell division. *Cancer Res.,* 33:3,239–3,249.
11. Smith, J. E., Borek, C., and Goodman, D. S. (1978): Regulation of retinol binding protein metabolism in cultured rat liver cell lines. *Cell,* 15:865–873.
12. Weinstein, I. B., Yamasaki, H., Wigler, M., Lee, L. S., Fisher, P. B., Jeffrey, A., and Grunberger, D. (1979): Molecular and cellular events associated with the action of initiating carcinogens and tumor promoters. In: *Carcinogens: Identification and Mechanisms of Action,* edited by A. C. Griffin and C. R. Shaw, pp. 399–418. Raven Press, New York.

Carcinogenesis, Vol. 7, edited by E. Hecker et al.
Raven Press, New York © 1982.

Modification of Epithelial Cell Differentiation *In Vivo* by Tumor-Promoting Diterpene Esters

Jürgen Schweizer

German Cancer Research Center, Institute of Experimental Pathology,
6900 Heidelberg, Germany

Recent observations indicate that the action of tumor-promoting phorbol esters on several cell lines *in vitro* is governed by two principles. The first is that tumor-promoting phorbol esters, but not their inactive analogues, are able to induce morphological alterations almost identical to those effected after transformation of the cells with either chemical carcinogens or tumor viruses (8,16,24, 48,61,62). The second principle is that tumor-promoting phorbol esters either reversibly inhibit terminal differentiation or enhance differentiation in a variety of cell lines (15,21,26,39,40,41,43,49,61,62,64). These observations have been explained in terms of a gene-modulating ability of tumor promoters *in vitro*.

Long before these results were known, an interference of tumor promoters with the genetic expression in epidermal cells *in vivo* had also been suggested to operate during experimental two-stage skin carcinogenesis (6). Faced with the intriguing fact that many substances can cause epidermal proliferation similar to that produced by tumor promoters without any observable tumor-promoting effect, it was assumed that tumor promoters, apart from their hyperplasiogenic ability, are able to specifically modify cellular gene expression, one consequence of this ability being the expression of the transformed phenotype (9,10,46).

Evidence which lent support to this view came from morphological observations indicating a tumor promoter-specific alteration of epidermal tissue differentiation. It was found that a single application of a tumor-promoting dose of 12-O-tetradecanoylphorbol-13-acetate (TPA) to the back skin of mice led to the development of morphological features in the epidermis that were not seen in epidermal hyperplasia produced by a nonpromoter (44,45). These very early effects—characterized mainly by a more embryonic appearance of the epidermis along with the induction of a phenotypically new "dark cell" population—were interpreted as being indicative of a tumor promoter-specific, reversible reprogramming of tissue differentiation (44,45,46).

Recently we were able to show that long-term application of the tumor-promoting phorbol esters phorbol-12,13-didecanoate (PDD), 12-O-(2E',4E') decadienoylphorbol-13-(2E,4E)decadienoate (PDD-dien), and TPA to noninitiated adult mouse tail epidermis led to the neogenesis of new functional hair follicles (Fig. 1 A to D) (50,54a). The degree of hair follicle neoformation could be correlated to both the hyperplasiogenic ability of the substances in tail and back epidermis and more importantly to their tumor-promoting capacity in back epidermis. In contrast, the highly hyperplasiogenic nonpromoter 4-O-methyl-12-O-tetradecanoylphorbol-13-acetate (4-O-methyl-TPA) did not lead to new hair follicle formation (Table 1; 50). Since normal hair follicle formation in mammals is a developmental event that is exclusively embryonic (42,54a), these findings indicate a mimetic property of tumor promoters that is distinctly organogenetic.

Due to the very particular structure of tail epidermis (27,52,54) (Fig. 1 A), an intimate relationship between tumor formation and hair neogenesis could be evidenced in dimethylbenz(a)anthracene (DMBA)-initiated and TPA-pro-

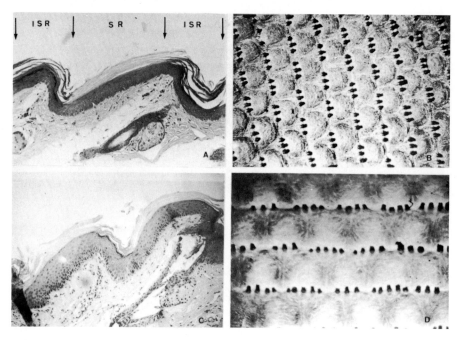

FIG. 1. Hair neogenesis in adult mouse tail epidermis. **A:** Vertical section of normal adult mouse tail skin showing the regularly alternating patterns of orthokeratotic interscale regions (ISR) and parakeratotic scale regions (SR). Note the different staining properties of the keratin layer in both regions. Hairs penetrate the epidermis in the interscale fold (H&E; × 110). **B:** Whole mount of separated tail epidermis viewed from the dermal side. The skin has been depilated prior to tissue separation. Note the follicular triplets associated with each scale (H&E; × 40). **C:** Vertical section of adult mouse tail skin treated twice weekly with 20 nmole TPA for 25 weeks. Note the maintenance of the differently keratinizing regions in the strongly hyperplastic epidermis (H&E; × 110). **D:** Whole mount of depilated tail epidermis treated twice weekly with 20 nmole TPA for 25 weeks. Note the sequences with more than three hairs per scale (H&E; × 80) (From Schweizer and Marks, ref. 54a.)

TABLE 1. *Hair neogenesis in adult mouse tail epidermis*[a]

Group	Substance	Number of samples	Mean values of scales associated with		Epidermal thickness μ	Promoting activity in back skin
			≦3 hairs	>3 hairs		
I	Acetone	20	979	21	30.68 ± 0.219	—
II	PDD	16	977	23	37.45 ± 0.305	+[b]
III	PDD-dien	16	961*	39*	40.15 ± 0.414	+[c]
IV	4-O-methyl-TPA	23	976	24	43.76 ± 0.430	−[b]
V	TPA	24	933*	67*	51.79 ± 0.313	++[b]

[a] Female NMRI-mice, 7 weeks old, were used in the experiment. Five groups, each consisting of 28 animals, were composed by random distribution, and each animal of the individual groups was treated twice weekly with a 100-μl acetone solution of the following substances: group II: 40 nmole PDD; group III: 40 nmole PDD-dien; group IV: 400 nmole 4-O-methyl-TPA; group V: 20 nmole TPA. (The phorbol esters were kindly provided by Dr. E. Hecker and co-workers). Group I served as control group and received only the solvent. Values indicated by * are statistically different from the control. For details, especially concerning Group II, see ref. 50.

[b] From E. Hecker (25).

[c] E. Hecker *(personal communication)*.

moted animals. Both phenomena, supposed to have a focal or clonal origin (10,42), seem to originate from the orthokeratinizing interscale region and particularly from the boundary region around the follicular orifices (Fig. 2 A,B) (54a). Interestingly, these infundibular epithelial areas have been shown to be particularly sensitive with regard to the induction of "dark keratinocytes" by tumor promoters (30).

Aside from these morphological evidences of a tumor promoter-specific interaction with epidermal cell differentiation, the existence of specific biochemical effects of tumor promoters in the epidermis is still a matter of conjecture. Despite much work in this direction, most biochemical reactions examined so far merely appear to reflect the ability of promoters to induce epidermal hyperplasia with the pleiotypic responses that usually proceed and accompany the cell division necessary for this process.

In the last decade considerable progress has been made with regard to the elucidation of epidermal differentiation and the characterization of proteins that are linked to keratinization. Histidine-rich (5,11,19,58–60) and cystine-rich proteins (19,20,38,39) have been identified as being distinctly localized (20,28,29) within epidermal keratohyalin granules (KHG) which, in turn, represent typical marker organelles of the integumental mammalian epidermis. There is evidence that both proteins contribute to the matrix portion of the fully differentiated epidermal cell (12,38,39). At least as far as the histidine-rich protein (HRP) is concerned, it has been shown that its biosynthesis begins with short-lived precursors (1,4,13,35) that probably polymerize in the cytoplasm of granular cells (1,3,4,59). Then, as polymerization proceeds, the material aggregates and finally leads to the formation of the relatively electron-lucent matrix portion of KHG. At the transition from the granular to the cornified layer, simultaneously with the decomposition of the granules, a processing of the polymers (4,5,51) gives rise to low molecular weight HRP species in the lowermost cornified layers. This class of high-level proteins represents a considerable part of the soluble protein fraction of mammalian epidermis (1–5, 11–14, 35).

In contrast, keratin polypeptides, the constituent proteins of epidermal tonofilaments, belong to the class of highly insoluble epidermal components. They represent by far the most abundant differentiation product in epidermis and as a rule show up as a protein family on denaturing gels within a MW range of 40,000 to 70,000 daltons (for review, see 33). There is convincing evidence that each keratin polypeptide is synthesized from its own messenger ribonucleic acid (mRNA) (18,22,53). Furthermore, a precursor-product relationship within the protein family, as well as the synthesis of precursor proteins larger than the extractable proteins, could be excluded (18,53).

Both KHG-associated and tonofilament-associated epidermal marker proteins should prove to be useful in the testing of a possible gene-modulating activity of tumor promoters in living epidermis. It is the aim of this chapter to review published data and to present new data on the effect of single and long-term application of tumor promoters on epidermal marker protein synthesis.

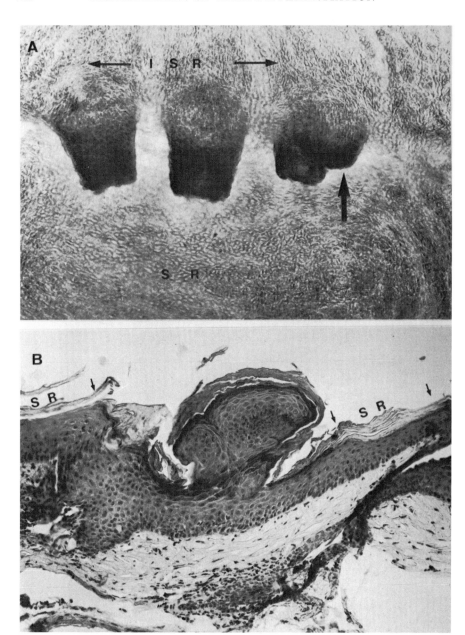

FIG. 2. Hair neogenesis and tumor formation in tail skin. **A:** Whole mount of epidermis of noninitiated tail skin treated twice weekly with 20 nmole TPA for 25 weeks. Adjacent to the right follicle of the triad, a small outgrowth of a newly forming follicular bud is visible (H&E; × 400) (From Schweizer and Marks, ref. 54a.) **B:** Vertical section of DMBA-initiated tail skin treated twice weekly with 20 nmole TPA for 9 weeks. A small papilloma rises from the orthokeratinizing interscale region (SR = Scale regions) (H&E; × 110).

SHORT-TERM EFFECTS OF TUMOR PROMOTERS AND NONPROMOTERS ON EPIDERMAL MARKER PROTEINS

Soluble Proteins

The first detailed study on the effects of the tumor promoter TPA on the biosynthesis of epidermal proteins stems from Balmain (2). He observed that the induction of hyperplasia by a single application of TPA to the back skin of adult mice led to the sequential and reversible appearance on polyacrylamide gels of two soluble proteins that were not detectable in the soluble protein fraction of untreated back epidermis (2). In a series of experiments (2–5) he was able to demonstrate that both proteins originated from KHG, one belonging to the class of crystine-rich proteins, the other to the class of HRP. The TPA-induced HRP could also be extracted in large amounts from newborn mouse epidermis, where it showed a considerable concentration at the transition of the granular and the cornified cell layers (2). The detection of this protein on gels was essentially facilitated by its particular staining properties. Whereas proteins normally stain blue with the Coomassie R 250 dye, the HRP clearly showed a red coloration (2).

The impressive synthesis of this protein in TPA-treated hyperplastic adult back epidermis, together with the fact that the same protein is abundantly present in neonatal mouse epidermis, inclines one to interpret these findings as a retrodifferentiation of the adult back epidermis under the influence of a tumor promoter.

As already stated by Balmain, however, another interpretation is that the protein is involved in normal keratinization of epidermis and that it is synthesized during the wave of differentiation that follows the epidermal proliferative phase without necessarily involving a return into a more embryonic stage (3). This is indeed the case as shown by the following experiments.

The morphology of the adult mouse back epidermis reveals an almost complete absence of a continuous granular layer (Fig. 3A). At most, KHG-containing cells are sporadically scattered throughout the suprabasal cell layers. If integumental epithelia of the adult mouse are arranged according to the histologically determinable prominence of their granular layer—for instance, in the sequence back, ear, tail, and footpad (Fig. 3 A to D)—and soluble proteins are extracted from these tissues, a clear-cut correlation between the thickness of the stratum granulosum and the intensity of the mouse HRP on gels becomes apparent (Fig. 4, slots A to E).[1] This would mean, however, that in an epidermis which under normal conditions contains a visible granular layer, the electrophoretic pattern of the HRP should not essentially be affected after treatment of this epidermis with TPA. That this is indeed the case could be demonstrated in adult guinea pig ear epidermis (49). Similar to neonatal mouse epidermis, guinea pig ear epidermis contains a pronounced granular layer (Fig. 5A), and the

---

[1] Experimental details will be reported elsewhere.

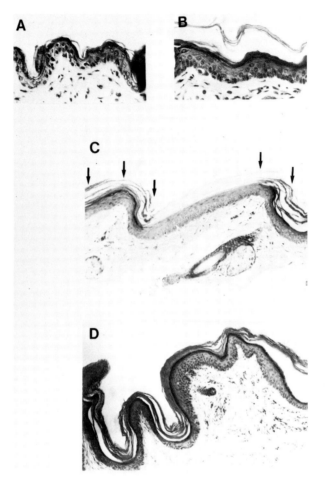

FIG. 3. Integumental epithelia from different anatomical regions of the adult mouse. **A:** Back; **B:** Ear; **C:** Tail; **D:** Footpad. **C** and **D** are only half the magnification (× 110) of **A** and **B** (× 220). Arrows in **C** indicate the granular layer-containing regions in tail epidermis (H&E).

tissue can also be subdivided at the transition of the living and dead cell layers after maceration of the epidermis in 1% acetic acid (Fig. 5B and C)—a manipulation that allows the exact localization of the HRP (3).

Extraction of the soluble proteins from whole ear epidermis leads to the complex electrophoretic protein pattern shown in slot 1 of Fig. 6 in which the prominent proteins A (MW = 65,000 daltons) and B (MW = 40,000 daltons) clearly show a red coloration after Coomassie staining. In accordance with Balmain's findings, these two proteins were almost the only extractable proteins from the keratinized layers (Fig. 6, slot 2) and, consequently, were lacking in the living layers (Fig. 6, slot 3). Thus, in the case of guinea pig ear epidermis,

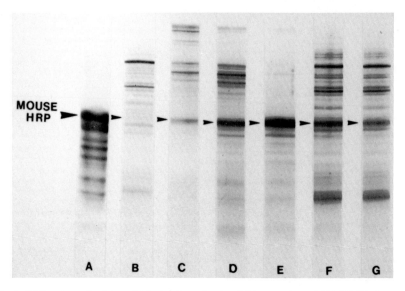

FIG. 4. SDS-polyacrylamide gel electrophoresis of soluble proteins of CH₃COOH-separated epithelia from different anatomical regions of the adult mouse. Arrows indicate the position of the 27,000 dalton MW-HRP (2–5). **A:** Newborn mouse epidermis; **B** Adult mouse back epidermis; **C:** Adult mouse ear epidermis; **D:** Adult mouse tail epidermis; **E:** Adult mouse footpad epidermis; **F:** Hyperplastic back epidermis of adult mouse, 72 hr after treatment with 20 nmole TPA: **G:** Hyperplastic back epidermis of adult mouse, 72 hr after treatment with 0.04 mmole EPP (10% PAA-gels according to Laemmli, ref. 31.)

one is obviously dealing with two stratum corneum-associated HRP species.

Unlike the situation in neonatal mouse epidermis (7), a strong and long-lasting hyperplasia can be induced by TPA in guinea pig ear epidermis. The time course of the hyperplasia is almost identical to that seen in adult mouse back epidermis and leads to a dramatic increase in the number of all cell layers above the basal layer (51). Despite this, the electrophoretic analysis of the soluble proteins during onset, peak, and decline of hyperplasia does not reveal any observable changes, either qualitative or quantitative, in the protein pattern (Fig. 7).

It can therefore be concluded that the remarkable appearance of the HRP in TPA-treated mouse back epidermis is due to the very special morphological situation in this anatomical region and does not generally apply to other epithelia. Furthermore, as already suggested by Balmain (3), the induction of the synthesis of this protein is not specific for tumors promoters. The same sequence of events can be brought about by any hyperplasiogenic stimulus; for example, removal of the horny layer by tape stripping (results not shown) or treatment of mouse back epidermis with the nonpromoting hyperplasiogen ethylphenylpropiolate (EPP) (47). Figure 4 shows that the electrophoretic protein patterns of the

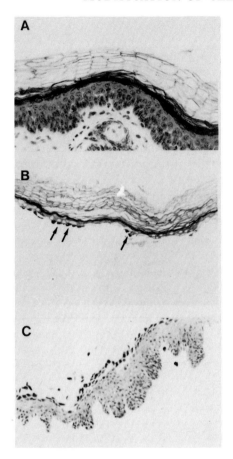

FIG. 5. Fractionation of adult guinea pig ear epidermis by means of cold 1% CH₃COOH. **A:** Whole ear skin; **B:** Stratum corneum fraction with few attached granular cells *(arrows);* **C:** Living cell layers containing the entire stratum granulosum (H&E; × 110).

soluble proteins of mouse back epidermis 72 hr after application of either TPA (slot F) or EPP (slot G) are essentially comparable to each other.[2]

---

[2] For completeness, three further papers dealing with the influence of TPA on the electrophoretic spectrum of soluble proteins of mouse back epidermis should be mentioned.

In 1972, Scribner and Boutwell (55) described the cycloheximide-sensitive induction of an extremely weak protein doublet 3 hr after TPA application. In 1973 and 1974, Scribner and Slaga (56,57) presented evidence for a TPA-induced small molecular weight protein 48 hr after treatment. The synthesis of this protein was suppressed or strongly reduced by concomitant application of steroid and nonsteroid antiinflammatory agents.

The interpretation of these results is generally hampered by the fact that no electrophoretic MW markers were used. However, if the size of the proteins is deduced from the acrylamide concentration and the position of the proteins on the gels, the protein doublet described by Scribner and Boutwell (55) has a MW > 200,000 daltons. The nature of these proteins is unknown; their induction is, however, not specific for TPA, since they can be also induced by acetic acid treatment, although the induction kinetics are different (55). The inducible low molecular weight protein described by Scribner and Slaga (56,57) appears to be identical to one of the proteins, probably the HRP, identified by Balmain (2,3). A relevance of these findings to tumor promoter specificity can therefore be excluded.

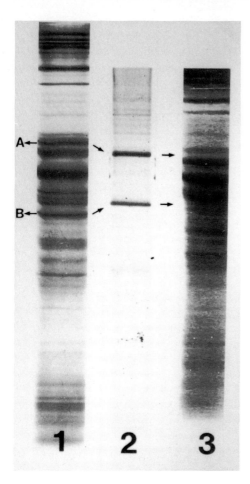

FIG. 6. SDS-polyacrylamide gel electrophoresis of soluble proteins of guinea pig ear epidermis. **Slot 1:** Soluble proteins of whole ear epidermis. Proteins A (65,000 daltons) and B (40,000 daltons) stain red with Coomassie R250; **Slot 2:** Soluble proteins of stratum corneum fraction; **Slot 3:** Soluble proteins of the living part of the epidermis (10% polyacrylamide gels according to Laemmli, ref. 31.)

Insoluble Proteins

It is especially apparent in the mouse that within the epithelia of one species, the keratin polypeptide spectrum, as well as the quantity of the particular polypeptides of the protein family, may vary in relation to the anatomical region (17,34,53,63). Slot A in Fig. 8 shows the polypeptide composition of keratins extracted from adult mouse tail epidermis which consists of nine discernible proteins in a MW range of 46,000 to 70,000 daltons. An essentially similar pattern, with only quantitative differences in the intensity of the intermediate-sized proteins 2 to 4, is encountered in footpad epidermis (not shown) and ear epidermis (Fig. 9, slot A). In contrast, as shown in slot B of Fig. 8, neonatal mouse epidermis—independent of the body site from which the keratins have been extracted—exhibits a pattern that differs qualitatively from the patterns described above, in that the largest member of the protein family (polypeptide 1) is completely absent. The adult back epidermis keratin polypeptide pattern

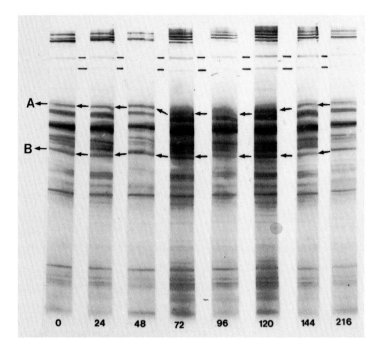

FIG. 7. SDS-polyacrylamide gel electrophoresis of soluble proteins of guinea pig ear epidermis after induction of hyperplasia by 20 nmole TPA. Arrows indicate the position of the red-staining proteins A and B. Figures at the bottom of the slots represent the time (in hr) after application of the promoter (10% polyacrylamide gels according to Laemmli, ref. 31.)

resembles the neonatal pattern, although the intermediate-sized proteins 2 to 4 are only faintly expressed (slot C, Fig. 8).

If back epidermis is treated by a single application of TPA and keratins are investigated during the period of hyperplasia, the same phenomenon as that observed for the soluble HRP occurs, namely the transient restoration of the embryonic pattern that is especially well visible between days 3 and 7 after TPA treatment (Fig. 8, slots F to H). However, and again in accordance with the situation found for soluble proteins, these effects are not specific for TPA but are produced in an identical manner by the nonpromoting agents 4-O-methyl-TPA, mezereine, and the Ca-Ionophore A 23187.

The transient restoration of an embryonic keratin pattern in adult back epidermis—although not specific for TPA—made it interesting to investigate the situation in an epidermis in which the keratin pattern differs qualitatively from that of newborn mouse epidermis, in that it contains the high molecular weight protein 1. As shown in Fig. 9 for ear epidermis, the keratin patterns during TPA-induced hyperplasia reveal only quantitative variations that concern the same keratin polypeptides as in back epidermis, whereas protein 1 is not at

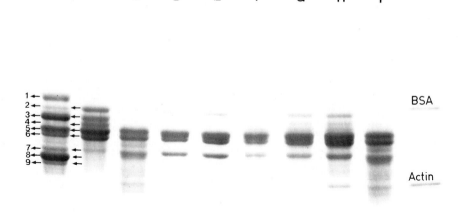

FIG. 8. SDS-polyacrylamide gel electrophoresis of keratins of adult and newborn mouse epidermis. Keratins were isolated as described by Franke et al., ref. 17. **Slot A:** Adult mouse tail epidermis. Proteins 1 to 9 have estimated MW (in daltons) of: 1 (70,000); 2 (67,000); 3 (64,000); 4 (62,000); 5 (60,000); 6 (58,000); 7 (51,000); 8 (48,000); 9 (46,000). Bovine serum albumin (BSA) and actin are run in MW markers. **Slot B:** Newborn mouse epidermis; **Slot C:** Adult mouse back epidermis; **Slots D to I** represent the keratin patterns of adult mouse back epidermis 1, 2, 3, 4, 7, and 14 days after induction of hyperplasia with 20 nmole TPA (9% polyacrylamide gels according to Laemmli, ref. 31.)

all affected. Again the same alterations were seen after induction of a hyperplasia by 4-O-methyl-TPA, mezereine, and the Ca-Ionophore.

LONG-TERM EFFECTS OF TUMOR PROMOTERS AND NONPROMOTERS ON EPIDERMAL MARKER PROTEINS

Long-term treatment of mouse back epidermis with TPA leads to the establishment of a sustained hyperplasia. From the morphological point of view, this new steady state of balanced epidermal growth is not different from the maximum hyperplasia that develops 3 to 5 days after a single application of the tumor promoter (23). Investigations with regard to the fate of the soluble proteins described by Balmain have not yet been undertaken. It is reasonable to assume, however, that the proteins as constituents of KHG are synthesized as long as the hyperplastic epidermis contains a granular layer.

The keratin polypeptide pattern of adult back epidermis during the peak of hyperplasia induced by a single application of TPA is not different from that after long-term treatment of back skin with the substance (Fig. 10, slots B

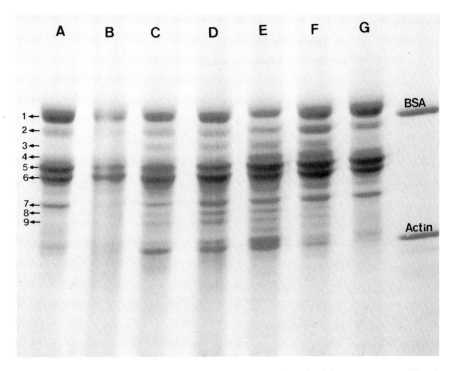

FIG. 9. SDS-polyacrylamide gel electrophoresis of keratins of adult mouse ear epidermis.
Slot A: Normal ear epidermis; **Slots B to G** represent the keratin patterns 1, 2, 3, 4, 7, and
14 days after induction of hyperplasia with 2 nmoles TPA (8.5% polyacrylamide gel according
to Laemmli, ref. 31.)

and C), both patterns essentially resembling that of the neonatal state (Fig.
10, slot D).

Surprisingly, TPA treatment of ear epidermis, i.e. an epidermal region in
which the keratin fraction normally contains protein 1 (Fig. 11, slot A), led
to a complete loss of this protein after long-term application, thus also restoring
the neonatal keratin pattern in this body site (Fig. 11, slot C). It should be
emphasized that this phenomenon is already detectable after 2 weeks of regular
treatment. There is, therefore, a fundamental difference in the keratin composition after single (Fig. 11, slot B) and after repeated application of TPA (Fig.
11, slot C) in those regions—although there are no morphological differences
between the induced and the sustained hyperplasia. It should be no surprise,
however, that this effect could also be brought about identically in the same
time period by application of pure hyperplasiogens, such as 4-O-methyl-TPA,
mezereine, and the Ca-Ionophore (Fig. 11, slot D).

More importantly, when tail epidermis (which also contains keratin polypeptide 1 Fig. 12, slot A) is treated for months with either TPA or 4-O-methyl-

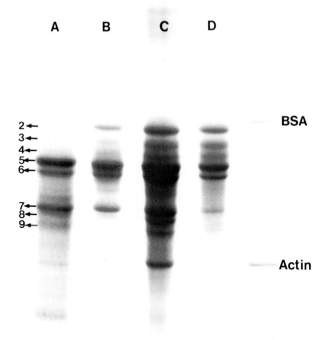

FIG. 10. SDS-polyacrylamide gel electrophoresis of keratins of adult mouse back epidermis. **Slot A:** Untreated adult mouse back epidermis; **Slot B:** Adult back epidermis 4 days after single application of 20 nmole TPA; **Slot C:** Adult back epidermis 2 weeks after daily application of 10 nmole TPA: **Slot D:** Newborn mouse epidermis (control) (9% polyacrylamide gels according to Laemmli, ref. 31.)

TPA, the morphological characteristics of this tissue, namely the alternating pattern of parakeratotic scales and the orthokeratotic interscale regions, are preserved (see Fig. 1 A and C) in the highly hyperplastic epidermis (50,54a). The resulting keratin polypeptide pattern can be interpreted as an approach to restore the neonatal keratin pattern, since the intensity of the typical neonatal keratin proteins 2 to 4 is clearly increased whereas protein 1 is diminished in intensity (Fig. 12, slots B and C). In contrast, daily treatment for 2 weeks with low doses of vitamin A acid is sufficient to transform the parakeratotic scale regions into orthokeratinizing regions (27,32,52,54), so that the strongly hyperplastic epidermis contains a continuous granular layer (Fig. 13). The keratin polypeptide pattern of this epidermis is then identical to that of the neonatal state (Fig. 12, slot D).

DISCUSSION

The integumental epithelia of the adult mouse show a broad spectrum of morphological variations in relation to their anatomical localization (53,63).

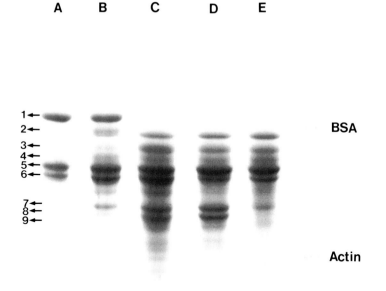

FIG. 11. SDS-polyacrylamide gel electrophoresis of keratins of adult mouse ear epidermis. **Slot A:** Untreated ear epidermis; **Slot B:** Ear epidermis 4 days after single application of 2 nmole TPA; **Slot C:** Ear epidermis 2 weeks after daily application of 2 nmole TPA; **Slot D:** Ear epidermis 2 weeks after daily application of 1.6 nmole mezerein; **Slot E:** Newborn mouse epidermis (control). (9% polyacrylamide gels according to Laemmli, ref. 31.)

These variations can also be demonstrated at the biochemical level by means of the electrophoretic behavior of marker proteins specifically involved in the process of epidermal differentiation.

The KHG-derived HRP is generally only subject to quantitative changes which can morphologically be directly related to the quantity of KHG in the granular layer of the epidermal tissue under consideration. In contrast, keratin polypeptides, the constituent proteins of tonofilaments, exhibit body site-specific alterations that are not detectable at the morphological level. Since each keratin polypeptide is encoded by its own mRNA (18,53), one can therefore speak of the existence of genetically determined local keratinization phenotypes in adult mouse epithelia that develop from a uniform embryonic keratinization phenotype. These findings offer an ideal starting point to investigate if tumor promoters exert specific influences on epidermal tissue differentiation, as in the case in *in vitro* cell lines.

The present study has demonstrated that a single application of a promoting dose of TPA to epithelia of various body sites of the adult mouse leads to reversible quantitative alterations of both the HRP and the keratin polypeptide patterns without, however, affecting the distinct local keratinization phenotype.

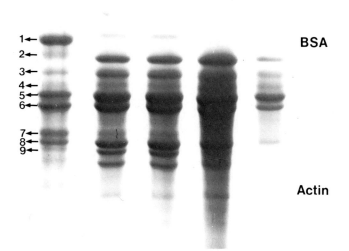

FIG. 12. SDS-polyacrylamide gel electrophoresis of keratins of adult mouse tail epidermis. **Slot A:** Untreated tail epidermis; **Slot B:** Tail epidermis 2 months after twice weekly application of 20 nmole TPA; **Slot C:** Tail epidermis 2 months after twice weekly application of 800 nmole 4-O-methyl-TPA; **Slot D:** Tail epidermis 20 days after daily application of 200 IU vitamin A acid; **Slot E:** Newborn mouse epidermis (control). (9% polyacrylamide gels according to Laemmli, ref. 31.)

The observed alterations may be explained by an enhanced metabolic activity following the hyperplasiogenic stimulus without any relevance to a tumor-promoting property of the stimulating agent.

Unlike induced hyperplasia—as visualized by the keratin polypeptide pattern—the establishment of a sustained hyperplasia by TPA leads to a reprogramming of adult tissue differentiation into the neonatal keratinization phenotype. This process is especially well visible in adult mouse ear epidermis since, in contrast to adult back epidermis, the keratinization phenotype in this tissue is qualitatively different from the neonatal phenotype.

Adult tail epidermis in which the keratin polypeptide composition is also different from the embryonic keratin pattern represents an unusual case. As shown, the establishment of a sustained hyperplasia by TPA does not lead to a loss of the alternating para- and orthokeratotic epidermal compartmentalization typical for this tissue. The incomplete restoration of the embryonic keratin pattern in this epidermis must therefore be traced back to a locally limited embryonic retrodifferentiation which, from the morphological point of view, can only have

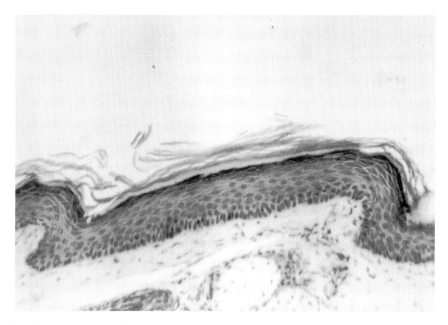

FIG. 13. Adult mouse tail epidermis, treated for 20 days with 200 i.u. vitamin A acid. Note the continuous granular layer throughout the epidermis and the uniformly staining keratin layer and compare with **FIG. 1 A** (H&E; × 110).

occurred in the orthokeratotic interscale region. This assumption is confirmed by the long-term vitamin A-effect on both tail epidermis morphology and keratin polypeptide pattern.

Recently we were able to show that keratins of mouse epidermis can be used as markers of the transformed state of epidermal cells (63). Whereas the keratin polypeptide pattern of the benign transformed state resembles the neonatal keratinization phenotype, the malignant state is characterized by a drastically reduced keratin polypeptide pattern in which the proteins above the 60,000 dalton level are no longer synthesized (63). On the basis of these findings, one may say that tumor promoters—at least after long-term application—are able to mimic the benign transformed state of epidermal cells *in vivo*.

Furthermore, since the reversal of the adult type of keratinization into the neonatal one in the course of a sustained hyperplasia shows up by the loss of a distinct keratin polypeptide, in a sense this event may be interpreted as an *in vivo* inhibition of the terminal differentiation of the local keratinization phenotype by tumor promoters.

As for TPA-induced hyperplasia, however, none of the alterations in epidermal marker protein synthesis observed in a sustained hyperplasia is specific for this most potent tumor-promoting diterpene ester. The kinetics of appearance and disappearance of protein alterations, in addition to their qualitative and quantitative changes seen in an epidermis, are identically brought about by nonpromoting hyperplasiogens, thus emphasizing that induction of hyperplasia, as well as reversal of the state of differentiation, are accompanying circumstances, but are not sufficient conditions for TPA-mediated tumor promotion in skin (36,37).

ACKNOWLEDGMENTS

I am grateful to my colleague Dr. Hermi Winter for valuable advice and helpful discussions, and to Mrs. Linda Berry for the expert correction of the manuscript.

REFERENCES

1. Ball, R. D., Walter, G. K., and Bernstein, I. A. (1978): Histidine-rich proteins as markers for epidermal differentiation. *J. Biol. Chem.,* 253:5,861–5,868.
2. Balmain, A. (1976): The synthesis of specific proteins in adult mouse epidermis during phases of proliferation and differentiation induced by the tumor promoter TPA, and in basal and differentiating layers of neonatal mouse epidermis. *J. Invest. Dermatol.,* 67:246–253.
3. Balmain, A. (1978): Synthesis of specific proteins in mouse epidermis after treatment with the tumor promoter TPA. In: *Carcinogenesis, Vol. 2: Mechanisms of Tumor Promotion and Cocarcinogenesis,* edited by T. J. Slaga, A. Sivak, and R. K. Boutwell, pp. 153–172. Raven Press, New York.
4. Balmain, A., Loehren, D., Alonso, A., and Goerttler, K. (1979): Protein synthesis during fetal development of mouse epidermis. II. Biosynthesis of histidine-rich and cystine-rich proteins *in vitro* and *in vivo. Dev. Biol.,* 73:338–344.
5. Balmain, A., Loehren, D., Fischer, J., and Alonso, A. (1977): Protein synthesis during fetal development of mouse epidermis. I. The appearance of "histidine-rich protein." *Dev. Biol.,* 60:442–452.
6. Berenblum, I. A. (1954): A speculative review: The probable nature of promoting action and its significance in the understanding of the mechanism of carcinogenesis. *Cancer Res.,* 14:471–477.
7. Bertsch, S., and Marks, F. (1974): Lack of an effect of tumor-promoting phorbol esters and of epidermal G_1 chalone on DNA synthesis in the epidermis of newborn mice. *Cancer Res.,* 34:3,283–3,288.
8. Blumberg, P. M., Driedger, P. E., and Rossow, P. W. (1976): Effect of a phorbol ester on a transformation-sensitive surface protein of chick fibroblasts. *Nature,* 264:446–447.
9. Boutwell, R. K. (1964): Some biological aspects of skin carcinogenesis. *Prog. Exp. Tumor Res.,* 4:207–250.
10. Boutwell, R. K. (1974): The function and mechanisms of promoters of carcinogenesis. *CRC Crit. Rev. Toxicol.,* 2:419–443.
11. Dale, B. A. (1977): Purification and characterization of a basic protein from the stratum corneum of mammalian epidermis. *Biochim. Biophys. Acta,* 491:193–204.
12. Dale, B. A., Holbrook, K. A., and Steinert, P. M. (1978): Assembly of stratum corneum basic protein and keratin filaments in macrofibrils. *Nature,* 276:729–731.
13. Dale, B. A., and Ling, S. Y. (1979*a*): Evidence of a precursor form of stratum corneum basic protein in rat epidermis. *Biochemistry,* 18:3,539–3,546.
14. Dale, B. A., and Ling, S. Y. (1979*b*): Immunologic cross-reaction of stratum corneum basic protein and a keratohyalin protein. *J. Invest. Dermatol.,* 72:257–261.
15. Diamond, L., O'Brien, T. G., and Rovera, G. (1977): Inhibition of adipose conversion of 3T3 fibroblasts by tumor promoters. *Nature,* 269:247–249.
16. Driedger, P. E., and Blumberg, P. M. (1977): The effect of phorbol diesters on chicken embryo fibroblasts. *Cancer Res.,* 37:3,257–3,265.
17. Franke, W. W., Weber, K., Osborn, M., Schmid, E., and Freudenstein, C. (1978): Antibody to prekeratin. Decoration of tonofilament-like arrays in various cells of epithelial character. *Exp. Cell Res.,* 116:429–445.

18. Fuchs, E., and Green, H. (1979): Multiple keratins of cultured human epidermal cells are translated from different mRNA molecules. *Cell,* 17:573–582.

19. Fukuyama, K., and Epstein, W. L. (1975): Heterogenous proteins in keratohyalin granules studied by quantitative autoradiography. *J. Invest. Dermatol.,* 65:113–117.

20. Fukuyama, K., and Epstein, W. L. (1978): Heterogenous ultrastructure of keratohyalin granules. A comparative study of adjacent skin and mucous membranes. *J. Invest. Dermatol.,* 61:94–100.

21. Gambarai, R., Fibach, E., Rifkind, R. A., and Marks, P. A. (1980): Inhibition of induced murine erythroleukemia cell differentiation by tumor promoters: Relation to the cell cycle. *Biochem. Biophys. Res. Commun.,* 94:867–874.

22. Gibbs, P. E. M., and Freedberg, I. M. (1980): Mammalian mRNA: Identification and characterization of the keratin messenger. *J. Invest. Dermatol.,* 74:382–388.

23. Goerttler, K., and Loehrke, H. (1976): Improved tumor yields by means of TPA-DMBA-TPA variation of the Berenblum-Mottram experiment on the back skin of NMRI mice. The effect of stationary hyperplasia without inflammation. *Exp. Pathol.,* 12:336–341.

24. Gottesman, M. M., and Sobel, M. E. (1980): Tumor promoters and Kirsten sarcoma virus increase synthesis of a secreted glycoprotein by regulating levels of translatable mRNA. *Cell,* 19:449–455.

25. Hecker, E. (1978): Structure-activity relationships in diterpene esters irritant and cocarcinogenic to mouse skin. In: *Carcinogenesis, Vol. 2: Mechanisms of Tumor Promotion and Cocarcinogenesis,* edited by T. J. Slaga, A. Sivak, and R. K. Boutwell, pp. 11–48. Raven Press, New York.

26. Huberman, E., and Callahan, M. F. (1979): Induction of terminal differentiation in human promyelotic leukemia cells by tumor-promoting agents. *Proc. Natl. Acad. Sci. USA,* 76:1,293–1,297.

27. Jarrett, A., and Spearman, R. I. C. (1964): *Histochemistry of the Skin—Psoriasis.* English University Press, London.

28. Jessen, H. (1972): Two types of keratohyalin granules. *J. Ultrastruct. Res.,* 38:16–26.

29. Jessen, H. (1973): Electron cytochemical demonstration of sulfhydryl groups in KHG and in the peripheral envelope of cornified cells. *Histochemie,* 33:15–29.

30. Klein-Szanto, A. J. P., Major, S. K., and Slaga, T. J. (1980): Induction of dark keratinocytes by 12-O-tetradecanoylphorbol-13-acetate and mezerein as an indication of tumor-promoting efficiency. *Carcinogenesis,* 1:399–406.

31. Laemmli, U. K. (1970): Cleavage of structural proteins during the assembly of bacteriophage T4. *Nature,* 227:680–685.

32. Lawrence, D., and Bern, H. A. (1958): On the specificity of the response of mouse epidermis to vitamin A. *J. Invest. Dermatol.,* 31:313–325.

33. Lazarides, E. (1980): Intermediate filaments as mechanical integrators of cellular space. *Nature,* 283:249–256.

34. Lee, L. D., Kubilus, J., and Baden, H. P. (1979): Intraspecies heterogeneity of epidermal keratin isolated from bovine hoof and snout. *Biochem. J.,* 177:187–196.

35. Lonsdale-Eccles, J. D., Hangen, J. A., and Dale, B. A. (1980): A phosphorylated keratohyalin-derived precursor of epidermal stratum corneum basic protein. *J. Biol. Chem.,* 255:2,235–2,238.

36. Marks, F., Bertsch, S., Grimm, W., and Schweizer, J. (1978): Hyperplastic transformation and tumor promotion in mouse epidermis: Possible consequences of disturbances of endogenous mechanisms controlling proliferation and differentiation. In: *Carcinogenesis, Vol. 2: Mechanisms of Tumor Promotion and Cocarcinogenesis,* edited by T. J. Slaga, A. Sivak, and R.K. Boutwell, pp. 97–116. Raven Press, New York.

37. Marks, F., Bertsch, S., and Schweizer, J. (1978): Homeostatic regulation of epidermal cell proliferation. *Bull. Cancer,* 2:207–222.

38. Matoltsy, A. G. (1975): Desmosomes, filaments, and KHG: Their role in the stabilization and keratinization of the epidermis. *J. Invest. Dermatol.,* 65:127–142.

39. Matoltsy, A. G., Lavker, R. M., and Matoltsy, M. N. (1974): Demonstration of cystine-containing protein in keratohyalin granules of epidermis. *J. Invest. Dermatol.,* 62:406–410.

40. Miao, R. M., Fieldsteel, A. H., and Fodge, D. W. (1978): Opposing effects of tumor promoters on erythroid differentiation. *Nature,* 274:271–272.

41. Mufson, R. A., Fisher, P. B., and Weinstein, I. B. (1979): Effect of phorbol ester tumor promoters on the expression of melanogenesis in B16 melanoma cells. *Cancer Res.,* 39:3,915–3,919.

42. Muller, A. S. (1971): Hair neogenesis. *J. Invest. Dermatol.,* 56:1–9.

43. Nakayasu, M., Shoji, M., Aoki, N., Sato, S., Miwa, M., and Sugimura, T. (1979): Enhancing

effect of phorbol esters on induction of differentiation of mouse myeloid leukemia cells by human urinary protein and lipopolysaccharide. *Cancer Res.,* 39:4,668–4,672.

44. Raick, A. N. (1972): Early effects of TPA on the incorporation of tritiated precursors into DNA and the thickness of the interfollicular epidermis and their relation to tumor promotion. *Cancer Res.,* 32:1,562–1,568.

45. Raick, A. N. (1973): Ultrastructural, histological, and biochemical alterations produced by TPA in mouse epidermis and their relevance to skin tumor promotion. *Cancer Res.,* 33:269–286.

46. Raick, A. N. (1974): Cell differentiation and tumor-promoting action in skin carcinogenesis. *Cancer Res.,* 34:2,915–2,925.

47. Raick, A. N., and Burdzy, K. (1973): Ultrastructural and biochemical changes induced in mouse epidermis by a hyperplastic agent, ethylphenylpropiolate. *Cancer Res.,* 33:2,221–2,230.

48. Rifkin, D. B., and Growe, R. M. (1979): Tumor promoters induce changes in the chick embryo fibroblast cytoskeleton. *Cell,* 18:361–368.

49. Rovera, G., O'Brien, T. G., and Diamond, L. (1979): Tumor promoters inhibit spontaneous differentiation of Friend erythroleukemia cells in culture. *Proc. Natl. Acad. Sci. USA,* 74:2,894–2,898.

50. Schweizer, J., (1979): Neogenesis of functional hair follicles in adult mouse skin selectively induced by tumor-promoting phorbol esters. *Experientia,* 35:1,651–1,653.

51. Schweizer, J. (1981*a*): Synthesis of histidine-rich proteins in embryonic, adult, and stimulated epidermis in different mammals. In: *Frontiers of Matrix Biology,* edited by M. Prunieras. S. Karger, Basel, vol. 9, pp. 127–141.

52. Schweizer, J. (1981*b*): Langerhans cells, epidermal growth control mechanisms, and types of keratinization. In: *The Epidermis in Health and Disease,* edited by E. Christophers and R. Marks. Medical Technical Press, Lancaster, pp. 481–499.

53. Schweizer, J., and Goerttler, K. (1980): *In vitro* synthesis of keratin polypeptides directed by mRNA isolated from newborn and adult mouse epidermis. *Eur. J. Biochem.,* 112:243–249.

54. Schweizer, J., and Marks, F. (1977): A developmental study of the distribution and frequency of Langerhans cells in relation to the formation of patterning in mouse tail epidermis. *J. Invest. Dermatol.,* 69:198–204.

54a. Schweizer, J., and Marks, A. (1977): Induction of formation of new hair follicles in mouse tail epidermis by the tumor promoter TPA. *Cancer Res.,* 37:4,195 4,201.

55. Scribner, J. D., and Boutwell, R. K. (1979): Inflammation and tumor promotion: Selective protein induction in mouse skin by tumor promoters. *Eur. J. Biochem.,* 8:617–621.

56. Scribner, J. D., and Slaga, T. J. (1973): Multiple effects of dexamethasone on protein synthesis and hyperplasia caused by a tumor promoter. *Cancer Res.,* 33:542–546.

57. Scribner, J. D., and Slaga, T. J. (1974): Influence of nonsteroid antiinflammatory agents on protein synthesis and hyperplasia caused by a tumor promoter. *J. Natl. Cancer Inst.,* 52:1,865–1,867.

58. Sibrack, L. A., Gray, R. H., and Bernstein, I. A. (1974): Localization of the histidine-rich protein in keratohyalin: A morphological and macromolecular marker of epidermal differentiation. *J. Invest. Dermatol.,* 62:394–405.

59. Sugawara, K., and Bernstein, I. A. (1971): Biosynthesis *in vitro* of HRP—A biochemical marker of epidermal differentiation. *Biochim. Biophys. Acta,* 238:129–138.

60. Tezuka, T., and Freedberg, I. M. (1974): Epidermal structural proteins. III. Isolation and purification of histidine-rich protein of the newborn rat. *J. Invest. Dermatol.,* 63:400–406.

61. Weinstein, I. B., Lee, L. S., Fisher, P. B., and Yamasaki, H. (1979): Action of phorbol esters in cell culture: Mimicry of transformation, altered differentiation, and effects on cell membranes. *J. Supramol. Struc.,* 12:195–208.

62. Weinstein, I. B., and Weigler, M. (1977): Cell culture studies provide new information on tumor promoters. *Nature,* 270:659–660.

63. Winter, H., Schweizer, J., and Goerttler, K. (1980): Keratins as markers of malignancy in mouse epidermal tumors. *Carcinogenesis,* 1:391–398.

64. Yamasaki, H., Fibach, E., Nudel, U., Weinstein, I. B., Rifkind, R. A., and Marks, P. A. (1977): Tumor promoters inhibit spontaneous and induced differentiation of murine erythroleukemia cells in culture. *Proc. Natl. Acad. Sci. USA,* 74:3,451–3,455.

Carcinogenesis, Vol. 7, edited by E. Hecker et al.
Raven Press, New York © 1982.

Quantitative Evaluation of Dark Keratinocytes Induced by Several Promoting and Hyperplasiogenic Agents: Their Use as an Early Morphological Indicator of Tumor-Promoting Action

A. J. P. Klein-Szanto, S. K. Major, and T. J. Slaga

Biology Division, Oak Ridge National Laboratory, Oak Ridge, Tennessee 37830

Dark basal keratinocytes (D cells) have been described in normal and hyperplastic epithelia (1–6). In an electron microscopic study, Raick and Burzdy (6) showed that topical treatment with 12-O-tetradecanoylphorbol-13-acetate (TPA) was much more effective in inducing D cells than either ethylphenylpropiolate (EPP) or wounding.

Since D cells can be effectively detected in 1-μm thick Epon sections stained with toluidine blue (4), and these sections offer a considerably larger sample size than the ultrathin sections used in transmission electron microscopy, we studied the percentage of D cells in epidermal hyperplasias induced by several compounds with varying tumor-promoting efficiencies.

MATERIALS AND METHODS

D cells were investigated in the normal and treated epidermis of Sencar mice. After a single topical application of TPA, mezerein, EPP, anthralin, 12-deoxyphorbol-13-2,4,6-decatrienate (tri-DPD), 12-deoxyphorbol-13-decanoate (DPD), 4-O-methyl-TPA, or the calcium ionophore A 23187, D cells were observed and quantified using procedures and materials described previously (3,8).

RESULTS

The light microscopic examination of the topically treated skin revealed a large number of D cells after treatment with the following compounds: TPA (Fig. 1, top), DPD, 4-O-methyl-TPA, and the calcium ionophore A 23187. On the other hand, the epidermis treated with mezerein, anthralin, EPP (Fig. 1, bottom), or tri-DPD exhibited a smaller number of D cells in the basal layer. Although very few D cells were seen in the normal epidermis, the quantitative analysis revealed that they constituted 2 to 3% of the total basal cell population.

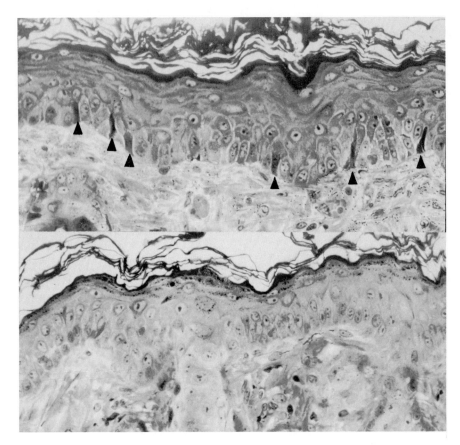

FIG. 1. Distribution of dark cells in the epidermis 48 hr after topical treatment with a single dose of either 4 μg TPA *(top)* or 14 mg EPP *(bottom)*. Note several dark cells in the TPA-treated epidermis *(arrowheads)* and no dark cells in the EPP-treated skin. One-μm thick Epon section stained with toluidine blue. × 550.

Table 1 summarizes the variations in D cell percentage found after topical treatment with the promoters and hyperplasiogenic agents. The best inducers of D cells were 4-O-methyl-TPA and DPD (more than 20% D cells after 24 to 48 hr). TPA and the calcium ionophore produced approximately 15 to 20% D cells, whereas mezerein and anthralin induced half that many D cells. EPP and, even to a smaller extent, tri-DPD induced a small increase in D cells.

DISCUSSION

The quantitative evaluation of D cells after topical application of several promoters and hyperplasiogenic agents showed good correlation between the

TABLE 1. *Percentage of dark cells in the epidermal basal layer after single topical application of several promoting and hyperplasiogenic compounds*

Time after application	TPA		Mezerein		EPP		Anthralin		tri-DPD		DPD		4-O-methyl-TPA		Calcium ionophore A 23187	
	2 µg	4 µg	2 µg	4 µg	1.4 µg	14 mg	40 µg	80 µg	5 µg	10 µg	5 µg	10 µg	250 µg	500 µg	40 µg	120 µg
12	9	11	8	8	3	4	2	11	—	—	—	—	10	12	8	9
24	15	27	14	3	4	4	8	5	3	5	5	6	20	30	9	18
48	18	13	5	9	6	8	3	4	2	4	10	30	9	23	10	12
72	11	9	6	7	—	—	—	—	—	—	—	—	—	—	—	—
96	10	12	5	10	7	3	7	9	1	2	3	6	8	20	4	4

D cell-inducing capacities of these compounds and their respective efficiencies as tumor promoters when applied to the skin after a subthreshold dose of a chemical carcinogen (Table 2). Of special interest was the astonishing difference between the promoting actions of two very closely related phorbol compounds, DPD and tri-DPD. Whereas DPD is a potent promoter, tri-DPD is extremely weak. This correlated very well with their respective dark cell-inducing capacities. The same could be said about TPA and mezerein; however, mezerein, which is effective if applied during the second part of a two-stage promotion protocol (7), is a moderate inducer of D cells, although always in a smaller percentage than TPA. The calcium ionophore A 23187 and 4-O-methyl-TPA in high doses are extremely good inducers of D cells (even more so than conventional tumor-promoting doses of TPA). The interesting fact about these compounds is that although ineffective as complete promoters, they are effective when applied prior to mezerein, in the first stage of a two-stage promotion protocol.

The D cell percentages mentioned in the present studies originated in the enumeration of these cells in the interfollicular epidermis, but it must be pointed out that these changes are also seen in the intrafollicular epidermis. In this portion of the epidermis, a larger number of D cells were observed in experimental conditions, making the differences beteween the potent and weak compounds slightly greater than in the interfollicular epidermis.

The presence of approximately 15% labeled dark cells, the evidence of ^{3}H-Tdr incorporation, and their ultrastructural characteristics (large nucleus, prominent nucleoli, cytoplasm occupied mainly by free ribosomes) indicate features of effective activity. Only a small percentage of dark cells (less than 10%) had features of necrobiotic or toxic injured cells. The different dark cell-inducing effects of the studied compounds indicate that the number of D cells is an adequate early indicator of their respective tumor-promoting abilities, and would

TABLE 2. *Dark cell induction and tumor-promoting abilities of several compounds*

	Dark cell induction	Tumor promotion
TPA	+ + + +	+ + + +
Mezerein	+ +	+
Anthralin	+/−	+
EPP	+/−	+/−
DPD	+ + + +	+ + +
Tri-DPD	−	
Calcium ionophore A 23187	+ + + +	−(Active first stage)
4-O-methyl TPA	+ + + + +	−(Active first stage)
Dimethylbenz(a)anthracene:		
Low initiating dose	−	−
High dose (complete		
carcinogen dose)	+ +	

point to the importance of the production of dedifferentiated dark cells during tumor promotion.

ACKNOWLEDGMENT

Research sponsored by the Office of Health and Environmental Research, U.S. Department of Energy, under contract W-7405-eng-26 with the Union Carbide Corporation.

REFERENCES

1. Breathnach, A. S. (1971): *An Atlas of the Ultrastructure of Human Skin,* p. 108. J. and A. Churchill, London.
2. Klein-Szanto, A. J. P. (1977): Clear and dark basal keratinocytes in human epidermis. A stereologic study. *J. Cutan. Pathol.,* 45:275–280.
3. Klein-Szanto, A. J. P., Major, S. K., and Slaga, T. J. (1980): Induction of dark keratinocytes by 12-O-tetradecanoylphorbol-13-acetate and mezerein as an indicator of tumor-promoting efficiency. *Carcinogenesis,* 1:399–406.
4. Klein-Szanto, A. J. P., Topping, D. C., Heckman, C. A., and Nettesheim, P. (1980): Ultrastructural characteristics of carcinogen-induced dysplastic changes in tracheal epithelium. *Am. J. Pathol.,* 98:83–100.
5. Raick, A. N. (1973): Ultrastructural, histological, and biochemical alterations produced by 12-O-tetradecanoylphorbol-13-acetate on mouse epidermis and their relevance to skin tumor promotion. *Cancer Res.,* 33:269–286.
6. Raick, A. N., and Burdzy, K. (1973): Ultrastructural and biochemical changes induced in mouse epidermis by a hyperplastic agent, ethylphenylpropiolate. *Cancer Res.,* 33:2,221–2,230.
7. Slaga, T.J., Fischer, S. M., Nelson, K., and Gleason, G. L. (1980): Studies on the mechanism of skin tumor promotion: Evidence for several stages in promotion. *Proc. Natl. Acad. Sci. USA,* 77:3,659–3,663.
8. Slaga, T. J., Klein-Szanto, A. J. P., Fischer, S. M., Nelson, K., and Major, S. (1980): Studies on the mechanism of action of anti-tumor-promoting agents: Their specificity in two-stage promotion. *Proc. Natl. Acad. Sci. USA,* 77:2,251–2,254.

Carcinogenesis, Vol. 7, edited by E. Hecker et al.
Raven Press, New York © 1982.

Patterns of Epidermal Cell Proliferation

I. C. Mackenzie and J. R. Bickenbach

Dows Institute for Dental Research, The University of Iowa, Iowa City, Iowa 52242

Mammalian epidermis shows an ordered alignment of the cells of the suprabasal strata (3,6). Examination of the position of mitotic (7) and of tritiated thymidine-labeled cells (4,9,11) indicates that cell division occurs preferentially in the region beneath columnar boundaries. The question arises as to the function of the centrally placed cells which are less proliferatively active. For the hemopoietic system and some other tissues, a two-compartment proliferative system has been proposed (5) and the existence of an analogous subpopulation of stem cells in epidermis, with one centrally placed stem cell beneath each column, has been suggested (10,12). Such stem cells would be self-regenerating and would also produce cells committed to differentiation but capable of a limited number of amplification divisions.

From what is known about stem cells in other tissues (5), epidermal stem cells might be expected to have a slow cell cycle, be relatively few in number, and act as "clonogens." Once labeled, they might be expected to retain incorporated nuclear label for a longer period of time than surrounding cells undergoing amplification division. A higher probability of labeling stem cells during a growth phase, when stem cells may divide to maintain population density, would also be expected. We have detected a subpopulation of epithelial cells that retains ^{3}H-TdR label for extended periods of time, and have undertaken some further investigations to identify such cells and to examine their ability to proliferate and their behavior in culture.

MATERIAL AND METHODS

Litters of C3H mice were injected subcutaneously with 0.05 ml ^{3}H-TdR (200 mCi/ml) at 8:00 A.M. and 8:00 P.M. on the 10th and 11th days after birth. Tissues were collected 1 hr and 10, 30, and 72 days following this labeling sequence. A few specimens were also examined 8 months after labeling. Specimens for light microscopic autoradiography were processed using Kodak NTB-2 Emulsion (13), with a standardized exposure time of 4 weeks. The tissues examined included ear, footpad, back, and tail skin, and palate, tongue, and buccal mucosa.

Specimens of ear epidermis for electron microscopic (EM) autoradiography were taken from mice labeled 1 hr, 30, and 72 days previously, embedded, sectioned and processed using Ilford L4 Emulsion by the loop method of Caro and van Tubergen (2).

Suspensions of ear epidermal cells for culture were prepared from mice labeled 30 days previously. The epidermis, separated from the connective tissue using buffered ethylenediaminetetraacetate (EDTA), was dissociated into cell suspensions by collagenase and cells centrally plated at a concentration of 2×10^6 cells/ml. Culture dishes with their attached cells were processed for autoradiography at various times after plating.

The ears of mice labeled 72 days previously were treated daily for 3 days with a 10^{-7} M solution of tetradecanoylphorbolacetate (TPA) in acetone to induce hyperplasia. Vinblastin was used to arrest dividing cells in metaphase and cells in mitosis were examined for labeling using dark-field illumination.

RESULTS

Light Microscopic Autoradiography

Mouse ear epidermis showed labeling of the majority of basal nuclei 1 hr following the labeling sequence (Fig. 1). Ten days later, basal nuclear labeling had been diluted by cell division and labeled nuclei were seen in differentiating suprabasal cells. Only slight residual labeling was present after 30 or 72 days, but occasional basal nuclei remained heavily labeled. Similar label-retaining basal cells (LRCs) were also seen in other epidermal regions and in the oral mucosa of these mice (Table 1). LRCs were still present in the few specimens examined 8 months after labeling.

Figure 2 shows the results of grain counts of LRCs 30 and 72 days after labeling. The modal grain count of LRCs was 11 to 15 grains per nucleus 30 days after labeling and had fallen to 6 to 10 grains per nucleus by 72 days after labeling.

EM Autoradiography

Specimens of mouse ear epidermis prepared for EM autoradiography 1 hr after labeling showed that the majority of the nuclei of basal keratinocytes were labeled. In 30- or 72-day specimens, a total of 73 LRCs was identified by the presence of 3 to 6 silver grains overlying the nucleus. Of these, 70 cells were identified as keratinocytes by the presence of cytoplasmic tonofilaments and desmosomal junctions with adjacent cells. Three cells had an appearance typical of Langerhans cells, although only one contained characteristic granules. No labeled melanocytes were identified.

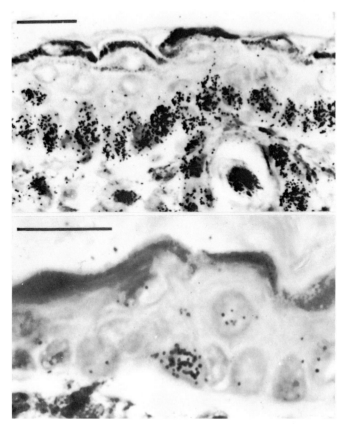

FIG. 1. Autoradiographs of mouse ear epidermis. One hr after the labeling sequence *(above)* the majority of basal nuclei are labeled. Thirty days later *(below)*, only slight residual nuclear label is seen, except for one nucleus that remains heavily labeled. (*Scale bars* = 30 μm.)

Effects of Induction of Hyperplasia

Autoradiographs of ear epidermis labeled 72 days previously and then treated with TPA for 1, 2, or 3 days showed development of a marked hyperplasia with 5, 9, and 11% of basal cells blocked in metaphase respectively. A small proportion (2.7, 6.6, 7.1%) of the label-retaining cells were also observed to be blocked in metaphase, indicating the ability of such cells at least to enter mitosis.

Behavior of Label-Retaining Cells in Culture

Three cell types were morphologically distinguishable in autoradiographs of cultured epithelial cells 3 days after plating: (a) large flattened cells with an

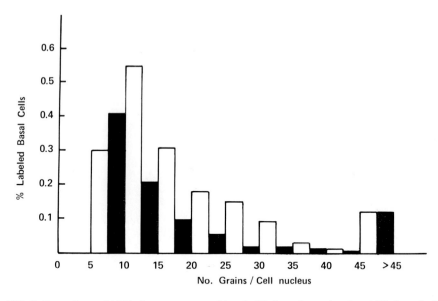

FIG. 2. Percentage of LRCs in mouse ear epidermis 30 days *(open bars)* and 72 days *(solid bars)* after labeling. Cells are grouped by degree of retained label assessed from the number of overlying silver grains.

appearance typical of epithelial cells in culture; (b) melanocytes; and (c) small, nonpigmented cells with a high nuclear/cytoplasmic ratio. The latter type of cell was frequently heavily labeled, suggesting correspondence with the label-retaining cells observed in the intact tissue. These three cell types were also seen in cultures at later stages when plaques of epithelial cells began to form. In such plaques, adjacent cells were observed to be labeled, suggesting a common origin from a labeled precursor or precursors. Counts of the labeled and unlabeled cells in such cultures are shown in Table 2. The 1:5 proportion of small cells to large cells remained approximately constant during a three- to fourfold increase in the total cell number, and the increasing proportion of labeled cells in both populations indicated cell division of both cell types.

TABLE 1. *Mean percentage of labeled basal cells ±SE*

Tissue	1 Hr postlabel (±SE)	30 Days postlabel (±SE)	72 Days postlabel (±SE)
Ear	90.7 ± 1.4	1.8 ± 0.12	1.0 ± 0.04
Palate	54.2 ± 2.6	0.1 ± 0.01	0.03 ± 0.01
Tongue	64.9 ± 2.0	0.1 ± 0.03	0.03 ± 0.02
Buccal mucosa	50.8 ± 4.9	0.1 ± 0.03	0.03 ± 0.01

TABLE 2. Cultures of epithelial cells dissociated 30 days after labeling in vivo (±SE)

Day	Cells/dish	% Small	% Large	% Melanocytes	% Labeled small	% Labeled large
3	721 ± 113	21.5 ± 2.8	76.9 ± 2.8	1.7 ± 0.4	10.2 ± 2.3	5.3 ± 1.2
4	1458 ± 120	13.2 ± 1.6	85.9 ± 1.8	1.4 ± 0.6	12.9 ± 1.3	4.9 ± 1.1
5	1691 ± 173	19.1 ± 1.5	79.1 ± 2.2	1.8 ± 0.9	20.8 ± 3.1	7.3 ± 1.4
6	1766 ± 111	21.1 ± 2.4	77.8 ± 2.4	1.4 ± 0.7	11.4 ± 2.1	9.0 ± 0.4
7	2576 ± 189	23.6 ± 0.2	74.1 ± 1.3	0.9 ± 0.2	20.3 ± 4.8	18.5 ± 2.7

DISCUSSION

The results show that in various epithelia, cells that retain label for extended periods of time can be identified, findings that suggest a very slow cell cycle or unusual pattern of division of these cells. The majority of LRCs examined by EM autoradiography were identified as keratinocytes. The presence of such cells does not appear to be an artifact of the incorporated radiation inhibiting the capacity for division, as label-retaining cells can be stimulated by TPA to enter mitosis and the pattern of grain loss from unstimulated tissue between 30 and 72 days is compatible with a slowly cycling cell population. The observations made in culture suggest that LRCs can complete division to produce clones of viable cells.

The role of such label-retaining cells in the maintenance of epithelial structure is uncertain. It is possible that they represent epithelial cells held out of the cell cycle in G_0 for extended periods of time. Alternatively, such label-retaining cells may correspond to epithelial stem cells. The existence of a subpopulation of stem cells within the epidermis would be of significance to studies of normal epithelial regeneration. The methods generally employed to examine epidermal proliferation would examine amplification divisions rather than the stem cell divisions that might ultimately be responsible for tissue regeneration. With a multistep mechanism of carcinogenesis (8), a stem cell is considered the main target cell for malignant transformation (5). The possibility of a protective mechanism of asymmetric separation of old and newly synthesized deoxyribonucleic acid (DNA) in stem cells, as proposed by Cairns (1), is of great interest. Demonstration of other properties of label-retaining cells, however, particularly amplification-division of committed daughter cells and a function as clonogens, is necessary before such cells may be considered evidence for a two-stage proliferative system. At present, therefore, the role in carcinogenesis of subpopulations of epithelial cells with unusual patterns of proliferation is undetermined. If, however, a correspondence between LRCs and epithelial stem cells can be established, the ability to mark such cells by a labeling technique would permit direct investigation of stem cell behavior.

REFERENCES

1. Cairns, J. (1975): Mutation selection and the natural history of cancer. *Nature,* 225:197.
2. Caro, L. G., and van Tubergen, R. P. (1962): High resolution autoradiography. *J. Cell Biol.,* 15:173–188.
3. Christophers, E. (1971): Cellular architecture of the stratum corneum. *J. Invest. Dermatol.,* 56:165–170.
4. Goerttler, K., Reuter, M., and Stahmer, H. E. (1973): Morphologische Untersuchungen zur Proliferationskinetik der Mausehaut. *Z. Zellforsch.,* 142:131–146.
5. Lajtha, L. G. (1979): Stem cell concepts. *Differentiation,* 14:2,324.
6. Mackenzie, I. C. (1969): The ordered structure of the stratum corneum of mammalian skin. *Nature,* 222:881–882.
7. Mackenzie, I. C. (1970): Relationship between mitosis and the structure of the stratum corneum in mouse epidermis. *Nature,* 226:653–655.

8. Peto, R. (1977): Epidemiology, multistate models, and short-term mutagenicity test. In: *Origins of Human Cancer,* edited by H. H. Hiatt, J. D. Watson, and J. A. Winsten, pp. 1,403–1,428. Cold Spring Harbor Laboratory, Cold Spring Habor, New York.
9. Potten, C. S. (1974): The epidermal proliferative unit: The possible role of the central basal cell. *Cell Tissue. Kinet.,* 7:77–78.
10. Potten, C. S. (1976): Identification of clonogenic cells in the epidermal proliferative unit (EPU). In: *Stem Cells of Renewing Cell Populations,* edited by A. B. Cairnie, P. K. Lala, and D. G. Osmond, pp. 91–102. Academic Press, New York.
11. Potten, C. S., and Allen, T. C. (1975): Control of epidermal proliferative units (EPU's). A hypothesis based on the arrangement of neighboring differentiated cells. *Differentiation,* 8:161–165.
12. Potten, C. S., and Hendry, H. H. (1973): Clonogenic cells and stem cells in epidermis. *Int. J. Radiat. Biol.,* 24:537–540.
13. Rogers, A. W. (1962): *Techniques of Autoradiography.* Elsevier Publishing Co., Amsterdam.

Carcinogenesis, Vol. 7, edited by E. Hecker et al.
Raven Press, New York © 1982.

Role of Differentiation in Determining Responses of Epidermal Cells to Phorbol Esters

*H. Hennings, *U. Lichti, †K. Holbrook, and *S. H. Yuspa

In Vitro Pathogenesis Section, Laboratory of Experimental Pathology, National Cancer Institute, Bethesda, Maryland 20205; and †Department of Biological Structure, University of Washington, Seattle, Washington 98104

In our laboratory, cultured mouse epidermal cells have been utilized for a variety of studies into the mechanisms of multistage carcinogenesis (4). Of primary importance is the determination of the types of cells in the complex epidermal tissue that are most responsive to tumor promoters. In this chapter, we describe conditions for the selective growth of epidermal basal cells, the presumed target cell for promoter action, and compare the 12-O-tetradecanoylphorbol-13-acetate (TPA)-responsiveness of these cells with epidermal cells induced to terminally differentiate in culture.

SELECTION OF BASAL CELLS WITH LOW CALCIUM MEDIUM

The usual pattern of epidermal cell growth in culture, characterized by limited proliferation, keratin synthesis, cell connections by desmosomes, stratification, and terminal differentiation, can be altered remarkably by lowering the ionic calcium concentration in the medium from the usual 1.2 to 2.0 mM to 0.02 to 0.1 mM. In low calcium medium, desmosome formation and stratification are prevented (Fig. 1B) and epidermal cells grow indefinitely as a monolayer (Fig. 1A) with a high proliferation rate (1). The synthesis of keratin proteins continues, but differentiating cells are shed into the medium instead of forming multilayers as they do in medium with standard calcium levels.

Attached cells maintain distinct intercellular spaces (Figs. 1A and B), with communication between cells only by microvilli and occasional gap junctions and tight junctions; desmosomes are absent (Fig. 1B). The numerous tonofilaments are arranged perinuclearly (Fig. 1B). Thus, low calcium growth selects for epidermal cells with the characteristics of basal cells: small polygonal cells with a rapid proliferation rate, which contain the pemphigoid antigen characteristic of basal cells, but lack the pemphigus antigen characteristic of superficial differentiating cells (4).

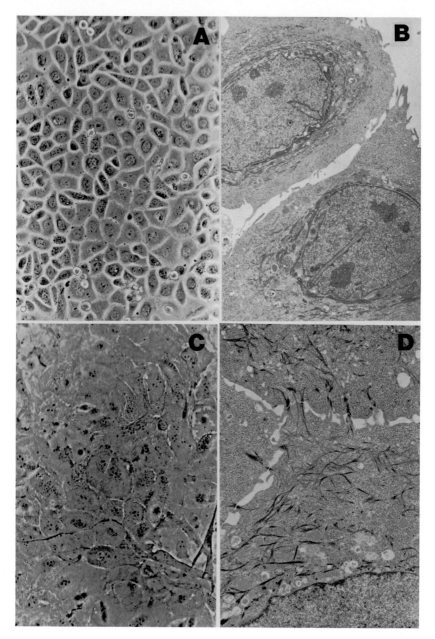

FIG. 1. Morphology and ultrastructure of epidermal cells in low calcium medium **(A,B)** and after calcium addition **(C,D)**. **A:** Epidermal cells maintained for 6 months in medium with 0.02 mM calcium (× 100). **B:** Epidermal culture after 7 days in medium with 0.07 mM calcium (× 18,500). **C:** Epidermal cells grown for 7 days in 0.07 mM calcium, then 2 days in 1.2 mM calcium (× 100). **D:** Epidermal cells grown for 7 days in 0.07 mM calcium, then 2 hr in 1.2 mM calcium (× 31,600).

INDUCTION OF TERMINAL DIFFERENTIATION
BY CALCIUM ADDITION

After the addition of calcium (1.20 mM) to epidermal cells growing in low calcium, desmosomes are formed within 1 to 2 hr (Fig. 1D), proliferation ceases by 36 hr (1), and the cells differentiate morphologically (Fig. 1C), stratify, and detach from the dish by 3 to 4 days (1). Thus, by restoring the calcium in the medium to standard levels, basal cells are rapidly committed to terminal differentiation.

INDUCTION OF ORNITHINE DECARBOXYLASE BY TPA IN BASAL
CELLS AND TERMINALLY DIFFERENTIATING CELLS

The induction of ornithine decarboxylase (ODC) by tumor promoters provides a characteristic response thought to be important in the tumor promotion process (3,5). In epidermal cells grown in medium with a standard level of calcium, ODC induction by TPA was found only in the first 36 hr after plating (2). The extent of this initial ODC induction by TPA could be increased several-fold by growing the cells in medium with 0.02 to 0.1 mM calcium (Table 1), levels which select for basal cells. In low calcium medium, the ODC response to TPA declined with time in culture, but a significant response remained after 7 days (Table 1) and as long as 4 weeks in culture (U. Lichti, *unpublished observations*).

Another important aspect of the tumor promotion process, induction of proliferation, has not been demonstrated in low calcium-selected basal cells. The high proliferation rate of low calcium epidermal cells, however, may preclude a further TPA-induced increase.

When low calcium cells are induced to terminally differentiate by calcium

TABLE 1. *Effect of medium calcium level on TPA induction of ODC at days 1 and 7 after plating epidermal cells*

Treatment time	Time after treatment (hr)	ODC activity in 0.07 mM Ca^{2+} (nmole CO_2/mg protein/hr)[a]		ODC activity in 1.20 mM Ca^{2+} (nmole CO_2/mg protein/hr)	
		DMSO[b]	TPA	DMSO	TPA
Day 1	4	1.9	9.4	1.2	5.4
	8	0.8	21.1	0.6	10.4
	12.5	0.4	25	0.4	6.3
Day 7	4	0.3	9.3	0.1	0.4
	8	0.02	4.7	0.04	0.13
	12.5	0.04	0.93	0.08	0.02

[a] ODC values are the average of duplicate samples that agreed to within ± 15%. TPA treatment was with 0.01 μg/ml.
[b] DMSO-Dimethylsulfoxide.

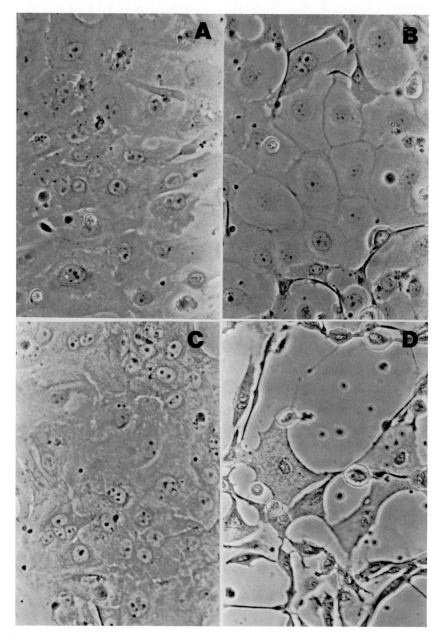

FIG. 2. Enhancement by TPA of calcium-induced terminal differentiation. Epidermal cells grown for 7 days in 0.07 mM calcium were switched to medium with 1.2mM calcium containing 0.01 µg TPA/ml **(B,D)** or DMSO solvent **(A,C)**. Microphotographs (× 200) were taken 10 hr **(A,B)** or 21 hr **(C,D)** later.

TABLE 2. *Reduced induction of ODC by TPA (0.01 µg/ml) in cells terminally differentiating after calcium addition*

Time of TPA treatment after calcium addition (hr)	ODC (percent of induction in low calcium medium)		Number of experiments
	Average	Range	
0	37.8	10–70	4
2	22.8	7.4–41	7
4	9.6	4.2–15	2
6	6.1	4.2–8.0	2

addition, responsiveness to TPA induction of ODC is rapidly lost. TPA responsiveness is reduced nearly 80% within 2 hr of calcium addition and 90 to 95% by 6 hr (Table 2). Thus, the ODC response to TPA in basal cells is much greater than in cells committed to differentiate.

TPA ENHANCEMENT OF CALCIUM-INDUCED TERMINAL DIFFERENTIATION

Morphological differentiation induced by calcium is enhanced by TPA treatment at the time of calcium addition (Fig. 2). Cells with thickened plasma membranes were apparent after 10 hr (Fig. 2B), and by 21 hr (Fig. 2D), squame-like cells with pycnotic nuclei were detaching from the plate. Although this population of committed cells is removed from the culture more rapidly in the presence of TPA, another population of cells is relatively unaffected by continued TPA treatment (not shown). This sort of selection process is likely to be important in the mechanism of action of tumor promoters.

ACKNOWLEDGMENT

We thank Mrs. Margaret Green for efficient secretarial assistance.

REFERENCES

1. Hennings, H., Michael, D., Cheng, C., Steinert, P., Holbrook, K., and Yuspa, S. H. (1980): Calcium regulation of growth and differentiation of mouse epidermal cells in culture. *Cell,* 19:245–254.
2. Lichti, U., Yuspa, S. H., and Hennings, H. (1978): Ornithine and S-adenosylmethionine decarboxylases in mouse epidermal cell cultures treated with tumor promoters. In: *Mechanisms of Tumor Promotion and Cocarcinogenesis,* edited by T. J. Slaga, A. Sivak, and R. K. Boutwell, pp. 221–232. Raven Press, New York.
3. O'Brien, T. G. (1976): The induction of ornithine decarboxylase as an early, possibly obligatory, event in mouse skin carcinogenesis. *Cancer Res.,* 36:2,644–2,653.
4. Yuspa, S. H., Hawley-Nelson, P., Stanley, J. R., and Hennings, H. (1980): Epidermal cell culture. *Transplant. Proc.,* 12:114–122.
5. Yuspa, S. H., Lichti, U., Ben, T., Patterson, E., Hennings, H., Slaga, T. J., Colburn, N., and Kelsey, W. (1976): Phorbol esters stimulate DNA synthesis and ornithine decarboxylase activity in mouse epidermal cell cultures. *Nature,* 262:402–404.

Carcinogenesis, Vol. 7, edited by E. Hecker et al.
Raven Press, New York © 1982.

Early Induction of the Arachidonic Acid Cascade and Stimulation of DNA Synthesis by TPA in Murine and Guinea Pig Epidermal Cells in Culture

G. Fürstenberger, C. Delescluse, S. M. Fischer, H. Richter, and F. Marks

Institute of Biochemistry, German Cancer Research Center, D-6900 Heidelberg, Federal Republic of Germany

Topical application of the tumor-promoting phorbol ester 12-O-tetradecanoyl-phorbol-13-acetate (TPA) to adult mouse skin *in vivo* exerts a strong hyperproliferative response in the epidermis which is mediated by an elevation of the epidermal prostaglandin E (PGE) content within the first 15 min (2). The dramatic increase of ornithine decarboxylase (ODC) activity preceding cell proliferation appears to be dependent on PGE (5). It was of interest to study the sequential and possibly obligatory relationship of the induction of the arachidonic acid cascade, ODC activity, and cell proliferation as observed *in vivo* after TPA treatment using an established murine epidermal cell line HEL/30 (for references, see ref. 3) and primary basal epidermal cells from adult guinea pigs (PGPBE cells, ref. 4).

MATERIALS AND METHODS

TPA was kindly supplied by Prof. Dr. E. Hecker, Heidelberg. PGE_2 and $PGF_{2\alpha}$ as well as arachidonic acid were purchased from Sigma, München; [1-^{14}C]arachidonic acid (55 mCi/mmole), D,L-(1-^{14}C) ornithine (60 mCi/mmole), and ^{3}H-thymidine (25 Ci/mmole) were purchased from Amersham Buchler, Braunschweig.

The murine epidermal cell line HEL/30 and the primary basal epidermal cells (PGPBE cells) from guinea pigs (Dunkins, Hartley strains) were grown following standard procedures (3,4). Four days (HEL/30) or 24 hr (PGPBE cells) after seeding, the culture medium was replaced by fresh medium containing 0.3 μCi [1-^{14}C]arachidonic acid (0.2 μCi/ml). After 9 or 15 hr, respectively, i.e., in the plateau phase of the labeling kinetics of the cellular phospholipids, the labeled medium was replaced with culture medium containing either acetone or dimethylsulfoxide (DMSO) (final concentration, 0.5%) and TPA ($1.6.10^{-6}$ M or 10^{-7} M, respectively), indomethacin (10^{-4} M), PGE_2 (10^{-6} M), or $PGF_{2\alpha}$ (10^{-6} M). After 24 hr the incubation medium was replaced by fresh medium or "indomethacin medium." For determination of the arachidonic acid and its metabolites released from prelabeled cells, the assay of ODC activity, and deoxyribonucleic acid (DNA) labeling see ref. 3.

RESULTS AND DISCUSSION

Figures 1 and 2 present the effect of TPA on the release of arachidonic acid, PGE_2, and $PGF_{2\alpha}$ into the culture medium of HEL/30 cells and PGPBE cells prelabeled with $[1-^{14}C]$arachidonic acid. After a lag phase of 10 to 15 min, levels of arachidonic acid and PGE_2 began to increase in the medium of TPA-treated HEL/30 cells, whereas the accumulation of $PGF_{2\alpha}$ did not start

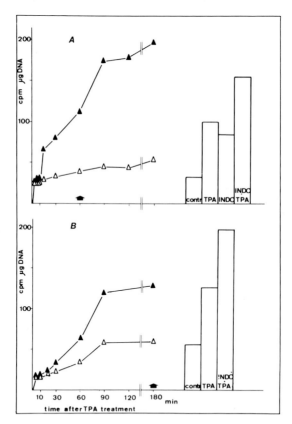

FIG. 1 Effect of TPA and indomethacin on the accumulation of arachidonic acid in the culture medium of HEL/30 **(A)** and of PGPBE cells **(B)**. Cultures prelabeled with $[1-^{14}C]$arachidonic acid were treated with 10^{-6} M or 10^{-7} M TPA (▲), indomethacin (10^{-4} M), respectively, or acetone or DMSO (△), respectively, at zero time and processed at the times indicated. For methodology see ref. 3. Radioactivity was determined by liquid scintillation counting. Each point is the mean of six assays **(A)** or the mean of three assays (one representative experiment of three; **B**).

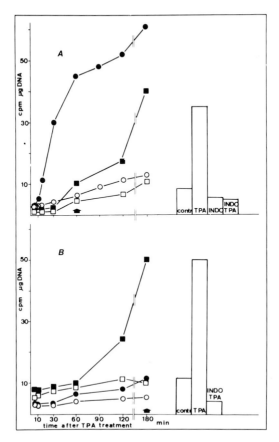

FIG. 2. Effect of TPA and indomethacin on the accumulation of prostaglandins E_2 (● ○) and $F_{2\alpha}$ (■ □) in the culture medium of HEL/30 **(A)** and of PGPBE cells **(B)**. For details, see Fig. 1. The arrows indicate the time point of the indomethacin experiment. Each point is the mean of six assays **(A)** or the mean of three assays (one representative of three assays).

earlier than 1 hr after TPA application (Figs. 1A and 2A). Following TPA treatment of PGPBE cells, arachidonic acid and $PGF_{2\alpha}$ accumulated in the medium with a lag phase of 30 to 60 min (Figs. 1B and 2B). After 120 min a slight increase of PGE_2 was observed.

TPA enhanced the ODC activity in HEL/30 cells, leading to a broad maximum (1,800% of the control) between 6 and 12 hr. In PGPBE cells the maximum of ODC activity (2,000% of the control) was reached 4 hr after TPA application (data not shown). On addition of TPA, a threefold stimulation of ^{3}H-thymidine incorporation into cellular DNA was observed in HEL/30 cells after 48 hr and a tenfold stimulation in PGPBE cells after 72 hr (Fig. 3).

Treatment of HEL/30 and PGPBE cells with indomethacin (10^{-4} M) inhibited the release of PGE_2 and $F_{2\alpha}$ induced by either medium change or TPA (Fig.

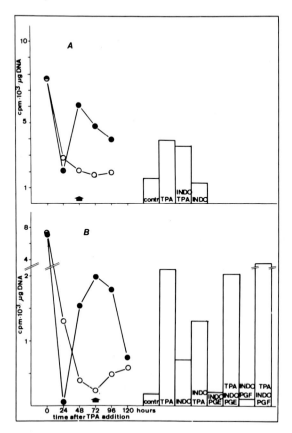

FIG. 3. Effect of TPA, indomethacin, and prostaglandins E_2 and $F_{2\alpha}$ on ³H-thymidine incorporation into DNA of HEL/30 **(A)** and PGPBE cells **(B).** At the time 30 min culture media were replaced by fresh medium or medium containing 10^{-4} M indomethacin. At zero time cultures were treated with 10^{-6} M TPA (●) or 10^{-7} M TPA (●), indomethacin (10^{-4} M), prostaglandins E_2 and $F_{2\alpha}$, or acetone or DMSO (○), and DNA was isolated at the times indicated (see Methods). The arrows indicate the time point of the indomethacin experiment. Each point is the mean of six assays (triplicate assays from two different experiments; **A**) or the mean of three assays (one representative experiment of three; **B**).

2). Accordingly, the release of free arachidonic acid into the media was enhanced (Fig. 1). Whereas in PGPBE cells no significant effect of indomethacin (10^{-4} M) on TPA-induced ODC activity could be observed, the stimulatory effect of TPA on the ODC activity in HEL/30 cells was, if anything, slightly enhanced in presence of the drug (data not shown). Indomethacin inhibited the TPA-induced stimulation of DNA labeling in PGPBE cells but not in HEL/30 cells (Fig. 3). The inhibition was reversed by simultaneous treatment of the cells with $PGF_{2\alpha}$ or PGE_2 (10^{-6} M).

Our results show that the stimulatory effect of TPA on prostaglandin synthesis characteristic for mouse epidermis *in vivo* (2) is also observed in epidermal cell cultures *in vitro.* In contrast to the *in vivo* situation, however, the experiments with the cyclooxygenase inhibitor indomethacin in the murine epidermal cell line did not reveal any relationship between prostaglandin synthesis and induction of ODC or cellular proliferation (HEL/30). Furthermore, in primary epidermal guinea pig cells, only TPA-stimulated DNA synthesis seems to be prostaglandin dependent. *In vitro* and *in vivo* (Delescluse et al., *unpublished results*), the inhibitory effect of indomethacin on guinea pig cell proliferation can be overcome by $PGF_{2\alpha}$ and—to a lesser extent—by PGE_2, whereas in mouse epidermis *in vivo,* such an effect is specifically restricted to PGE_2 (1).

This means that by switching over from the living animal to *in vitro* systems, not only may the specificity of the prostaglandin effect be lost, but the whole sequence of events leading to TPA-induced cellular hyperproliferation may be "uncoupled" from prostaglandin synthesis. Such a result would be consistent with the general view that prostaglandins are "modifiers" of regulatory effects rather than being autonomous effectors. Whether or not such modification (amplification, mediation) of the stimulatory effect of TPA is necessary may entirely depend on the accompanying circumstances of the experiment.

ACKNOWLEDGMENTS

We thank Eva Besemfelder, Heidi Trumpfheller, and Ingeborg Vogt for expert technical assistance. This work was supported by the Deutsche Forschungsgemeinschaft and the Wilhelm- und Maria-Meyenburg Foundation.

REFERENCES

1. Fürstenberger, G., and Marks, F. (1978): Indomethacin inhibition of cell proliferation induced by the phorbolester TPA is reversed by prostaglandin E_2 in mouse epidermis *in vivo. Biochem. Biophys. Res. Commun.,* 84:1,103–1,111.
2. Fürstenberger, G., and Marks, F. (1980): Early prostaglandin E synthesis in an obligatory event in the induction of cell proliferation in mouse epidermis *in vivo* by the phorbol ester TPA. *Biochem. Biophys. Res. Commun.,* 92:749–756.
3. Fürstenberger, G., Richter, H., Fusenig, N. E., and Marks, F. (1981): Arachidonic acid and prostaglandin E_2 release and enhanced cell proliferation induced by the phorbol ester TPA in a murine epidermal cell line. *Cancer Letters,* 11:191–198.
4. Prunieras, M., Delescluse, C., and Regnier, M. (1978): A cell culture model for the study of epidermal (chalone) homeostasis. *Pharm. Ther.,* 9:271–295.
5. Verma, A. K., Ashendel, L. C., and Boutwell, R. K. (1980): Inhibition of prostaglandin synthesis inhibitors of the induction of ornithine decarboxylase activity, the accumulation of prostaglandins, and tumor promotion caused by 12-O-tetradecanoylphorbol-13-acetate. *Cancer Res.,* 40:308–315.

Carcinogenesis, Vol. 7, edited by E. Hecker et al.
Raven Press, New York © 1982.

On the Relationship Between Epidermal Hyperproliferation and Skin Tumor Promotion

Friedrich Marks, David L. Berry, Stefan Bertsch, Gerhard Fürstenberger, and Hartmut Richter

Institut für Biochemie, Deutsches Krebsforschungszentrum, German Cancer Research Center, D-6900 Heidelberg, Federal Republic of Germany

SOME GENERAL IDEAS ON THE ROLE OF CELL PROLIFERATION AND TISSUE MATURATION IN THE PROCESS OF TUMOR PROMOTION

In skin, tumor promotion seems to be inseparably linked to epithelial hyperproliferation, since all promoting agents and manipulations studied thus far have strong mitogenic effects. The question is whether or not enhanced cell proliferation is a sufficient condition of tumor promotion, as has been repeatedly suggested in the past. The discovery of "two-stage promotion" (7,34) now enables us to subdivide two-stage carcinogenesis into three subsequent steps: (a) initiation by means of a carcinogen; (b) expression of the tumor phenotype by the promoter; and (c) generation of visible tumors by means of continuous growth stimulation, which can be brought about by the promoter itself or by a nonpromoting mitogen (Fig. 1).

As we have recently postulated (22), the expression of the tumor phenotype is an essential event of two-stage skin carcinogenesis since, in epidermis, initiation has occurred in a tissue that under normal conditions seems to be strictly committed to a special type of function, i.e., formation of dead horny scales (suicide maturation pathway). Such a tissue will probably not be allowed to realize a new functional program such as "tumor growth" unless the genetic readout is reprogrammed. Taking into consideration the metaplasiogenic effects of tumor-promoting manipulations such as 12-O-tetradecanoylphorbol-13-acetate (32,33) or wounding (26,28) as well as the striking similarities between promoter-treated and embryonic epidermis (22), we have postulated that a promoter brings about the expression of the tumor phenotype in the course of a metaplastic reaction (i.e., alteration of tissue commitment) possibly via a transient relapse of the whole system into an ontogenetically more "primitive" state (22).

There is indeed a steadily increasing body of evidence that tumor promoters such as TPA exert pronounced effects on cell and tissue differentiation in a wide variety of systems *(this volume)*. Whereas in certain tissues the obligatory

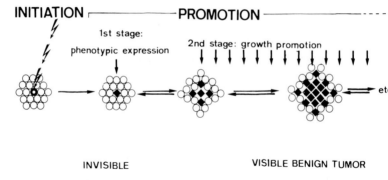

FIG. 1. The concept of two-stage promotion. For details, see text.

role of cell divisions for functional programming has been quite firmly established (concept of "quantal cell division," see ref. 19), as far as epidermis is concerned a similar conclusion is based on deduction by analogy rather than on experimental facts. Under normal conditions epidermal cell maturation (keratinization) proceeds via several steps of cell multiplication. So, although unable to get direct experimental proof, at present, we might at least assume that for a promoter-induced alteration of tissue commitment (i.e., the expression of the tumor phenotype), cell proliferation is obligatory.

The role of cell proliferation in the second stage of promotion is possibly a rather trivial one. In the classic experimental approach of two-stage skin carcinogenesis, the great majority of tumors are benign papillomas (8). Since their growth patterns are reversible, they will become visible to the naked eye and thus countable only if continuous exogenous growth stimulation is applied. Therefore, the second stage of promotion is possibly inherent in our assay system rather than a biologically important condition of promotion.

THE PROBLEM OF "PROMOTION-SPECIFIC" TPA EFFECTS

The most potent and most widely used skin tumor promoter TPA has a chemical structure and physiochemical properties that make it a strong membrane-active agent. As such, TPA would be expected—and has been found—to interfere with many biological events that are somehow related to membrane structure, membrane permeability, and the signal transfer across membranes. It is not too surprising, therefore, that TPA has been shown to either mimic or antagonize the actions of hormones and other agents, especially of those acting via membrane receptors. Since hormone effects depend entirely on the target tissue and its functional program, the prodigous variety of TPA effects on different cell types is easily understood, as is the influence of TPA on cell and tissue differentiation, because hormones are by definition biochemical signals that control tissue function.

Perhaps the most important question of today's phorbol ester research is, then, whether the investigation of those pleiotypic effects of TPA may lead us to a better understanding of the phenomenon of tumor promotion, or whether such studies—although certainly of interest for basic research in cell biology—have to be considered as "l'art pour l'art" as far as cancer research is concerned. This problem is becoming even more critical in view of the fact that in most systems used for research on the biological effects of TPA, tumor promotion has not been demonstrated at all, or has not been proven so conclusively as in mouse skin *in vivo*.

THE PROBLEM OF THE NEGATIVE CONTROL

When considering tumor promotion in skin, it can be stated that all promoting agents or manipulations evoke both an inflammatory response and epidermal hyperproliferation. On the other hand, not every mitogenic irritant is a promoter. This discrepancy again gives rise to the question of which of the many biological effects of TPA observed in skin or other systems are indicative for promotion, and which are merely related to its irritating and mitogenic activities. A related question is whether epidermal hyperproliferation always proceeds via the same sequence of biochemical events or whether we can perhaps differentiate between a "normal" and a "promotion-specific" pathway to epidermal hyperproliferation.

It is now a well-established fact that epidermal hyperproliferation not only can be evoked by different means, but in addition can be approached on different biochemical routes. If the stimulus (skin massage, for example) does not damage the tissue, the hyperproliferative response is not accompanied by inflammatory processes and does not lead to an immediate multiplication of cell number, i.e., hyperplasia (4). The reason for this is probably that endogenous mechanisms of growth regulation, such as chalone control (23), are preserved so that an increase of the rate of cell proliferation is automatically and precisely matched by an increase of the rate of cell maturation and cell loss. This kind of hyperproliferative response must be considered as nothing but an amplification of the normal, everyday tissue regeneration process.

If the tissue is *damaged* by mechanical or chemical means, some sort of an "SOS response" enters the game. In the case of mouse epidermis, this is characterized by the rapid development of a hyperplastic state which strikingly resembles neonatal epidermis and is always accompanied by more or less pronounced symptoms of skin inflammation. This "hyperplastic transformation" has been shown to be associated with a temporary breakdown of a special endogenous growth control device, i.e., the G_1 chalone mechanism (4,22,23). As will be shown below, it is accompanied by several biochemical events that are not seen when a nondamaging stimulus is applied. Since TPA induces hyperplastic transformation, the problem of the negative control becomes important for every study devoted to the search for true biochemical parameters of tumor promotion. Nonmitogenic compounds such as phorbol are, of course, quite useless in this respect, and so are hyperplasiogenic irritants of high toxicity, such as acetic acid, which probably kill the initiated cells before they can be promoted (27). What we have to look for is a control compound that induces hyperplastic transformation via essentially the same mechanism as TPA, without being a promoter and without being more toxic than TPA.

IS 4-O-METHYL-TPA A USEFUL NEGATIVE CONTROL?

The almost nonpromoting 4-O-methyl-ether of TPA (21) is presently widely used as a negative control in promoter research. In a dose about 50-fold higher, it induces epidermal hyperproliferation as powerful as TPA and may also bring about a weak or moderate epidermal hyperplasia without showing visible signs of toxicity (21).

The mitotic effect is, however, all that 4-O-methyl-TPA has in common with TPA. In every other aspect these phorbol esters behave completely differently. Thus 4-O-methyl-TPA is not an irritant and does not induce biochemical reactions that normally accompany hyperplastic transformation such as prostaglandin synthesis (16), ornithine decarboxylase activity (21), catecholamine refractoriness (F. Marks et al., *unpublished results*), and desensitization to epidermal G_1 chalone (H. Richter and F. Marks, *unpublished results*). Since, in contrast to TPA, the mitogenic effect of the methyl ether is apparently not mediated by prostaglandin synthesis, it is also resistant to indomethacin inhibition (16).

As a whole, the mitogenic effect of 4-O-methyl-TPA resembles that of a nondamaging stimulus such as skin massage (4) rather than that of TPA. Therefore, the compound can no longer be regarded as a useful control for TPA studies.

NONPROMOTING AGENTS THAT INDUCE HYPERPLASTIC TRANSFORMATION OF EPIDERMIS ALONG THE SAME PATHWAY AS TPA

Divalent Cation Ionophore A 23187

We have recently shown that the antibiotic A 23187 (Fig. 2), known as divalent cation ionophore (29), is a potent irritant mitogen for mouse skin (25). The compound is not a tumor promoter and apparently is nontoxic in long-term experiments. When locally applied in a proper dose (50- to 100-fold that of TPA) it provokes in mouse epidermis exactly the same responses as TPA. These include a strong increase of ornithine decarboxylase and cyclic nucleotide phosphodiesterase activities, catecholamine refractoriness, and prostaglandin E release (25). The latter reaction is obligatory for the hyperplastic response, as has been shown by means of inhibitors of prostaglandin synthesis (refs. 15 and 25; see also below). These results indicate that A 23187 and TPA share the same mechanism of action, thus lending support to the conclusion that all the responses mentioned above are indicative for hyperplastic transformation rather than for tumor promotion.

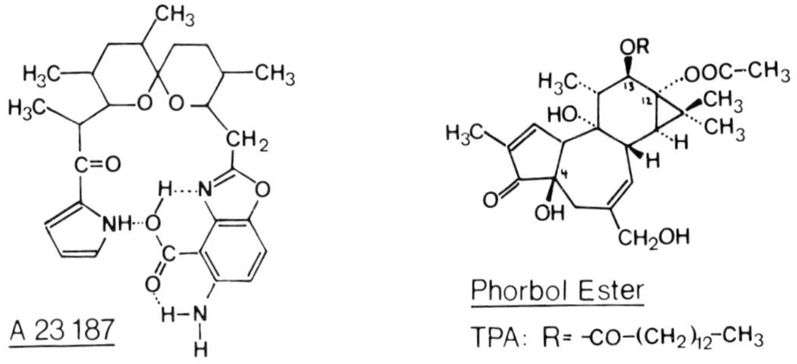

FIG. 2. Chemical structure of ionophore A23187 as compared with that of phorbol ester TPA.

TPA Derivatives with an Unsaturated Fatty Acid Side Chain

There is an increasing body of evidence for the existence of specific binding sites for TPA on target cells *(this volume)*. Since A 23187 and TPA are compounds of quite different chemical structures, it could be argued that the ionophore is not a suitable negative control because it may bypass the supposed receptor mechanism, for instance, by facilitating the membrane transport of ions that are perhaps the "second messengers" of TPA-receptor interaction. Although it is difficult to see how such a bypass could abolish just the tumor-promoting properties of a compound (since a second messenger is generally capable of evoking all the responses of its primary signal), this argument has to be taken seriously as long as the molecular mechanism of promotion is unknown.

Our argument that most of the biological effects of TPA on skin are indicative for hyperplastic transformation rather than for tumor promotion would be considerably strengthened if nonpromoting irritant mitogens with an intact phorbol moiety, regarded as critical for any receptor interaction, would become available. Such compounds can indeed be synthesized by introducing double bonds into the long chain fatty acid residue of TPA (13). We have recently described the biological properties of $C_{14:4}$-phorbol acetate ("Ti8", see Fig. 3), a phorbol ester naturally occurring in *Euphorbia tirucally* (13; courtesy of Prof. Hecker, Heidelberg). On a molar base this compound provokes skin inflammation, epidermal hyperproliferation, and epidermal hyperplasia nearly as strong as TPA, whereas its tumor-promoting activities are negligible (21). $C_{14:4}$-phorbol acetate is also a strong inducer of epidermal ornithine decarboxylase activity and catecholamine refractoriness (21; F. Marks et al., *unpublished results*).

Recently, we have synthesized a TPA analogue in which the tetradecanoyl side chain is replaced by a retinoyl residue (12-O-retinoylphorbol-13-acetate, RPA; see Fig. 3). This compound combines the tumor-promoting principle of a phorbol ester with the antipromoting principle of retinoic acid. As an irritant mitogen, RPA is at least as powerful as TPA (Fig. 4); it also induces ornithine decarboxylase activity as well as catecholamine refractoriness (F. Marks et al.,

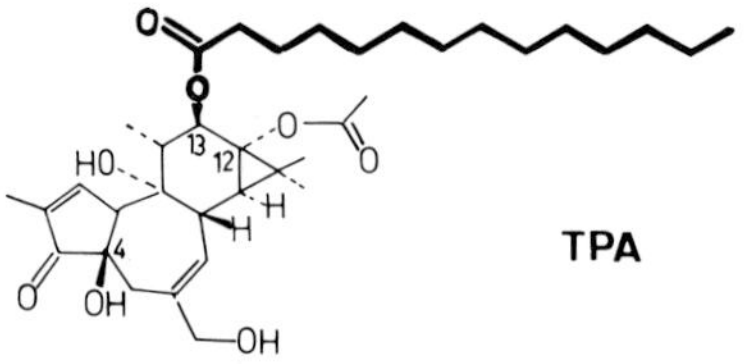

FIG. 3. Tumor promoter TPA and nonpromoting TPA analogues with an unsaturated long chain fatty acid residue. The transconfiguration of double bonds 6,7 and 8,9 of $C_{14:14}PA$ is not yet definitely proven.

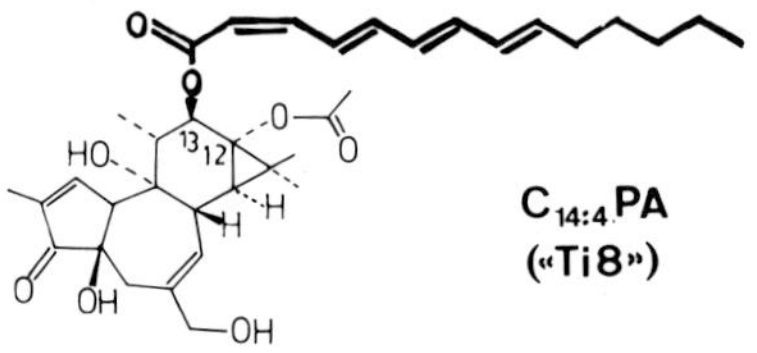

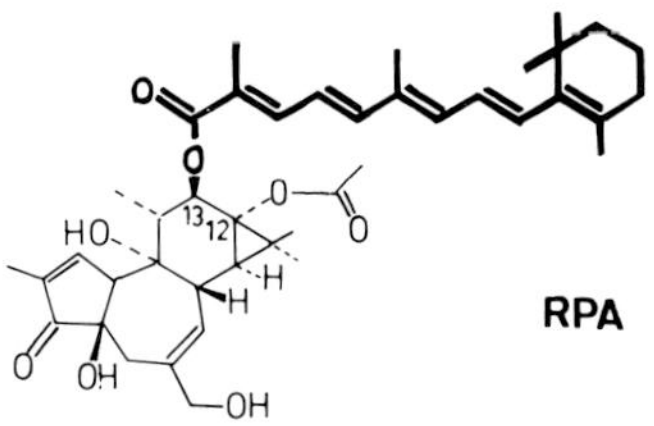

unpublished results). Its hyperplasiogenic effect is mediated by prostaglandin E_2 (PGE$_2$) synthesis and is thus sensitive to indomethacin inhibition. One has to conclude, therefore, that as a hyperplasiogenic agent, RPA, has the same mechanism of action as TPA. Nevertheless, RPA completely lacks tumor-promoting efficacy, although the compound has turned out to be the most potent "second stage promoter" (see above) when applied in combination with TPA (Table 1). In this respect it is much more powerful than the second stage promoter mezerein (34), which is in addition a weak full promoter (Table 1).

Although not yet proven, one may easily assume that both $C_{14:4}$-phorbol acetate and RPA are able to interact with the supposed phorbol ester receptor due to the integrity of their phorbol moiety. Since these nonpromoting agents evoke in skin biological and biochemical responses identical to those caused by TPA, these responses cannot be true parameters of tumor promotion, but are merely indicators of hyperplastic transformation, which may be an essential process in the second stage of promotion but which is most probably not the only reason for the first stage, i.e., the expression of the tumor phenotype (see above).

THE ROLE OF PROSTAGLANDINS IN HYPERPLASTIC TRANSFORMATION

Although specific binding sites for TPA have been found in epidermis (11), it is not known yet if these are involved in the mitogenic effect. Thus, the

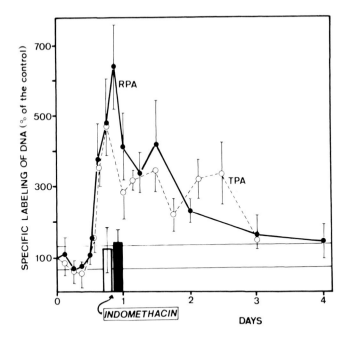

FIG. 4. Deoxyribonucleic acid (DNA) labeling in mouse epidermis *in vivo* after topical application of TPA (--○--; 10 nmole/0.1 ml acetone) or RPA (—●—; 10 nmole/0.1 ml acetone) at zero time. The columns show the inhibition achieved by topical application of indomethacin (1.1 µmole/0.1 ml acetone) 30 min prior to mitogen treatment (*empty column,* TPA; *black column,* RPA). The horizontal lines represent the average standard deviation of the controls. For DNA labeling, ^{3}H-thymidine was injected i.p. 45 min prior to sacrifice. For other experimental details see ref. 20.

very first in the chain of events leading to hyperplastic transformation is still a matter of conjecture. All that can be asserted is that the phorbol ester most probably interacts with the cell membrane, possibly via specific sites. The immediate consequence of such an interaction has been more precisely described in the last few years. In mouse epidermis this consequence is the biosynthesis of PGE$_2$, which can be observed almost immediately after application of TPA, RPA, A 23187, and—to a lesser extent—C$_{14:4}$-phorbol acetate (Fig. 5). By means of proper tissue culture systems, we could show that the prostaglandin release is preceded by a liberation of arachidonic acid from membrane phospholipids (probably mainly from phosphatidylinositol) and that the whole sequence of events can occur in epidermis (see ref. 17 and *this volume*). *In vivo* the PGE$_2$ level reaches a peak about 10 to 20 min after stimulation (Fig. 5 and refs. 16, 25). If this early response is prevented by inhibitors of prostaglandin biosynthesis, such as indomethacin or 5, 8, 11, 14-eicosatetraynoic acid (ETYA), neither epidermal hyperproliferation (16,25) nor induction of ornithine decarboxylase (36,37) will occur, whereas other responses such as increase of phosphodiesterase activity (24), catecholamine refractoriness (F. Marks, *unpublished results*), and inflammation (25) will remain unaffected. This and the fact that the indomethacin

TABLE 1. Effect of RPA as full promoter and second stage promoter as compared with the tumor-promoting effects of TPA and mezerein[a]

Treatment	After 12 weeks		After 15 weeks		After 18 weeks	
	Rate (%)[b]	Yield[c]	Rate (%)	Yield	Rate (%)	Yield
Acetone	0	0	0	0	0	0
Mezerein	0	0	7	0.7	7	0.7
RPA	0	0	0	0	0	0
TPA	100	4.6	100	7.6	100	7.4
Four applications of TPA, treatment continued with mezerein	13	0.13	13	0.13	20	0.27
Four applications of TPA, treatment continued with RPA	60	1.9	67	3.3	80	5.2

[a] For each group 16 female NMRI mice (7 weeks old) were initiated by topical application of 100 nmole dimethylbenz(a)anthracene (dissolved in 0.1 ml acetone) onto the shaved back skin. One week later, the treatments with either acetone (controls), mezerein, or the phorbol esters were started. For this purpose, the compounds were dissolved in 0.1 ml acetone and applied twice weekly. The doses per application were: 0.1 ml acetone, 5 nmole TPA, 8 nmole mezerein, and 10 nmole RPA.
[b] Tumor-bearing animals/survivors (100% survival in all groups).
[c] Number of tumors/survivor.

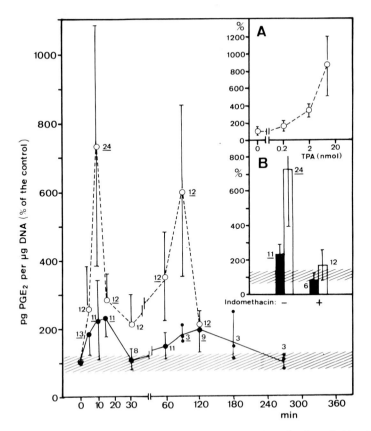

FIG. 5. Level of PGE_2 in mouse epidermis *in vivo* after topical application of either TPA (10 nmole/0.1 ml acetone; --○--) or A23187 (200 nmole/0.1 ml acetone; —●—) at zero time. The hatched zone represents the average SD of the control values (treatment with acetone only) as obtained from 34 acetone-treated animals (7.3 ± 2.0 pg PGE_2/μg DNA = 100%). **Insert A:** The dose-response curve for TPA as measured 10 min after application (n ≥ 12, SD). **Insert B:** Results when 1.1 μmole indomethacin was applied topically 30 min prior to TPA or A23187 treatment, and the PGE_2 content was measured 10 min after TPA *(open columns)* or 15 min after A23187 application *(black columns)*. Each point or column represents a mean value (± SD). The number of experiments is given beside each point or column. *Underlined number:* value different from the control at a level of significance of $\alpha = 0.05$ (statistical evaluation by means of the Kruskal-Wallis test). For further details, see ref. 25.

inhibition of hyperproliferation can be specifically overcome by low doses of PGE_2 but not by $PGF_{2\alpha}$ (15,25) strongly indicate that E-prostaglandins selectively mediate the mitogenic stimulus, whereas accompanying reactions such as those mentioned above follow different pathways.

Indomethacin given 15 min or later after stimulation does not interfere with epidermal hyperproliferation, thus excluding the possibility of nonspecific toxic effects of the inhibitor and indicating that the very early pulse of PGE_2 synthesis is the key event (25). As TPA or A23187 is not able to induce epidermal hyperproliferation in the absence of PGE_2 (or when endogenous PGE_2 synthesis is inhibited by indomethacin), PGE_2 does not exhibit any distinct mitogenic effect on epidermis in the absence of TPA or A23187 (16,25). In addition, indomethacin is unable to inhibit normal epidermal cell proliferation to a visible extent (15,16,25). This synergistic action of PGE_2 and the mitogenic stimulus means that PGE_2 synthesis is a necessary but not a sufficient "trigger event" in the course of hyperplastic transformation.

As mentioned above and discussed in more detail elsewhere (4,22,23), hyperplastic transformation of mouse epidermis is accompanied by a temporary refractoriness of the tissue for a tissue-specific endogenous growth control signal, the G_1 chalone. This breakdown of chalone control can also be prevented by indomethacin, i.e., it is most probably prostaglandin dependent (H. Richter and F. Marks, *unpublished results*). Since neonatal mouse epidermis is also refractory to the chalone and, as compared with adult epidermis, has a "hyperplastic" morphology, it is tempting not only to interpret hyperplastic transformation as a temporary relapse in an earlier state of tissue development, but also to speculate on a causal relationship between chalone mechanism and hyperplasia. There is some evidence that the inhibitory effect of G_1 chalone is restricted to a certain cell population of the proliferative compartment of epidermis and that this population disappears after hyperplastic stimulation (22,23). As a consequence, epidermal cell proliferation is then taken over by a chalone-insensitive stem cell population. It is easily conceivable that such a far-reaching change of the homeostatic equilibrium of the tissue depends on specific endogenous signals, one of which is PGE_2.

Hyperplastic transformation is not a pathological situation but is the normal response of (mouse) epidermis to injury. It can be evoked not only by mitogenic agents, but also by removal of the uppermost horny layer (sandpaper rubbing; see ref. 4). In this case the hyperproliferative response is again sensitive to indomethacin inhibition (14); i.e., it is most probably mediated by prostaglandins and accompanied by chalone refractoriness (4). Thus, prostaglandin-mediated epidermal hyperplasia may be regarded as an essential part of a self-defense mechanism of an epithelium. Within this frame, PGE_2 fulfills the requirements of a local "SOS signal" in that it is a specific epidermal factor released upon tissue damage, being obligatory for the induction of the regenerative process.

Since PGE_2 cannot by itself induce epidermal cell proliferation but acts synergistically with a mitogen (see above), one has to wonder whether epidermal damage by itself is a sufficient mitogenic trigger or whether endogenous growth factors are released upon injury. Such a question is consistent with the general view that, with some exceptions, prostaglandins play a role as local modifiers (amplifiers, integrators, feedback inhibitors) of hormone action rather than acting as "autonomous" hormones.

THE ROLE OF PROSTAGLANDINS IN TUMOR PROMOTION

Provided that prostaglandin E-mediated hyperplastic transformation of epidermis is obligatory for at least stage 2 of tumor promotion, promotion as a whole

TABLE 2. *Effect of indomethacin and prostaglandins on TPA-induced tumor promotion*[a]

Treatment	After 12 weeks		After 15 weeks		After 18 weeks	
	Rate (%)	Yield	Rate (%)	Yield	Rate (%)	Yield
Acetone	0	0	0	0	0	0
TPA	100	5.2	100	8.6	100	8.4
TPA + indomethacin	40	1.1	40	2.0	47	1.2
TPA + indomethacin + PGE_2	33	1.3	36	2.2	36	1.5
TPA + indomethacin + $PGF_{2\alpha}$	73	3.1	85	4.1	85	4.6
PGE_2	0	0	0	0	0	0
$PGF_{2\alpha}$	0	0	0	0	0	0

[a] The doses per application (twice a week) were: 5 nmole TPA, 0.5 μmole indomethacin, 30 nmole prostaglandin (each dissolved in 0.1 ml acetone). Indomethacin was applied 30 min prior to and prostaglandins simultaneously with each TPA application. For other details, see Table 1.

should be sensitive to inhibition by indomethacin and related inhibitors of prostaglandin synthesis. That this is indeed the case has been reported recently (35, 36,38) and is shown in Table 2. Surprisingly, the effect of the inhibitor could not be overcome by $PGE_{2\alpha}$, but only by PGF_2, which in turn cannot release indomethacin inhibition of hyperplastic transformation after a single TPA application as PGE_2 is able to do (see above). This means that either the prostaglandin responsiveness of epidermis is qualitatively altered during long-term treatment with the promoter or that F-prostaglandins are involved in an event that is absolutely essential for promotion, while E-prostaglandin-mediated cell proliferation plays only a permissive role. A further investigation of the function of prostaglandins in skin tumor promotion promises, therefore, a deeper insight into the nature of endogenous regulatory mechanisms which are expected to be disturbed by a phorbol ester tumor promoter.

THE DIFFERENCE BETWEEN NONPROMOTING AND PROMOTING HYPERPLASIOGENS MAY REFLECT THE DIFFERENCE BETWEEN THE RESPONSES TO SUPERFICIAL DAMAGE OF EPIDERMIS VERSUS WHOLE SKIN WOUNDING

As we have seen PGE_2-mediated hyperplastic transformation *per se* seems to be unable to promote tumor development. On the other hand, whole skin wounding, for example by cutting the skin with a scalpel down to the subcutaneous tissue, has been shown to exhibit a pronounced tumor-promoting effect (1,9,12,18). Since nonpromoting hyperplastic transformation can be evoked by superficial damage of epidermis (removal of the horny layer, see above), a difference between the response to epidermal wounding as compared with that to full skin wounding may be expected.

That such a difference really exists can be clearly seen when neonatal mouse skin is injured. Whereas, under these conditions, epidermal damage as well as other treatments that cause hyperplastic transformation of the adult tissue do not show a mitogenic effect (5,22), deep skin wounding induces a proliferative response that is almost as strong as in the adult animal (6; Fig. 6). This observation rules out the possibility that neonatal epidermis does not respond by hyperplastic transformation because its proliferative capacities are exhausted.

Interestingly, the proliferative response to deepskin wounding is sensitive to indomethacin inhibition in adult epidermis, whereas in the neonatal tissue it is not (6). This would mean that epidermal hyperproliferation induced by deep skin wounding *can* at least partially be mediated by prostaglandins but that prostaglandins are not obligatory for the response. It is easily conceivable that deep skin wounding of adult epidermis evokes prostaglandin-dependent hyperplastic transformation *in addition* to the "wound-specific" hyperproliferation, whereas neonatal tissue, which is already hyperplastically transformed *per se,* exhibits only the latter response.

We propose, therefore, that mouse epidermis can exist in at least three different

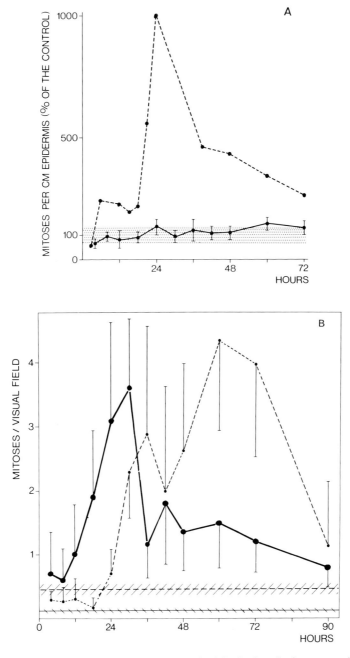

FIG. 6. Mitotic activity in neonatal *(solid line)* and adult *(broken line)* mouse epidermis *in vivo* after removal of the horny layer (sandpaper rubbing, **A**) and deep skin wounding (**B**) at zero time. In **B**, maximal mitotic activity 1–5 mm adjacent to a skin wound (cutting by means of a scalpel) is plotted against time. For details, see refs. 5, 6.

proliferative states (which perhaps resemble certain states of tissue differentiation): (a) the "mature" state, which is under G_1-chalone control and characteristic for the adult animal; (b) the "neonatal" state of hyperplasia, which is not under G_1-chalone control; and (c) the "state of wound healing" (see Fig. 7).

As mentioned above, the rate of cell proliferation in the mature state can be increased by certain nondamaging stimuli such as skin massage or application of 4-O-methyl-TPA; this kind of stimulation does not result in hyperplastic transformation. When the epidermis is damaged, a PGE_2-mediated transformation of the mature into the neonatal state takes place via a burst of cell proliferation (hyperplastic transformation).

For reaching the state of wound healing, an additional endogenous stimulus may be postulated. Since deep skin wounding differs from epidermal wounding by a damage of connective tissue and blood vessels, such a stimulus may be provided by certain growth factors, alias "wound hormones," either blood-born or of mesenchymal origin. There are several candidates for such a role. They include epidermal growth factor, which has been shown to stimulate neonatal and wounded tissue rather than intact adult epidermis (3,10,30) or platelet-derived growth factor (31), which is locally released upon platelet aggregation and thus fulfills the requirements of a "wound hormone" in an ideal fashion. There is some indirect evidence that platelet-derived growth factor has a stimulatory effect not only on mesenchymal (31) but also on epidermal cells (2).

Since full skin wounding has a tumor-promoting effect whereas epidermal damage does not, the key event of promotion may be sought in the different responses to both kinds of injury. Provided nonepidermal growth factors are involved in wound healing, one may assume that TPA somehow mimics the effect of a "wound hormone" or augments—perhaps via some special kind of membrane interaction—the cellular responsiveness to such a factor. Nonpromot-

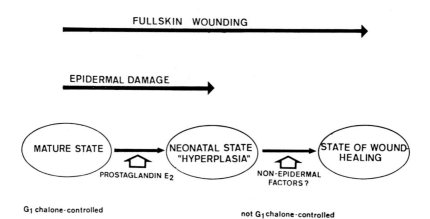

FIG. 7. An attempt to interpret the observed differences between the proliferative behavior of epidermis of normal, neonatal, and wounded skin. For details, see text.

ing hyperplasiogenic agents such as RPA, ionophore A23187, and others should not be able to do this. In other words: whereas nonpromoting mitogens make epidermis "believe" to be superficially damaged, a promoter such as TPA simulates deep skin wounding.

REFERENCES

1. Argyris, T. S. (1979): Tumor promotion by abrasion-induced epidermal hyperplasia in the skin of mice. *Fed. Proc.,* 38:1,073; and *Proc. Am. Assoc. Cancer Res.,* 20:4.
2. Aso, K., Kondo, S., and Amano, M. (1980): Platelet-dependent serum factor that stimulates the proliferation of epidermal cells *in vitro.* In: *Biochemistry of Normal and Abnormal Epidermal Differentiation,* edited by I. A. Bernstein and M. Seiji, pp. 83–89. University of Tokyo Press, Tokyo.
3. Bem, J. L., and Richardson, C. B. (1972): Stimulation of mouse epidermis by epidermal growth factor. *J. Invest. Dermatol.,* 58:265.
4. Bertsch, S., Csontos, K., Schweizer, J., and Marks, F. (1976): Effect of mechanical stimulation on cell proliferation in mouse epidermis and on growth regulation by endogenous factors (chalones). *Cell Tissue Kinet.,* 9:445–457.
5. Bertsch, S., and Marks, F. (1978): Removal of the horny layer does not stimulate cell proliferation in neonatal mouse epidermis. *Cell Tissue Kinet.,* 11:651–658.
6. Bertsch, S., and Marks, F. (1982): A comparative study on wound healing in neonatal and adult mouse epidermis *in vivo. Cell Tissue Kinet.* 15 *(in press).*
7. Boutwell, R. K. (1964): Some biological aspects of skin carcinogenesis. *Prog. Exp. Tumor Res.,* 4:207–250.
8. Burns, F. J., Vanderlaan, M., Snyder, E., and Albert, R. E. (1978): Induction and progression kinetics of mouse skin papillomas. In: *Carcinogenesis, Vol. 2,* edited by T. J. Slaga, A. Sivak, and R. K. Boutwell, pp. 91–96. Raven Press, New York.
9. Clark-Lewis, I., and Murray, A. W. (1978): Tumor promotion and the induction of epidermal ornithine decarboxylase in mechanically stimulated mouse skin. *Cancer Res.,* 38:494–497.
10. Cohen, S. (1971): Studies on the mechanism of action of epidermal growth promoting factor (EGF). In: *Hormones in Development,* edited by M. Hamburgh and E. J. W. Burrington, p. 753. Meredith Company, New York.
11. Delclos, K. B., Magle, D. S., and Blumberg, P. M. (1980): Specific binding of phorbol ester tumor promoters in mouse skin. *Cell,* 19:1,025–1,032.
12. Deelman, H. T. (1924): Die Entstehung des experimentellen Teerkrebses und die Bedeutung der Zellregeneration. *Z. Krebsforsch.,* 21:220–226.
13. Fürstenberger, G. (1976): Über die Isolierung sowie die chemische und biologische Charakterisierung der hautreizenden Wirkstoffe aus Euphorbia tirucalli L. Ph.D. Thesis, University of Heidelberg.
14. Fürstenberger, G., DeBravo, M., Bertsch, S., and Marks, F. (1979): The effect of indomethacin on cell proliferation induced by chemical and mechanical means in mouse epidermis *in vivo. Res. Commun. Chem. Pathol. Pharmacol.,* 24:533–541.
15. Fürstenberger, G., and Marks, F. (1978): Indomethacin inhibition of cell proliferation induced by the phorbol ester TPA is reversed by prostaglandin E_2 in mouse epidermis *in vivo. Biochem. Biophys. Res. Commun.,* 84:1,103–1,110.
16. Fürstenberger, G., and Marks, F. (1980): Early prostaglandin E synthesis is an obligatory event in the induction of cell proliferation in mouse epidermis *in vivo* by the phorbol ester TPA. *Biochem. Biophys. Res. Commun.,* 92:749–756.
17. Fürstenberger, G., Richter, H., Fusenig, N. E., and Marks, F. (1980): Arachidonic acid and prostaglandin E_2 release and enhanced cell proliferation induced by the phorbol ester TPA in a murine epidermal cell line. *Cancer Letters,* 11:191–198.
18. Hennings, H., and Boutwell, R. K. (1970): Studies on the mechanism of skin tumor promotion. *Cancer Res.,* 30:312–325.
19. Holtzer, H. (1978): Cell lineages, stem cells, and the quantal cell cycle concept. In: *British Society of Cell Biology, Symp. 2: Stem Cells and Tissue Homeostasis,* edited by B. I. Lord, C. S. Potten, and R. J. Cole, pp. 1–27. Cambridge University Press, New York.

20. Krieg, L., Kühlmann, I., and Marks, F. (1974): Effect of tumor-promoting phorbol esters and of acetic acid on mechanisms controlling DNA synthesis and mitosis (chalones) and on biosynthesis of histidine-rich protein in mouse epidermis. *Cancer Res.,* 34:3,135–3,146.
21. Marks, F., Bertsch, S., and Fürstenberger, G. (1979): Ornithine decarboxylase activity, cell proliferation, and tumor promotion in mouse epidermis *in vivo. Cancer Res.,* 39:4,183–4,188.
22. Marks, F., Bertsch, S., Grimm, W., and Schweizer, J. (1978): Hyperplastic transformation and tumor promotion in mouse epidermis: Possible consequences of disturbances of endogenous mechanisms controlling proliferation and differentiation. In: *Carcinogenesis, Vol. 2,* edited by T. J. Slaga, A. Sivak, and R. K. Boutwell, pp. 97–116. Raven Press, New York.
23. Marks, F., Bertsch, S., and Schweizer, J. (1978): Homeostatic regulation of epidermal cell proliferation. *Bull. Cancer (Paris),* 65:207–222.
24. Marks, F., and Fürstenberger, G. (1980): Effect of phorbol ester application and other mitogenic treatments on 3′,5′-cyclic-nucleotide phosphodiesterase activity in mouse epidermis *in vivo. Hoppe Seylers Z. Physiol. Chem.,* 361:1,641–1,650.
25. Marks, F., Fürstenberger, G., and Kownatzki, E. (1981): Prostaglandin E-mediated mitogenic stimulation of mouse epidermis *in vivo* by divalent cation ionophore A23187 and by tumor promoter TPA. *Cancer Res.,* 41:696–702.
26. Muller, S. A. (1971): Hair neogenesis. *J. Invest. Dermatol.,* 56:1–9.
27. Murray, A. W. (1978): Acetic acid pretreatment of initiated epidermis inhibits tumor promotion by a phorbol ester. *Experientia (Basel),* 34:1,507–1,508.
28. Pinkus, H. (1971): Embryology and anatomy of skin. In: *The Skin,* edited by E. B. Helwig and F. K. Mostofi, pp. 1–28. The Williams and Wilkins Co., Baltimore.
29. Pressman, B. C. (1976): Biological application of ionophores. *Annu. Rev. Biochem.,* 45:501–530.
30. Savage, C. R., and Cohen, S. (1973): Proliferation of corneal epithelium induced by epidermal growth factor. *Exp. Eye Res.,* 15:361.
31. Scher, C. D., Shepard, R. C., Antoniades, H. N., and Stiles, C. D. (1979): Platelet-derived growth factor and the regulation of the mammalian fibroblast cell cycle. *Biochem. Biophys. Acta,* 560:217–241.
32. Schweizer, J. (1979): Neogenesis of functional hair follicles in adult mouse skin selectively induced by tumor-promoting phorbol esters. *Experientia (Basel),* 35:1,651–1,653.
33. Schweizer, J., and Marks, F. (1977): The tumor promoter TPA induces the formation of new hair follicles in the epidermis of the mouse tail. *Cancer Res.,* 37:4,195–4,201.
34. Slaga, T. J., Fischer, S. M., Nelson, K., and Gleason, G. L. (1980): Studies on the mechanism of skin tumor promotion: Evidence for several stages of promotion. *Proc. Natl. Acad. Sci. USA,* 77:3,659–3,663.
35. Slaga, T. J., and Scribner, J. D. (1973): Inhibition of tumor initiation and promotion by antiinflammatory agents. *J. Natl. Cancer Inst.,* 51:1,723–1,725.
36. Verma, A. K., Ashendel, C. L., and Boutwell, R. K. (1980): Inhibition by prostaglandin synthesis inhibitors of the induction of epidermal ornithine decarboxylase activity, the accumulation of prostaglandins, and tumor promotion caused by TPA. *Cancer Res.,* 40:308–315.
37. Verma, A. K., Rice, H. M., and Boutwell, R. K. (1977): Prostaglandins and skin tumor promotion: Inhibition of tumor promoter-induced ornithine decarboxylase activity in epidermis by inhibitors of prostaglandin synthesis. *Biochem. Biophys. Res. Commun.,* 79:1,160–1,166.
38. Viaje, A., Slaga, T. J., Wigler, M., and Weinstein, I. B. (1977): Effects of antiinflammatory agents on mouse skin tumor promotion, epidermal DNA synthesis, phorbol ester-induced cellular proliferation, and production of plasminogen activator. *Cancer Res.,* 37:1,530–1,536.

Carcinogenesis, Vol. 7, edited by E. Hecker et al.
Raven Press, New York © 1982.

TPA Reversibly Blocks the Differentiation of Chick Myogenic, Chondrogenic, and Melanogenic Cells

H. Holtzer, M. Pacifici, R. Payette, J. Croop, A. Dlugosz, and Y. Toyama

Department of Anatomy, School of Medicine, University of Pennsylvania, Philadelphia, Pennsylvania 19104

The major theme of this chapter is that 12-O-tetradecanoylphorbol-13-acetate (TPA) preferentially but reversibly blocks the terminal differentiation program of normal chick myogenic, chondrogenic, and melanogenic cells. This preferential, but reversible, blocking of the differentiation programs of these cell types does not cancel or alter the status of the affected cell in its particular lineage. A minor theme of this chapter is that the pp60[src] protein kinase synthesized by cells infected with RSV mimics the effects of TPA.

These two themes are consistent with the view that some event associated with transforming one type of normal cell into a particular type of neoplastic cell probably involves lesions in the cell's differentiation program. Two important corollaries derive from this view: (a) the specific metabolic lesion(s) that transforms a normal chondrogenic cell into a chondrosarcoma cell may be quite different from that involved in the transformation of a normal melanogenic cell into a melanoma cell or of a normal hepatocyte into a hepatoma cell; and (b) neoplastic cells do not become "undifferentiated" but retain to varying degrees their lineage affiliations, i.e., chondrosarcoma, melanoma, and hepatoma cells have more in common with their normal chondrogenic, melanogenic, and hepatogenic precursors than they have with each other or with neoplastic cells derived from other lineages.

EFFECTS OF TPA ON PRESUMPTIVE MYOBLASTS, DEFINITIVE POSTMITOTIC MYOBLASTS, AND MYOTUBES

The differentiation programs of cells in the ultimate and penultimate compartments of the myogenic lineage are qualitatively very different. The presumptive myoblasts are replicating cells, synthesizing "constitutive" contractile proteins and incapable of fusing to form multinucleated myotubes. Their daughters, the definitive myoblasts, are postmitotic and the only type of cell capable of fusing with other postmitotic myoblasts to form multinucleated myotubes. The cell membrane of the definitive myoblasts must differ from the cell membranes of all other cells since they (a) "recognize" other myoblast membranes, and (b) undergo local restructuring or melding of their lipid bilayers when juxtaposed to other myoblast membranes. Fusion-competent myoblasts fuse with each other within 1 hr following a period of protracted juxtaposition (12,13,16).

The most unequivocal biological evidence that one major target of TPA is the cell surface is the observation that TPA blocks fusion of chick and quail myogenic cells (5; Pacifici & Holtzer *unpublished observations*). Multinucleated myotubes normally appear in day 2 primary cultures. In TPA, fusion is blocked even if the cultures are maintained for 5 days. In some experiments, however, myotubes do "break through" in the TPA-treated cultures. This breakthrough varies with different lots of the tumor promoter and with different lots of horse serum and embryo extract. Even in the absence of cells, embryo extract and horse serum degrade the tumor promoter (T. G. O'Brien and H. Holtzer, *unpublished observations*), requiring higher concentrations of TPA and/or feeding twice a day to achieve maximal inhibition (see also 6).

The ongoing differentiation program of the definitive myoblasts and/or myotubes involves the synthesis of muscle-specific myosin heavy and light chains, alpha actin, and muscle-type intermediate filaments (1,2,9,12). TPA preferentially, but reversibly, blocks the accumulation of the muscle-specific contractile proteins, but has no obvious effect on the accumulation of the "constitutive" contractile proteins in presumptive myoblasts or fibroblasts (6,12,35). Day 5 myogenic cultures consist of thousands of multinucleated myotubes, each containing huge numbers of striated myofibrils (Fig. 1). These myotubes contract spontaneously. Large numbers of 10-nm filaments course parallel to, and between, the myofibrils. Eighteen hr after TPA is added to these cultures, spontaneous contractions cease. Within 48 hr, TPA selectively, but reversibly, dismantles the formed myofibrils in most of the myotubes. This effect of TPA has been demonstrated by electron micrographic (EM) studies (35) and by staining the TPA-treated myotubes with fluorescein-labeled antibodies against muscle-specific light meromyosin (anti-LMM). After 72 hr in TPA, the majority of myotubes are largely depleted of myofibrils (Fig. 2). The finding that TPA actively degrades and/or selectively inhibits the synthesis of the muscle-specific myosin and actin is particularly provocative, because the "constitutive" proteins that make up the microfilaments subtending the sarcolemma are not grossly disturbed by TPA (6). Furthermore, TPA does not deplete the constitutive contractile proteins in presumptive myoblasts, fibroblasts, or other types of nonmuscle cells. In brief, TPA, by preferentially degrading the muscle-specific contractile protein but sparing the constitutive contractile proteins, appears to act selectively on the differentiation program of the cell.

Nothing is known of the way in which TPA selectively degrades myofibrils. Recently, we have shown that Ca^{2+} fails to accumulate in TPA-treated myotubes whereas the behavior of Mg^{2+} is not affected. It will be interesting to determine if this failure to accumulate Ca^{2+} is responsible for the loss of integrity of the

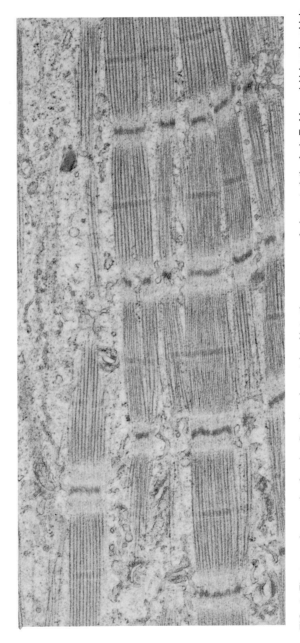

FIG. 1. Electron micrograph of a day 5 cultured myotube. Note the presence of characteristic A, I, Z, M, and H bands which form by interdigitation of thick and thin filaments. A few microtubules and intermediate filaments run parallel to the myofibrils. ×25,000.

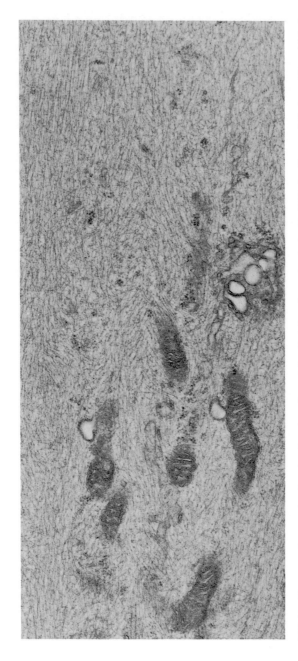

FIG. 2. Electron micrograph of a day 8 cultured myotube that has been treated with TPA for the past 3 days. The striated myofibrils present in day 5 myotubes have been completely dismantled. Note the remarkable density of intermediate filaments (10 nm). ×31,000.

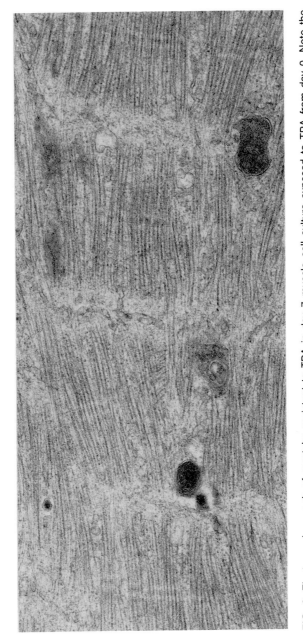

FIG. 3. Electron micrograph of myotube resistant to TPA in day 7 muscle cell culture exposed to TPA from day 0. Note the atypical myofibrils lacking Z bands. ×34,000.

myofibrils by activating intracellular proteases and whether or not TPA alters Ca^{2+} homeostasis in other types of cells.

After protracted exposure to the tumor promoter (e.g. 6 to 7 days), a population of TPA-resistant myotubes appeared in these cultures (6). These myotubes resistant to TPA often contained atypical myofibrils which lacked Z-bands (Fig. 3). The TPA-resistant myotubes degenerated after another 4 to 5 days in TPA, but the remaining mononucleated cells in these cultures continued to replicate. We are attempting to learn more about these actively replicating cells that have been cultured in the presence of TPA for over 2 weeks, but which no longer evidence readily detectable myogenic properties.

The selective but reversible blocking by TPA of the differentiation program of the definitive myogenic cell is mimicked by infection with ts-RSV (8,14,22). Ts-RSV-infected myogenic cells reared at permissive temperature are indistinguishable from RSV-transformed chondroblasts or fibroblasts. At the end of each subculture (6 to 8 days), approximately 2% of the cells have withdrawn from the cell cycle and terminally differentiated. If, however, these transformed cells are shifted from permissive to nonpermissive temperature, within 24 to 48 hr roughly half the cells withdraw from the cell cycle and initiate the differentiation program characteristic of the definitive myotube. Recently, we found the percentage of cells that at permissive temperature withdraw from the cell cycle and terminally differentiate varies from 2% to 15%, depending on unknown factors in the growth medium. Operationally, we cannot determine whether these factors in the growth medium enhance the expression of the transformed cell's normal differentiation program, or reciprocally, whether these factors depress the expression of the RSV-transformed phenotype.

Given the fact that TPA blocks distinct phases of skeletal myogenesis—fusion of mononucleated cells into myotubes and the maintenance of striated myofibrils and acetylcholine (Ach)-receptors (21)—we expected TPA to block various aspects of cardiac myogenesis. Thus far, over a wide range of concentrations, TPA has had no detectable effect on (a) the spontaneous contraction of developing cardiac myoblasts, or (b) the assembly and maintenance of cardiac myofibrils.

EFFECTS OF TPA ON CHONDROBLASTS AND FIBROBLASTS

Chondroblasts from chick embryos readily grow in suspension as "floaters" (4,10). If such floaters are plated in plastic dishes after 3 days, less than 50% will attach to the substrate, where they form colonies of polygonal cells. In sister cultures treated with TPA, 100% of the cells adhere to the substrate within 24 hr. Clearly, TPA rapidly alters some properties of the chondroblast cell surface, allowing the cells to bind to plastic. TPA also rapidly alters the polygonal morphology of those chondroblasts that adhere to the substrate. Upon removal of TPA, most of these cells reexpress their polygonal morphology. The tumor promoter acts as a mitogen on cultured chondroblasts (17).

Normal chondroblasts are readily differentiated from all other cell types by their unique capacity to synthesize Type IV sulfated proteoglycans (14,26) and Type II collagen chains (19,33,36). TPA rapidly inhibits the synthesis of the cartilage-unique Type IV sulfated proteoglycan. This inhibition is reversible. The proteoglycan molecules synthesized by TPA-treated chondroblasts differ from those synthesized by normal chondroblasts in monomer size, polysaccharide chain length, hyaluronic acid-binding ability, and ratio of 6S/4S disaccharides (29). TPA also greatly depresses the synthesis of the cartilage-specific Type II procollagen chains.

The reversibility of the blocking effects of TPA on the "luxury molecules" (10) synthesized by chondroblasts is progressively lost with continued exposure. When chondroblasts reared in TPA for over 2 weeks are returned to normal medium, they will replicate at a higher rate than control chondroblasts but fail to reexpress their most salient morphological and biochemical properties. It is important now to learn more about the kinds of molecules that these cells synthesize and if they have any properties of chondrosarcoma cells.

The response to TPA of chondroblasts and fibroblasts has been compared, as these two cell types are derived from a common ancestral cell (9,13,18). TPA induces normal chick fibroblasts to form long, fine processes, similar to those induced in chondroblasts. TPA does not inhibit fibroblasts from synthesizing their characteristic Type III sulfated proteoglycan, however, nor does it act as a mitogen on fibroblasts (17). It is not yet clear whether TPA does or does not block the differentiation program of fibroblasts.

We are curious about the effects of TPA on cells earlier in the chondrogenic lineage: specifically on (a) penultimate cells in the lineage, the presumptive chondroblasts; (b) antepenultimate cells in the lineage, the cells yielding presumptive chondroblasts and fibroblasts; and (c) the still earlier "mesenchyme cells," etc. (9). Organ cultures of late chick limb buds (stage 23 to 24) form morphologically definitive chondroblasts and myoblasts which synthesize their unique Type IV sulfated proteoglycan and skeletal muscle-specific myosins and actin. Chondroblasts and myoblasts do not emerge if such late limb buds are exposed to TPA (9). This blocking effect can be reversed by removing TPA. Of greater theoretical interest, however, is the consequence of treating younger limb buds (e.g., stage 18 to 20) with TPA. These cells are in earlier stages of the chondrogenic and myogenic lineages. When organ-cultured, some of these cells yield progeny that develop into definitive chondroblasts and definitive striated myoblasts and myotubes. Reared in TPA, they do not yield chondroblasts or striated myoblasts or myotubes (9,11). If TPA is removed from these cells, they continue to replicate, but do not produce progeny that differentiate into recognizable chondroblasts or myoblasts. Apparently, the blocking effects of TPA on the chondroblasts and presumptive myoblasts are reversible, but its effects on cells in earlier compartments of the chondrogenic lineage (or myogenic lineage) are more complex.

Similar results to those reported above with TPA have been obtained by transforming definitive chondrogenic cells with a temperature-sensitive mutant of RSV (11,27,28,31).

EFFECT OF TPA ON MELANOBLASTS AND NEUROBLASTS

TPA preferentially but reversibly blocks melanogenesis and the assembly of premelanosomes in chick melanoblasts derived from the neural crest and in chick retinal pigment epithelial cells. There are, however, differences in the response of trunk and retinal pigment cells to TPA, and these responses also vary depending on breed of chicken and culture conditions.

Dispersed chick neural crest cells replicate and after 5 to 7 days in culture yield pigmented melanoblasts with their typical dendritic morphology. In our standard culture medium—70% minimum essential medium (MEM), 20% horse serum, 10% embryo extract—between 15 and 30% of the cells in 10-day cultures are pigmented melanoblasts. If TPA is present when the cultures are established, pigmented cells do not appear, though the cultures are maintained for 6 to 8 weeks. If TPA is removed during the first 15 days of culture, within the next 4 days melanoblasts will appear and comprise 15 to 30% of the population. If TPA is added to cultures containing dendritic melanoblasts, almost all the melanoblasts will disappear within 3 to 4 days. The nonpigmented cells continue to replicate in TPA, but TPA is not a mitogen in this medium. If the TPA is removed from such cultures, again large numbers of melanoblasts reappear within 4 days. We have not determined whether the loss of melanoblasts is due to selective cell death or whether the cells shed their pigment granules and are converted into amelanotic melanoblasts. If cultured in TPA for longer than 14 days and then subcultured into normal medium, melanoblasts do not appear, though the cells continue to replicate. Protracted exposure of chick neural crest cells to TPA appears to deplete the replicating population of a subset of cells in relatively late compartments of the melanogenic lineage.

One-hundred percent of the retinal pigment epithelial cells of day 6 chick embryos are pigmented. When trypsinized and cultured, they replicate and lose their pigment granules. In control cultures, epithelial sheets are formed within 5 to 6 days. Virtually 100% of the epithelioid cells pigment. If, however, TPA is added prior to the formation of epithelial colonies, the cells assume a "fibroblastic" morphology and not a single cell pigments. If left in TPA, these cells form a confluent sheet, then multi-layer, but never pigment. On the other hand, in contradistinction to the response of pigmented trunk melanoblasts, pigmented retinal cells show no response to the tumor promoter if it is added after the cells have pigmented; the cells do not lose their pigment nor lose their epithelioid morphology.

Sieber-Blum and Sieber (34) have reported that TPA not only failed to block quail neural crest from differentiating into melanoblasts, but increased the number of pigmented colonies over controls. They used a culture medium rich in amino acids and nucleosides. We have confirmed their findings with quail neural crest in enriched medium. Clearly, the response of trunk melanocytes to TPA is influenced by unknown factors in growth media and species differences. In contrast, the response of retinal pigment epithelial cells to TPA is the same for both quail and chick melanoblasts in either medium: melanogenesis is totally blocked if cells are exposed to the tumor promoter prior to epithelioid organization and pigmentation.

Differences in the response of melanoma cells to TPA have also been reported. In the B-16 murine melanoma, TPA delays pigmentation, after which the cells "escape" from the block and pigment (23). In a line of human melanoma cells, TPA and dimethylsulfoxide (DMSO) both decrease the growth rate, stimulate melanogenesis, but kill the cells (15). DMSO has no discernible effect on chick pigmenting cells (30).

Chick retinal pigment cells have been infected with ts-RSV. When reared at permissive temperatures they replicate, lose their pigment, and assume the morphology of transformed cells. If, after 15 to 20 generations, these ts-transformed cells are shifted to nonpermissive temperature, within 4 to 5 days colonies of pigmented, epithelioid cells appear (3,11, 31). Both TPA and active pp60^{src} protein kinase selectively but reversibly block melanogenesis. Both agents permit cell replication for many generations, but preferentially block those few metabolic events required for terminal differentiation. Blocking pigmentation, however, does not derange the genetic mechanisms that generation after generation maintain these replicating cells in the retinal melanogenic lineage.

In addition to consisting of precursors to melanoblasts, trunk neural crest contains precursors to nerve, Schwann, and adrenal chromaffin cells. Neither TPA nor mezerein blocks the emergence of neurons in our cultures of chick neural crest. The neurons that appear in these TPA-treated cultures of neural crest cells morphologically are indistinguishable from controls. Whether TPA affects the transmitter content of these neurons or the differentiation of Schwann or chromaffin cells is still unknown. Obviously it will be of interest to learn why some of the descendants of the neural crest do terminally differentiate in TPA, whereas others do not.

DISCUSSION

At this time no generalization regarding the mode of action of TPA on different cell types is possible (7). If TPA augments the activity of ornithine decarboxylase and the frequency of cell cycling in one line of fibroblasts, it has different effects on other lines of fibroblasts (25). If TPA blocks the induction of hemoglobin (Hb) synthesis in Friend erythroleukemic cells (32,37), it does not do so with Rauscher erythroleukemic cells (20). Even here, where the blocking of the differentiation program of several cell types has been deliberately emphasized, the failure of TPA to interfere with the differentiation program of fibroblasts, nerve cells, cardiac cells, as well as the enhancement of pigmentation in quail trunk melanoblasts, has also been stressed.

Any effort to reconcile these seemingly contradictory observations will not be convincing until some of the pleiotropic effects of TPA are better understood. This is not an unusual situation, either in the area of cell differentiation or in tumorigenesis. Often many unrelated molecules "induce" precursor cells to differentiate terminally; likewise carcinogens and viruses transform some cell types but are ineffective on related cell types. The variable responses to TPA with respect to differentiation may be due to the availability of TPA-receptors, to differences in the capacities of various cell types to inactivate the tumor promoter, or to as yet unknown molecules in the growth medium. On a biological level, the blocking of pigmentation in chick trunk melanoblasts, the fusion of myoblasts, or the destruction of formed myofibrils is a near-threshold phenomenon. In most systems in which TPA blocks differentiation, this effect is not only readily reversed upon removal of TPA, but reversal often occurs even in the presence of TPA. Thus, although TPA degrades the myofibrils after acting on myotubes for 3 days, continued exposure to the drug for a total of 6 to 7 days does not prevent the "escape" of some cells that are able to assemble new, though defective, myofibrils.

These experiments with TPA and ts-RSV transformed cells, as well as other experiments in which transformed cells have been induced to differentiate terminally with a corresponding loss in their tumorigenicity, support the notion of some type of inverse relationship between the neoplastic state and the expression of a cell's differentiation program. They encourage a reexamination of the idea that other tumorigenic agents, such as chemical carcinogens, irradiation, etc., may also act via blocking in whole, or in part, the differentiation program of the responding cells.

The visualization of the emergence of neoplastic cells as arising due to lesions in their differentiation program has far-reaching theoretical implications. It requires, for example, recognizing that there is no such entity as a "tumor cell," any more than there is such an entity as a "normal undifferentiated cell" (9, 10,14). There are chondrosarcoma, melanoma, hepatoma etc. cells, but they differ as much among themselves as their normal counterparts differ among themselves. Similarly, an embryonal carcinoma cell has more in common with normal, early, differentiated morula cells than with neoplastic cells of any sort. The fact that the normal differentiation program of early morula cells can be activated in embryonal carcinoma cells, with a corresponding loss of their tumorigenicity, is similar to the reactivation of the differentiation programs observed when ts-RSV infected cells are shifted to nonpermissive temperature. This view also renders unlikely the notion that tumors derived from different types of normal cells display a common set of tumor antigens.

ACKNOWLEDGMENTS

This research was supported in part by National Institutes of Health grants HL-18535 (to the Pennsylvania Muscle Institute), HL-18708, CA-18194, GM-07170, by the Muscular Dystrophy Association, and a fellowship from the John A. Hartford Foundation to Dr. Payette.

REFERENCES

1. Bennett, G. S., Fellini, S. A., and Holtzer, H. (1978): *Differentiation,* 12:71–82.
2. Bennett, G. S., Fellini, S. A., Toyama, Y., and Holtzer, H. (1979): *J. Cell Biol.,* 82:577–584.
3. Boettiger, D., Roby, K., Brumbaugh, J., Bichl, J., and Holtzer, H. (1977): *Cell,* 11:881–890.
4. Chacko, S., Abbott, J., Holtzer, S., and Holtzer, H. (1969): *J. Exp. Med.,* 130:417–430.
5. Cohen, R., Pacifici, M., Rubinstein, N., Biehl, J., and Holtzer, H. (1977): *Nature,* 266:538–540.
6. Croop, J., Toyama, Y., Dlugosz, A., and Holtzer, A. (1980): *Proc. Natl. Acad. Sci. USA,* 77:5,273–5,277.
7. Diamond, L., O'Brian, T. G., and Baird, W. M. (1980): *Adv. Cancer Res.,* 32:1–73.
8. Holtzer, H., Yeoh, G., and Kaji, A. (1975): *Proc. Natl. Acad. Sci. USA,* 72:513–517.
9. Holtzer, H. (1978): In: *Stem Cells and Tissue Homeostasis,* edited by B. Lord, C. Potten, and R. Cole, pp. 1–28. Cambridge University Press, Cambridge.
10. Holtzer, H., and Abbott, J. (1968): In: *The Stability of the Differentiated State,* edited by H. Ursprung, pp. 1–16. Springer-Verlag, New York.
11. Holtzer, H., Biehl, J., Pacifici, M., Boettiger, D., Payette, R., and West, C. (1980): In: *Results and Problems in Cell Differentiation, Vol. II, Differentiation and Neoplasia,* edited by R. G. McKinnell, pp. 166–177. Springer-Verlag, Heidelberg.
12. Holtzer, H., Croop, J., Toyama, Y., Bennett, G., Fellini, S., and West, C. (1980): In: *Plasticity of Muscle,* edited by D. Pette, pp. 133–146. Walter de Gruyter, New York.
13. Holtzer, H., Sanger, J., Ishikawa, H., and Strahs, K. (1973): In: *Cold Spring Harbor Symposium of Quantitative Biology,* 37:549–566.
14. Holtzer, H., Rubinstein, N., Fellini, S., Yeoh, G., Chi, S., Birnbaum, J., and Okayama, M. (1975): *Q. Rev. Biophys.,* 8:523–557.
15. Huberman, E., Heckman, C., and Langenbach, R. (1979): *Cancer Res.,* 39:2,618–2,624.
16. Knudsen, K., and Horwitz, A. F. (1978): *Dev. Biol.,* 58:238–338.
17. Lowe, L. E., Pacifici, M., and Holtzer, H. (1978): *Cancer Res.,* 38:2,350–2,356.
18. Mayne, R., Schiltz, J., and Holtzer, H. (1974): In: *The Biology and Biochemistry of the Fibroblast,* edited by J. Pikkarainen, pp. 61–78. Academic Press, New York.
19. Mayne, R., Vail, M. S., and Miller, E. J. (1975): *Proc. Natl. Acad. Sci. USA,* 72:4,511–4,516.
20. Miao, R., Fieldsteel, A., and Fodge, D. (1978): *Nature,* 274:271–272.
21. Miskin, R., Easton, T. G., Maelicke, A., and Reich, E. (1978): *Cell,* 15:1,287–1,300.
22. Moss, P. S., Honeycutt, T., Pawson, T., and Martin, G. S. (1979): *Exp. Cell Res.,* 123:95–105.
23. Mufson, R. A., Fisher, P. B., and Weinstein, I. B. (1979): *Cancer Res.,* 39:3,915–3,919.
24. O'Brien, T. G., and Diamond, L. (1977): *Cancer Res.,* 37:3,895–3,900.
25. O'Brien, T. G., Lewis, M. A., and Diamond, L. (1979): *Cancer Res.,* 39:4,477–4,480.
26. Okayama, M., Pacifici, M., and Holtzer, H. (1976): *Proc. Natl. Acad. Sci. USA,* 73:3,224–3,228.
27. Pacifici, M., Adams, S., Boettiger, D., and Holtzer, H. (1980): *J. Cell Biol.* (Abstract CD–149).
28. Pacifici, M., Boettiger, D., Roby, K., and Holtzer, H. (1977): *Cell,* 11:891–899.
29. Pacifici, M., and Holtzer, H. (1980): *Cancer Res.,* 40:2,461–2,464.
30. Payette, R., Biehl, J., Toyama, Y., Holtzer, S., and Holtzer, H. (1980): *Cancer Res.,* 40:2,465–2,474.
31. Roby, K., Boettiger, D., Pacifici, M., and Holtzer, H. (1976): *Am. J. Anat.,* 147:401–405.
32. Rovera, G., O'Brien, T. G., and Diamond, L. (1977): *Proc. Natl. Acad. Sci. USA,* 74:2,894–2,898.
33. Schiltz, J. R., Mayne, R., and Holtzer, H. (1973): *Differentiation,* 1:97–108.
34. Sieber-Blum, M., and Sieber, F. (1980): *Eur. J. Cell Biol.,* 22:407 (abstract).
35. Toyama, Y., West, C. M., and Holtzer, H. (1979): *Am. J. Anat.,* 156:131–137.
36. von der Mark, K., and Conrad, M. (1979): *Clin. Orthop.,* 139:185–205.
37. Yamasaki, H., Fibach, E., Nudel, E., Weinstein, I. B., Rifkind, R. A., and Marks, P. A. (1977): *Proc. Natl. Acad. Sci. USA,* 74:3,451–3,455.

Carcinogenesis, Vol. 7, edited by E. Hecker et al.
Raven Press, New York © 1982.

In Vitro Studies on the Mechanism of Tumor Promoter-Mediated Inhibition of Cell Differentiation

Hiroshi Yamasaki, Cécile Drevon, and Nicole Martel

International Agency for Research on Cancer, 69372 Lyon Cédex 2, France

Among the biological effects of the phorbol ester tumor promoters on cultured cells (58,59), their modulating action on various programs of cell differentiation has drawn considerable attention (11,59,62), since it has long been postulated that aberrant differentiation is involved in the process of carcinogenesis. These compounds inhibit differentiation of many types of cells but also induce or stimulate certain types of cell differentiation (Table 1). At first sight, these dual effects of tumor promoters appear confusing for an interpretation of the mechanism of tumor promotion in terms of aberrant differentiation; however, we believe that the inhibitory effect is directly responsible for carcinogenesis. Most of the types of differentiation affected by the phorbol ester tumor promoters are of terminal program for a given type of cells. Therefore, when, on the one hand, phorbol esters induce cell differentiation, what one observes is merely a hastening of cell death in that population; thus, one would not expect to see accumulation of the cells. This effect of tumor promoters may partially explain why some of them have an antileukemic action. On the other hand, when terminal cell differentiation is blocked, there would be a rapid accumulation of undifferentiated cells, which may represent the origin of a tumor (62). Such accumulation can be attained in a shorter time by the hyperplasminogenic action of these compounds. A similar hypothesis was presented in 1954 by Dr. Berenblum (1). Figure 1 illustrates his view of the mechanism of two-stage mouse skin carcinogenesis; we consider that our results obtained *in vitro* strongly support his hypothesis (62).

One of the best differentiation systems *in vitro* is that consisting of Friend erythroleukemia cells (FELC) established by Friend et al. (20), in which it is possible to observe reversible inhibition of spontaneous and induced differentiation by tumor promoters (51,64). We employ the FELC system as a model to study the mechanism by which the phorbol ester tumor promoters reversibly inhibit cell differentiation, taking advantage of the fact that biochemical and biological events associated with the expression of this differentiation program are being studied extensively at the cellular and molecular levels (36). Furthermore, clones of FELC have been isolated that are completely resistant to phorbol

TABLE 1. *Modulation of cell differentiation by tumor-promoting phorbol esters*

Cell type	Phenotype affected	Reference
A. *Inhibition or delay of differentiation*		
Murine erythroleukemia	Hemoglobin synthesis	51,64
Murine 3T3 fibroblasts[a]	Lipid accumulation	10
Murine neuroblastoma	Neurite formation	30
Murine ganglia[a]	Neurite formation	29
Murine melanoma[a]	Melanin synthesis	40
Murine myeloid leukemia[b]	Morphology, phagocytic activity	31
Murine C3H 10T½ cells	Morphology	38
Mouse epidermal cultures	Keratinization	22
Chick embryo myoblasts	Myotube formation	9
Chick embryo chondroblasts	Sulfated proteoglycan synthesis	45
Chick embryo melanogenic cells	Melanin synthesis	46
Rat mammary carcinoma	Dome formation	15
Hamster epidermal cultures	Keratinization	53
Nematode *(C. elegans)*	Early development	c
Sea urchin	Embryogenesis	7
B. *Induction or stimulation of differentiation*		
Murine erythroleukemia	Hemoglobin synthesis	37
Murine myeloid leukemia[b]	Morphology, phagocytosis, etc.	43
Chick myeloid leukemia	Morphology, phagocytosis	48
Human myeloid leukemia	Morphology, phagocytosis, etc.	27,34,52
Human melanoma	Dendrite formation	28
Human T lymphoblasts	E-rosette formation	42

[a] Differentiation is delayed, but not completely blocked, by phorbol esters.
[b] Inhibition was observed when calf serum was used in culture medium; however, TPA induces differentiation in the presence of fetal calf serum (Hozumi, *personal communication*).
[c] Miwa et al., submitted for publication.

ester-mediated inhibition of differentiation and yet retain the capacity to differentiate normally in response to various inducers (19). These variant clones have been characterized and compared with tumor promoter-sensitive clonal FELC (19,61,63,65,66,68).

REVERSIBILITY OF 12-O-TETRADECANOYLPHORBOL-13-ACETATE-MEDIATED INHIBITION OF INDUCED DIFFERENTIATION OF FELC

Reversibility is one of the most striking features of the tumor promotion process on mouse skin (2,6,56). Most of the biological and biochemical effects of 12-O-tetradecanoylphorbol-13-acetate (TPA) on cell cultures are reversible when TPA is removed from the culture medium (58,59). In order to determine to what extent the inhibitory effect of TPA on FELC differentiation is reversible, the long-term effects of TPA were followed.

Although FELC lose their ability to divide a few divisions after induction of differentiation (19,20), they continue to grow if TPA is present, since their terminal differentiation is inhibited (65,67). FELC were maintained in the presence of hexamethylene bisacetamide (HMBA) plus TPA for about 8 months

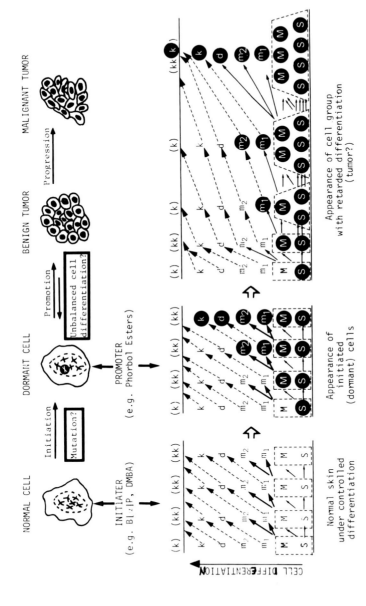

FIG. 1. Schematic diagram of a possible mechanism for two-stage chemical carcinogenesis. ●: Initiated cells; ⬤: Cells with dividing capacity; →: Differentiation by division; ⇢: Differentiation by movement to the surface; S: Stem cell; M, m₁, m₂, d: Differentiating cells; k: Keratin. (Modified from Berenblum, ref. 1.)

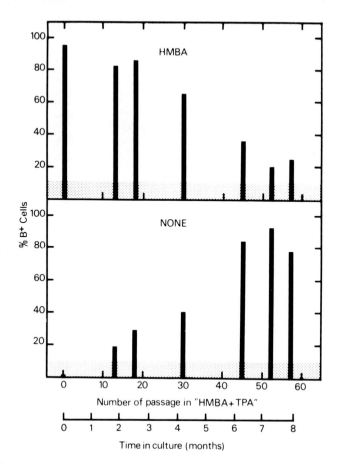

FIG. 2. Differentiation of FELC clone Ts19-8 after release from long-term blockage by TPA. Cells of clone TS19-8 were grown in the presence of 4mM HMBA and 100 ng TPA per ml. The cells were transferred twice a week at approximately 10^5 cells/ml into culture medium containing fresh HMBA and TPA. After the indicated number of passages, FELC were washed four times with culture medium (including 30 min of incubation in the medium at 37° between the third and fourth washings) and were resuspended at 10^5 cell/ml in control medium or medium containing 4mM HMBA, 100 ng TPA per ml, or HMBA plus TPA. After 4 and 5 days in culture, the extent of differentiation was scored, and the higher percentage of B⁺ from 4- and 5-day cultures was recorded. **Top:** Cells were removed from HMBA and TPA after various numbers of passages and resuspended in the presence of HMBA alone or in the presence of HMBA and TPA *(stippled area)*. **Bottom:** Cells were suspended in control medium or in TPA-containing medium *(stippled area)*.

by transferring the cells twice weekly to fresh medium containing those compounds. During that period, differentiation, scored by the appearance of benzidine-positive cells, was always less than 5% and usually less than 1%, indicating that there was no significant escape of cells from the TPA blockage during that time. FELC were periodically released from the TPA blockage by thorough washing, and their response to freshly added HMBA, an inducer of differentiation, and TPA, an inhibitor, was examined (Fig. 2). When cells cultured with HMBA and TPA for as long as 2.5 months were transferred to fresh medium containing HMBA alone, they were induced to differentiate to an extent (80 to 90%) similar to that observed in cells not previously cultured with TPA (Fig. 2 (top)). This confirms and extends our previous reports that TPA-mediated inhibition of HMBA-induced differentiation is reversible (64,65).

As shown in Fig. 2 (top), if cells are maintained for a longer period of time in the presence of HMBA and TPA, they tend to lose their ability to differentiate when transferred to HMBA-containing medium. After 7 months of continuous growth in HMBA and TPA, only about 20% of the cells were induced to differentiate by addition of HMBA. Thus, TPA-mediated inhibition of HMBA-induced differentiation is reversible for as long as 2.5 months, but later becomes partially irreversible. As shown in Fig. 2 (bottom), however, FELC do differentiate when released from TPA blockage into medium that does not contain HMBA: more than 80% of cells underwent differentiation in control medium upon release from 8 months of continuous culture in HMBA plus TPA. It appears, therefore, that TPA never erases the ability of FELC for erythroid differentiation, and in this sense, TPA-mediated inhibition of differentiation is reversible during the 8-month period. These results suggest that the apparent irreversibility of HMBA-induced differentiation of FELC after long-term culture with HMBA plus TPA is due to the paradoxical fact that HMBA inhibits some process of differentiation in these cells (see below).

STAGES OF FELC DIFFERENTIATION BLOCKED BY TPA

FELC undergo a program of erythroid differentiation when various chemicals, including dimethylsulfoxide (DMSO), HMBA, and butyric acid, are added to the culture medium (20,36,44). We have shown previously that during the process of induction of differentiation, one specific stage is sensitive to the inhibitory effect of TPA (64,65). When FELC are exposed to inducers, an increasing proportion become committed to differentiate, i.e., they are capable of undergoing differentiation even after the inducer is washed out. If HMBA is used as the inducer, for example, committed FELC are detectable as early as 24 hr after exposure to HMBA, and commitment is complete by 48 hr (18).

The relationship between commitment and TPA-mediated inhibition of differentiation was studied by HMBA-induced FELC differentiation. In order to obtain maximum inhibition of differentiation, it was necessary to add TPA to the culture within 24 hr of exposure to HMBA (64,65). If the addition was delayed beyond this time, the percentage of inhibition decreased; there is little inhibition when TPA is added later than 48 hr after the addition of HMBA. Thus, the decrease in inhibitory effect is related inversely to the proportion of the cells committed to differentiate. These results suggest that TPA inhibits the differentiation of cells that have not yet passed a critical step necessary for commitment or the expression of commitment (64). Our results (Fig. 2) suggest that TPA exerts its inhibitory effects at two different stages in the process of FELC differentiation: (a) at cell entry into commitment, and (b) at expression of the committed state to differentiate (see below).

When FELC that have been cultured for 13 passages (about 2 months) in HMBA plus TPA are transferred to control medium, about 20% undergo differentiation; similarly, after 18 passages, about 30% of the cells undergo differentiation (Fig. 2, bottom). These results imply that only 20% and 30% of the cells were committed to differentiate after 12 and 18 passages, respectively, in medium containing HMBA plus TPA. Since the majority of FELC are committed within 48 hr after exposure to HMBA (18), TPA appears to inhibit the commitment of FELC to differentiate.

When the cells were grown for a longer time in the presence of HMBA and TPA, the percentage of committed cells gradually increased (Fig. 2, bottom). After a 7-month incubation of FELC in the presence of HMBA and TPA, for example, 90% of the cell population underwent differentiation when the cells were released from TPA blockage into unsupplemented control medium, implying that 90% of the cells were committed to differentiate.

In order to determine if cells thus presumed to be committed after long-term culture in HMBA and TPA can be maintained in a state of commitment in the absence of HMBA, they were transferred to medium containing only TPA and grown for many generations. Two FELC clones, TS19-8 and TS19-

TABLE 2. *TPA-mediated maintenance of HMBA-induced commitment of FELC[a]*

	Number of passages after transfer to TPA alone	% B+ cells
TS19-8 cells (after	0	84
	3	81
45 passages in	7	78
	12	52
HMBA + TPA)	43	66
TS19-10 cells (after	0	87
	6	96
36 passages in	18	81
	37	77
HMBA + TPA)	60	75

[a]TS19-8 and TS19-10 cells were grown in HMBA and TPA, as described in the legend to Fig. 1 for 45 and 36 passages, respectively. The cells were then washed four times with culture medium and transferred to a medium containing TPA only (100 ng/ml); cells were transferred twice a week at approximately 10^5 cells/ml into medium containing fresh TPA. At the indicated number of passages, the cells were washed four times and resuspended in control medium. The percentage of benzidine-positive (B+) cells was determined 3, 4, and 5 days later, and the highest number was recorded.

10, were maintained in HMBA plus TPA for 4 to 5 months, were washed and grown in TPA only for the indicated number of passages, and were periodically released from TPA blockage. A high percentage of cells in each cell line underwent differentiation upon removal of TPA, even after 43 or 60 passages, respectively (Table 2).

These results suggest that TPA inhibits the entry of FELC into commitment but that, because this inhibition is leaky, FELC are eventually committed to differentiate. TPA also inhibits the expression of commitment, however, so that HMBA-induced committed cells gradually accumulate in the cell population.

Although FELC undergo very long-term inhibition of spontaneous and induced differentiation, escape from TPA inhibition was observed in 3T3 preadipose and melanoma cells (10,41); the escape could not be prevented by frequent additions of fresh TPA to the culture medium. This phenomenon may be related to the stage of commitment in the differentiation program at which inhibition takes place: it may be that these cells are blocked by TPA before commitment but that the expression of commitment is not blocked and, therefore, TPA blockage appears to be "leaky." Another possible explanation for the phenomenon is down regulation of TPA receptors during the culture of these cells with TPA. The long-term suppression of FELC differentiation by TPA indicates that no significant "down regulation" of TPA receptors occurs in FELC.

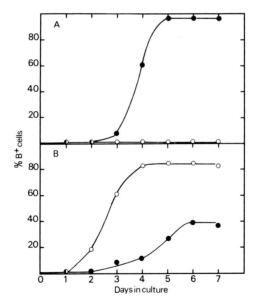

FIG. 3. Time course of differentiation of TS19-10 cells before and after long-term growth in HMBA plus TPA. **A:** TS19-10 cells were grown in the presence of 100 ng TPA per ml for four passages, washed thoroughly, as described in the legend to Fig. 2, and then incubated in control medium (0) or in medium containing 4 mM HMBA (●). **B:** TS19-10 cells underwent 46 serial passages in HMBA plus TPA and then were washed and allowed to differentiate in control medium (0) or medium containing HMBA (●).

CHARACTERIZATION OF FELC PRESUMED TO BE COMMITTED BY TPA ACCUMULATION

Figure 3 shows the time course of differentiation of TS19-10 cells presumed to be committed by TPA accumulation after their release from TPA blockage in control medium (Fig. 3B), as compared with the usual HMBA-induced differentiation of TS19-10 (Fig. 3A). When TS19-10 cells that had been grown in HMBA and TPA for 6 months were washed and grown in control medium, they started to differentiate after 2 days and reached a maximum on day 4 (Fig. 3B). Induction of differentiation of TS19-10 cells by HMBA started on day 3 and was complete by day 5 (Fig. 3A). Thus, cells grown in HMBA plus TPA for a long time can differentiate at least 24 hr earlier than usual, further suggesting that FELC cultured in HMBA and TPA are blocked after their commitment to differentiate.

Although after 4 to 5 months of culture in HMBA and TPA and most cells were presumably committed and therefore underwent differentiation when washed and released from TPA into control medium, fewer cells differentiated when they were released into HMBA-containing medium (Fig. 3A). This indicates that HMBA, a potent inducer of FELC differentiation, inhibits the expression of commitment to differentiate.

HMBA indeed inhibited the expression of differentiation of HMBA-induced committed cells (Table 3). Another inducer of FELC differentiation, DMSO, also almost completely inhibited this process. Butyric acid partially inhibited it; however, hemin failed to inhibit it at a concentration that can induce differentiation in untreated TS19-10 cells.

TABLE 3. *Effects of various inducers of FELC differentiation on the expression of commitment[a]*

Compound added	B[+] cells (%)
None	70
HMBA, 4 mM	11
DMSO, 1.5%	2
1.0%	1
Butyric acid, 0.8 mM[b]	< 1
0.6 mM	40
Hemin, 0.1 mM	71
0.03 mM	59

[a] TS19-10 cells were grown in the presence of 4 mM HMBA plus 100 ng/ml TPA for 48 passages and were washed as described in the legend to Fig. 1, then grown in fresh medium containing the compounds indicated. Differentiation was scored on day 5.

[b] This concentration of butyric acid was also toxic to cell growth.

Figure 4 shows the growth curve of TS19-8 cells grown in HMBA plus TPA for 45 passages, washed, then incubated in control medium or medium containing TPA, HMBA, or HMBA plus TPA. When the cells are released from TPA blockage, they lose their ability to divide. Regardless of the number of cells inoculated (10^3, 10^4, or 10^5 cells/ml), they stop dividing after only three or four divisions in control medium, whereas in the presence of TPA they continue to multiply. These results indicate that FELC not only become benzidine-positive, but also undergo terminal differentiation upon removal of TPA.

Accumulation of globin messenger ribonucleic acid (mRNA) in the cytoplasm precedes the appearance of benzidine-positive cells in the process of FELC differentiation (44). TPA inhibits the accumulation of globin mRNA induced by HMBA (64), and it appears that globin-specific mRNA synthesis remains suppressed as long as TPA is present in the culture medium. Only a background amount of globin mRNA was detected in FELC cultured in HMBA plus TPA

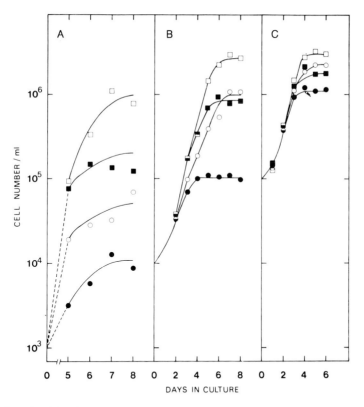

FIG. 4. Growth of FELC clone TS19-8 after continuous culture in HMBA plus TPA for 45 passages. Cells maintained in HMBA and TPA were washed four times in control medium, as described in the legend to Fig. 2. The cells were then resuspended in control medium (●), medium containing 4 mM HMBA (0), 100 ng TPA per ml (■), or HMBA plus TPA (□). The numbers of cells per ml originally inoculated were: **A,** 10^3; **B,** 10^4; **C,** 10^5.

for 45 passages, although mRNA synthesis resumed upon release from TPA blockage (W. Ostertag et al., *unpublished observations*). While such gene expression specific for cell differentiation is inhibited by TPA, other housekeeping genes necessary for cell proliferation are apparently normally expressed, since FELC grow for many generations in the presence of TPA. Thus, we conclude that TPA is a potent modulator of specific types of gene expression in FELC.

CHARACTERIZATION OF TPA-RESISTANT FELC CLONES

When a cell line of FELC, DS19, was randomly cloned using methyl cellulose, the isolated clones varied in their response to TPA (19,65). Several clones of FELC which are resistant to TPA-mediated inhibition of differentiation retain their ability to differentiate in response to various inducers (19). These variant cells have been characterized extensively in studies to elucidate the mechanism of tumor promoter-mediated inhibition of cell differentiation (61,63).

In all cases of TPA-mediated inhibition of differentiation studied so far, a good positive correlation has been observed between the ability of various phorbol esters and their congeners to promote mouse skin tumors and their ability to inhibit differentiation (62). Table 4 summarizes the effects of various plant diterpenes and other compounds on the differentiation of TPA-sensitive and TPA-resistant FELC. The resistance of TR19-9 clonal FELC to TPA extends to related compounds, such as phorbol-12,13-didecanoate (PDD), mezerein, and ingenol dibenzoate. These TPA-resistant clones are sensitive, however, to inhibition of differentiation by dexamethasone and the anesthetics procaine and tetracaine. These results indicate that the mechanism of resistance to the plant diterpene tumor promoters is selective. Table 4 also shows the effect of nonphorbol-type tumor promoters, cocarcinogens, and suspected promoters on the differentiation of FELC. None of these compounds inhibited the HMBA-induced differentiation of FELC, even at doses much higher than those of TPA and its derivatives. The finding that phorbol ester-type tumor promoters do not share common effects with nonphorbol promoters is consistent with several other reports (12,60). It is likely that tumor promoters are organ specific. Indeed, when we added phenobarbital (0.3 mg/ml) to one of the rat liver epithelial cell lines (IAR6-1) established by Montesano et al. (39), the cells showed morphological changes relatively similar to those obtained by incubation with TPA (H. Yamasaki et al., *unpublished observations*). These findings may partially explain the organospecificity of tumor promoters; phenobarbital might be a tumor promoter specific to liver cells, whereas TPA has broader organ specificity for its promoting activity. This implies that one should be careful when attempting to develop a short-term screening test for tumor promoters: such a test might not be found if only one kind of cell is used.

TPA and related compounds exert various biological and biochemical effects on FELC that are associated with inhibition of cell differentiation (61). Such

TABLE 4. *Inhibition of differentiation of TPA-sensitive and TPA-resistant FELC by various plant diterpenes and other compounds*[a]

Compound tested	Reference for biological activities of compounds	% Inhibition of differentiation	
		TPA-sensitive (TS19-10)	TPA-resistant (TR19-9)
Diterpenes (100 ng/ml)			
TPA		99	6
PDD		99	5
Mezerein	24, 25, 41, 52, 54, 55	99	6
Ingenol dibenzoate		78	1
Phorbol		0	1
4-α-PDD		0	4
Local anesthetics			
Procaine (5 × 10⁻⁴ M)	3	45	57
Tetracaine (5 × 10⁻⁵ M)		33	61
Dexamethasone (10⁻⁸ M)	33	72	85
Nonditerpene promoters (or cocarcinogens)			
Iodoacetate (1 mg/ml)	23	<5	<5
Anthralin (0.1 mg/ml)	5	<5	<5
Limonene (1 mg/ml)	50	<5	<5
Phenobarbital (1 mg/ml)	47	<5	<5
Saccharin (1 mg/ml)	26	<5	<5
Undecane (1 mg/ml)	57	<5	<5
Catechol (1 mg/ml)	57	<5	<5
Pyrogallol (1 mg/ml)	57	<5	<5
Tween 60 (0.3 mg/ml)	21	<5	<5

[a] Differentiation was induced by 4 mM HMBA; the compounds were added at the same time as HMBA. The extent of differentiation was scored on day 4 and/or day 5, and the % inhibition was calculated.

TABLE 5. *Effects of TPA on TPA-sensitive and TPA-resistant FELC*

Effect	TPA-sensitive clonal cells	TPA-resistant clonal cells	Reference
Inhibition of differentiation	+	−	19,64
Induction of cell adhesion	+	−	64,67
Morphological changes in cell surface	+	−	62
Changes in surface membrane protein	+	−	62
Transient cell growth inhibition	+	−	19,64
Induction of plasminogen activator	+	−	64
Induction of prostaglandin synthesis	+	−	65
Specific binding of phorbol-12,13-dibutyrate	+	?	

effects on TPA-sensitive and TPA-resistant FELC have been compared (Table 5). None of the pleiotropic effects of TPA on TPA-sensitive clonal FELC were observed with TPA-resistant cells. However, TPA-sensitive and TPA-resistant clones metabolized ^{3}H-TPA at the same rate (50% of a dose of 30 ng/ml ^{3}H-TPA was metabolized within 17 hr by 10^5 cells per ml), and the highest percentage of the metabolites was accounted for by phorbol-13-acetate, as identified by thin-layer chromatography and high-pressure liquid chromatography (61,66). When phorbol-13-acetate was tested for its ability to inhibit cell differentiation and induce cell adhesion of FELC, it was inactive (66). Thus, differences in the metabolism of TPA are not the reason for the different susceptibilities of these clones to TPA.

Several recent studies have suggested that an early and possibly primary site of action of tumor-promoting phorbol esters is the cell membrane (4,8,14,32, 59,63,68). Comparison of the effects of TPA on TPA-sensitive and TPA-resistant FELC also suggests that the primary action of phorbol esters is on cell membranes and that this may be essential for inhibition of differentiation. The earliest changes caused by TPA in FELC are morphological alterations of the cell surface as revealed by interference microscopy (Fig. 5) and by the induction of cell adhesion to the culture flasks (68). Neither of these effects was observed with TPA-resistant FELC (63,68).

Since the induction of cell adhesion to the surface of culture flasks is rapid, and since quantitative assay of the effect is relatively simple, various compounds have been screened in this way. As with FELC inhibition, only the phorbol ester-type tumor promoters induced cell adhesion. When quantitative data on cell adhesion induction with various plant diterpenes were compared with data obtained *in vivo,* there was, in general, a good qualitative correlation with mouse skin tumor-promoting activity, and a better quantitative correlation with inflammatory activity on mouse ear (H. Yamasaki et al., *unpublished observations*). It has also been reported that the potency of phorbol derivatives in producing membrane-related effects in chicken embryo fibroblasts (such as increased deoxyglycose transport and loss of the large external transformation-sensitive glyco-

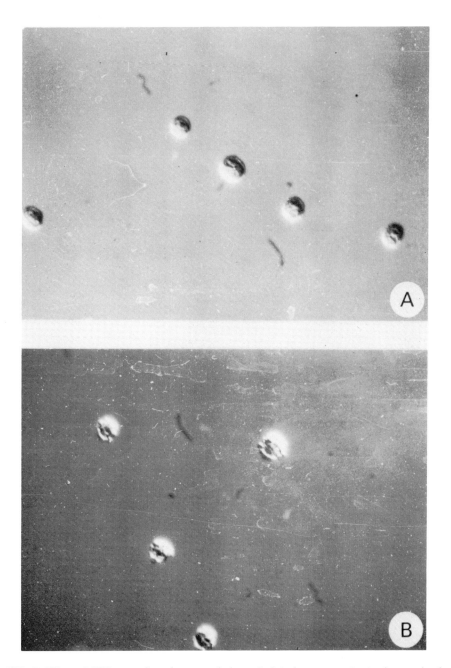

FIG. 5. Effect of TPA on cell surface morphology. **A:** Interference contrast micrograph of TPA-sensitive FELC clone TS19-10 in control medium. **B:** Interference contrast micrograph of TS19-10 cells exposed to TPA (30 ng/ml) for 24 hr in a bacterial Petri dish.

protein) also correlates better with their inflammatory potency than with their promoting potency in mice (13). The effects of phorbol ester derivatives on cell culture systems and on mouse ear may reflect the intrinsic action of these compounds in biological reactions, which is presumably an interaction with cell surface membranes, although tumor-promoting ability must be the result of a more complex interaction with mouse skin tissue. Nevertheless, the FELC adhesion assay may provide a simple and rapid method for studying the quantitative structure-activity relationships of the plant diterpene derivatives.

In order to demonstrate the biochemical effect of TPA on cell surface membranes, lactose peroxidase-catalyzed iodination of the external surface of FELC membrane was carried out. ^{125}I-labeled proteins of FELC surface membrane were analysed by sodium dodecyl sulfate polyacrylamide gel electrophoresis. When TPA-sensitive FELC (TS19-10) were incubated with TPA and the iodinated surface protein pattern compared with those of cells incubated with solvent only, several changes could be seen. For example, after the cells had been incubated with TPA for 24 hr, a protein band of approximate MW 1×10^5 disappeared, and two new proteins appeared, with MW of approximately 4×10^4 and 1×10^4. In contrast, there were essentially no qualitative change in the iodinated surface protein pattern of TPA-resistant FELC (TR19-9aR) before or after the incubation of the cells with TPA (63).

The fact that early effects of TPA on FELC are seen on cell membranes and that these membrane effects are absent in TPA-resistant clonal FELC indicates that the primary and essential interaction of TPA with FELC takes place on the cell surface membrane and that such interaction cannot take place in TPA-resistant cells. The receptors for TPA were recently demonstrated by Blumberg and his colleagues in various types of cells (14,16). We have started to look at the receptors on FELC employing their method. We can demonstrate a specific, saturable binding of ^{3}H-phorbol-12,13-dibutyrate in the particular fractions of TS19-101 (Fig. 6). We are now comparing TPA receptors of TPA-sensitive and TPA-resistant clones of FELC; our preliminary results suggest that some but not all TPA-resistant clonal cells have fewer receptors than TPA-sensitive cells.

CONCLUSIONS AND IMPLICATIONS

Inhibition or induction of differentiation by TPA has been demonstrated in a variety of cell culture systems (Table 1), and there are several indications that TPA also inhibits cell differentiation *in vivo* (35,49). In cell culture systems, TPA exerts its modulating effect on cell differentiation at a dose that is not toxic to cells. For example, in this study, FELC continued to grow in the presence of TPA for 8 months, during which the differentiation of FELC was suppressed. Thus, TPA selectively modulates gene expression that is participating in cell differentiation. Although the TPA-induced modulation of gene expression is selective, however, various programs of cell differentiation are affected; these

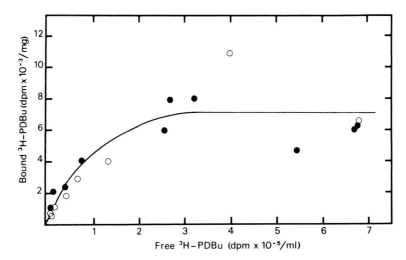

FIG. 6. Specific binding of ³H-phorbol-12,13-dibutyrate (³H-PDBu) to particulate preparations of FELC (TS19-10) as a function of ligand concentration. Particulate fractions prepared from undifferentiated (●) or differentiating (0) TS10-101 Friend cells were incubated with increasing concentrations of ³H-PDBu for 30 min at 39°, and specific binding was determined as described by Driedger and Blumberg (14). Differentiation was induced by incubating the cells with 4 mM HMBA for 4 days; differentiation, scored by benzidine staining, was approximately 80%.

include hemoglobin synthesis, neurite formation, lipid synthesis, melanin synthesis, myosin synthesis, proteoglycan synthesis, etc., all of which are obviously expressions of different genes.

How can TPA recognize this variety of gene expressions without affecting most of the other housekeeping ones? We believe that TPA does not recognize gene expressions, but rather recognizes a common triggering step that is necessary for a variety of cell differentiation programs. One possible such signal for cell differentiation might be the appearance of a class of histone, H_1^0, which has been shown to be involved in the commitment of a number of different programs of cell differentiation (17). If TPA indeed modulates the appearance of H_1^0 or other such signals common to many cell differentiation, this may provide a clue to how TPA can modulate so many types of cell differentiation (or gene expressions). This approach is important not only for understanding the mechanism of action of tumor promoters, but also for understanding fundamental problems of cell differentiation.

Phorbol ester tumor promoters also reversibly inhibit the normal development of a nematode, *C. elegans* (Miwa et al., *submitted for publication*). If similar effects occur in higher animals, these tumor promoters might be expected to act as teratogens. To our knowledge, no such effect has been reported.

Our long-term experiments on TPA-mediated inhibition of HMBA-induced FELC differentiation have indicated that although TPA never erases the erythroid character of FELC, HMBA-inducible differentiation is apparently irreversibly inhibited by TPA; this effect is due to the paradoxical inhibitory effect of HMBA on the differentiation of FELC. HMBA, a potent inducer of FELC differentiation, actually inhibits the differentiation of FELC cultured for a long time in the presence of HMBA and TPA, suggesting that the response of FELC to HMBA changes completely during the culture period.

We attempted to use this phenomenon to elucidate the transition from the reversible stage of tumor growth to the irreversible and independent growth of tumors. During two-stage mouse skin carcinogenesis, the skin must be painted with TPA over a long period of time before the tumor attains independent growth. If it is assumed that mouse skin cell differentiation is a phenomenon inducible by some endogenous factor, repeated painting of TPA provides a situation very similar to long-term FELC culture with a differentiation inducer, HMBA, and TPA. Therefore, perhaps treatment of mouse skin with TPA inhibits the initiated cells from differentiating, and they therefore continue to multiply and form a mass of undifferentiated cells (tumor ?). Since this TPA-mediated inhibition of differentiation is reversible over a certain period, the cells undergo normal differentiation if TPA application is discontinued too soon; thus, this mass of cells would disappear. After prolonged treatment with TPA, cells can no longer differentiate in response to an inducer of differentiation, and they finally achieve irreversible growth even if TPA treatment is stopped. This hypothesis implies that the role of TPA in stimulating tumor growth can be taken over by some endogenous factor that controls normal cell differentiation and thus achieves "lock-in" of the TPA effect. Further understanding of the control of normal skin cell differentiation as well as its interaction with tumor promoters is necessary to clarify this hypothesis.

ACKNOWLEDGMENTS

The authors wish to thank Dr. I. B. Weinstein for his continuous interest in and helpful discussions of the work. The keen interest of Drs. R. Montesano and L. Tomatis in our work is deeply appreciated. We are indebted to Mrs. L. Saint-Vincent for her assistance in the laboratory, to Mrs. E. Heseltine for editing the manuscript, and to Ms. C. Dériol for her secretarial aid.

REFERENCES

1. Berenblum, I. (1954): A speculative review: The probable nature of promoting action and its significance in the understanding of the mechanisms of carcinogenesis. *Cancer Res.,* 14:471–474.
2. Berenblum, I. (1975): Sequential aspects of chemical carcinogenesis. In: *Cancer, A Comprehensive Treatise, Vol. 1,* edited by F. F. Becker, pp. 323–344. Plenum Press, New York.
3. Bernstein, A., Boyd, A. S., Crichley, V., and Lamb, V. (1976): Induction and inhibition of Friend leukemia cell differentiation—The role of membrane-active compounds. In: *Biogenesis and Turnover of Membrane Macromolecules,* edited by J. S. Cook, pp. 145–159. Raven Press, New York.
4. Blumberg, P. M., Driedger, P. E., and Rossow, P. W. (1976): Effect of a phorbol ester on transformation-sensitive surface protein of chick fibroblasts. *Nature,* 264:446–447.

5. Bock, F. G., and Burns, R. (1963): Tumor-promoting properties of anthralin (1,8,9-anthratriol). *J. Natl. Cancer Inst.*, 30:393–397.
6. Boutwell, R. K. (1974): The function and mechanisms of promoters of carcinogenesis. *CRC Crit. Rev. Toxicol.*, 2:419–443.
7. Bresch, H., and Arendt, U. (1978): Disturbances of early sea urchin development by the tumor promoter TPA (phorbol ester). *Naturwissenschaften*, 65:660–662.
8. Castagna, M., Rochette-Egly, C., and Rosenfeld, C. (1979): Tumour-promoting phorbol diester induces substrate-adhesion and growth inhibition in lymphoblastoid cells. *Cancer Letters*, 6:227–234.
9. Cohen, R., Pacifici, M., Rubenstein, N., Biehl, J., and Holtzer, H. (1977): Effect of a tumor promoter on myogenesis. *Nature*, 266:538–540.
10. Diamond, L., O'Brien, T. G., and Rovera, G. (1977): Inhibition of adipose conversion of 3T3 fibroblasts by tumor promoters. *Nature*, 269:247–248.
11. Diamond, L., O'Brien, T. G., and Rovera, G. (1978): Tumor promoters: Effects on proliferation and differentiation of cells in culture. *Life Sci.*, 23:1,979–1,988.
12. Driedger, P. E., and Blumberg, P. M. (1978): Nonphorbol mouse skin tumour promoters do not mimic phorbol myristate acetate in its effects on chick embryo fibroblasts. *Int. J. Cancer*, 22:63–69.
13. Driedger, P. E., and Blumberg, P. M. (1979): Quantitative correlation between *in vitro* and *in vivo* activities of phorbol esters. *Cancer Res.*, 39:714–719.
14. Driedger, P. E., and Blumberg, P. M. (1980): Specific binding of phorbol ester tumor promoters. *Proc. Natl. Acad. Sci. USA*, 77:567–571.
15. Dulbecco, R., Bologna, M., and Unger, M. (1980): Control of differentiation of a mammary cell line by lipids. *Proc. Natl. Acad. Sci. USA*, 77:1,551–1,555.
16. Dunphy, W. G., Delclos, K. B., and Blumberg, P. M. (1980): Characterization of specific binding of [³H]phorbol-12,13-dibutyrate and [³H]phorbol 12-myristate-13-acetate to mouse brain. *Cancer Res.*, 40:3,635–3,641.
17. Eisen, H., Hasthorpe, S., Gjerset, R., Nasi, S., and Keppel, F. (1980): Distribution and behaviour of the chromosomal protein IP₂₅ *in vivo* and in tissue culture. In: *In Vivo and in Vitro Erythropoiesis: The Friend System*, edited by G. B. Rossi, pp. 289–296. Elsevier/North Holland Biomedical Press, Amsterdam.
18. Fibach, E., Reuben, R., Rifkind, R. A., and Marks, P. A. (1977): Effect of hexamethylene bisacetamide on the commitment to differentiation of murine erythroleukemia cells. *Cancer Res.*, 37:440–444.
19. Fibach, E., Yamasaki, H., Weinstein, I. B., Marks, P. A., and Rifkind, R. A. (1978): Heterogeneity of murine erythroleukemia cells with respect to tumor promoter-mediated inhibition of cell differentiation. *Cancer Res.*, 38:3,685–3,688.
20. Friend, C., Scher, W., Holland, J. G., and Sato, T. (1971): Hemogulobin synthesis in murine virus-induced leukemic cells *in vitro:* Stimulation of erythroid differentiation by dimethylsulfoxide. *Proc. Natl. Acad. Sci. USA*, 68:378–382.
21. Fukushima, S., Tatematsu, M., and Takahashi, M. (1974): Combined effects of various surfactants on gastric carcinogenesis in rats treated with *N*-methyl-*N'*-nitro-*N*-nitrosoguanidine. *Gann*, 65:371–376.
22. Fusenig, N. E., Breitkreutz, P., Boukamp, P., Lueder, M., Ormscher, G., and Worst, P. K. M. (1979): Chemical carcinogenesis in mouse epidermal cell cultures: Altered expression of tissue-specific functions accompanying cell transformation. In: *Neoplastic Transformation in Differentiated Epithelial Cell Systems in vitro*, edited by L. M. Franks and C. B. Wigley, pp. 37–98. Academic Press, London.
23. Gwynn, R. H., and Salaman, M. H. (1953): Studies on cocarcinogenesis. SH-reactors and other substances tested for cocarcinogenic action in mouse skin. *Br. J. Cancer*, 7:482–489.
24. Hecker, E. (1975): Cocarcinogens and cocarcinogenesis. In: *Handbuch der Allgemeinen Pathologie, Vol. 4*, edited by E. Grundmann, pp. 651–676. Springer Verlag, Berlin.
25. Hecker, E. (1978): Structure-activity relationship in diterpene esters irritant and carcinogenic to mouse skin. In: *Carcinogenesis—Mechanisms of Tumor Promotion and Cocarcinogenesis, Vol. 2*, edited by T. J. Slaga, A. Sivak, and R. K. Boutwell, pp. 11–48. Raven Press, New York.
26. Hicks, R. M., Wakefield, J. St J., and Chowaniec, J. (1973): Cocarcinogenic action of saccharin in the chemical induction of bladder cancer. *Nature*, 243:347–349.
27. Huberman, E., and Callahan, M. (1979): Induction of terminal differentiation in human promy-

elocytic leukemia cells by tumor-promoting agents. *Proc. Natl. Acad. Sci. USA,* 76:1,293–1,297.

28. Huberman, E., Heckman, C., and Langenbach, R. (1979): Stimulation of differentiated functions in human melanoma cells by tumor-promoting agents and dimethylsulfoxide. *Cancer Res.,* 39:2,618–2,624.

29. Ishii, D. N. (1978): Effect of tumor promoters on the response of cultured embryonic chick ganglion to nerve growth factor. *Cancer Res.,* 38:3,886–3,893.

30. Ishii, D. N., Fibach, E., Yamasaki, H., and Weinstein, I. B. (1978): Tumor promoters inhibit morphological differentiation in cultured mouse neuroblastoma cells. *Science,* 200:556–559.

31. Kasukabe, T., Honma, Y., and Hozumi, M. (1979): Inhibition of functional and morphological differentiation of cultured mouse myeloid leukemia cells by tumour promoters. *Gann,* 70:119–123.

32. Lee, L. S., and Weinstein, I. B. (1978): Tumor-promoting phorbol esters inhibit binding of epidermal growth factor to cellular receptors. *Science,* 202:313–315.

33. Lo, S. C., Aft, R., Ross, J., and Mueller, G. C. (1978): Control of globin gene expression by steroid hormones in differentiating Friend leukemia cells. *Cell,* 15:447–453.

34. Lotem, J., and Sachs, L. (1979): Regulation of normal differentiation in mouse and human myeloid leukemic cells by phorbol esters and the mechanism of tumor promotion. *Proc. Natl. Acad. Sci. USA,* 76:5,158–5,162.

35. Marks, F., Bertsch, S., Grimm, W., and Schweizer, J. (1978): Hyperplastic transformation and tumor promotion in mouse epidermis: Possible consequences of disturbances of endogenous mechanisms controlling proliferation and differentiation. In: *Carcinogenesis, Vol. 2,* edited by T. J. Slaga, A. Sivak, and R. K. Boutwell, pp. 91–116. Raven Press, New York.

36. Marks, P. A., and Rifkind, R. A. (1978): Erythroleukemic differentiation. *Annu. Rev. Biochem.,* 47:419–448.

37. Miao, R. M., Fiedsteel, A. H., and Fodge, D. W. (1978): Opposing effects of tumor promoters on erythroid differentiation. *Nature,* 274:271–272.

38. Mondal, S., and Heidelberger, C. (1980): Inhibition of induced differentiation of C3H/10T½ clone 8 mouse embryo cells by tumor promoters. *Cancer Res.,* 40:334–338.

39. Montesano, R., Saint-Vincent, L., and Tomatis, L. (1973): Malignant transformation *in vitro* of rat liver cells by dimethylnitrosamine and *N*-methyl-*N'* -nitro-*N*-nitrosoguanidine. *Br. J. Cancer,* 28:215–220.

40. Mufson, R. A., Fisher, P. B., and Weinstein, I. B. (1979): Effects of phorbol ester tumor promoters on the expression of melanogenesis in B-16 melanoma cells. *Cancer Res.,* 39:3,915–3,919.

41. Mufson, R. A., Fisher, S. M., Slaga, T. J., Gleason, G. L., Venma, A. K., and Boutwell, R. K. (1979): Effects of 12-O-tetradecanoylphorbol-13-acetate and mezerein on epidermal ornithine decarboxylase activity, isoproterenol-stimulated levels of cyclic adenosine 3':5'-monophosphate, and induction of mouse skin tumors *in vivo. Cancer Res.,* 39:4,791–4,795.

42. Nagasawa, K., and Mak, T. W. (1980): Phorbol esters induce differentiation in human malignant T lymphoblasts. *Proc. Natl. Acad. Sci. USA,* 77:2,964–2,968.

43. Nakayasu, M., Shoji, M., Aoki, N., Sato, S., Miwa, M., and Sugimura, T. (1979): Enhancing effect of phorbol esters on induction of differentiation of mouse myeloid leukemia cells by human urinary protein and lipopolysaccharide. *Cancer Res.,* 39:4,668–4,672.

44. Ostertag, W., Melderis, H., Steinheider, G., Kluge, N., and Dube, S. (1972): Synthesis of mouse hemoglobin and globin mRNA in leukemia in DBA/2 mice. *Nature New Biol.,* 239:231–234.

45. Pacifici, M., and Holtzer, H. (1977): Effects of tumor-promoting agent on chondrogenesis. *Am. J. Anat.,* 150:207–212.

46. Payette, R., Biehl, J., Toyama, Y., Holtzer, H. (1980): Effects of 12-O-tetradecanoylphorbol-13-acetate on the differentiation of avian melanocytes. *Cancer Res.,* 40:2,465–2,474.

47. Peraino, C., Fry, R. J. M., Staffeldt, E., and Christopher, J. P. (1975): Comparative enhancing effects of phenobarbital, amobarbital, diphenylhydantoin, and dichlorodiphenyltrichloroethan on 2-acetylaminofluorene-induced hepatic tumorigenesis in the rat. *Cancer Res.,* 35:2,884–2,890.

48. Pessano, S., Gazzolo, L., and Moscovici, C. (1979): The effect of a tumor promoter on avian leukemia cells. *Microbiologia,* 2:379–383.

49. Raick, A. N. (1973): Ultrastructural, histological, and biochemical alterations produced by 12-O-tetradecanoylphorbol-13-acetate on mouse epidermis and their relevance to skin tumor promotion. *Cancer Res.,* 33:269–286.

50. Roe, F. J. C., and Pierce, W. E. H. (1960): Tumor promotion by citrus oil: Tumours of the skin and urethral orifice in mice. *J. Natl. Cancer Inst.,* 24:1,389–1,403.

51. Rovera, G., O'Brien, T. G., and Diamond, L. (1977): Tumor promoters inhibit spontaneous differentiation of Friend erythroleukemia cells in culture. *Proc. Natl. Acad. Sci. USA,* 74:2,894–2,898.

52. Rovera, G., O'Brien, T. G., and Diamond, L. (1979): Induction of differentiation in human promyelocytic leukemia cells by tumor promoters. *Science,* 204:868–870.

53. Scribner, J. D., and Suss, R. (1978): Tumor initiation and promotion. *Int. Rev. Exp. Pathol.,* 18:137–198.

54. Sisskin, E., and Barrett, J. C. (1979): Inhibition of differentiation of Syrian hamster epidermal cells in culture by TPA. *Proc. Am. Assoc. Cancer Res.* (Abstract), 20:197.

55. Slaga, T. J., Klein-Szanto, A. J. P., Fischer, S. M., Weeks, C. E., Nelson, K., and Major, S. (1980): Studies on mechanisms of action of antitumor-promoting agents: Their specificity in two-stage promotion. *Proc. Natl. Acad. Sci. USA,* 77:2,251–2,254.

56. Van Duuren, B. L. (1969): Tumor-promoting agents in two-stage carcinogenesis. *Prog. Exp. Tumor Res.,* 11:31–68.

57. Van Duuren, B. L., and Goldschmidt, B. M. (1976): Cocarcinogenic and tumor-promoting agents in tobacco carcinogenesis. *J. Natl. Cancer Inst.,* 56:1,237–1,242.

58. Weinstein, I. B., Wigler, M., and Pietropaolo, C. (1977): The action of tumor-promoting agents in cell culture. In: *Origins of Human Cancer, Vol. 4,* edited by H. H. Hiatt, J. D. Watson, and J. A. Winsten, pp. 751–772. Cold Spring Harbor Laboratory, New York.

59. Weinstein, I. B., Yamasaki, H., Wigler, M., Lee, L. S., Fisher, P. B., Jeffrey, A. M., and Grundberger, D. (1979): Molecular and cellular events associated with the action of initiating carcinogens and tumor promoters. In: *Carcinogens–Identification and Mechanisms of Action,* edited by A. C. Griffin and C. R. Shaw, pp. 399–418. Raven Press, New York.

60. Wigler, M., DeFeo, D., and Weinstein, I. B. (1978): Induction of plasminogen activator in cultured cells by macrocyclic plant diterpene esters and other agents related to tumour promotion. *Cancer Res.,* 38:1,434–1,437.

61. Yamasaki, H. (1980a): Biological and biochemical effects of phorbol ester-type tumour promoters on Friend cells. In: *In Vivo and in Vitro Erythropoiesis: The Friend System,* edited by G. B. Rossi, pp. 593–602. Elsevier/North Holland Biomedical Press, Amsterdam.

62. Yamasaki, H. (1980b): Reversible inhibition of cell differentiation by phorbol esters as a possible mechanism of promotion step in chemical carcinogenesis. In: *Molecular and Cellular Aspects of Carcinogen Screening Tests,* edited by R. Montesano, H. Bartsch, and L. Tomatis, pp. 91–111. IARC, Lyon.

63. Yamasaki, H., and Drevon, C. (1980): Tumour promoter-induced membrane changes associated with inhibition of differentiation in Friend erythroleukemia cells. In: *Biology of the Cancer Cell Proceedings of the Fifth Meeting of the European Association for Cancer Research, 1979,* pp. 317–325. Kugler Publications, Amsterdam.

64. Yamasaki, H., Fibach, E., Nudel, U., Weinstein, I. B., Rifkind, R. A., and Marks, P. A. (1977): Tumor promoters inhibit spontaneous and induced differentiation of murine erythroleukemia cells in culture. *Proc. Natl. Acad. Sci. USA,* 74:3,451–3,455.

65. Yamasaki, H., Fibach, E., Weinstein, I. B., Nudel, U., Rifkind, R. A., and Marks, P. A. (1979): Inhibition of Friend leukemia cell differentiation by tumor promoters. In: *Oncogenic Viruses and Host Cell Genes,* edited by T. Ikawa and T. Odaka, pp. 365–376. Academic Press, New York.

66. Yamasaki, H., Mufson, R. A., and Weinstein, I. B. (1979): Phorbol ester-induced prostaglandin synthesis and [³H] TPA metabolism by TPA-sensitive and TPA-resistant Friend erythroleukemia cells. *Biochem. Biophys. Res. Commun.,* 89:1,018–1,025.

67. Yamasaki, H., Saint-Vincent, L., and Martel, N. (1980): Long-term effect of a tumor promoter, 12-O-tetradecanoylphorbol-13-acetate, on induced differentiation of Friend leukemia cells. *Cancer Res.,* 40:3,780–3,785.

68. Yamasaki, H., Weinstein, I. B., Fibach, E., Rifkind, R. A., and Marks, P. A. (1979): Tumor promoter-induced adhesion of the DS-19 clone of murine erythroleukemia cells. *Cancer Res.,* 39:1,989–1,994.

Carcinogenesis, Vol. 7, edited by E. Hecker et al.
Raven Press, New York © 1982.

Modification of Growth and Differentiation of Myeloid Leukemia Cells by Tumor Promoters

Motoo Hozumi, Takashi Kasukabe, and Yoshio Honma

*Department of Chemotherapy, Saitama Cancer Center Research Institute,
Saitama 362, Japan*

The mouse myeloid leukemia cell line M1 can be induced to differentiate into macrophages and granulocytes by treatment with proteinous factors in conditioned media from various cell sources, various body fluids, and some chemicals (2,3,7).

Although we found that 12-O-tetradecanoylphorbol-13-acetate (TPA) and other tumor-promoting plant diterpenes could inhibit induction of differentiation of M1 cells into macrophages and granulocytes by dexamethasone or proteinous inducer (4), Lotem and Sachs (5) and Nakayasu et al. (6) reported recently that tumor promoters scarcely affected, or rather enhanced, the induction of cell differentiation by some inducers. Therefore, we reexamined these conflicting findings. We now present data showing that the response of M1 cells to TPA depends on the type of serum in the medium and that some fractions of the serum are responsible for modification of the actions of TPA.

EFFECT OF TPA ON INDUCTION OF DIFFERENTIATION OF M1 CELLS

In our laboratory, M1 cells have been cultured in Eagle's minimum essential medium with twice concentrations of amino acids and vitamins and supplemented with 10% heat-inactivated calf serum for more than 5 years (2). Induction of the phagocytic activity of the cells, a typical functional marker of differentiated M1 cells, by dexamethasone (4×10^{-8} M) was markedly inhibited dose-dependently by TPA in 10% calf serum medium (Fig. 1), as we reported previously (4). Induction of phagocytic activity, however, was not inhibited but rather enhanced when the cells were washed twice with phosphate-buffered saline and transferred from medium containing 10% calf serum to medium containing 10% fetal calf serum and treated with dexamethasone and TPA (Fig. 1). Phorbol had no effect on the induction of phagocytic activity of the cells in medium with calf serum or fetal calf serum (Fig. 1).

These different responses of M1 cells to TPA in media with different serum were confirmed with three lots each of calf serum (lots 11778 and 746: Chiba

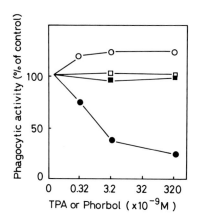

FIG. 1. Effects of TPA and phorbol on induction of phagocytic activity of M1 cells by dexamethasone in medium with calf serum and fetal calf serum. M1 cells were incubated with 4×10^{-8} M dexamethasone and various concentrations of TPA for 24 hr in medium with calf serum (●) or fetal calf serum (○) and with various concentrations of phorbol in medium with calf serum (■) or fetal calf serum (□). The phagocytic activities of M1 cells treated with 4×10^{-8} M dexamethasone alone were 59.6% in calf serum medium and 71.5% in fetal calf serum medium.

Kessei Laboratories, Ichikawa, Japan, and A381012: GIBCO) and fetal calf serum (lots A283619 and C480122: GIBCO, and 4055890: Flow Laboratories). It was also found that TPA inhibited the induction of phagocytic activity by dexamethasone in 10% horse serum medium (lot 3376: Pel-Freez Biological Inc.) as well as in calf serum medium. These serum-dependent inductions of phagocytic activity of M1 cells by TPA were observed in all clones of M1 cells examined (DS-3, DS-4, T-22, and B24) (2). Therefore, these results suggest that the response of M1 cells to TPA varies with the serum, but not with the clone of cells used. TPA also inhibited induction of phagocytic activity of M1 cells by other inducers such as lipopolysaccharide (*Salmonella typhimurium,* Difco Laboratories) or proteinous inducer in ascitic fluid (2) when the cells were cultured in calf serum medium, and enhanced it when they were cultured in fetal calf serum medium.

In addition, TPA significantly inhibited morphological differentiation of M1 cells to mature macrophages and granulocytes induced by the proteinous inducer in calf serum medium (Table 1), whereas it increased the proportion of differentiated cells in intermediate stages between myeloblastic cells and mature cells in fetal calf serum medium (Table 1). Thus TPA inhibited the inductions by various inducers of both functional and morphological differentiation of M1 cells in calf serum medium, but had the opposite effect in fetal calf serum medium.

EFFECT OF TPA ON SYNTHESIS OF PROSTAGLANDIN E_2 OF M1 CELLS

To obtain information on how TPA modified differentiation of M1 cells, we examined its effect on synthesis of prostaglandin E_2 by the cells, because we have found that the syntheses of E-type prostaglandins are involved in the mechanism of induction of differentiation of M1 cells (1,2). TPA alone did not significantly affect the synthesis of prostaglandin E_2 of M1 cells in calf

TABLE 1. *Effect of TPA on morphological differentiation of M1 cells in medium with calf serum or fetal calf serum[a]*

Serum	Protein inducer (%)	TPA (3.2 × 10⁻⁸ M)	Differentiation (%)		
			Myeloblastic cells	Intermediate stages	Macrophages and granulocytes
Calf serum	−	−	92.5	7.5	0
	+	−	55.5	40.0	4.5
	+	+	79.0	20.5	0.5
Fetal calf serum	−	−	56.5	43.5	0
	+	−	46.0	47.0	7.0
	+	+	21.0	72.0	7.0

[a]M1 cells were cultured with 1% proteinous inducer from ascitic fluid of rats bearing hepatoma AH-130 (2) with or without 3.2 × 10⁻⁸ M TPA for 3 days in medium with 10% calf serum or 10% fetal calf serum.

serum medium, although it slightly enhanced formation of total metabolites of arachidonate (Table 2). On the other hand, proteinous inducer from ascitic fluid markedly enhanced production of total metabolites of arachidonate and synthesis of prostaglandin E_2, as previously reported (1) (Table 2). TPA markedly inhibited the production of the total metabolites and the synthesis of prostaglandin E_2 with the inducer in calf serum medium. On the contrary, in fetal calf serum medium, TPA alone did not inhibit the production of total metabolites of arachidonate or the synthesis of prostaglandin E_2, and it significantly enhanced the production of total metabolites and the synthesis of prostaglandin E_2 in the presence of lipopolysaccharide. These results show that modification by TPA of synthesis of prostaglandin E_2 is closely associated with changes in differentiation of M1 cells.

It is unknown, however, whether TPA is directly involved in the mechanisms of modification of prostaglandin synthesis during induction of differentiation of M1 cells; its modification of prostaglandin synthesis could result from its inhibition of induction of cell differentiation.

PROPERTIES OF THE SERUM FACTOR(S) MODIFYING THE EFFECT OF TPA ON DIFFERENTIATION OF M1 CELLS

TPA also had different effects on M1 cells in medium with dialysed calf serum and dialysed fetal calf serum. Therefore, the factor(s) in these sera that modifies the effect of TPA is nondialyzable and macromolecular.

Next we fractionated calf serum (lot 11778) and fetal calf serum (lot A283619) on a Sephadex G-200 column and examined the effects of the fractions on the effect of TPA on dexamethasone-induced differentiation of M1 cells in medium

TABLE 2. *Effect of TPA on synthesis of prostaglandin E_2 from ^{14}C-arachidonate in M1 cells in medium with calf serum or fetal calf serum[a]*

Serum	Inducer	TPA (10^{-7} M)	Total metabolites of arachidonate (cpm/10^6 cells)	Prostaglandin E_2 (cpm/10^6 cells)
Calf serum	—	—	355	20
	—	+	426	26
	Protein inducer	—	1,371	263
	Protein inducer	+	609	125
Fetal calf serum	—	—	743	59
	—	+	696	53
	Lipopolysaccharide	—	4,360	550
	Lipopolysaccharide	+	5,500	700

[a] M1 cells were cultured with 5% proteinous inducer from ascitic fluid of rats bearing hepatoma AH-130 (2) with or without 10^{-7} M TPA in calf serum medium for 3 days, or with 0.5 µg/ml of lipopolysaccharide from *Salmonella typhimurium* with or without 10^{-7} M TPA in fetal calf serum medium for 4 days. ^{14}C-Arachidonate (Radiochemical Center, Amersham, U.K.) was added for 18 hr and total metabolites of arachidonate and synthesis of prostaglandin E_2 were determined as reported previously (1).

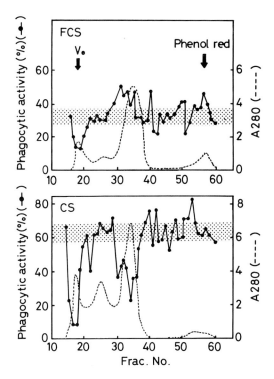

FIG. 2. Sephadex G-200 gel filtration patterns of material in calf serum and fetal calf serum modifying the response to TPA of induction of differentiation of M1 cells by dexamethasone. Five ml of calf serum or fetal calf serum was applied to a Sephadex G-200 column (1.5 × 87 cm) and eluted with phosphate-buffered saline. Fractions of 2.8 ml were collected. The amount of protein was determined from the absorbance at 280 nm. The effects of the fractions of calf serum (CS) and fetal calf serum (FCS) on modification of induction of differentiation of M1 cells by 1.6 × 10⁻⁷ M TPA were determined with 1 × 10⁻⁸ M dexamethasone for calf serum and 4 × 10⁻⁹ M dexamethasone for fetal calf serum. The shaded areas represent the range of the standard deviation of phagocytic activity induced by dexamethasone alone.

containing 1% calf serum (Fig. 2). The large molecular fractions of calf serum and fetal calf serum recovered in the void volume both inhibited differentiation of M1 cells (Fig. 2), but the inhibitory activity of this fraction of calf serum was much higher than that of the fraction of fetal calf serum. Moreover, fractions number 25 to 35 of fetal calf serum significantly stimulated differentiation of M1 cells, and no other fractions were inhibitory, whereas no fractions of calf serum were stimulatory (Fig. 2), and fractions number 30 to 36 were strongly inhibitory (Fig. 2).

These results suggest that the different responses of M1 cells to TPA in different sera depend on the presence of these fractions in the sera. Further characterization of these fractions and investigations on their mechanisms of action are under way.

SUMMARY

The tumor promoter TPA inhibited both functional and morphological differentiation of mouse myeloid leukemia M1 cells cultured in medium containing calf serum or horse serum, but enhanced these inductions in medium containing fetal calf serum.

The metabolic processes of prostaglandin E_2 synthesis were associated with modification by TPA of differentiation of M1 cells.

The factor(s) in the sera affecting the differentiation of M1 cells with TPA was nondialyzable and macromolecular. Upon Sephadex G-200 gel filtration, much more inhibitory activity was found in calf serum than in fetal calf serum, and stimulatory activity was found only in fetal calf serum.

ACKNOWLEDGMENT

This work was partly supported by a Grant-in-Aid for Scientific Research from the Ministry of Education, Science, and Culture of Japan.

REFERENCES

1. Honma, Y., Kasukabe, T., Hozumi, M., and Koshihara, Y., (1980): Regulation of prostaglandin synthesis during differentiation of cultured mouse myeloid leukemia cells. *J. Cell Physiol.,* 104:349–357.
2. Hozumi, M. (1982): A new approach to chemotherapy of myeloid leukemia: Control of leukemogenicity of myeloid leukemia cells by induction of normal differentiation. In: *Cancer Biology Reviews.* Marcel Dekker, New York *(in press).*
3. Ichikawa, Y. (1969): Differentiation of a cell line of myeloid leukemia. *J. Cell Physiol.,* 74:223–234.
4. Kasukabe, T., Honma, Y., and Hozumi, M. (1979): Inhibition of functional and morphological differentiation of cultured mouse myeloid leukemia cells by tumor promoters. *Gann,* 70:119–123.
5. Lotem, J., and Sachs, L. (1979): Regulation of normal differentiation in mouse and human myeloid leukemic cells by phorbol esters and the mechanism of tumor promotion. *Proc. Natl. Acad. Sci. USA,* 76:5,158–5,162.
6. Nakayasu, M., Shoji, M., Aoki, N., Sato, S., Miwa, M., and Sugimura, T. (1979): Enhancing effect of phorbol esters on induction of differentiation of mouse myeloid leukemia cells by human urinary protein and lipopolysaccharide. *Cancer Res.,* 39:4,668–4,672.
7. Sachs, L. (1978): Control of normal differentiation and the phenotypic reversion of malignancy in myeloid leukemia. *Nature,* 274:535–539.

Carcinogenesis, Vol. 7, edited by E. Hecker et al.
Raven Press, New York © 1982.

Regulation of Growth and Differentiation by Phorbol Esters and the Mechanism of Tumor Promotion

Joseph Lotem and Leo Sachs

Department of Genetics, Weizmann Institute of Science, Rehovot, Israel

SUMMARY

Our studies on the growth and differentiation of normal and malignant myeloid cells have shown that tumor-promoting, but not nonpromoting, phorbol esters can induce the production of and specifically increase cell susceptibility to the normal myeloid inducers of growth and differentiation, the macrophage- and granulocyte-inducing proteins MGI. In some clones of myeloid leukemic cells, the tumor promoters induced cell differentiation via the production of MGI. In other clones that were not inducible by adding only the tumor promoters or MGI, the tumor promoters induced differentiation by increasing cell susceptibility to externally added MGI. Normal myeloid progenitor cells, unlike leukemic cells, require MGI for cell viability and multiplication. Our studies with these normal cells have shown, that tumor promoters can also induce cell multiplication both by the induction of MGI and by increasing cell susceptibility to externally added MGI. We suggest that by the above mechanisms of inducing the production and increasing cell susceptibility to normal regulators of cell multiplication and differentiation, tumor-promoting phorbol esters can exert pleiotropic effects, the nature of these effects depending on which molecules are being regulated in the treated cells.

INTRODUCTION

Studies on tumor development in animals have led to the isolation of different chemicals that can promote the formation of tumors after their initiation. Among the most potent tumor promoters are plant diterpenes such as 12-O-tetradecanoylphorbol-13-acetate (TPA) (4), that promote tumor development by increasing cell multiplication of initiated cells. This allows the occurrence and eventual selection of cells with other changes required for malignancy, such as specific chromosome changes (7). Experiments with TPA and many different cell types *in vitro* have indicated that increased cell multiplication may be obained by blocking cell differentiation (1,3), although in other cell types, including myeloid leukemic cells (1,5,6), TPA induces cell differentiation. The present experiments using genetically different types of myeloid leukemic cells that differ in their competence to differentiate *in vitro* by the macrophage- and granulocyte-inducing protein MGI (6) and normal bone marrow myeloblasts were undertaken, to elucidate the mechanism by which TPA regulates cell multiplication and differentiation. Experimental details have been described elsewhere (5).

CLONAL DIFFERENCES IN INDUCTION OF DIFFERENTIATION IN MOUSE MYELOID LEUKEMIC CELLS BY TPA

Mouse myeloid leukemic clones inducible for differentiation by MGI (MGI^+D^+), clones that were only partially inducible (MGI^+D^-), and clones that were not inducible for differentiation by MGI (MGI^-D^-) were used (5,6). Incubation of MGI^+D^+ clone 7-M18 and MGI^-D^- clone 6 with TPA resulted in cell attachment to the Petri dish, followed by induction of Fc and C3 rosettes, phagocytosis of these rosettes (immune phagocytosis), lysozyme (only in clone 7-M18), and morphological differentiation to macrophages (5). Induction of these properties was detectable with 1 ng/ml TPA (1.6 nM) and optimal at 1 μg/ml (Fig. 1). There was, however, no induction of cell attachment or differentiation by TPA in another MGI^+D^+ clone (Fig. 1), in two MGI^+D^- clones, or two other MGI^-D^- clones. One of these MGI^-D^- clones (clone 1) showed inducibility by TPA plus MGI (5). Substitution of MGI by bacterial lipopolysaccharide (LPS) or dexamethasone did not induce differentiation in MGI^-D^-

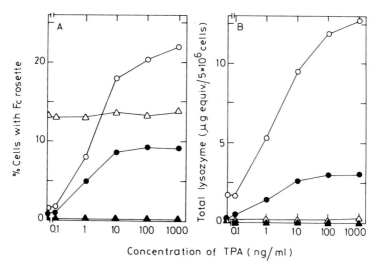

FIG. 1. Differences in mouse MGI^+D^+ leukemic clones 7-M18 and 11 in inducibility for Fc rosettes and lysozyme by TPA. Cells were incubated for 4 days with different concentrations of TPA without *(black symbols)* or with *(white symbols)* 1% mouse MGI and then assayed for **A:** Fc rosettes, and **B:** lysozyme. Clone 7-M18 *(circles)*; clone 11 *(triangles)*.

clone 1 together with TPA. The use of phorbol esters that differ in their tumor-promoting activity on mouse skin (4) has shown that induction of differentiation parallels tumor-promoting ability (5).

INDUCTION OF DIFFERENTIATION IN HUMAN MYELOID LEUKEMIC CELLS BY TPA

Incubation of the human HL-60 myeloid leukemic cells with TPA induced cell attachment (starting at about 12 hr), rosettes (mainly C3), phagocytosis of these rosettes, lysozyme, and differentiation to mature macrophages. Optimum induction of these properties was obtained with 0.5 ng/ml TPA. Induction of macrophages was also obtained with these cells by the addition of human MGI in 25 to 50% conditioned medium from phytohemagglutinin-treated human lymphocytes. Addition of 0.1 ng/ml TPA and 5% MGI together, each at a noninducing concentration, resulted in strong cell attachment and induction of the other differentiation associated properties (5).

MECHANISM OF INDUCTION OF DIFFERENTIATION BY TPA

It has been shown that some clones of mouse myeloid leukemic cells can be induced to differentiate by LPS, and that this differentiation is due to the induction of MGI activity by LPS in the cells that then differentiated (6). We have also found MGI activity, detected by the ability to induce the formation of macrophage or granulocyte colonies or clusters from normal mouse bone marrow myeloblasts, in the culture medium of MGI^+D^- clone 7-M18 cells already 1.5 hr after treatment with TPA. This induction of MGI activity was much earlier than the induction of Fc rosettes (12 hr) or lysozyme (2 days) after treatment with TPA. The human HL-60 cells were induced to differentiate to macrophages only by TPA or by human MGI, and as with clone 7-M18, TPA also induced MGI activity in the culture medium of HL-60 cells. TPA did not induce any detectable MGI activity in the culture medium in any of the other mouse myeloid leukemic cell clones. The combined effect of TPA and added MGI on MGI^-D^- clone 1 indicates that in this clone TPA induces cell susceptibility to externally added MGI.

EFFECT OF TPA ON COLONY AND CLUSTER FORMATION FROM NORMAL MYELOBLASTS

The seeding of normal mouse bone marrow cells for colony formation in agar with 1 µg/ml TPA without added MGI induced about 80 clusters of 4 to 16 myeloid cells per 5×10^4 cells at 3 days after seeding, most of which degenerated at 7 days. The use of conditioned medium from normal bone marrow cells incubated with TPA (Table 1) indicates that this cluster formation was due to the induction of MGI activity by TPA. Therefore, when seeding a higher

TABLE 1. *Induction of MGI activity by TPA in normal mouse bone marrow cells*

Source of externally added MGI	TPA in agar (0.4 μg/ml)	No. of bone marrow cells seeded in agar	MGI activity	
			No. of colonies	No. of clusters
—	—	5×10^4–5×10^5	0	0
—	+	5×10^4	0	7
—	+	1.5×10^5	10	52
—	+	5×10^5	94	160
CM from TPA-treated bone marrow cells[a]	+	5×10^4	32	62

[a]Normal bone marrow cells were incubated for 1 day in mass culture at 10^6 cells/ml with 1 μg/ml TPA. The culture supernatant (CM) was then assayed for MGI activity at a final concentration of 40%.

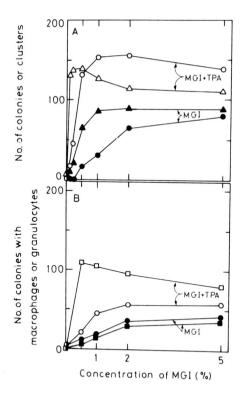

FIG 2. TPA enhancement of MGI induction of cluster and colony formation by normal bone marrow cells. 5×10^4 nucleated mouse bone marrow cells were seeded with different concentrations of mouse MGI with *(white symbols)* or without *(black symbols)* 1 μg/ml TPA, and colonies and clusters were counted 7 days after seeding. **A:** Total number of colonies ($\circ$-$\circ$) and clusters ($\triangle$-$\triangle$); **B:** Number of macrophage ($\square$-$\square$) or granulocyte ($\circ$-$\circ$) colonies.

number of cells in the agar plates, TPA by itself could induce the formation of colonies (Table 1), as has also been reported by others (2), via the production of MGI activity. The addition of TPA together with MGI has shown that TPA can increase the number of macrophage and granulocyte colonies and clusters at 7 days after seeding, and that the highest increases were obtained with the lower concentrations of MGI (Fig. 2). The colonies with TPA were also larger and there was a higher increase in the number of macrophages than of granulocyte colonies (10-fold higher at 0.5% MGI).

DISCUSSION

The present results have shown that TPA induced normal cell differentiation in one clone of mouse myeloid leukemic cells (MGI^+D^+ clone 7-M18) by inducing the production of MGI activity, and in another clone (MGI^-D^- clone 1) by inducing cell susceptibility to externally added MGI, but not to LPS or dexamethasone. TPA also induced differentiation in the human myeloid leukemic cell line HL-60 with the induction of MGI activity and enhanced susceptibility to externally added MGI (5). This indicates that TPA can induce differentiation by two different mechanisms. With normal mouse bone marrow cells, TPA also induced the synthesis of MGI, and increased their susceptibility for the formation of colonies by externally added MGI. However, other MGI^+D^+, MGI^+D^-, or MGI^-D^- clones did not show the above effects of TPA alone or together with MGI.

We suggest that the above clonal differences in induction of MGI activity and increased susceptibility to MGI by TPA may be associated with differences in receptors for TPA and the ability of TPA to modify receptors for MGI.

Clonal variation in susceptibility to inhibition or induction of differentiation by TPA has also been found with erythroleukemic cells (3), which may be due to a similar mechanism in relation to regulators of erythropoiesis. TPA also increased the susceptibility of normal T lymphocytes to the normal T cell colony protein inducer (TCI) (Gerassi and Sachs, *unpublished observations*). There thus appears to be a general mechanism of action of TPA by modulating cellular interactions with normal regulators of multiplication and differentiation. Induction or increased susceptibility to normal inducers of cell multiplication can stimulate multiplication of initiated cells in tumor promotion. This multiplication can then permit the occurrence and eventual selection of the other cellular changes that are required for malignancy.

REFERENCES

1. Diamond, L., O'Brien, T. G., and Baird, W. M. (1980): Tumor promoters and the mechanism of tumor promotion. In: *Advances in Cancer Research, Vol. 32,* edited by G. Klein and W. Weinhouse, pp. 1–74. Academic Press, New York.
2. Fibach, E., Marks, P. A., and Rifkind, R. A. (1980): Tumor promoters enhance myeloid and erythroid colony formation by normal mouse hemopoietic cells. *Proc. Natl. Acad. Sci. USA,*

77:4,152–4,155.

3. Fibach, E., Yamasaki, H., Weinstein, I. B., Marks, P. A., and Rifkind, R. A. (1978): Heterogeneity of murine erythroleukemia cells with respect to tumor promoter-mediated inhibition of cell differentiation. *Cancer Res.,* 38:3,685–3,688.

4. Hecker, E. (1971): Isolation and characterization of the cocarcinogenic principles from Croton oil. In: *Methods in Cancer Research, Vol. 6,* edited by H. Busch, pp. 439–484. Academic Press, New York.

5. Lotem, J., and Sachs, L. (1979): Regulation of normal differentiation in mouse and human myeloid leukemic cells by phorbol esters and the mechanism of tumor promotion. *Proc. Natl. Acad. Sci. USA,* 76:5,158–5,162.

6. Sachs, L. (1978): Control of normal cell differentiation and the phenotypic reversion of malignancy in myeloid leukemia. *Nature,* 274:535–539.

7. Sachs, L. (1980): Constitutive uncoupling of pathways of gene expression that control growth and differentiation in myeloid leukemia. A model for the origin and progression of malignancy. *Proc. Natl. Acad. Sci. USA,* 77:6,152–6,156.

Carcinogenesis, Vol. 7, edited by E. Hecker et al.
Raven Press, New York © 1982.

Effects of Tumor Promoters on the Differentiation of C3H/10T1/2 Mouse Embryo Fibroblasts

Charles Heidelberger and Sukdeb Mondal

*University of Southern California Comprehensive Cancer Center,
Los Angeles, California 90033*

SUMMARY

The discovery by Jones that 5-azacytidine (5-AzCR) induces C3H/10T1/2 mouse embryo fibroblasts to differentiate into muscle cells, adipocytes, and chondrocytes opened the way to study the effects of tumor promoters on differentiation in this cell culture system, in which initiation and promotion have been clearly demonstrated. 5-AzCR-induced differentiation into muscle cells was significantly inhibited by the following tumor promoters: 12-0-tetradecanoylphorbol-13-acetate (TPA) phorbol dibutyrate, phorbol dibenzoate, mezerein, saccharin, epidermal growth factor, and iodoacetic acid. This differentiation was not affected by phorbol, phorbol diacetate, 4α-phorbol didecanoate, anthralin, acetic acid, and phenobarbital. The following inhibitors of promotion also inhibited 5-AzCR-induced muscle cell formation and did not affect the inhibition produced by TPA: antipain, retinoic acid, fluocinolone acetonide, and dexamethasone. In the induction of differentiation into adipocytes, dexamethasone, fluocinolone acetonide, antipain, and indomethacin, inhibitors of promotion were active, in addition to 5-AzCR. TPA, mezerein, Tween 60, and retinoic acid inhibited dexamethasone-induced adipocyte formation, and iodoacetic acid, epidermal growth factor, and anthralin did not. Differentiation into muscle cells and adipocytes was affected in opposite directions by anthralin, iodoacetic acid, saccharin, and epidermal growth factor (EGF), whereas both processes were inhibited by TPA, mezerein, and epidermal growth factor. Hence there is no consistent effect on these differentiative processes produced by tumor promoters of several chemical classes or by various inhibitors of promotion.

INTRODUCTION

(a) Initiation and promotion have been demonstrated in C3H/10T1/2 mouse embryo fibroblasts (3,6).

(b) Tumor promoters affect in different ways (inhibit or stimulate) a variety of differentiative processes.

(c) Jones and colleagues have discovered that 5-AzCR induces differentiation of C3H/10T1/2 fibroblasts into muscle cells and adipocytes (2).

(d) 5-AzCR also produces oncogenic transformation of C3H/10T1/2 cells (1).

(e) Phorbol esters, but not all other chemical classes of tumor promoters, inhibit the 5-AzCR-induced differentiation of C3H/10T1/2 fibroblasts into muscle cells (4).

(f) Several inhibitors of tumor promotion also inhibit 5-AzCR-induced differentiation of C3H/10T1/2 fibroblasts into muscle cells (4).

(g) These inhibitors of tumor promotion do not affect (reverse or increase) the inhibition by TPA of 5-AzCR-induced differentiation of C3H/10T1/2 fibroblasts into muscle cells (4).

(h) Since 5-AzCR also induces C3H/10T1/2 cells to differentiate into adipocytes (2), we have investigated the effects of various tumor promoters and other substances on this process (5).

MATERIALS AND METHODS

(a) C3H/10T1/2 cells were cultured as previously described (6).

(b) Cells were plated and 1 day later were treated for 24 hr with 5-AzCR. Two days later, the promoters or inhibitors of promotion were added and kept in the medium for 18 to 20 days.

(c) Dishes were fixed and stained. Muscle cells were counted after Giemsa staining (4). Adipocytes were counted after oil red 0 staining.

(d) Initiation and promotion were assayed as previously described (3).

CONCLUSIONS

(a) Corticosteroids strongly induce, and tumor promoters chemically unrelated to phorbol esters weakly induce, differentiation of C3H/10T1/2 fibroblasts into adipocytes (data not shown).

(b) Phorbol ester-related tumor promoters inhibit dexamethasone- and 5-AzCR-induced differentiation of C3H/10T1/2 fibroblasts into adipocytes. Other classes of tumor promoters and/or inhibitors of tumor promotion either stimulate or inhibit this process (Table 1).

(c) 5-AzCR is an initiator of oncogenic transformation of C3H/10T1/2 cells with TPA as promoter. Inhibitors of tumor promotion inhibit this process (data not shown).

(d) The inconsistent effects of various chemical classes of tumor promoters on 5-AzCR-induced differentiation of C3H/10T1/2 fibroblasts into either muscle cells or adipocytes preclude the use of this system as a short-term test for tumor promoters (Tables 1 and 2).

(e) If effects on differentiation are essential in the mechanism of tumor promotion, such effects are too complex and inconsistent in this system to be used as a critical means to establish mechanisms.

TABLE 1. A. *Effects of compounds on dexamethasone-induced adipocyte formation*

Compounds	Concentration (μg/ml)	Colonies relative to dexamethasone alone	Promoter or inhibitor of promotion in C3H/10T½ cells
Dexamethasone	1.0	100	Inhibitor
" + TPA	0.1	7	Promoter
" + Phorbol	0.1	100	Inactive
" + Mezerein	1.0	7	Promoter
" + Tween 60	0.1	7	Promoter
" + Iodoacetic acid	0.05–0.1	110	Promoter
" + Anthralin	0.1	110	Promoter
" + Epidermal growth factor	0.001	100	Promoter
" + Antipain	1.0	140	Inhibitor
" + Retinoic acid	0.05	1	Inhibitor
" + Fluocinolone acetonide	0.5	130	Inhibitor
" + Indomethacin	10	130	Inhibitor

B. *Effects on 5-AzCR-induced differentiation of C3H/10T1/2 cells into muscle cells and adipocytes in the same dish*

Compound	Concentration (μg/ml)	Average no. muscle cells	Average no. adipocyte colonies	Average no. cells/ adipocyte colony
5-AzCR	0.5	240	4	100–200
" + TPA	0.1	124	3	10–20
" + Dexamethasone (DM)	1.0	86	40	100–200
" + Fluocinolone acetonide (FA)	0.5	32	42	100–200
" + TPA + DM		81	24	10–15
" + TPA + FA		45	28	10–15

TABLE 2. *Effects of various compounds on promotion and on muscle cell and adipocyte formation in C3H/10T1/2 cells*

Compound	Promoter or inhibitor of transformation of C3H/10T½ cells[a]	Effect on:	
		muscle cells	adipocytes
TPA	P	−	−
Phorbol	No effect	No effect	No effect
Anthralin	P	±	+
Iodoacetic acid	P	−	+
Tween 60	P	−	−
Epidermal growth factor	P	−	+
Mezerein	P	−	−
Saccharin	P	−	+
Dexamethasone	I	−	+ +
Fluocinolone acetonide	I	−	+ +
Antipain	I	−	+ +
Indomethacin	I	−	+ +
Retinoic acid	I	−	−
Phenobarbital	No effect	No effect	No effect

[a] P = Promoter; I = inhibitor; − = inhibition; + = stimulation.

ACKNOWLEDGMENTS

Supported by Contract N01-CP-65831 from the National Cancer Institute and Grant R-80-5208 from the Environmental Protection Agency.

REFERENCES

1. Benedict, W. F., Banerjee, A., Gardner, A., and Jones, P. A. (1977): Induction of morphological transformation in mouse C3H/10T1/2 clone 8 cells and chromosomal damage in hamster A (Ti) Cl-3 cells by cancer chemotherapeutic agents. *Cancer Res.*, 37:2,202–2,208.
2. Constantinides, P. G., Taylor, S. M., and Jones, P. A. (1978): Phenotypic conversion of cultured mouse embryo cells by azapyrimidine nucleosides. *Dev. Biol.*, 66:57–71.
3. Mondal, S., Brankow, D. W., and Heidelberger, C. (1976): Two-stage chemical oncogenesis in cultures of C3H/10T1/2 cells. *Cancer Res.*, 36:2,254–2,260.
4. Mondal, S., and Heidelberger, C. (1980a): Inhibition of induced differentiation of C3H/10T1/2 clone 8 mouse fibroblasts by tumor promoters. *Cancer Res.*, 40:334–338.
5. Mondal, S., and Heidelberger, C. (1980b): Cell differentiation and tumor promotion. *Proc. Am. Assoc. Cancer Res.*, 21:96.
6. Reznikoff, C. D. A., Brankow, D. W., and Heidelberger, C. (1973): Establishment and characterization of a cloned line of C3H mouse embryo cells sensitive to postconfluence inhibition of division. *Cancer Res.*, 33:3,231–3,238.

Carcinogenesis, Vol. 7, edited by E. Hecker et al.
Raven Press, New York © 1982.

The Tumor Promoter PMA Reversibly Inhibits Chondrogenesis—Influence on the Expression of Collagen Types and Fibronectin

Joachim Sasse and Klaus von der Mark

*Max-Planck-Institut für Biochemie, Department of Connective Tissue Research, D-8033
Martinsried bei München, Federal Republic of Germany*

High density cultures of undetermined chick limb bud mesenchymal cells differentiate into cartilage *in vitro.* We have shown recently by immunofluorescence studies that a dense fibrous extracellular network of type I collagen and fibronectin is deposited in these cultures before onset of chondrogenesis (J. Sasse and K. von der Mark, *in preparation*). Here we report that the tumor promoter phorbol-12-myristate-13-acetate (PMA) inhibits cartilage differentiation and prevents the formation of the extracellular matrix.

EXPERIMENTAL RESULTS

If cultured in medium containing PMA (10^{-7} M), cartilage differentiation is completely inhibited (Fig. 1). PMA-treated mesenchymal cells deposit little type I collagen (Fig. 2a) and fibronectin (not shown); the cultures do not stain for the cartilage-specific type II collagen (Fig. 2b).

If returned to normal medium after 3 days of exposure to PMA, extracellular type I collagen (Fig. 2c) and fibronectin (not shown) are arranged in the form of a dense network similar to that of untreated cultures. Four days later, staining with antibodies against the cartilage-specific type II collagen (Fig. 2d) marks the onset of chondrogenesis.

When released from hyaline cartilage by trypsin and plated onto culture dishes at clonal densities, chick chondrocytes reaccumulate cartilage matrix consisting of type II collagen and chondroitin sulfate proteoglycan. Recently we have shown that under these conditions chondrocytes synthesize and deposit fibronectin in an extracellular, strandlike pattern (1). Here we report that the tumor promoter PMA reversibly modulates the synthesis and deposition of collagen types and fibronectin.

If cultured in medium containing PMA (5×10^{-8} M), chondrocytes are modulated into multilayered, fibroblastic cells (2) (Fig. 3). Synthesis of cartilage-specific type II collagen decreases 15-fold. By immunofluorescence studies, little type II collagen can be detected (Fig. 4b), whereas type I collagen is located

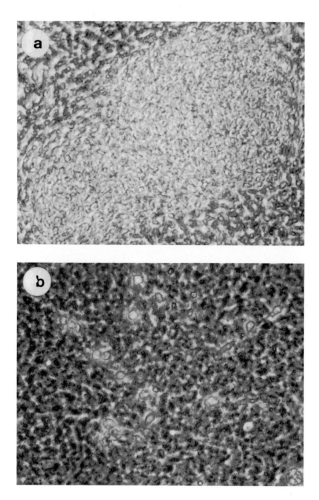

FIG. 1. a: Phase micrograph of a 4-day-old culture of chick limb bud mesenchymal cells forming a large cartilage nodule. **b:** A sister culture to that shown in **a,** but reared in medium containing PMA, fails to develop cartilage nodules. ×120.

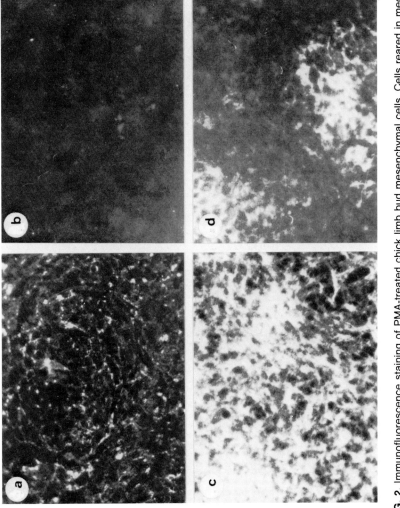

FIG. 2. Immunofluorescence staining of PMA-treated chick limb bud mesenchymal cells. Cells reared in medium containing PMA for 3 days deposit little type I collagen **(a)** and fibronectin (not shown), and no type II collagen **(b)**. Sister cultures, returned to normal medium after 3 days, show a dense extracellular network of type I collagen **(c)** and fibronectin (not shown). Two days later, cartilage nodules, staining for type II collagen, form **(d)**. ×150.

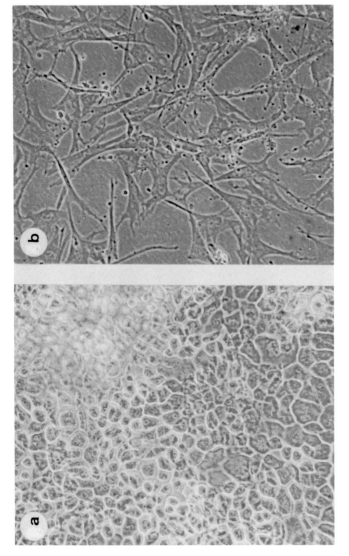

FIG. 3. a: Phase micrograph of a control—living 5-day-old chondrocyte culture. **b:** A sister culture to that shown in **(a)**, but reared in medium containing PMA. ×250.

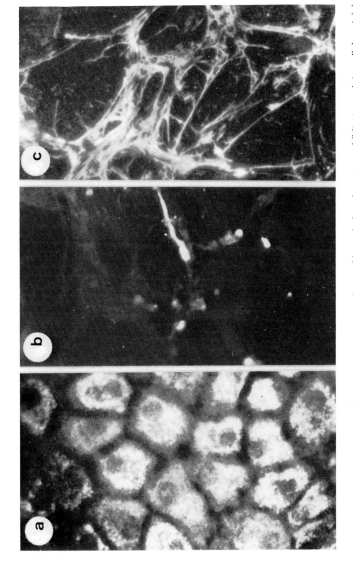

FIG. 4. Immunofluorescence labeling of chondrocyte cultures. Normal chondrocytes exhibit strong intracellular staining for the cartilage-specific type II collagen (**a**). In contrast, cells treated for 3 days with PMA show little type II collagen (**b**) while depositing an extracellular network of type I collagen (**c**). ×820.

extracellularly (Fig. 4c). Short intercellular fibronectin strands, which are typical for cartilage cells, extend in length and acquire fibroblast-like appearance in PMA-treated chondrocytes, but the amount of extracellular fibronectin is reduced, as determined by lactoperoxidase-mediated labeling of the cell surface with ^{131}I. If returned to normal medium after 1 to 6 days exposure to PMA, the chondrocytes reacquire polygonal morphology and switch back to the chondrocyte-like pattern of synthesis and deposition of type II collagen and fibronectin.

CONCLUSIONS

In contrast to other factors causing inhibition of chondrogenesis and modulation of the chondrocyte phenotype, the effect of PMA is reversible and thus offers advantages for studying the regulation of the synthesis of collagen types and fibronectin and—in general—for evaluating the mode of action of a tumor promoter.

ACKNOWLEGMENTS

The antibodies to the collagen types and fibronectin were kindly provided by Drs. W. Dessau, H. von der Mark, and R. Timpl.

REFERENCES

1. Dessau, W., Sasse, J., Timpl, R., Jilek, F., and von der Mark, K. (1978): Synthesis and extracellular deposition of fibronectin in chondrocyte cultures. Response to the removal of extracellular cartilage matrix. *J. Cell Biol.,* 79:342–355.
2. Lowe, M. E., Pacifici, M., and Holtzer, H. (1978): Effects of phorbol-12-myristate-13-acetate on the phenotypic program of cultured chondroblasts and fibroblasts. *Cancer Res.,* 38:2,350–2,356.

Carcinogenesis, Vol. 7, edited by E. Hecker et al.
Raven Press, New York © 1982.

Phorbol Esters Stimulate Protease Production by Human Endothelial Cells

*David Moscatelli, †Eric A. Jaffe, and *Daniel B. Rifkin

Department of Cell Biology, New York University Medical Center, New York, New York, 10016; and †Division of Hematology-Oncology, Department of Medicine, Cornell University Medical College, New York, New York 10021

It has often been proposed that proteases are involved in invasive processes. There is indirect evidence that proteolytic activity may be associated with the invasive process in neovascularization. New capillaries form by sprouting from existing blood vessels. In the area of the developing sprout, there is a fragmentation of the blood vessel basement membrane (1). Since basement membrane is rich in collagen and collagen is resistant to most proteases except collagenase, this observation suggested that blood vessel endothelial cells produce a collagenase during neovascularization. The production of a collagenase during neovascularization is also suggested by the ability of capillaries to grow into areas that are rich in collagen (3,8).

We have investigated whether cultured endothelial cells can produce a collagenase and whether the amount produced can be modulated. As a modulating agent, we chose 12-O-tetradecanoylphorbol-13-acetate (TPA). TPA is known to stimulate protease production by a variety of normal cells, including collagenase production by rabbit synovial fibroblasts (2) and plasminogen activator production by rabbit and bovine endothelial cells (5,6).

Using a sensitive radioactive assay for collagenase (7), we tested the serum-free culture medium from confluent cultures of human umbilical cord vein endothelial cells for the presence of collagenase. No active collagenase could be detected. However, most cells that produce a collagenase secrete it in an inactive form. Inactive or latent collagenase can be converted to active enzyme by treatment with certain proteases or certain sulfhydryl reagents. When the serum-free culture medium from endothelial cells was assayed after first treating it with trypsin and then inactivating the trypsin with Trasylol, small amounts of active collagenase could be detected. Likewise, treatment of the conditioned medium with the mercurial compound mersalyl allowed detection of collagenase.

Since we established that endothelial cells can produce collagenase, we investigated if the amount produced could be modulated. TPA stimulated the collagenase production by cultured endothelial cells in a dose-dependent manner (Table 1). Concentrations of TPA below 10^{-9} M had no effect on collagenase production. TPA stimulated collagenase production at 10^{-9} M, and maximal stimulation

TABLE 1. *Effect of phorbol esters on collagenase production by endothelial cells[a]*

Phorbol ester concentration	Relative collagenase activity			
	TPA	PDD	4-0-Me TPA	4α-PDD
0	1.0	1.0	1.0	1.0
10^{-11} M	1.0	1.1	1.3	0.9
10^{-10} M	1.0	1.2	1.3	1.1
10^{-9} M	3.3	2.2	1.4	1.4
10^{-8} M	12.0	10.8	1.4	1.1
10^{-7} M	12.7	9.7	1.7	1.2

[a] Human endothelial cells were grown to confluency in 35-mm tissue culture dishes in Medium 199 containing 20% human serum. The cultures were then washed and incubated for 18 hr in Medium 199 containing 10% tryptose phosphate broth and the indicated concentrations of phorbol ester. The culture fluids were collected, concentrated 10-fold, activated with trypsin, and assayed for collagenase.

was obtained with 10^{-8} to 10^{-7} M TPA. 90 to 95% of the collagenase produced by these cells was in a latent form and could be detected only after first treating the conditioned medium with trypsin.

To determine if the stimulation of collagenase production by endothelial cells is a general property of phorbol esters, analogs of TPA were tested for their ability to stimulate collagenase production. Phorbol didecanoate (PDD), an analog of TPA that is a potent tumor promoter, also stimulated collagenase production at the same concentrations that were effective for TPA (Table 1). 4-0-methyl TPA (4-0-Me TPA) and 4α-PDD, two analogs of TPA that are inactive as tumor promoters, did not stimulate collagenase production at concentrations up to 10^{-7} M (Table 1). Thus, the stimulation of collagenase production seems to be limited to phorbol esters that are active as tumor promoters.

The stimulation of collagenase production by TPA was rapid. Increased accumulation of collagenase could be detected in cultures of endothelial cells by 3 hr after the addition of 10^{-7} M TPA (Table 2). Endothelial cells produced collagenase at an elevated rate as long as TPA was present in the medium. When TPA-stimulated cells were changed to TPA-free medium, they continued to produce collagenase at the stimulated rate for 24 hr and then returned to basal levels of production over the next 24 hr, demonstrating that the effect of TPA is reversible.

Synthesis of both new ribonucleic acid (RNA) and new protein was necessary for the stimulation of collagenase production by TPA. Addition of the protein synthesis inhibitor cycloheximide (3 μg/ml) to endothelial cell cultures inhibited the stimulation of collagenase production by TPA and also inhibited basal levels of production in unstimulated cells (Table 2). Likewise, the RNA synthesis inhibitor actinomycin D (0.1 μg/ml) inhibited both the stimulation of collagenase production by TPA and the basal levels of production in unstimulated cells (Table 2).

TABLE 2. *Time course of the effects of TPA, cycloheximide, or actinomycin D on collagenase production by endothelial cells*[a]

Additions to the medium	Collagenase activity mU/10^5 cells					
	0 hr	3 hr	5.5 hr	11 hr	14 hr	24 hr
None	0	0.05	0.09	0.21	0.25	0.65
10^{-7} M TPA	0	0.24	1.17	4.30	10.4	17.3
3 μg/ml cycloheximide	0			0.09		0.16
10^{-7} M TPA + 3 μg/ml cycloheximide	0			0.14		0.24
0.1 μg/ml actinomycin D	0			0.08		0.10
10^{-7} M TPA + 0.1 μg/ml actinomycin D	0			0.11		0.13

[a] Human endothelial cells were grown to confluency in T-75 flasks in Medium 199 containing 20% human serum. The medium was removed, the cells were washed, and the wash fluid was replaced with Medium 199 containing tryptose phosphate broth and the indicated concentrations of TPA, cycloheximide, and actinomycin D. Aliquots of the culture media were collected at the indicated times, were concentrated 20-fold, activated with trypsin, and assayed for collagenase. One unit (U) of collagenase is the amount of collagenase required to degrade 1 μg of collagen in 1 hr at 25°C.

The production of collagenase by several other cell types can be inhibited by glucocorticoids (4,9). In contrast to the findings with other cells, dexamethasone at concentrations up to 10^{-6} M did not affect collagenase production by either TPA-stimulated or unstimulated endothelial cells.

The collagenase produced by human endothelial cells was further characterized. The endothelial cell collagenase has the same inhibitor specificity as all other known vertebrate collagenases and was inhibited by ethylenediaminetetraacetate (EDTA) and serum but not by inhibitors of serine, thiol, or aspartate proteases. The endothelial cell collagenase cleaves collagen at one site, producing fragments that are three-quarters and one-quarter of the length of the intact molecule. These fragments correspond to the TC_A and TC_B fragments characteristic of the cleavage of collagen by vertebrate collagenases. Thus, the endothelial cell collagenase seems to be a typical vertebrate collagenase.

The latent endothelial cell collagenase could be activated by plasmin as well as by trypsin. If human endothelial cells produced plasminogen activator (PA), their PA could convert plasminogen, which is abundant in the plasma and in tissue spaces, to plasmin. The plasmin would activate the latent collagenase produced by the endothelial cells and serve as a general protease in the invasive process. Therefore, we investigated if the human endothelial cells produce PA in response to TPA.

Initially we could not detect PA activity in TPA-treated human endothelial cells. This was due to the presence of a potent inhibitor of PA that was produced by these cells. If human endothelial cells were extracted with 2 M NaSCN, however, PA activity could be separated from the inhibitor. NaSCN extracts of TPA-treated cultures yielded three times as much PA activity as NaSCN extracts of untreated cultures. Although the levels of PA detected were very low, there may have been enough to generate local high concentrations of plasmin around the endothelial cells.

We have shown that endothelial cells respond to TPA by producing two proteases, collagenase and plasminogen activator, which may be important in the invasive process. This suggests that TPA mimics the action of the physiological regulator of neovascularization. It may be possible to use stimulation of collagenase production in endothelial cell cultures as an assay system in the purification of the physiological molecule.

ACKNOWLEDGMENTS

This work was supported by grants from the National Institutes of Health HL-18828 and CA-23753, the American Cancer Society CD77, and the Arnold R. Krakower Hematology Foundation. DM was supported by a training grant from the NIH (CA-09161).

REFERENCES

1. Ausprunk, D. H., and Folkman, J. (1977): Migration and proliferation of endothelial cells in preformed and newly formed blood vessels during tumor angiogenesis. *Microvasc. Res.,* 14:53–65.
2. Brinckerhoff, C. E., McMillan, R. M., Fahey, J. V., and Harris, E. D. (1979): Collagenase production by synovial fibroblasts treated with phorbol myristate acetate. *Arthritis Rheum.,* 22:1,109–1,116.
3. Folkman, J. (1975): Tumor angiogenesis. In: *Cancer—A Comprehensive Treatise, Vol. 3,* edited by F. F. Becker, pp. 355–388. Plenum Press, New York.
4. Koob, T. J., Jeffrey, J. J., and Eisen, A. Z. (1974): Regulation of human skin collagenase activity by hydrocortisone and dexamethasone in organ culture. *Biochem. Biophys. Res. Commun.,* 61:1,083–1,088.
5. Levin, E. G., and Loskutoff, D. J. (1979): Comparative studies of the fibrinolytic activity of cultured vascular cells. *Thromb. Res.,* 15:869–878.
6. Loskutoff, D. J., and Edgington, T. S. (1977): Synthesis of a fibrinolytic activator and inhibitor by endothelial cells. *Proc. Natl. Acad. Sci. USA,* 74:3,903–3,907.
7. Moscatelli, D., Jaffe, E. A., and Rifkin, D. B. (1980): Tetradecanoylphorbol acetate stimulates latent collagenase production by cultured human endothelial cells. *Cell,* 20:343–351.
8. Reddi, A. H., and Huggins, C. B. (1972): Biochemical sequences in the transformation of normal fibroblasts in adolescent rats. *Proc. Natl. Acad. Sci. USA,* 69:1,601–1,605.
9. Werb, Z. (1978): Biochemical actions of glucocorticoids on macrophages in culture. Specific inhibition of elastase, collagenase, and plasminogen activator secretion and effects on other metabolic functions. *J. Exp. Med.,* 147:1,695–1,712.

Carcinogenesis, Vol. 7, edited by E. Hecker et al.
Raven Press, New York © 1982.

Cell Differentiation, Alterations in Polyamine Levels, and Specific Binding of Phorbol Diesters in Cultured Human Cells

*Eliezer Huberman, Charles Weeks, Virendra Solanki,
*Michael Callaham, and Thomas Slaga

Biology Division, Oak Ridge National Laboratory, Oak Ridge, Tennessee 37830

The concept of chemical carcinogenesis is that of a multistage process that is probably initiated by a somatic mutation caused by the carcinogen. Indeed, various studies have demonstrated the capacity of a large number of chemical carcinogens to induce mutations (7,20,23,25,26,31). It is also presumed that in human or animal cells, these mutations may involve the genes controlling the expression of malignant transformations (3,6,19,24). Other studies, however, have indicated that certain environmental agents may act during the subsequent stages of the carcinogenesis process to promote tumor formation (2,4,16,42,45). The action of these tumor promoters may be a rate-limiting determinant in carcinogenesis since mutagens are ubiquitous in nature. In view of this, it is important to elucidate the mode of action and to identify environmental chemicals that may act as tumor promoters. Although we do not know the exact mechanism by which these environmental chemicals promote tumor formation, it is known that many of these agents are devoid of mutagenic activity in the various bacterial and mammalian mutagenesis assays. These chemicals, most likely, promote tumor formation not by a mutational mechanism but rather by another process, such as altering cellular differentiation processes. Indeed, phorbol-12-myristate-13-acetate (PMA) and related phorbol diesters, which are tumor promoters in a two-stage skin carcinogenesis system, were found to alter cell differentiation in some avian and murine cells (8,9,28,29,33,35,47).

INDUCTION OF CELL DIFFERENTIATION IN HUMAN MELANOMA AND MYELOID LEUKEMIA CELLS

It was, therefore, of interest to determine if human cells will respond in a similar way. To accomplish this we studied the effect of tumor promoters such as the phorbol diesters in cultured human HO melanoma (18) and human HL-60 promyelocytic leukemia cells (17). These cells were chosen since they display

* Present address: Division of Biological and Medical Research, Argonne National Laboratory, Argonne, Illinois 60439

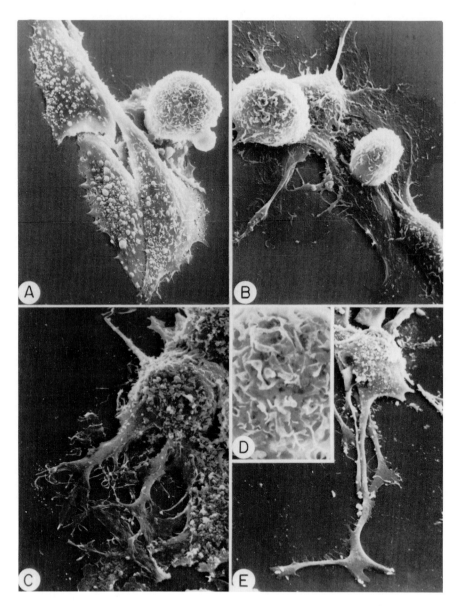

FIG. 1. Scanning electron microscopic morphology of human HO melanoma cells. **A:** An untreated control; **B:** 4-hr treatment with 4×10^{-8} PMA: **C:** 8-hr treatment with PMA; **D:** high magnification view of ridges on the surface of an 8-hr cell; and **E:** 24-hr treatment with PMA. **A** to **C** $\times$ 1,600 **D** $\times$ 3,530; and **E** $\times$ 1,115. From Huberman et al., ref. 18.

useful markers of cell differentiation and allow the study of the mode of action of chemicals that can induce or inhibit cell differentiation.

Our studies with the HO melanoma cells indicated that PMA, at doses of 5×10^{-10} to 5×10^{-7} M, caused a stimulation of various markers of cell differentiation (18). These included inhibition of cell growth, stimulation of melanin synthesis, and formation of dendrite-like structures (Fig. 1). Phorbol-12, 13-dibutyrate (PDBu), which is less active than PMA in the mouse skin, required higher doses to produce an effect comparable to that of PMA. Whereas phorbol-12, 13-diacetate (PDA), and 4-O-methyl PMA (4-O-mPMA), both of which lack tumor-promoting activity, were either inactive or elicited a poor response. In the HL-60 leukemia cells, PMA induced cell differentiation at doses as low as 6×10^{-11} M (17). In this cell system, differentiation was characterized by an inhibition of cell growth and by increases in the percent of morphologically mature cells, phagocytosis (Fig. 2), and lysozyme activity (17,28,36,37). In analyzing the effect of 10 different phorbol esters, we found that, as in the case of HO melanoma cells, their ability to induce differentiation in the HL-60 leukemia cells correlated with their tumor-promoting activity in the mouse skin (Fig. 3) (17).

These results suggest that some human cell types that can be induced to differentiate by chemical agents may represent a useful tool by which some known tumor-promoting agents can be studied and new ones may perhaps be detected.

ALTERATION IN POLYAMINE LEVELS INDUCED BY PHORBOL DIESTERS AND OTHER AGENTS THAT PROMOTE DIFFERENTIATION IN THE HL-60 CELLS

The physiologically occurring polyamines, putrescine, spermidine, and spermine, have been shown to be involved in the regulation of cell growth and in tumor promotion (22,38,40,44,46). It was also suggested that they may play a role in the control of cell differentiation (11,14,15,41). It was therefore of interest to determine the possible involvement of these polyamines in the control of cell growth and differentiation in human HL-60 leukemia cells.

Treatment of the HL-60 cells with either PMA or phorbol-12,13-didecanoate (PDD) resulted in increased levels of putrescine (Fig. 4 and Table 1) (21). Furthermore, no increase in putrescine could be detected after PMA treatment of a HL-60 cell variant, designated as R-20, which exhibited a reduced susceptibility to PMA-induced differentiation (Fig. 5) (21). These cells were isolated after subculturing the HL-60 cells for 20 subcultures (5- to 8-day intervals) in the presence of 5×10^{-10} M PMA. Similarly, no increase in putrescine was observed with two non-tumor promoters, PDA and 4-O-mPMA, or with anthralin, a non-phorbol-type tumor promoter (Table 1). The increase in putrescine levels, after PMA treatment preceded the expression of the induced PMA differentiation markers (Figs. 4 and 5). In addition to enhancing putrescine levels, PMA also increased the amount of spermidine and decreased the amount of spermine

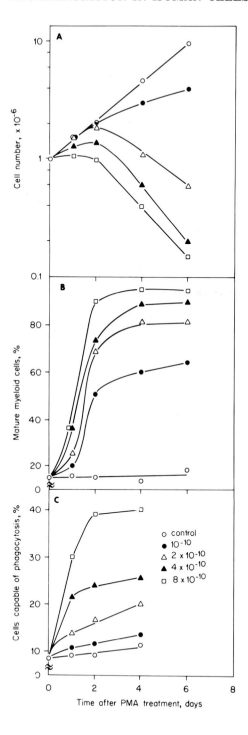

(Fig. 4). Unlike these changes the activities of ornithine decarboxylase (ODC) and S-adenosylmethionine decarboxylase (SAMD) (22,40), which are polyamine biosynthetic enzymes, did not significantly change. α-Methylornithine (MO) (1, 34), α-difluoromethylornithine (DFMO) (30), and methylglyoxal bis-(guanyl-hydrazone) (MGBG) (34), which are inhibitors of the polyamine biosynthetic enzymes, also did not affect differentiation in control or PMA-treated cells. Furthermore, the addition of exogenous polyamines did not affect cell differentiation in either control or PMA-treated HL-60 cells.

Because of these observations, we suggest that the changes in polyamine levels may involve biochemical pathways other than the known biosynthetic ones. Furthermore, these pathways, or their byproducts, may be involved in the control of cell growth and differentiation in the HL-60 cells. Transglutaminase(s) may be an example of such a case, since they use polyamines as their physiological substrates (12). It is interesting to note that transglutaminases were found to be involved in membrane and receptor functions which are critical targets for the control cell growth and differentiation (27, 43).

SPECIFIC BINDING OF [³H]PDBu in HL-60 CELLS

The mechanism of induction of differentiation in susceptible cells, including HL-60, is yet unknown. Changes in cell morphology, however, and in lipid biosynthesis (5,17,36) lend themselves to the suggestion that the primary site of PMA action in the HL-60 cells is the cell surface. Blumberg and his associates (10) have demonstrated specific binding of PDBu, an active phorbol derivative that is less lipophilic than PMA, to chicken embryo fibroblasts, mouse skin, and nerve cells. It was therefore of interest to determine if this binding is associated with the induction of differentiation in HL-60 cells by phorbol diesters. To accomplish this, we have analyzed specific [³H]PDBu binding in susceptible and resistant HL-60 cells (39). As resistant cells we used the HL-60 R-35 variant cells which were the R-20 cells (Fig. 5) (21) after 15 additional subcultures in the presence of 5×10^{-10} M PMA. These R-35 cells were not susceptible to the induction of differentiation by either PMA or PDBu at doses up to 3×10^{-7} M. We found that the variance in the response of HL-60 and R-35 cells to PMA- or PDBu-induced cell differentiation was not due to either the number of binding sites or the affinity of [³H]PDBu specific binding sites (Fig. 6), but

---

FIG. 2. Cell growth **(A)**, percent of morphologically mature cells **(B)**, and phagocytosis **(C)** in HL-60 cells at different times after treatment with different concentrations of PMA. The cultures were treated a day after seeding 5×10^5 cells in 5 ml of growth medium in 60-mm Petri dishes. Cells were counted to determine cell growth and stained with Wright-Giemsa stain to determine the percent of mature and phagocytizing cells. The mature cells were composed mainly of myelocytes and metamyelocytes. A small fraction of banded and segmented cells was also observed. Phagocytosis was determined after the HL-60 cells were incubated for 30 min with 4×10^6 cells per ml of the diploid *S. cervisiae* strain XY 664. Control: ○, PMA: ●, 10^{-10} M; △, 2×10^{-10} M; ▲, 4×10^{-10} M; □, 8×10^{-10} M. From Huberman and Callaham, ref. 17.

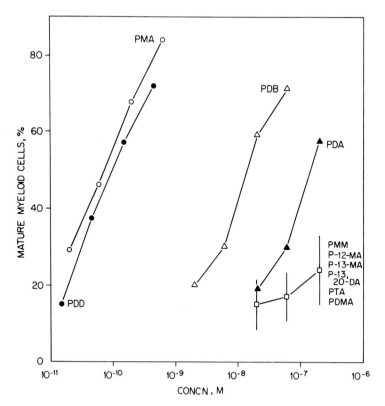

FIG. 3. Percent morphologically mature HL-60 cells at 2 days after treatment with different phorbol esters. The percent of morphologically mature cells was determined after cells were stained with Wright-Giemsa. The control cultures contained about 15% mature cells. ○, PMA; ●, PDD; △, PDBu; ▲, PDA; □, phorbol-12-monomyristate, phorbol-12-monoacetate, phorbol-13-monoacetate, phorbol-13,20-diacetate, phorbol-12,13,20-triacetate, and phorbol-20-oxo-12-myristate-13-acetate. From Huberman and Callaham, ref. 17.

rather to the down regulation (i.e., loss of PDBu bound to the cells) of bound PDBu following maximal specific binding. This was deduced from the fact that the down regulation of bound [^{3}H]PDBu seen in HL-60 was not observed in R-35 cells (Fig. 7 and Table 2). This down regulation was temperature dependent, as no loss of radiolabel occurred by 1 hr at 4°C. This apparent down regulation of [^{3}H]PDBu could result from conformational changes in the PDBu binding sites or perhaps, more likely, from internalization of the phorbol ester binding sites and their degradation by lysosomal enzymes (13,32). It must be emphasized at this point, however, that we do not have any data to prove either case.

Based on these and other studies, we can suggest that down regulation of specific PDBu binding is an important phenomenon involved in the mechanism of action of phorbol esters and may lead to the modification of the various biological and biochemical events involved in cellular differentiation and perhaps also in tumor promotion.

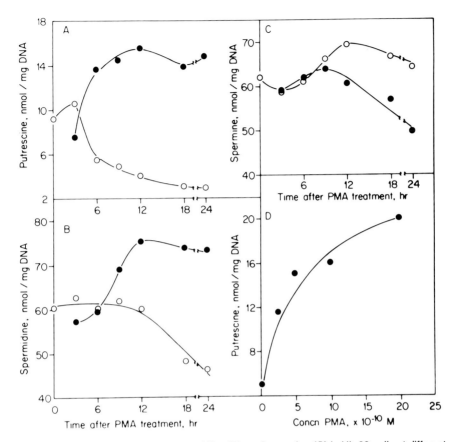

FIG. 4. The level of putrescine **(A)**, spermidine **(B)**, and spermine **(C)** in HL-60 cells at different times after treatment with 5×10^{-10} M PMA. **D:** Amount of putrescine at 12 hr after treatment with PMA at different concentrations. ●, PMA; ○ control. From Huberman et al., ref. 21.

Based on the present results we can conclude that human HO melanoma and HL-60 leukemia cells may be useful for the study of the mode of action of some known tumor promoters and may also be helpful in the identification of some unknown classes of tumor-promoting agents.

ACKNOWLEDGMENTS

This research was sponsored jointly by the National Cancer Institute under Interagency Agreement 40-636-77; Environmental Protection Agency under Interagency Agreement 79-D-X0533; and the Office of Health and Environmental Research, U.S. Department of Energy, under contract W-7405-eng-26 with the Union Carbide Corporation. V. S. was a postdoctoral investigator supported by subcontract no. 3322 from the Biology Division of Oak Ridge National Laboratory to the University of Tennessee.

TABLE 1. *The relationship between percent morphologically mature HL-60 cells and putrescine levels after treatment with anthralin and phorbol diesters*

Treatment[a]	Tumor-promoting activity	Morphologically mature cells (%)[b]	Putrescine level nmole/mg DNA[c]
Anthralin	+	11	3
PDA	−	12	3
4-O-mPMA	−	15	4
PDD	+++	70	10
PMA	+++	85	13

[a] The HL-60 cells were treated with 5×10^{-10} M of the phorbol esters and 4×10^{-4} M anthralin.

[b] The percent of the morphologically mature cells was determined 2 days after incubation with phorbol diesters and 5 days after incubation with anthralin. The control contained 12 and 15% mature cells after 2 and 5 days, respectively.

[c] Putrescine levels were determined 12 hr after treatment with the inducer. The control value was 4 nmole of putrescine per mg of cellular deoxyribonucleic acid (DNA). The differences in putrescine values between treated and control were highly reproducible in four separate experiments. From Huberman et al. (21).

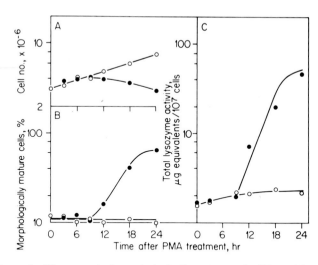

FIG. 5. Cell growth **(A)**, percent of morphologically mature cells **(B)**, and lysozyme activity **(C)** in HL-60 and R-20 cells at different times after treatment with 5×10^{-10} M PMA. The cultures were treated 1 day after seeding 1×10^6 cells in 10 ml of growth medium in 100-mm Petri dishes. The morphologically mature cells were composed mainly from myelocyte and metamyelocyte-like cells. A small fraction of cells with banded and segmented-like nuclei was observed. ●, HL-60; ○, R-20. From Huberman et al., ref. 21.

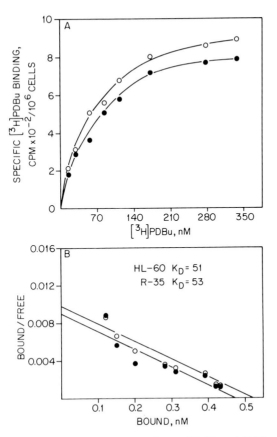

FIG. 6. **A:** Equilibrium of specific [³H]PDBu binding to HL-60 and R-35 cells as a function of ligand concentration. Incubation was carried out at 4°C in the absence and presence of 30 μM unlabeled PDBu for 45 min. **B:** Specific binding of [³H]PDBu represented by the method of Scatchard. ○, HL-60; ●, R-35. From Solanki et al., ref. 39.

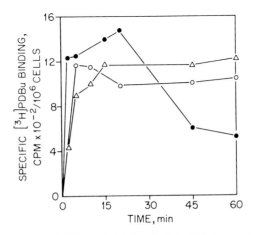

FIG. 7. Time course of specific [³H]PDBu binding to intact HL-60 cells at 37°C (●) and at 4°C (○), and to R-35 cells at 37°C (△). From Solanki et al., ref. 39.

TABLE 2. *Effect of prior exposure of HL-60 and R-35 cells with PMA on specific* [³H]PDBu binding[a]

	Specific [³H]PDBu binding (%)			
	HL-60		R-35	
Pretreatment with	~27 nM	~82 nM	~27 nM	~82 nM
Saline	100	150	100	147
PMA (1 μM)	22	33	97	150

[a] Specific binding was measured at 27 nM and 82 nM labeled PDBu at 4°C, following 90-min exposure of the cells with saline or 1 μM PMA at 37°C. The amount of specific binding at 27 nM [³H]PDBu without PMA pretreatment was considered as 100%. Cells were washed with 2 × 1 ml cold physiological buffered saline (PBS) (pH 7.4) before incubation at 4°C. From Solanki et al. (39).

REFERENCES

1. Abdel-Monem, M. M., Newton, N. E., and Weeks, C. E. (1974): Inhibitors of polyamine biosynthesis. I. α-Methylornithine, an inhibitor of ornithine decarboxylase. *J. Med. Chem.,* 17:447–451.
2. Berenblum, I. (1969): A reevaluation of the concept of cocarcinogenesis. *Prog. Exp. Tumor Res.,* 11:21–30.
3. Bouck, N., and DiMayorca, G. (1976): Somatic mutation as the basis for malignant transformation of BHK cells by chemical carcinogens. *Nature (Lond.),* 264:360–361.
4. Boutwell, R. K. (1974): Function and mechanism of promoters of carcinogenesis. *CRC Crit. Rev. Toxicol.,* 2:419–447.
5. Cabot, M., Welsh, C. J., Callaham, M. F., and Huberman, E. (1980): Alteration in lipid metabolism induced by 12-O-tetradecanoylphorbol-13-acetate in differentiating human myeloid leukemia cells. *Cancer Res.,* 40:3,674–3,679.
6. Cairns, J. (1975): Mutation selection and the natural history of cancer. *Nature (Lond.),* 255:197–200.
7. Clive, D., Johnson, K. O., Spector, J. F. S., Batson, A. G., and Brown, M. M. M. (1979): Validation and characterization of the L5178YTK[+−] mouse lymphoma mutagen assay system. *Mutat. Res.,* 59:61–108.
8. Cohen, R., Pacifici, M., Rubenstein, N., Biehl, J., and Holtzer, H. (1977): Effect of a tumor promoter on myogenesis. *Nature (Lond.),* 266:538–540.
9. Diamond, L., O'Brien, T. G., and Rovera, G. (1977): Inhibition of adipose conversion of 313 fibroblasts by tumor promoters. *Nature (Lond.),* 269:247–248.
10. Driedger, P. E., and Blumberg, P. M. (1980): Specific binding of phorbol ester tumor promoters. *Proc. Natl. Acad. Sci. USA,* 77:576–581.
11. Emanuelsson, H., and Heby, O. (1978): Inhibition of putrescine synthesis blocks development of the polychete *Ophryotrocha labronica* at gastrulation. *Proc. Natl. Acad. Sci. USA,* 75:1,039–1,042.
12. Folk, J. E., Park, M. H., Chung, S. I., Schrode, J., Lester, E. P., and Cooper, H. L. (1980): Polyamines as physiological substrates for transglutaminases. *J. Biol. Chem.,* 255:3,695–3,700.
13. Fox, C. F., and Das, M. (1979): Internalization and processing of the EGF receptor in the induction of DNA synthesis in cultured fibroblasts: The endocytic activation hypothesis. *J. Supramol. Struct.,* 10:199–214.
14. Fozard, J. R., Part, M-L., Prakash, N. J., Grove, J., Shechter, P. J., Sjoerdsma, A., and Koch-Weser, J. (1980): L-ornithine decarboxylase: An essential role in early mammalian embryogenesis. *Science,* 208:505–508.
15. Gazitt, Y., and Friend, C. (1980): Polyamine biosynthesis enzymes in the induction and inhibition of differentiation in Friend erythroleukemia cells. *Cancer Res.,* 40:1,727–1,732.

16. Hecker, E. (1978): Structure-activity relationships in diterpene esters irritant and cocarcinogenic to mouse skin. In: *Mechanisms of Tumor Promotion and Cocarcinogenesis,* edited by T. J. Slaga and R. K. Boutwell, pp. 11–48. Raven Press, New York.

17. Huberman, E., and Callaham, M. (1979): Induction of terminal differentiation in human promyelocytic leukemia cells by tumor-promoting agents. *Proc. Natl. Acad. Sci. USA,* 76:1,293–1,297.

18. Huberman, E., Heckman, C., and Langenbach, R. (1979): Stimulation of differentiated functions in human melanoma cells by tumor-promoting agents and dimethylsulfoxide. *Cancer Res.,* 39:2,618–2,624.

19. Huberman, E., Mager, R., and Sachs, L. (1976): Mutagenesis and transformation of normal cells by chemical carcinogens. *Nature,* 264:360–361.

20. Huberman, E., and Sachs, L. (1976): Mutability of different genetic loci in mammalian cells by metabolically activated carcinogenic polycyclic hydrocarbons. *Proc. Natl. Acad. Sci. USA,* 731:188–192.

21. Huberman, E., Weeks, C. E., Herrmann, A., Callaham, M., and Slaga, T. J. (1981): Alterations in polyamine levels induced by phorbol diesters and other agents that promote differentiation in human promyelocytic leukemia cells. *Proc. Natl. Acad. Sci. USA,* 78:1,062–1,066.

22. Janne, J., Poso, H., and Raina, A. (1978): Polyamines in rapid growth and cancer. *Biochim. Biophys. Acta,* 473:241–293.

23. Jones, C. A., and Huberman, E. (1980): A sensitive hepatocyte-mediated assay for the metabolism of nitrosamines to mutagens for mammalian cells. *Cancer Res.,* 40:406–411.

24. Knudsen, A. G., Jr., Hetchcote, H. W., and Brown, B. W. (1975): Mutation and childhood cancer: A probabilistic model for the incidence of retinoblastoma. *Proc. Natl. Acad. Sci. USA,* 72:5,166.

25. Krahn, D. F., and Heidelberger, C. (1977): Liver homogenate-mediated mutagenesis in Chinese hamster V79 cells by polycyclic aromatic hydrocarbons and aflatoxins. *Mutat. Res.,* 46:27–44.

26. Kuroki, T., Drevon, C., and Montesano, R. (1977): Microsome-mediated mutagenesis in V79 Chinese hamster cells by various nitrosamines. *Cancer Res.,* 37:1,044–1,050.

27. Levitzki, A., Willingham, M., and Pastan, I. (1980): Evidence for participation of transglutaminase in receptor-mediated endocytosis. *Proc. Natl. Acad. Sci. USA,* 77:2,706–2,710.

28. Lotem, J., and Sachs, L. (1979): Regulation of normal differentiation in mouse and human myeloid leukemia cells by phorbol esters and the mechanism of tumor promotion. *Proc. Natl. Acad. Sci. USA,* 76:5,158–5,162.

29. Lowe, M. E., Pacifico, M., and Holtzer, H. (1978): Effects of phorbol-12-myristate-13-acetate on the phenotypic program of cultured chondroblasts and fibroblasts. *Cancer Res.,* 38:2,350–2,356.

30. Mamont, P., Duchesne, M-C., Grove, J., and Bey, P. (1978): Antiproliferative properties of *DL-α*-difluoromethylornithine in cultured cells. A consequence of the irreversible inhibition of ornithine decarboxylase. *Biochem. Biophys. Res. Commun.,* 81:59–66.

31. McCann, J. B., and Ames, B. N. (1976): Detection of carcinogens as mutagens in the Salmonella microsome test: Assay of 300 chemicals. Discussion. *Proc. Natl. Acad. Sci. USA,* 73:950–954.

32. McKanna, J. A., Haigler, H. T., and Cohen, S. (1979): Hormone receptor topology and dynamics: Morphological analysis using ferritin-labeled epidermal growth factor. *Proc. Natl. Acad. Sci. USA,* 76:5,689–5,693.

33. Miao, R. M., Fieldsteel, A. H., and Fodge, D. W. (1978): Opposing effects of tumor promoters on erythroid differentiation. *Nature,* 274:271–272.

34. Newton, N. E., and Abdel-Monem, M. M. (1977): Inhibitors of polyamine biosynthesis. 4. Effects of α-methyl(±) ornithine and methylglyoxal bis(guanylhydrazone) on growth and polyamine content of L1210 leukemic cells of mice. *J. Med. Chem.,* 20:249–253.

35. Rovera, G., O'Brien, T. A., and Diamond, L. (1977): Tumor promoters inhibit spontaneous differentiation of Friend erythroleukemia cells in cultures. *Proc. Natl. Acad. Sci. USA,* 74:2,894–2,898.

36. Rovera, G., O'Brien, T. G., and Diamond, L. (1979): Induction of differentiation in human promyelocytic leukemia cells by tumor promoters. *Science,* 204:868–870.

37. Rovera, G., Santoli, D., and Damsky, C. (1979): Human promyelocytic leukemia cells in culture differentiate into macrophage-like cells when treated with a phorbol diester. *Proc. Natl. Acad. Sci. USA,* 76:2,779–2,783.

38. Rupniak, H. T., and Paul, D. (1978): Regulation of the cell cycle by polyamines in normal

and transformed fibroblasts. In: *Advances in Polyamine Research, Vol. 1,* edited by R. A. Campbell, D. R. Morres, D. Bartos, G. D. Daves, and F. Bartos, pp. 117–126. Raven Press, New York.

39. Solanki, V., Slaga, T. J., Callaham, M., and Huberman, E. (1981): The down regulation of specific binding of [20-³H]phorbol-12,13-dibutyrate- and phorbol ester-induced differentiation of human promyelocytic leukemia cells. *Proc. Natl. Acad. Sci. USA,* 78:1,722–1,725.
40. Tabor, C. W., and Tabor, H. (1976): 1,4-Diaminobutane (putrescine), spermidine, and spermine. *Annu. Rev. Biochem.,* 45:285–306.
41. Takigawa, M., Ishida, H., Teruko, T., and Suzuki, F. (1980): Polyamine and differentiation: Induction of ornithine decarboxylase by parathyroid hormone is a good marker of differentiated chondrocytes. *Proc. Natl. Acad. Sci. USA,* 77:1,481–1,485.
42. Van Duuren, B. L. (1969): Tumor-promoting agents in two-stage carcinogenesis. *Prog. Exp. Tumor Res.,* 11:31–38.
43. Van Leuven, F., Cassiman, J. J., and Van Den Berghe, H. (1980): Primary amines inhibit recycling of α₂M receptors in fibroblasts. *Cell,* 20:37–43.
44. Weeks, C. E., and Slaga, T. J. (1979): Inhibition of phorbol ester polyamine accumulation in mouse epidermis by antiinflammatory steroid. *Biochem. Biophys. Res. Commun.,* 91:1,488–1,496.
45. Weinstein, I. B., Wigler, M., Fisher, P. B., Sisskin, E., and Pietropaolo, C. (1978): Cell culture studies on biological effects of tumor promoters. In: *Carcinogenesis, Mechanism of Tumor Promotion and Cocarcinogenesis, Vol. 2,* edited by T. J. Slaga, A. Sivak, and R. K. Boutwell, pp. 313–333. Raven Press, New York.
46. Yuspa, S. H., Lichti, U., Ben, T., Patterson, E., Hennings, H., Slaga, T., Colburn, N., and Kelsey, W. (1976): Phorbol esters stimulate DNA synthesis and ornithine decarboxylase activity in mouse epidermal cell cultures. *Nature,* 262:402–404.
47. Yamasaki, H., Fibach, E., Nudel, U., Weinstein, I. B., Rifkind, R. A., and Marks, P. A. (1977): Tumor promoters inhibit spontaneous and induced differentiation of murine erythroleukemia cells in cultures. *Proc. Natl. Acad. Sci. USA,* 74:3,451–3,456.

Carcinogenesis, Vol. 7, edited by E. Hecker et al.
Raven Press, New York © 1982.

How Can Altered Differentiation Induced by 12-O-Tetradecanoylphorbol-13-acetate Be Related to Tumor Promotion?

Manfred Schwab

Genetisches Institut der Justus-Liebig-Universität, D-6300 Giessen,
Federal Republic of Germany

There exist a number of reports dealing with 12-O-tetradecanoylphorbol-13-acetate (TPA)-induced alteration of differentiation of normal and of transformed cells. In certain systems TPA induces further differentiation, whereas in others it inhibits this process (for comprehensive review, see ref. 5.). But the crucial question of what role TPA-induced alteration of differentiation plays in tumor promotion is far from being answered yet. This chapter attempts to relate in *Xiphophorus*, using pigment cell neoplasia as the experimental system, TPA-altered differentiation and tumor promotion. It furthermore intends to stimulate continued experimentation on the two-step concept of carcinogenesis under the perspective of "initiation" as genetic change in its broadest sense (point mutation, chromosome rearrangement) and "promotion" as a process affecting cellular differentiation, thereby putting together the two often mutually exclusive cancer etiologies decribed as processes of "somatic mutation" and "altered differentiation."

Xiphophorus was introduced to cancer research in 1927 by Myron Gordon (New York), Curt Kosswig (Münster), and Georg Häussler (Heidelberg). The feature originally attracting attention was that all species can be mated to each other to yield fully fertile hybrids. The combination of the distantly evolved genomes confers to the hybrids in a Mendelian fashion either the capacity for development of "spontaneous" pigment cell neoplasia (2,6) or the susceptibility for a large spectrum of neoplasms to be induced by carcinogens, notably by the direct acting nitrosamide N-methyl-N-nitrosourea (MNU) or X-rays. This is in contrast to the nonhybrid species that are highly resistant (9–11; for last comprehensive presentation, see ref. 2).

This chapter will first give a short introduction to genetic control of pigment cell neoplasia in *Xiphophorus* as relevant to "initiation" and "promotion." It will then report some preliminary data on biological effects of TPA in pigment cell neoplasia, and finally will set up a system that might be useful in further

---

Dr. Schwab's present address is Department of Microbiology and Immunology, School of Medicine, University of California, San Francisco, California 94143.

analyzing *in vivo* "initiation" and "promotion" (for promotion, see also Schartl et al., *this volume,* describing more advanced studies on the action of hormones).

GENES CONTROLLING PIGMENT CELL NEOPLASIA

This study focuses on neoplastic pigment cells encoded by the corresponding genes of *Xiphophorus maculatus.* Three loci are of relevance: *tumor (Tu), differentiation (Diff),* and *golden (g).*[1]

Tu

The simplest dermal pigment cell phenotype of wildtype *Xiphophorus* consists of melanophores, pterinophores (xanthophores and "erythrophores"), and guanophores (iridophores), distributed more or less uniformly. Observed pigment cell mosaicism (4) would suggest that the three types differentiate from neural crest-derived chromatoblasts (7).

The differentiation of melanophores, on which this chapter focuses, proceeds via the melanoblasts, which have been recently subdivided into the three types (stem, intermediate, and advanced melanoblast) (Fig. 1; 3), to the melanocyte, and eventually the melanophore, earlier described as micromelanophore (6). Certain populations exhibit, in addition, giant melanophores (macromelanophores). These are, according to a recent hypothesis of Anders and Anders (2), due to expression of *Tu,* which is part of the macromelanophore-gene com-

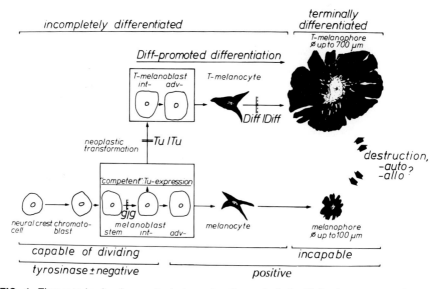

FIG. 1. Elements in development of pigment cell neoplasia in *Xiphophorus,* and action of *Tu, Diff,* and *g.* Stages of pigment cell differentiation and their characteristics are according to ref. 3. Substages of the melanoblast are hypothetical. int-: intermediate; adv-: advanced; T-: neoplastically transformed (neoplastic).

---

[1] These should be regarded as operational terms until molecular data on their structure and function are available.

plexes. Normally *Tu* is controlled by regulating genes *(R)* that are nonlinked and/or linked to *Tu* (2). In case R genes are eliminated by interspecific hybridizations (in the case of nonlinked *R*), or are inactivated by mutagens (in case of linked *R*), *Tu* may transform a "competent" melanoblast (Fig. 1) into a neoplastic one. The result is malignant pigment cell neoplasia (melanoma) consisting predominantly of incompletely differentiated dividing cells, or benign neoplasia consisting predominantly of terminally differentiated, nondividing neoplastic melanophores (12; Fig. 2d,f, and h, versus a,c,e, and g).

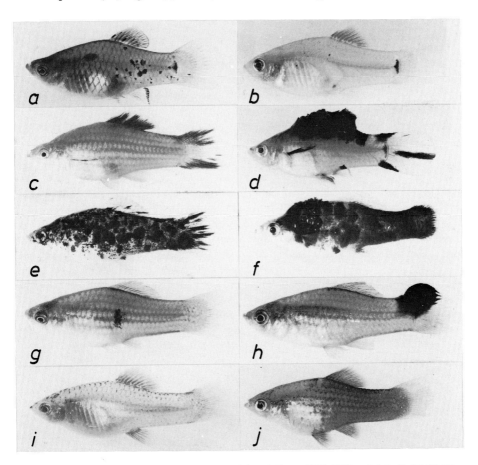

FIG. 2. Influence of *Diff* and *g* on the expressivity of *Tu*. **a:** $Diff^+/Diff^+$, g^+/g^+, Tu^{Sp+}/Tu^{Sd+}; **b:** $Diff^+/Diff^+$, g/g, Tu^{Sp+}/Tu^{Sd+}; **c:** $Diff^+/Diff$, g^+/g^+, Tu^{Sd+}/Tu^{Sd}; **d:** $Diff/Diff$, g^+/g^+, Tu^{Sd+}/Tu^{Sd}; **e:** $Diff^+/Diff$, g^+/g^+, Tu^{Sp+}/Tu^{Sp}; **f:** $Diff/Diff$, g^+/g^+, Tu^{Sp+}/Tu^{Sp}; **g:** $Diff^+/Diff$, g^+/g^+, Tu^{Sd}/Tu^{Sd}; **h:** $Diff/Diff$, g^+/g^+, Tu^{Sd}/Tu^{Sd}; **i:** $Diff^+/Diff$, g/g, Tu^{Sd+}/Tu^{Sd}; and **j:** $Diff/Diff$, g/g, Tu^{Sd+}/Tu^{Sd}. The abbreviation Tu^{Sd+} refers to *Tu* as part of the macromelanophore-complex locus "spotted dorsal." In accordance, Sp stands for "spotted body side" (see footnote on p. 420). Neoplasia in **a** and **c–f** are "spontaneous," due to interspecific hybridizations; **g** and **h** are "induced" by MNU (from ref. 11). Lack of *Diff* causes malignant phenotype **(d,f,h)**; single doses, benign phenotype **(c,e,f)**; double doses, extremely benign phenotype **(a)**. Homozygosity for *g* protects from development of neoplasia (compare **b** with **a**, and **c–h** with **i–j**).

Deletions of *Tu*, due to translocations (2), lead to loss of capacity for development of neoplastic cells (Fig. 1).

Altogether, *Tu*, which is normally controlled by *R* genes, is thought to transform "competent" melanoblasts in case regulation of *Tu* is impaired or dismantled.

Diff

Genetic analyses revealed the chromosomal gene complex *Diff* (12), in the presence of which neoplastic pigment cells are stimulated to differentiate terminally. Double doses of *Diff* induce nearly all neoplastic melanoblasts to differentiate terminally; in case of a single dose, this effect is less pronounced, leading in both cases to benign neoplasia (Fig. 2a, c,e, and g). Lack of *Diff* causes the neoplastic cells to remain in their incompletely differentiated stage (Fig. 1) and results in malignant neoplasia (Fig. 2d, f, and h). A marker isozyme locus, *Esterase-1 (Est-1)*, chromosomally linked to *Diff* (Fig.3; 1,11) permits the identification of the presence of the *Diff*-carrying chromosome in nearly any genotype.

Mechanistically, the benign state is secondary to the malignant one, and is not a "preneoplastic lesion" as, for instance, papilloma of the rat from which carcinoma gradually may develop. Consequently, benign neoplasia never becomes malignant, except for the rare cases in which neoplastic stem cells are still present and *Diff* undergoes mutation or the effect of *Diff* is overcome by epigenetic modulation (induction or inhibition) of differentiation (2,3,11). In animals carrying *Diff*, carcinogen-induced neoplastic melanophores may eventually be degraded by host mechanisms or degenerate (Fig. 1), resulting in regression of neoplasia (for epigenetic terminal differentiation and regression see Schartl et al., *this volume*.

g

In *X. maculatus* homozygous for the autosomal recessive *g*, dermal melanophores are virtually absent except for a few (compare Fig. 2a and b). In contrast, pterinophores and guanophores develop normally. A feasible hypothesis for the lack of melanophores is that differentiation of the dermal *X. maculatus* melanophores is blocked behind the chromatoblast, according to earlier studies (3) behind the stem melanoblast (Fig. 1; this block may be less effective in other species as described in Schartl et al., *this volume*). Consequently, in *gg* individuals, elimination or mutation of *R* genes controlling *Tu* does not, except for rare cases, lead to pigment cell neoplasia, due to the "precompetent" differentiation block (Fig. 1; e.g. compare 2f, g^+g^+, with 2j, *gg*).[2]

The general feasibility of these genotypes lies in the fact that they clearly

---

[2] The + sign is used for the normal allele with reference to *X. maculatus* in cases of interspecific homozygosity or heterozygosity. This is with the formal assumption that the heterozygous interspecific hybrids *(X. maculatus* × *X. helleri)* have different alleles at the genetic loci in their homologous chromosome segments.

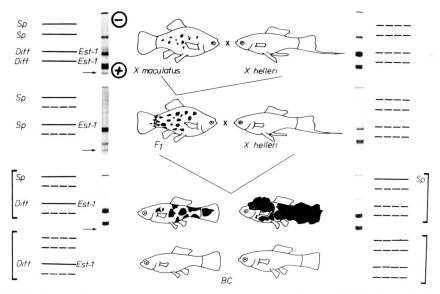

FIG. 3. Means of identification of the *Diff*-carrying chromosome by assaying in polyacrylamide gel electrophoresis for *Est*-1. *Est*-1-locus is chromosomally linked to *Diff* (according to refs. 1 and 11).

demonstrate that genetic change and aberrant differentiation are not, as often discussed, mutually exclusive etiologies of cancer, but, at least in certain cases, are essential elements of the multistep nature of carcinogenesis that only in combination with each other lead to the neoplastic phenotype.

BIOLOGICAL EFFECTS OF TPA IN PIGMENT CELL NEOPLASIA

In the Fish

In order to test if TPA has any effects at all in pigment cell neoplasia of *Xiphophorus,* in a screening experiment approximately 250 fish from 14 different genotypes arbitrarily taken from our breeding colony were exposed to aqueous solution of TPA (1 ng per ml aquarium water; TPA predissolved in acetone). The genotypes are characterized by rigidity of control of *Tu,* i.e., in some genotypes *Tu* is controlled rigidly, in others weakly (details shall be published elsewhere). So far in one genotype, 2 fish individuals characterized by weakly controlled *Tu* developed neoplasia after about 2 months of treatment (Fig. 4). The other genotypes have proved to be resistant so far.

In Cultured Tissue and Cells

In order to test if TPA influences differentiation of pigment cells, total malignant melanoma (from fish as shown in Fig. 2d and f) as well as cultivated

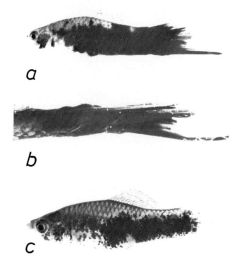

FIG. 4. Pigment cell neoplasia occurring after 2 months continued treatment of fish with TPA (1 ng per ml aquarium water). **a** and **b**: experimentals; **c**: control.

melanophore stem cells, which can be brought to differentiate to neoplastic melanophores upon injection into suitable hosts (M. Schartl, *personal communication*), were treated in culture with TPA (100 ng per ml medium 199; details shall be published elsewhere).

In melanoma, which can be cultivated for up to 24 hr without detectable cellular dysfunction, the activity of tyrosinase, the key enzyme of melanogenesis used as differentiation marker, is increased within that time up to approximately 150% over that of controls (Fig. 5). Concomitantly, synthesis of DNA and of

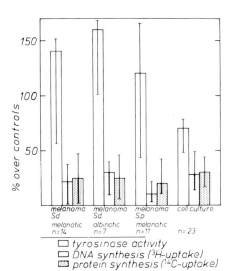

FIG. 5. Effects of TPA (100 ng/ml) on tyrosinase activity, DNA, and protein synthesis in *in vitro* cultivated malignant melanoma (see Fig. 2d and f) and cultivated pigment cell precursors. Time of exposure: melanoma, 24 hr; cells, 15–20 passages.

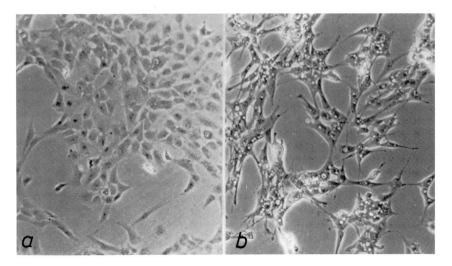

FIG. 6. Long-term effects of TPA (100 ng/ml) on morphology of pigment cell precursors during 15–20 passages. **a:** controls; **b:** exposed cells showing highly dendritic morphology with fine elongated processes.

protein is increased, although to a much lower degree. In cultivated cells a somewhat lower increase of tyrosinase, deoxyribonucleic acid (DNA), and protein synthesis is observed. These cultivated cells change their morphology from spindle-shaped or epithelial to highly dendritic with fine elongated processes upon prolonged exposure throughout 15 to 20 passages (Fig. 6). Melanogenesis was not detected, however.

Interpretation

The apparently narrow host range of TPA induction of melanoma, restricted possibly to genotypes with very weak control of *Tu*, would suggest genetic control of the tumor-promoting activity of TPA. A feasible working hypothesis is that these genotypes transmit "initiation" as an inherited character through their germ line.

An interpretation with respect to "promotion" by TPA might take into account the observed increase of tyrosinase activity and the morphological changes of cultivated cells. Increase of tyrosinase activity could be due to three mechanisms, either alone or in combination with each other: (a) increase of specific activity of the enzyme while the fraction of tyrosinase-positive cells remains constant (Fig. 1); (b) increase of the fraction of tyrosinase-positive cells by mitogenic stimulation, a process that may be indicated by elevated DNA synthesis; and (c) increase of the fraction of tyrosinase-positive cells via TPA-stimulated further differentiation of tyrosinase-negative cells. Although further experiments are required to find out the actual mechanism, the change of morphology of cultivated cells, which may be interpreted as further differentiation, gives some support to the working hypothesis that TPA stimulates further differentiation of pigment cell precursors. Accordingly, "promotion" by TPA might consist of stimulated further differentiation of stem cells to the "competent" stage, in which they can be transformed by Tu (Fig. 1). This hypothesis follows in essence the idea described in Schartl et al. *(this volume)* with respect to the action of hormones in tumor promotion. Thus, TPA seems to mimic hormone action.

The hypothesized action of TPA in tumor promotion shall be further studied in a genetic set-up, making use of the action of Tu, $Diff$, and g, which might be suitable to generate further necessary experimental data.

GENETIC SET-UP TO STUDY INITIATION AND PROMOTION

With the knowledge of the action of Tu, $Diff$, and g in control of neoplasia and the results on TPA, a system is being set up consisting of an array of defined genotypes in which "initiation" by carcinogens can be studied under the perspective of genetic change (point mutation, chromosome rearrangement), and "promotion" under the perspective of aberrant differentiation. This system consists of two groups of genotypes (a) for testing sensitivity, and (b) for testing resistance.

For testing sensitivity, the genotypes should lack $Diff$, which might interfere with the expected alteration of differentiation. In this group four classes of genotypes shall be constructed and subsequently tested (Fig. 7).

(a) Tu^+R/TuR, g^+/g^+; does develop neoplasia "spontaneously," due to derepressed Tu and lack of g (for phenotype, see Fig. 2a,c–f).

(b) Tu^+R^+/TuR, g/g; (phenotype as in Fig. 2i,j); does not develop neoplasia "spontaneously." "Initiation," i.e. carcinogen-inactivation of R leads to derepressed Tu (2,8,11). The neoplastic phenotype can only be expressed in

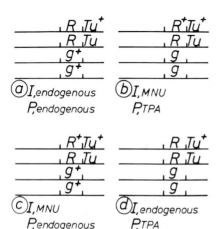

FIG. 7. Genetic set-up for testing carcinogenesis under the two-step concept. I: "Initiation" by MNU leading to mutation of R controlling Tu-expression. P: "Promotion" by TPA overcoming the differentiation block gg resulting in generation of cells "competent" for Tu expression. See Fig. 1 and footnote on p. 420.

case the differentiation block exerted by *gg* is overcome by "promotion," i.e., by TPA-induced stimulation of differentiation of stem cells to "competence" (Fig. 1).

(c) Tu^+R^+/TuR, g^+/g^+; does develop neoplasia simply after "initiation" with carcinogens, due to apparent somatic mutation of R (2). These functional heterozygotes shall also be used as a more direct test for the hypothesized recombinogenic activity of TPA. Recently Kinsella and Radman (8) proposed that the tumor-promoting activity of TPA might result from enhancement of mitotic recombination which, when followed by cell division, would lead to segregation of recessive chromosomal lesions produced by a carcinogen. If this hypothesis is correct, the heterozygotes Tu^+R^+/TuR should develop neoplasia simply following treatment with TPA.

(d) Tu^+R/TuR, g/g; (phenotype as in Fig. 2i,j); should develop neoplasia due to derepressed Tu simply by "promotion," i.e., differentiation to "competence" (Fig. 1).

For testing resistance, genotypes should be employed that are Tu^+R^+/Tu^+ R^+, g/g. Because the corresponding counterparts g^+/g^+ are resistant to primary carcinogens (MNU, X-rays; 8,11), it would be expected that g/g genotypes are also resistant to both "initiators" and "promoters" in conditions under which genotypes a to d are sensitive.

CONCLUSIONS

An understanding of the data, including those in this chapter, on "initiation" and "promotion" as elements in the multistep nature of carcinogenesis might be best obtained by looking at the levels of genetic change (point mutation, chromosome rearrangement) and of aberrant cellular differentiation. TPA action relevant to tumor promotion is likely to be explained on the basis of altering gene expression or gene products, thereby disrupting the normal growth controls. This chapter sets up a genetic system *in vivo* with the potential to contribute further to the role of genetic change and aberrant differentiation in carcinogenesis.

ACKNOWLEDGMENTS

This research was supported by Deutsche Forschungsgemeinschaft (Schw 251/1), and by DFG-Sonderforschungsbereich 103 "Zellenergetik und Zelldifferenzierung," Marburg, by project C11 given to A. and F. Anders. I am indebted to Prof. E. Hecker, Deutsches Krebsforschungszentrum, for generously supplying me with TPA. The concept for this manuscript was largely developed during the exciting symposium at the Castle of Elmau.

REFERENCES

1. Ahuja, M. R., Schwab, M., and Anders, F. (1980): Linkage between a regulatory locus for melanoma cell differentiation and an esterase locus in *Xiphophorus. J. Hered.* 71:403–410.
2. Anders, A., and Anders, F. (1978): Etiology of cancer as studied in the platyfish-swordtail system. *Biochim. Biophys. Acta-Rev. Cancer,* 516:61–95.
3. Anders, F., Diehl, H., Schwab, M., and Anders, A. (1979): Contributions to an understanding of the cellular origin of melanoma in the Gordon-Kosswig xiphophorine fish tumor system. In: *Pigment Cell,* edited by S. N. Klaus, pp. 142–149. Karger, Basel.
4. Bagnara, J. T., Matsumoto, J., Ferris, W., Frost, S. K., Turner, W. T., Tchen, T. T., and Taylor, J. D. (1979): Common origin of pigment cells. *Science,* 203:410–415.
5. Diamond, L., O'Brien, T. G., and Baird, W. M. (1980): Tumor promoters and the mechanism of tumor promotion. In: *Advances in Cancer Research,* edited by G. Klein and S. Weinhouse, pp. 1–75. Academic Press, New York.
6. Gordon, M. (1959): The melanoma cell as an incompletely differentiated pigment cell. In: *Pigment Cell Biology,* edited by M. Gordon, pp. 215–236. Academic Press, New York.
7. Humm, D. C., and Young, R. S. (1956): The embryological origin of pigment cells in platyfish-swordtail hybrids. *Zoologica,* 41:1–10.
8. Kinsella, A. R., and Radman, M. (1978): Tumor promoter induces sister chromatid exchanges: Relevance to mechanisms of carcinogenesis. *Proc. Natl. Acad. Sci. USA,* 75:6,149–6,153.
9. Schwab, M., and Anders, A. (1981): Carcinogenesis in *Xiphophorus* and the role of the genotype in tumor susceptibility. In: *Neoplasms—Comparative Pathology of Growth in Animals, Plants, and Man,* edited by H. E. Kaiser. Williams and Wilkins, Baltimore, pp. 451–459.
10. Schwab, M., Kollinger, G., Haas, J., Ahuja, M. R., Anders, A., and Anders, F. (1979): Genetic basis of susceptibility for neuroblastoma following treatment with N-methyl-N-nitrosourea (MNU) and X-rays in *Xiphophorus. Cancer Res.,* 39:519–526.
11. Schwab, M., and Scholl, E. (1981): Neoplastic pigment cells induced by N-methyl-N-nitrosourea (MNU) in *Xiphophorus,* and genetic control of their terminal differentiation. *Differentiation* 19:77–83.
12. Vielkind, U. (1976): Genetic control of cell differentiation in platyfish-swordtail melanomas. *J. Exp. Zool.,* 196:197–204.

Carcinogenesis, Vol. 7, edited by E. Hecker et al.
Raven Press, New York © 1982.

Promotion and Regression of Neoplasia by Testosterone-Promoted Cell Differentiation in *Xiphophorus* and *Girardinus*

A. Schartl, M. Schartl, and F. Anders

*Genetisches Institut, Justus-Liebig-Universität Giessen, D-6300 Giessen,
Federal Republic of Germany*

The precursors of the melanin-producing pigment cells of *Xiphophorus,* like those of other vertebrates, originate from the neural crest and migrate to their final location (2). They divide and undergo differentiation through the stages of chromatoblasts, stem(S)-melanoblasts, intermediate(I)-melanoblasts, advanced(A)-melanoblasts, melanocytes, and finally differentiate to melanophores, which are incapable of dividing. At a certain age the melanophores are removed by macrophages. Supply comes from S-melanoblasts. Depending on the genotype and the developmental stage of the fish, certain fish show a delay or even an arrest of differentiation in the stage of S-melanoblasts (1).

Studies on melanoma formation have shown that the only stage of differentiation in which the pigment cells are competent for neoplastic transformation is the stage of the I-melanoblasts (2). If a certain gene, the "tumor gene" *(Tu),* that mediates neoplastic transformation becomes derepressed by hybridization-conditioned elimination or mutation-conditioned impairment of *Tu*-specific regulating genes *(R),* the I-melanoblasts become transformed to TI-melanoblasts (T = transformed), which continue to differentiate to TA-melanoblasts, T-melanocytes, and finally T-melanophores, which are incapable of dividing.

Differentiation and division of the T-cells result in melanoma formation. The degree of malignancy of the melanoma depends on the ratio of incompletely differentiated, dividing T-cells to terminally differentiated, nondividing T-melanophores. The more incompletely differentiated T-cells are present in the melanoma, the higher is the degree of malignancy. Melanoma that consist predominantly of terminally differentiated cells are benign. The findings suggest that melanoma development, including initial tumor formation and further tumor growth, is a problem of cell differentiation rather than of cell division.

The objective of our experiments was to find out if substances that influence pigment cell differentiation may also influence melanoma formation. For this purpose we used the steroid 17-methyltestosterone, which was recently found to be a strong promoter of pigment cell differentiation in *Xiphophorus* (8,9).

This chapter contains part of the dissertation of A. Schartl.

To show a more general significance of our results, we used *Girardinus* besides *Xiphophorus* as experimental animals.

MATERIAL AND METHODS

Certain genotypes of the genera *Xiphophorus* HECKEL 1848 and *Girardinus* POEY 1854 (Pisces: Poeciliidae), which are all characterized by a derepressed *Tu* due to crossing conditioned elimination of *R* genes (see introduction), served as experimental animals. They can roughly be divided into (a) fish that had not developed melanoma due to a genetic and developmentally conditioned delay of pigment cell differentiation in the stage of the S-melanoblasts, and (b) fish that bore melanoma, which predominantly consisted of poorly differentiated transformed cells.

The genotypes out of which the experimental animals were chosen are as follows:

(a) *Xiphophorus Tu-Sp^e:* Backcross hybrids, produced by introgression of the *Tu*-containing gene complex *Tu-Sp^e* (spotted extended) of *X.maculatus* from the Rio Jamapa into the genome of *X.helleri* wild fish stock from the Rio Lancetilla (Mexico).

(b) *Xiphophorus Tu-Li (a/a):* Backcross hybrids, produced by introgression of the *Tu*-containing gene complex *Tu-Li* (Lineatus) of *X.variatus,* originating presumably from the Rio Panuco, into the genome of the albino *X.helleri (a/a).*

(c) *Xiphophorus Tu-Li (g/g):* Backcross hybrids like (b), however, nonalbino and homozygous for the golden gene *(g/g).*

(d) *Girardinus Tu-Vn:* Animals derived from *G. metallicus* wild fish stock from Cuba carrying the *Tu*-containing gene complex *Tu-Vn* (Ventral nigra), the origin of which is unknown.

All stocks were raised in our laboratory under standard conditions (25°C, 12-hr artificial light/24 hr) and were fed a standard diet (TETRA, Melle, FRG).

Testosterone Treatment

The fish were treated by adding an ethanolic solution of 17-methyl-testosterone[1] (1 mg/ml; EGA-Chemie, Steinheim, FRG) to the aquarium water. The treatment was carried out continuously during periods up to 8 to 12 weeks and with different dosages ranging from 2 to 20 μl/l aquarium water per day. Adult females of the guppy *(Poeclia reticulata),* which are known to respond to testosterone by the development of male secondary sex characteristics, served as a test system for the biological activity of the hormone. Controls were kept under the same conditions and treated with the appropriate dosages of pure ethanol.

---

[1] 17 β-hydroxy-17-methylandrost-4-en-3-one

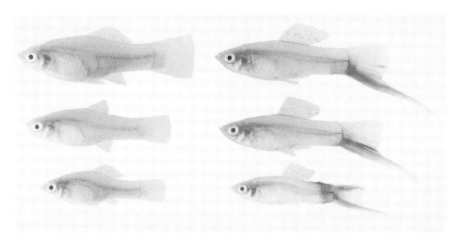

FIG. 1. 17-Methyltestosterone-induced malignant melanoma (2 µg/l aquarium water and per day). Untreated fish of *Xiphophorus Tu-Li (a/a) (left);* fish of the same genotype after 3 months of treatment *(right).*

Determination of Malignancy

The degree of malignancy of each melanoma was determined macroscopically and/or histologically according to the criteria given in ref. 2.

RESULTS

Tumor Promotion

In the first series of experiments we investigated the effect of testosterone on fish that, due to a delay of the differentiation of S-melanoblasts, had either not yet developed or normally do not develop melanoma.

In the *Xiphophorus Tu-Li (a/a)* an extremely benign amelanotic melanoma normally develops spontaneously at the age of 3 months on the side of the body. When treated continuously with testosterone[2] starting at birth, 72 out of 96 individuals (75%) developed at the age of 1 month malignant amelanotic melanoma. This melanoma, however, developed at the peduncle of the tail fin (Fig. 1). In the controls ($N = 104$) no melanoma was observed at that age.

In another experiment of this series, 317 animals of *Xiphophorus Tu-Sp[e]*, which normally develop melanotic melanoma spontaneously at the age of 4 to 5 weeks on the whole body including the fins and occasionally the eyes, were treated from birth. All of the treated fish developed melanoma at the age of

---

[2] Further effects of testosterone, which will not be discussed in this chapter, were the development of male secondary sex characteristics in immature fish of both sexes and in adult females, and an increase of the expression of male secondary sex characteristics in adult males.

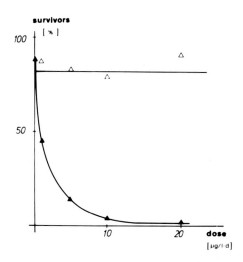

FIG. 2. Dosage dependency of cancer mortality in *Xiphophorus Tu-Sp*ᵉ treated continuously from birth. Survivors after 3 weeks of treatment with 17-methyltestosterone: △: non-tumorous fish lacking *Tu-Sp*ᵉ; ▲: fish carrying *Tu-Sp*ᵉ.

3 days. The melanomas were extremely malignant and led to a testosterone dosage-dependent increase in cancer mortality as compared to the controls (Fig. 2).

In *Girardinus Tu-Vn,* melanotic melanoma develop normally in males older than 6 months after sexual maturation in the ventral region of the belly and of the operculi. Females of this genotype normally do not develop melanoma although carrying *Tu-Vn.* Testosterone-treated animals developed melanoma in 8-day-old fish of both sexes ($N = 20$) when treated from birth. Treatment of adult females ($N = 16$) resulted in melanoma formation within 5 to 7 days. In about 6 weeks the melanomas reached a phenotype similar to that of untreated males. The growth and malignancy of these melanomas were enhanced by further testosterone treatment, and these exceeded the spontaneous melanoma of untreated males (Fig. 3). Adult tumor-bearing males showed only a slight increase of neoplasia following treatment.

Tumor Regression and Tumor Suppression

In the second series of experiments, those fish that bore the type of melanoma that consisted predominantly of poorly differentiated transformed cells were treated. In 162 out of 208 individuals (78%) of those adult fish of *Xiphophorus Tu-Sp*ᵉ which bore malignant melanoma on the whole body, the amount of terminally differentiated T-melanophores was increased after 3 to 4 weeks of testosterone treatment. The promotion of cell differentiation resulted in a benignization of the melanoma. T-melanophores were removed by macrophages, thus leading to tumor regression in the fins, the abdominal part of the body, and

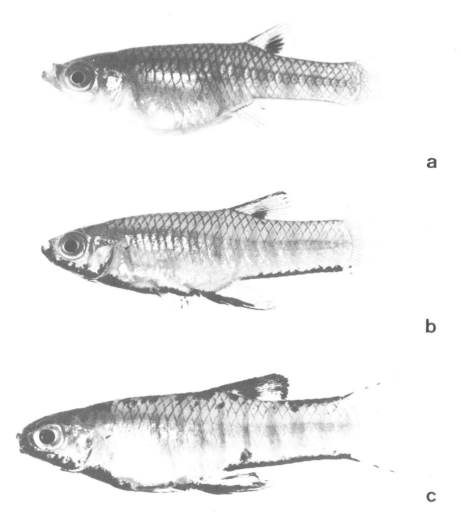

FIG. 3. 17-Methyltestosterone-induced melanoma (20 μg/l aquarium water and per day). **a:** Untreated female of *Girardinus Tu-Vn;* **b:** female after 6 weeks of treatment; **c:** female after 3 months of treatment.

the caudal part of the trunk. No regression was observed in the peduncle of the tail. After a further treatment of 3 months, all tumors were reduced to small benign melanoma in the peduncle of the tail (Fig. 4). In controls, 17 of 198 animals (8.6%) showed a regression of the melanoma, which, however, was never as prominent as in the treated fish.

In *Xiphophorus Tu-Li (g/g)*, normally benign melanotic melanoma develop spontaneously in adults at the age of 4 months on the side of the body. If these animals ($N = 24$) were treated from the onset of melanoma formation,

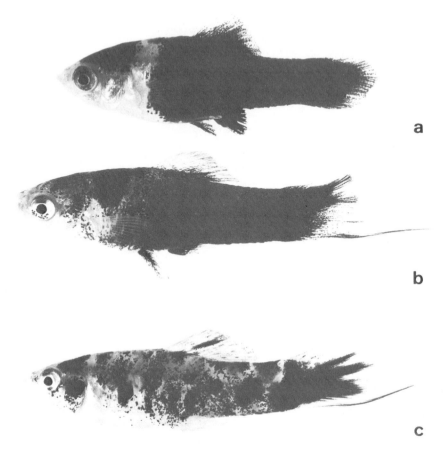

FIG. 4. Regression of malignant melanoma following treatment with 17-methyltestosterone (2 μg/l aquarium water and per day). **a:** Untreated fish of *Xiphophorus Tu-Sp^e*; **b:** same animal after 3 weeks of treatment; **c:** same animal after 8 weeks of treatment.

they developed only small T-cell colonies consisting of terminally differentiated T-melanophores. In these fish the formation of melanoma was suppressed (Fig. 5).

DISCUSSION

In one group of the *Xiphophorus* genotypes including *Girardinus,* testosterone has promoted melanoma formation, and in the other group it has suppressed melanoma formation. The dual effects can be explained by a promotion of cell differentiation mediated by the steroid hormone (9).

In one group, the majority of the pigment cell precursors are arrested in a

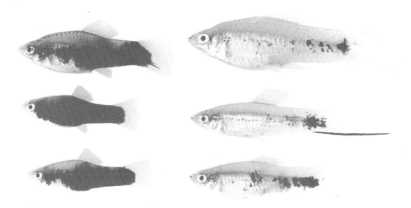

FIG. 5. Suppression of melanoma formation following treatment with 17-methyltestosterone (4 μg/l aquarium water and per day). Untreated fish of *Xiphophorus Tu-Li (g/g) (left)*; fish of the same genotype after 3 months of treatment *(right)*.

precompetent stage (see introduction) and may become competent via testosterone-promoted differentiation. Concerning melanoma development, two different situations have to be considered: First, melanoma does not yet develop because the majority of the pigment cells is arrested in the precompetent stage. Under the influence of testosterone, they differentiate to the competent stage. Thus testosterone appears to be an inducer of melanoma. Second, melanoma formation starts because some of the precompetent cells reach the competent stage due to an endogenous promotion of cell differentiation. Under the influence of testosterone, an increased amount of these cells reach the competent stage. In this case, testosterone appears as an enhancer of melanoma growth.

In the other group, the majority of the pigment cell precursors reach the competent stage for neoplastic transformation autonomously, and melanoma develops. Due to the influence of testosterone, the incompletely differentiated T-cells complete differentiation. The terminally differentiated T-cells that are incapable of dividing are removed by macrophages. Thus testosterone (a) may convert malignant melanoma to a benign phenotype, (b) may cause regression, and (c) may even prevent tumor formation. Testosterone, therefore, appears in these fish as a tumor suppressor.

According to the initiation-promotion model of carcinogenesis proposed by Berenblum (4), 17-methyltestosterone can be considered a tumor promoter or cocarcinogen. In the experiments presented here, "initiation" is represented by the derepression of *Tu*, whereas "promotion" is represented by the testosterone-induced differentiation of cells from a precompetent stage to a stage where the derepressed *Tu* can become active. Thus initiation means a genetic change, namely derepression of *Tu*, whereas promotion means an epigenetic shift in the stage of differentiation of the cells.

On the basis of our results one can also explain the cocarcinogenic effect of "classic" tumor promoters like the 12-O-tetradecanoylphorbol-13-acetate (TPA) (5) as well as the cocarcinogenic effect of substances such as diethylstilbestrol (11), many androgens (6), and retinoids (10), which are also known to promote cell differentiation. These compounds also require a genetic change as a precondition for their cocarcinogenicity. We assume that the genetic change may correspond to the derepression of *Tu*, whereas the cocarcinogenicity may correspond to the differentiation-promoting effect of methyltestosterone in our experiments.

Androgens, retinoids, and other compounds have also shown both carcinogenic and anticarcinogenic activity in certain experiments (3,7). We assume that the dual effect corresponds to that of testosterone reported here. Our results, including the findings on cocarcinogenic and anticarcinogenic effects of the compounds mentioned above, suggest that depending on the stage of differentiation of the target cells, "classic" tumor promoters like TPA may also act as anticarcinogens.

ACKNOWLEDGMENTS

We thank R. Palmer for critical reading and E. Silomon-Pflug for typing the manuscript.

REFERENCES

1. Anders, A., and Anders, F. (1978): Etiology of cancer as studied in the platyfish-swordtail system. *Biochim. Biophys. Acta—Rev. Cancer,* 516:61–95.
2. Anders, F., Diehl, H., Schwab, M., and Anders, A. (1979): Contributions to an understanding of the cellular origin of melanoma in the Gordon-Kosswig xiphophorine fish tumor system. In: *Biological Basis of Pigmentation, Vol. 4: Pigment Cell,* edited by S. N. Klaus, pp. 142–149. Karger, Basel.
3. Becci, P. J., Thompson, H. J., Sporn, M. B., and Moon, R. C. (1980): Retinoid inhibition of highly invasive urinary bladder carcinomas induced in mice by N-butyl-N-(4-hydroxybutyl)-nitrosamine (OH-BBN). *Proc. Am. Assoc. Cancer Res.,* 21:88.
4. Berenblum, I., editor (1974): *Carcinogenesis as a Biological Problem.* North Holland Publishing Company, Amsterdam.
5. Diamond, L., O'Brien, T. G., and Baird, W. M. (1980): Tumor promoters and the mechanism of tumor promotion. In: *Advances in Cancer Research,* edited by G. Klein and S. Weinhouse, pp. 1–75. Academic Press, New York.
6. Jull, J. W. (1976): Endocrine aspects of carcinogenesis. In: *Chemical Carcinogens,* edited by E. Searle, pp. 87–96. American Chemical Society Monographs, Washington.
7. Martz, G., editor (1968): *Die hormonale Therapie maligner Tumoren.* Springer, Berlin.
8. Schartl, A. (1980): *Experimentelle Beeinflussung der Zelldifferenzierung durch Testosteron-Promotion und Regression von Melanomen bei lebendgebärenden Zahnkarpfen (Poeciliidae).* Diplomarbeit, Giessen.
9. Schartl, M., Schartl, A., and Anders, F. (1981): Phenotypic conversion of malignant melanoma to benign melanoma and vice versa in *Xiphophorus.* In: *Biological Basis of Pigmentation, Vol. 6: Pigment Cell,* edited by K. Seji, pp. 493–500. Karger, Basel (in press).
10. Stinson, F. F., and Donahoe, R. (1980): Effects of three retinoids on tracheal carcinogenesis in hamsters. *Proc. Am. Assoc. Cancer Res.,* 21:122.
11. Sumi, C., Yokoro, K., Kajitani, T., and Ito, A. (1980): Synergism of diethylstilbestrol and other carcinogens in concurrent development of hepatic, mammary, and pituitary tumors of castrated male rats. *J. Natl. Cancer Inst.,* 65:169–175.

Carcinogenesis, Vol. 7, edited by E. Hecker et al.
Raven Press, New York © 1982.

Early Changes in the Cell Cycle Traverse of HeLa Cells Induced by Tumor Promoter TPA Resemble Irradiation Effects

Volker Kinzel, Michael Stöhr, and James Richards

Institute of Experimental Pathology, German Cancer Research Center, D-6900 Heidelberg, Federal Republic of Germany

The mechanism by which tumor-promoting agents like 12-O-tetradecanoyl-phorbol-13-acetate (TPA) convert initiated cells into tumor cells and into tumors is little understood. Often the mitogenic capacity of promoters has been thought to be the responsible activity. Indeed most of the biochemical parameters measured so far after application of TPA seem to be related to mitogenesis. There are indications, however, that the mitogenic capacity of promoters alone is not sufficient to explain the phenomenon of promotion. Since mitogenesis is presumably a result of the interaction of promoters with G_0 or G_1 cells, it is necessary to ask therefore: How does the promoter TPA interact with proliferating cells?

Actively proliferating cells are known to be a prerequisite for transformation by a variety of carcinogens; cells in the S phase of the cell cycle are most susceptible, whereas resting cells are very little affected. For the case of tumor promoters, the corresponding question is open. For technical reasons this problem is more difficult to approach since promoters, unlike carcinogens, have to be applied repeatedly. The question can be raised, however, whether small non-toxic doses of TPA interfere with the cell cycle, thus possibly highlighting susceptible phases in the cell cycle; an approach well known, for example, in irradiation studies with cell cultures. In this case the phase most sensitive for the mutagenic activity of X-rays coincides with that influenced in terms of cell cycle kinetics.

The effects to be looked at should occur early after administration of TPA, since critical events seem to be switched on immediately after application of the promoter (as experiments with antipromoting compounds have indicated). In order to dissect out the stimulatory activity of TPA, the cellular system to be used should not respond to mitogenesis, i.e., it should be already fully proliferative. The cells should nevertheless respond through some parameters to a large series of phorbol derivatives in a manner closely related to the biological activity of these in mouse skin. HeLa cells have been shown to fulfill these requirements (2,7), and their replication is diminished in the presence of TPA.

PROCEDURES

The responses of asynchronous and of monolayer HeLa cells synchronized by Amethopterin-blockage and thymidine release to small nontoxic doses of TPA (10^{-7} or 10^{-8} M final concentration) or 4-O-methyl-TPA (10^{-6} M final concentration) in dimethylsulfoxide (0.05%) or acetone (0.2%) were measured by a variety of independent methods. During the 24 hr after application, the following parameters were evaluated in asynchronous cultures: incorporation rates of ^{3}H-thymidine into deoxyribonucleic acid (DNA) (30-min periods); autoradiographic analysis of cells labeled with thymidine; number of cells in mitosis; and DNA-histogram through flow cytometry, by which last method experiments with synchronized cells were exclusively analyzed. Details of the procedures have been published elsewhere (3,4,5). The donation of phorbol derivatives by Dr. E. Hecker and members of the Institute of Biochemistry (DKFZ, Heidelberg) is gratefully acknowledged.

RESULTS

The changes induced by small nontoxic doses of TPA on HeLa cells were transient and dependent on the phase in which the first contact with TPA occurred. Cells in G_1 were inhibited from entering the S phase as is evident (a) from a decrease of cells in S phase (Fig. 1A; autoradiography), (b) from the fact that almost no cells pass from G_1 to early S phase (DNA histograms), and (c) from an increased percentage of cells in G_1 (Fig. 2; DNA histograms). Cells in S phase were delayed as evident (a) from an overproportional decrease of thymidine incorporation rates when compared with the percentage of cells in S phase (Fig. 1B), (b) from a delayed flow of cells out of S phase (DNA histograms), and (c) from a delayed passage through S phase of synchronized cells (5). A rather transient blockage of cells in G_2 is indicated by a rapid decrease of cells undergoing mitosis from which cells have recovered to some degree after approximately 8 to 12 hr (Fig. 1C). A delay of a portion of cells in G_2 which were in S phase at the addition of TPA is indicated (a) by a disproportionally high percentage of cells in G_2 between 8 and 12 hr (Fig. 2), and (b) by experiments with synchronous cultures treated at different times during S phase (5). None of these results was obtained with a high concentration (10^{-6} M) of the hyperplasiogenic but rarely promoting agent 4-O-methyl-TPA (Figs. 1 A, C, and 2).

DISCUSSION

The question raised initially, how the tumor promoter TPA interacts with proliferating cells, has been partially answered in terms of cell cycle kinetics. The transient changes in the cell cycle traverse of HeLa cells induced by TPA resemble those described for irradiated cultures. For a detailed discussion of

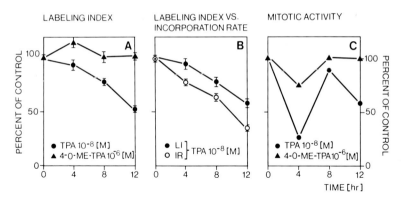

FIG. 1. Responses of asynchronous monolayer HeLa cells to TPA versus 4-O-methyl-TPA given at zero time. **A:** Labeling index of cells incubated for 30 min with ^{3}H-thymidine prior to the times indicated. **B:** Comparison of labeling index (LI) versus incorporation rate (IR) of ^{3}H-thymidine into DNA in the presence of TPA. **C:** Mitotic activity.

the data, see refs. 3, 4, 5. A few general remarks may point to further similarities between the action of promoters and that of X-rays. Alterations in skin induced by TPA including edema, inflammation, and hyperkeratosis in mice as well as hyperpigmentation and melanosis in hamsters (1) and in C57 black mice (K. Goerttler and H. Loehrke, *personal communication*) have several properties in common with the radiation dermatitis observed in humans. With regard to mechanistic aspects, data by W. Troll et al. (see this volume) that indicate an involvement of free radicals in TPA action should be noted. T. J. Slaga et al. (see this volume) were even able to demonstrate the capacity of free radical-

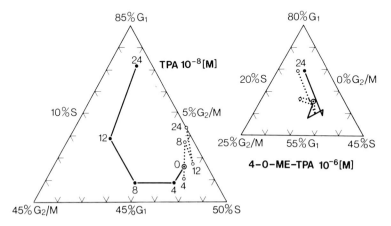

FIG. 2. Three parameter plots of the cell cycle staging of HeLa cells developing during 24 hr in the presence of TPA or 4-O-methyl-TPA *(solid lines)* or solvent *(dotted lines)* given at zero time. Shown are the data derived from histograms as obtained by computerized flow cytometry.

producing compounds to promote tumors. Since the tumor promoter TPA is believed not to interact directly with genomic material, these observations may inversely lead to an understanding of the significance of nongenomic targets for X-rays and thereby possibly to an elucidation of the way in which X-rays may promote tumorigenesis.

The relevance of the cell cycle changes induced by TPA to the mechanism of promotion remains to be established. The observations by A. R. Peterson et al. (6) that an initially inhibited incorporation of thymidine into DNA of C3H/10T1/2 cells—a measure reflecting inhibited activity and/or smaller number of cells in S phase—was a prerequisite for promotion, at least *in vitro,* may point to the significance of the interaction of TPA with proliferating cells. If there is a critical phase in the replication cycle for the interaction with TPA, it can probably be narrowed down by the use of TPA analogs having similar biological potencies other than promoting capacity, and by the use of compounds known to counteract the action of phorbol promoters as well as those that protect from X-ray-induced lesions.

CONCLUSION

The problem of how the tumor promoter TPA interacts with proliferating cells was approached by studying its influence on the cell cycle of HeLa cells. A variety of transient changes were detected that mimic those reported for irradiated cultures.

ACKNOWLEDGMENT

We thank N. König for excellent technical assistance.

REFERENCES

1. Goerttler, K., Loehrke, H., Schweizer, J., and Hesse, B. (1980): Two-stage tumorigenesis of dermal melanocytes in the back skin of the Syrian golden hamster using systemic initiation with 7,12-dimethylbenz(a)anthracene and topical promotion with 12-O-tetradecanoylphorbol-13-acetate. *Cancer Res.,* 40:155–161.
2. Kinzel, V., Kreibich, G., Hecker, E., and Süss, R. (1979): Stimulation of choline incorporation in cell cultures by phorbol derivatives and its correlation with their irritant and tumor-promoting activity. *Cancer Res.,* 39:2743–2750.
3. Kinzel, V., Richards, J., and Stöhr, M. (1980): Tumor promoter TPA mimics irradiation effects on the cell cycle of HeLa cells. *Science,* 210:429–431.
4. Kinzel, V., Richards, J., and Stöhr, M. (1981a): Early effects of the tumor-promoting phorbol ester 12-O-tetradecanoylphorbol-13-acetate on the cell cycle traverse of asynchronous HeLa cells. *Cancer Res.,* 41:300–305.
5. Kinzel, V., Richards, J., and Stöhr, M. (1981b): Responses of synchronized HeLa cells to the tumor-promoting phorbol ester 12-O-tetradecanoylphorbol-13-acetate as evaluated by flow cytometry. *Cancer Res.,* 41:306–309.
6. Peterson, A. R., Mondal, S., Brankow, D. W., Thon, W., and Heidelberger, C. (1977): Effects of promoters on DNA synthesis in C3H/10T1/2 mouse fibroblasts. *Cancer Res.,* 37:3223–3227.
7. Süss, R., Kreibich, G., and Kinzel, V. (1972): Phorbol esters as a tool in cell research? *Eur. J. Cancer,* 8:299–304.

Carcinogenesis, Vol. 7, edited by E. Hecker et al.
Raven Press, New York © 1982.

Effects of 12-O-Tetradecanoylphorbol-13-acetate on Lymphocyte Proliferation

Andrea M. Mastro and Karen G. Pepin

Department of Microbiology, Cell Biology, Biochemistry, and Biophysics, The Pennsylvania State University, University Park, Pennsylvania 16802

The tumor promoter 12-O-tetradecanoylphorbol-13-acetate (TPA) has a variety of effects on mammalian cell differentiation and division in culture. We have found with bovine lymph node lymphocytes that TPA modulates the morphological and proliferative responses of the cells to mitogens. The particular effect depends on the length of exposure to TPA relative to the mitogenic stimulus. Normally, unstimulated lymphocytes do not divide in culture. Addition of a mitogenic lectin such as phytohemagglutinin (PHA) or placement of the cells in mixed lymphocyte culture (MLC) brings about morphological changes, i.e., blast formation and cell proliferation.

TPA is only weakly mitogenic for bovine lymph node lymphocytes (3). At 10^{-7} M, it causes about a threefold increase ($\bar{X} = 2.7 \pm 1.4$; range = 0.9 − 4.9) in ^{3}H-thymidine incorporation compared with unstimulated cells (Fig. 1A); whereas, the addition of an optimal concentration of PHA results in stimulation indices ranging from 10 to 230 depending on the experiment ($\bar{X} = 73 \pm 55$). The TPA response is typically 5 to 10% of the PHA response. Also, while the proliferative response to TPA is at a maximum on day 1, the response to PHA is greatest on day 2 or 3 (Fig. 1A, B). Although we originally observed that the mitogenic response to TPA was more evident in freshly isolated cells than in those incubated overnight at 37°C, we have since tested cells from over 100 animals and have seen many cases of weak mitogenic activity with either treatment. The variation in the degree of the mitogen response to TPA may be due to the animal's immune activity at the time of cell isolation. TPA may act synergistically with endogenous mitogens. We have found it to act synergistically with exogenous ones.

When TPA and PHA are added simultaneously to lymphocytes, a comitogenic activity is seen. ^{3}H-Thymidine incorporation is greater than the additive incorporation in cells treated separately with TPA or PHA (3). The enhancing activity is due to an increase in the number of responding cells in the culture. This synergistic activity is amplified when cells are stimulated with suboptimal doses of PHA (1; Fig. 1B). In cells from animals tested over the past several months, we have found that on the average the comitogen stimulation is about 8.0-

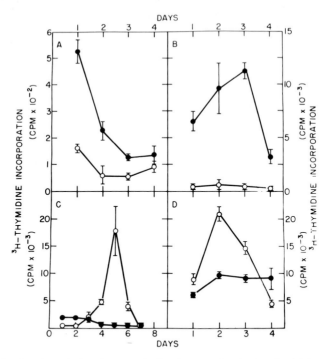

FIG. 1. Bovine lymph node lymphocytes, isolated as previously described (4), were cultured at 5×10^6 viable cells/ml of RPMI 1640 medium containing 10% calf serum and 50 μg/ml gentamycin. For assays of DNA synthesis, the cells were plated in replicate in microwell cultures, 1×10^6 per well. Triplicate cultures were pulsed for 2 hr with ^{3}H-thymidine (6.7 Ci/mM, 1 μCi/ml). The pulse was ended by harvesting with a Skatron cell harvester onto filter paper. The pads were dried and counted in a liquid scintillation spectrometer. The data are presented as cpm incorporated $\bar{X} \pm$ SD. Note the difference in scale for **A. A:** Mitogenic effect of TPA: (○) control cells; (●) lymphocytes plus 10^{-7} M TPA. **B:** Comitogenic effect of TPA: (●) cells with a suboptimal dose of PHA (1/10,000 dilution) plus 10^{-7} M TPA; (○) control cells with PHA alone. **C:** Effect of TPA on the MLR: (●) mixture of cells from 2 animals plus TPA (10^{-7} M) added at the beginning of culture; (○) control mixture of cells. **D:** Effect of TPA pretreatment on the response to PHA: (●) lymphocytes incubated for 42 hr with 10^{-7} M TPA, washed, resuspended, and stimulated with an optimal dose (1/1,000 dilution) of PHA; (○) control cells treated the same way except with no TPA.

fold over the additive responses of PHA and TPA alone (range 2 to 20). We have also found a similar result with bovine spleen lymphocytes (Table 1). With these cells, TPA is a weak mitogen but it is comitogenic with PHA, a T-cell mitogen, and with lipopolysaccharide (LPS), a B-cell mitogen.

In contrast to its mitogenic and comitogenic activity, TPA inhibits deoxyribonucleic acid (DNA) synthesis in the MLC (4; Fig. 1C). This effect is also seen morphologically. Very few blast cells form in the MLC in the presence of TPA (2). The mixed lymphocyte response (MLR) takes longer to occur than does the response to PHA (Fig. 1B and C). Addition of TPA during the first 2 days of the MLC blocks the subsequent response. Adding it late or to an ongoing response, however, does not stop DNA synthesis. In order to look at the effects

TABLE 1. *Effect of TPA on mitogenic responses of bovine spleen cells[a]*

	Pretreatment[b]	Additions	^{3}H-Thymidine incorporation (cpm, $\bar{X} \pm SD$)
Experiment	—	None	69 ± 23
	—	PHA (1/10,000)	$2,740 \pm 866$
	—	TPA (10^{-8} M)	247 ± 52
	—	PHA + TPA	$4,970 \pm 424$
Experiment 2	—	None	121 ± 32
	—	LPS (10 μg/ml)	207 ± 68
	—	TPA (10^{-7} M)	$1,384 \pm 262$
	—	LPS + TPA	$3,148 \pm 1,169$
Experiment 3	No additions	None	97 ± 32
	No additions	PHA (1/1,000)	$13,053 \pm 1,297$
	+ TPA (10^{-7} M)	None	78 ± 9
	+ TPA (10^{-7} M)	PHA (1/1,000)	810 ± 38

[a] Spleen cells were isolated by pushing small pieces of bovine spleen through a stainless steel screen into culture medium. After centrifugation the cells were exposed for 10 sec to a hypotonic solution to lyse the red blood cells. The lymphocytes were washed and resuspended in RPMI 1640 medium with 10% calf serum and treated exactly as the lymph node lymphocytes (2–6). ^{3}H-Thymidine pulses, 2 hr long, were done with triplicate cultures each day for 4 days, as described in the legend to Fig. 1. Maximum incorporations are shown: day 3 for experiment 2; day 4 for experiments 1 and 3.

[b] Cells in Exps. 1 and 2 were not pretreated. In Exp. 3 the cells were incubated for 42 hr in medium $\pm$ 10^{-7} M TPA before they were washed and treated as described in column 2.

of TPA on a one-way MLR, cells were pretreated for 2 days before they were mixed (2). The subsequent MLR was prevented. The inhibitory activity was associated with both responding and stimulating cells. In addition, we found that TPA-pretreated cells gave a depressed response to lectins (5; Fig. 1D). This was in contrast to TPA's synergistic activity if added simultaneously with the lectins. Inhibition was seen if TPA-treated lymph node cells were stimulated with PHA, concanavalin A, or pokeweed mitogen. The response of spleen lymphocytes to PHA was depressed (Table 1). The inhibitory activity was reversible. If the treated cells were incubated overnight in fresh medium before they were stimulated with lectins or placed in the MLC, they responded as well as untreated cells. Thus, if inhibition is due to the suppression of a subpopulation of TPA-sensitive cells, they can recover. A short (2-hr) pretreatment was sufficient to depress the MLC, whereas a longer (1 to 2 day) pretreatment was necessary to depress the lectin response (5). This result may reflect the difference in sensitivity to the stimuli. None of these effects was seen with phorbol or the solvent dimethylsulfoxide. We also checked to see if they were caused by metabolites of TPA. Even during the relatively long pretreatment periods, TPA is degraded less than 15% (6). The major hydrolysis products, phorbol-13-acetate and 12-O-tetradecanoylphorbol, are not responsible for the effects of TPA.

We tested the possibility that TPA's inhibitory effects were due to a block in ^{3}H-thymidine transport. Isotope-dilution experiments and the use of another label for DNA (^{3}H-deoxycytidine) ruled out this effect as well as the possibility that cold thymidine was being produced by the TPA-treated cells. The treated cultures do produce increased amounts of plasminogen activator (5), but this may be incidental to the effects of TPA treatment.

In summary, TPA is a powerful agent in modulation of lymphocyte responses. Whether its activities can be explained by direct action on the responding cell population or through intermediate lymphokine activity or both remains to be determined.

ACKNOWLEDGMENT

This work was supported by grant CA-24385 from the National Cancer Institute.

REFERENCES

1. Kensler, T. W., and Mueller, G. C. (1978): Retinoic acid inhibition of the comitogenic action of mezerein and phorbol esters in bovine lymphocytes. *Cancer Res.,* 38:771–775.
2. Mastro, A. M., Krupa, T. A., and Smith, P. (1979): Interaction of the tumor promoter 12-O-tetradecanoylphorbol-13-acetate with cells in mixed lymphocyte culture. *Cancer Res.,* 39:4,078–4,082.
3. Mastro, A. M., and Mueller, G. C. (1974): Synergistic action of phorbol esters in mitogen-activated bovine lymphocytes. *Exp. Cell Res.,* 88:40–46.
4. Mastro, A. M., and Mueller, G. C. (1978): Inhibition of the mixed lymphocyte proliferation response by phorbol esters. *Biochim. Biophys. Acta,* 517:246–254.
5. Mastro, A. M., and Pepin, K. G. (1980a): Suppression of lectin-stimulated DNA synthesis in bovine lymphocytes by the tumor promoter 12-O-tetradecanoylphorbol-13-acetate. *Cancer Res.,* 40:3,307–3,312.
6. Mastro, A. M., and Pepin, K. G. (1980b): The interaction of [^{3}H]TPA with bovine lymph node lymphocytes *in vitro. Chem. Biol. Interact.,* 30:171–179.

Carcinogenesis, Vol. 7, edited by E. Hecker et al.
Raven Press, New York © 1982.

Epidermal Growth Factor Receptors Interact with Transforming Growth Factors Produced by Certain Human Tumor Cells and Are Distinct from Specific Membrane Receptors for Phorbol and Ingenol Esters

George J. Todaro, Joseph E. De Larco, and Mohammed Shoyab

Laboratory of Viral Carcinogenesis, National Cancer Institute, Frederick, Maryland 21701

A growth-promoting transforming polypeptide is characterized by the following properties: it is a strong mitogen which causes loss of density-dependent inhibition of cell growth in monolayer culture; and it causes morphologic transformation of normal cells and anchorage-independent growth (a property in cell culture that correlates best with tumorigenicity *in vivo*) (7,18). Polypeptides that cause phenotypic transformation of indicator cells and meet the above criteria for a transforming protein have been isolated from a number of human and animal carcinoma and sarcoma cells. These polypeptides have been termed transforming growth factors (TGFs) (38). The first TGF to be recognized as such was sarcoma growth factor (SGF) (11).

It was observed that murine sarcoma virus (MSV)-transformed cells are characterized by a loss of measurable cell surface receptors for the growth-stimulating polypeptide epidermal growth factor (EGF) (12,43). The apparent loss of cell surface receptors occurs in both fibroblastic and epithelioid cells transformed by MSV and can be demonstrated with cells derived from various species (10,12). The effect is seen with transforming ribonucleic acid (RNA) viruses but not with deoxyribonucleic acid (DNA) virus transformation nor with most chemical carcinogen-induced transformation. Over the years we have accumulated cells transformed by a variety of agents, including DNA viruses such as simian virus 40 (SV40) and polyoma, RNA viruses such as murine and avian sarcoma viruses, chemical carcinogens, and radiation, as well as cells that have become transformed spontaneously during passage in cell culture. These have been obtained from Swiss 3T3, Balb/3T3, and other mouse and rat cell systems. In collaboration with Stanley Cohen, these transformed cells were tested for their ability to bind ^{125}I-labeled EGF (43). Of 47 independently isolated, chemically transformed cells, five show a pattern like the MSV-transformed cells, i.e., almost complete loss of EGF receptors with normal levels of other receptors maintained. The chemically transformed cells without detectable EGF receptors have not yet been further characterized for the growth factors they may be producing. They represent a minority of chemically transformed cells that, with respect to this phenotype, behave like the MSV-transformed cells. The basis for this finding appears to be the production by the sarcoma virus-transformed cells of a family of growth factors called SGFs (11). Sufficient quantities are released into serum-free medium of Moloney MSV-infected mouse 3T3 cells to allow for their partial purification and characterization (11).

The growth factors that are produced by the sarcoma virus-transformed cells are a family of heat- and acid-stable transforming polypeptides. Addition of these SGFs to the culture medium of normal cells results in rapid and reversible changes. They cause normal rat fibroblasts to grow and form large colonies in soft agar (induction of anchorage-independent cell growth). They also have a pronounced morphologic effect on normal fibroblasts, converting them to transformed cells that pile up and are virtually indistinguishable from those genetically transformed by sarcoma viruses (Fig. 1). Thus, these polypeptides have the property of reversibly conferring the transformed phenotype on normal cells *in vitro* and, in this sense, can tentatively be considered proximate effectors of the malignant phenotype (11). The SGFs are specific for murine or feline sarcoma virus-transformed cells in that supernatants from untransformed cells or DNA tumor virus-transformed cells do not contain detectable quantities of these factors (11).

One of these SGFs has been further purified and shown to specifically bind to EGF membrane receptors (13). The ability to bind to and be eluted from EGF receptors provides an important purification step in the isolation and characterization of EGF-like growth factors. SGF binding to EGF receptors can be completely blocked by mouse salivary gland EGF. The chemical properties of radiolabeled SGF that has been purified using this method give further support to the idea that SGF and EGF are distinctly different molecules. The SGFs have been shown to compete with EGF for available membrane receptors, yet they do not crossreact with antibodies to EGF and their biological activity is distinct from that of EGF. Cells lacking EGF receptors are unable to respond to the growth-stimulating effects of this partially purified SGF. We concluded, therefore, that SGF released by MSV-transformed cells elicits its biologic effects via specific interaction with EGF membrane receptors.

Polypeptides characterized by their ability to confer a transformed phenotype on an untransformed indicator cell have also been isolated directly from tumor cells growing both in culture and in the animal using an acid-ethanol extraction procedure (30). The properties of these intracellular polypeptides from both virally and chemically transformed cells are similar to those described for the SGFs isolated from the conditioned medium of sarcoma virus-transformed mouse 3T3 cells, suggesting the definition of a new class of transforming growth factors common to tumor cells of different origin. Thus, the TGFs represent a new class of polypeptides common to cells transformed either by chemicals or by sarcoma viruses and possess biological activity distinct from that of EGF.

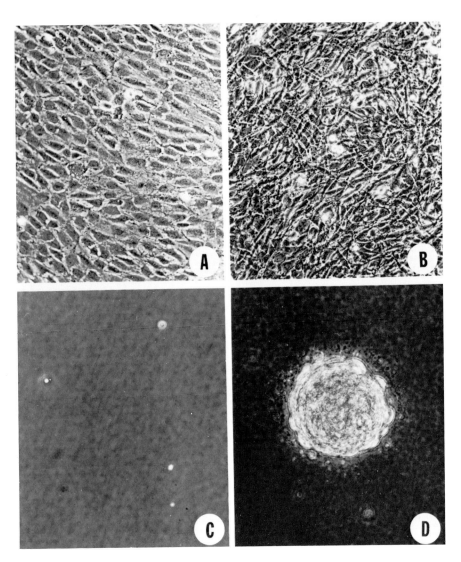

FIG. 1. A: Untreated NRK cells. × 83. **B:** NRK cells treated with an aliquot of SGF at 10 μg/ml and photographed 6 days later. The cells have grown to considerably higher cell density and display a morphology similar to that of virus-transformed cells. × 83. **C:** Untreated NRK cells plated in 0.3% soft agar. × 165. **D:** NRK cells plated in 0.3% soft agar, treated with an aliquot of SGF at 10 μg/ml and photographed 2 weeks after treatment. The untreated cultures show primarily single cells with two or three cell colonies, but none of larger size. In the treated cultures, many colonies contained well over 500 cells. × 165.

Murine sarcoma virus-transformed cells lack available receptors for EGF. We have shown that this altered phenotype is the result of the endogenous production of growth factors by the MSV-transformed cells themselves. There is no evidence that SGF acts as a complete carcinogen itself, producing permanent cell transformation; its properties resemble classic chemical promoters of carcinogenesis like 12-O-tetradecanoylphorbol-13-acetate (TPA) (3,37,46), the highly active component of croton oil. Whereas TPA is an exogenous plant derivative acting on an animal or a cell, SGF is an endogenous, virally induced growth promoter.

Several biochemical and biological studies provide evidence that the initial site of action of tumor-promoting phorbol esters may be the membrane of target cells (3,31,34,35,36,37,39,47). The tumor-promoting phorbol esters have been found to modulate the interaction between EGF and its membrane receptors in a variety of cells in culture (4,21,33). The pleiotypic effects of TPA and related tumor promoters *in vivo* as well as *in vitro* seem to mimic the several actions of growth-stimulating polypeptide hormones such as EGF (8) and SGF (11). The effect, however, though rapid for modulating the EGF receptors, is indirect as it cannot be shown using low temperatures (33) and/or fixed cells or in isolated cell membranes *(unpublished results)*. This would suggest that TPA produces its membrane effects through an interaction distinct from the EGF-receptor interaction.

[3]H-TPA has been reported to bind to HeLa cells in a nonsaturable, noncompetitive, and nonspecific fashion (22). We found that ^{3}H-TPA binds to a variety of fibroblastic and epithelioid cells in a saturable and reversible manner, but these binding sites for TPA seem to be numerous (30×10^6 per cell) and of low affinity ($K_d = 10^{-7}$ M). We have used ^{3}H-phorbol-12,13-dibutyrate (PDBu) to characterize the binding sites of phorbol and ingenol esters. PDBu is a phorbol ester which is highly active *in vivo* and *in vitro* but is comparatively less lipophilic than TPA (20,37). Thus, PDBu would partition in membrane lipids much less than TPA and lead to less nonspecific binding. Recently, ^{3}H-PDBu binding to a particulate fraction of chicken embryo fibroblasts has been reported (14).

The ability of ^{3}H-PDBu (19.7 ng/ml, specific activity 6.4 C_i/mmole, Life System Co., Newton, Massachusetts) to bind to live and fixed mink lung cells (CCL 64) (16) and Balb/3T3 clone A31 cells (CCL 163) (2) at 23°C and the competition of binding of labeled PDBu to cells with unlabeled PDBu was tested. The live and fixed mink cells bound 2,155 and 1,987 cpm, respectively, whereas live and fixed A31 cells bound 3,605 and 3,419 cpm, respectively, of ^{3}H-PDBu per 10^6 cells in the absence of unlabeled PDBu. As the concentration of unlabeled PDBu was increased, the binding of ^{3}H-PDBu to both types of cells decreased. Viable and glutaraldehyde-fixed mink cells required 30 to 35 ng/ml of PDBu for 50% inhibition of binding; the A31 cells showed ID_{50}s of 65 to 70 ng/ml and, again, no difference between viable and fixed cells.

The extent of binding of ^{3}H-PDBu to mink lung cells at various temperatures as a function of incubation time was tested. The binding increased linearly for

15 min at 4°C, whereas binding at 23°C and 37°C was linear for only a few min. Maximal binding was achieved within 7.5 min at 37°C and started to decrease with the increasing incubation time. The saturation of the binding of labeled PDBu to cells at 23 or 4°C was observed between 20 to 40 and 90 to 120 min, respectively. When ^{3}H-PDBu-labeled mink lung cells (23°C, 30-min incubation) containing bound ^{3}H-PDBu were incubated in only binding buffer at 4, 23, or 37°C, bound radioactivity dissociated from cells and was released into the medium in a time- and temperature-dependent manner.

The optimum binding of PDBu was achieved at pH 6.7. The binding was linear up to 12×10^6 cells/ml (23°C, 20-min incubation). It was not significantly affected by hydroxyurea (10 mM), actinomycin D (10 μg/ml), cycloheximide (10 μg/ml), or sodium fluoride (1 mM). Thus, it seems that PDBu binding to its receptors does not require DNA, RNA, protein synthesis, or metabolic energy. We did not find any absolute requirements of metal ions for PDBu binding to cells; however, metal chelating agents, ethylenediamine tetraacetate (EDTA) and ethylene glycol-bis-β-aminoethylethane-N,N^1-tetraacetic acid (EGTA), at 5 mM concentration reduced the binding to approximately 50%. Mg^{2+}, Co^{2+}, Na^+, and K^+ did not significantly affect the binding although Mn^{2+}, Ca^{2+}, and Zn^{2+} significantly stimulated the binding of ^{3}H-PDBu to mink cells.

Subcellular distribution of bound ^{3}H-PDBu to mink cells (4°C for 30 min or 23°C for 10 min) revealed that approximately 80% of labeled PDBu bound to the membranous fraction. This result and the comparable binding of ^{3}H-PDBu to fixed or live cells suggest that the binding sites are located on the plasma membranes of cells.

We have shown that there is a wide distribution of PDBu binding sites in cell cultures and various murine tissues. Table 1 shows the specific binding of ^{3}H-PDBu to various normal cell lines from different species in culture and murine cell lines transformed by RNA tumor viruses, DNA tumor viruses, SV40 and polyoma, or by chemical carcinogens, benzopyrene (BP), and methylcholanthrene (MC). PDBu bound to murine (normal or transformed), rat, cat, mink, hamster, rabbit, bat, dog, monkey, human, and chicken cells. The transformed murine cells were found to bind more PDBu than their normal counterparts. ^{3}H-PDBu also bound to Kirsten sarcoma virus-transformed murine cells as well as to Swiss/3T3 clone NR-6; both cell lines lack EGF receptors (28,43). The specific binding sites are also present in murine brain, spleen, thymus, lung, skin, kidney, heart, thigh muscle, liver, and intestine in decreasing order. The murine brain, which lacks EGF receptors, and spleen have an exceptionally high number of receptors for PDBu. Neither human or mouse erythrocytes bound detectable amounts of ^{3}H-PDBu. Thus, the PDBu binding sites are widely distributed and are distinct from EGF binding sites.

The effect of PDBu concentration on PDBu binding to mink lung cells and murine Balb/3T3-A31 cells is shown in Fig. 2. PDBu binding was found to be linear up to a PDBu concentration of about 5 ng/ml for both cell types. As the concentration of PDBu was increased beyond 5 ng/ml, the binding of

TABLE 1. *Binding of ³H-PDBu to cells of various species*

Species	Cells	³H Binding (cpm per 10^6 cells)[a]
Chicken	Embryo fibroblasts	4,273
Mouse	Balb/3T3-A31	3,506
	MSV-transformed A31	4,995
	BP-transformed A31	5,790
	SV40-transformed A31	5,505
	MC-transformed A31	7,983
	NIH/3T3 Cl 142	3,285
	Polyoma virus-transformed NIH/3T3 (Cl 4A)	6,729
	Swiss/3T3 CL 8	3,635
	Swiss/3T3-NR6 (no EGF receptors)	3,342
	Swiss/3T3 Cl Ll (preadipocytes)	1,560
	129/J F9 (teratocarcinoma)	487
	Swiss mouse erythrocytes (fresh)	6
Rat	NRK (fibroblasts) clone 49F	2,824
	NRK (epithelial) VB-4	1,928
Hamster	Ovary CHO	3,357
Mink	Lung (epithelial Mv1Lu (CCL 64)	2,074
Bat	Lung (fibroblastic) Tb1Lu (CCL 88)	2,498
Cat	Embryo (FEC) Cl 60	3,362
Dog	Thymus cf2Th	1,626
Monkey	Rhesus RBS	1,407
Human	Fibroblast (CCL 1553)	4,360
	Cervical carcinoma HeLaS3	864
	Epidermal carcinoma of vulva A431	2,250
	Acute myelogenous leukemia HL60	2,114
	Erythrocytes	12

[a] The binding assays were performed and the nonspecific binding was corrected as described in Fig. 2.

PDBu to cells gradually began to deviate from linearity and started to level off. PDBu binding sites were almost saturated at a PDBu concentration of 200 ng/ml (Fig. 2, insets). Figure 2 also includes Scatchard plots of PDBu binding to mink lung cells and to Balb/3T3 cells. These data produced almost linear plots for both cell types. At the saturating concentration of PDBu, approximately 2.0×10^5 molecules bound to mink lung cells and 5.1×10^5 molecules to Balb/3T3 cells. The apparent K_d values were calculated to be 1.3×10^{-9} M for mink lung cells (Fig. 2A) and 0.9×10^{-9} M for Balb/3T3 cells (Fig. 2B). The apparent K_d value for EGF interaction to its receptors on both cell types has been reported to be 0.5×10^{-9} M (33). Thus, the affinity of PDBu for its receptors is in the same range as that of EGF receptors for its ligands and other ligands for their receptors (33).

Several natural and synthetic analogs of phorbol and ingenol with various degrees of promoting activity in the two-stage tumorigenesis model are now available (3,15,34,37,45). We studied their effects on the inhibition of the binding of ³H-PDBu to mink lung cells (Fig. 3 and Table 2). TPA was the most potent competitor of PDBu binding among the phorbol, ingenol, and mezerein derivatives tested. The relative potency of these agents in competing for EGF binding was: TPA>DPTD>IHD>MZ>PDBu>PDD>PDB>PDA>ITA>Me-TPA> 4α-PDD>phorbol>ingenol (see Table 2 for abbreviations and data). The inhibition of PDBu binding to its receptors by different phorbol and ingenol derivatives correlated well with their tumor-promoting activity. Table 2 also summarizes the dose required for 50% inhibition of EGF binding for various phorbol derivatives, ingenol derivatives, and mezerein *(unpublished data)*. 2 ng/ml of ^{125}I-EGF and 19.7 ng/ml of ^{3}H-PDBu were used in these binding experiments. Table 2 shows that ID values for PDBu binding and for the indirect effect on EGF binding, as well as calculated K_1 values for PDBu binding and EGF binding for the various agents correlated well with each other and with their tumor-promoting potential. The relative values (ID_{50}/K_1) for various agents were found to be almost similar.

Nonditerpene ester tumor-promoting agents such as phenol, iodoacetic acid, iodoacetamide, bile acids, barbiturate, oleate, laurate, limonene, canthraidin, anthradin, saccharin, or cyclamate (3,15,34,37,45) did not affect the binding of ^{3}H-PDBu to its receptors even up to a concentration of 10 μg/ml. However, anthralin, another tumor promoter, actually enhanced the binding of PDBu to mink lung cells (Table 3). Thus it seems that nonditerpene ester tumor-promoting agents do not exert their biological effect through these membrane receptors. Retinoic acid, dexamethasone, prostaglandins, and disulfiram are reported to inhibit tumor promotion (3,15,34,37,45). None of these reagents significantly modulated the binding of PDBu to mink lung cells (Table 3). These results suggest that these reagents inhibit tumor promotion by acting at some site other than the receptors for phorbol or ingenol esters. In addition, cholera toxin, diphtheria toxin, oxytocin, vasopressin, gramicidin, mohesin, melittin, digitonin, fillipin, amphotericin, kanacidin, ganglioside, nystatin, cholesterol, and lysophosphocholine, up to a concentration of 10 μg/ml, did not significantly affect the binding of labeled PDBu to its receptors.

The binding of PDBu to mink lung cells is not inhibited by EGF even up to a concentration of 10 μg/ml (Table 3). Although biologically active diterpene esters efficiently modulate EGF-receptor interaction in this cell (33), PDBu binds to cells lacking EGF receptors (Table 1). The binding of PDBu to cells does not correlate with their EGF receptor numbers. These experiments clearly demonstrate that membrane receptors that specifically interact with phorbol or ingenol diterpene esters are structurally and functionally distinct from EGF membrane receptors.

These experiments demonstrate the existence of high affinity sites on avian, mammalian, and primate cells in culture that specifically interact with biologically active phorbol and ingenol derivatives but not with biologically inert analogs of these diterpenes. PDBu binding to its receptors exhibits specificity, saturability, and reversibility. PDBu binding sites in cell membranes are different from EGF membrane receptors as PDBu also binds to cells that lack EGF receptors. In contrast to the modulation of EGF binding to its receptors by biologically active

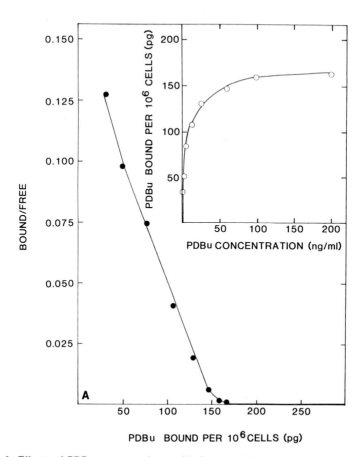

PDBu BOUND PER 10^{6}CELLS (pg)

FIG. 2. A: Effects of PDBu concentration on binding to mink lung cells and Scatchard plot. The cells were grown in 850-cm^2 roller culture bottles (RCB) in Dulbecco's minimum essential medium (DMEM) containing 10% calf serum (CS). Approximately 70% confluent cells were used for the binding assays. The medium was aspirated from bottles, cells were washed twice with 50 ml of binding buffer (BB) consisting of DMEM containing bovine serum albumin (BSA, 1 mg/ml) and N-bis-(2-hydroxyethyl)-2-amino-ethane-sulfonic acid (BES, 5 mM N), ad-justed to pH 6.8. The cells were scraped in 25 ml of BB per RCB and transferred to plastic tubes and pelleted in a refrigerated centrifuge. The cell pellets were suspended in BB and an aliquot was used to determine cell number in a Coulter counter. The binding assays were performed in duplicate in 12 × 75-mm disposable culture glass tubes (Kimax). The binding mixture contained 5 ng ^{3}H-PDBu (~4 × 10^4 cpm), 0–5 μg of unlabeled PDBu, 0.5% final concentration of dimethylsulfoxide (DMSO), and 1 × 10^6 cells in a total volume of 0.25 ml BB. After incubation for 30 min at 23°C, 4 ml cold BB was added to each tube, the contents mixed, and the tubes were centrifuged for 4 min at 4°C at 1,000 × *g* to pellet the cells. The supernatant solution was carefully drained off, the pellet was suspended in 4 ml of cold BB, and transferred to other tubes. Tubes were again centrifuged as earlier, supernatant solution was again removed, and cell pellets were solubilized in 0.7 ml of lysing buffer (0.01 M Tris-HCl, pH 7.4, containing 0.5% SDS and 1 mM EDTA). The mixture was transferred to counting vials and 10 ml of Optigel (Meloy Laboratories) was added to each vial. The vials were vigorously shaken and radioactivity was determined using a Beckman beta counter. For binding assays with fixed cells, the medium was aspirated, cells were washed twice with cold PBS, scraped from RCB, and transferred to plastic tubes and pelleted. The pellet was suspended in 2%

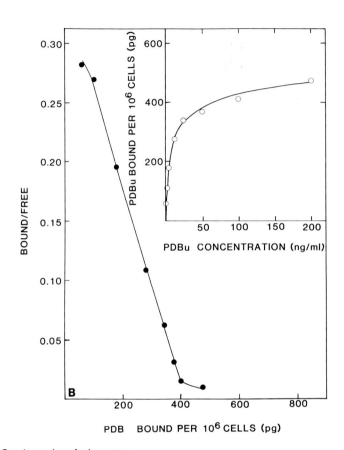

PDB BOUND PER 10⁶ CELLS (pg)

FIG. 2 B. See legend on facing page.

gluteraldehyde, pH 7.4 (1 ml per 10^6 cells) for 2 hr at 4°C. After this period, cells were pelleted and washed twice with cold PBS and the final pellet was suspended in BB. The binding with fixed cells was performed as described for the live cells. The radioactivity bound to cells in the presence of 20 μg/ml unlabeled PDBu was considered to be nonspecific binding and all data were corrected accordingly. ○, PDBu binding as a function of PDBu concentration; ●, Scatchard plot of the data in inset. **B:** Effect of PDBu concentration on PDBu binding to Balb/3T3-A31 cells and Scatchard plot. The experiment was performed in **A.** ○, PDBu binding as function of PDBu concentration; ●, Scatchard plot of the data in inset.

TABLE 2. *Correlation between the potency of phorbol and ingenol derivatives for promoting skin tumors and their ability to inhibit the binding of* ^3H-*PDBu or* ^{125}I-*EGF to cells*

Compound (with abbreviation)	Dose required for 50% inhibition (mg/ml)		K_1 values (M)[c]		Tumor-promoting activity[d]
	PDBu binding to its receptor[a]	EGF binding to its receptor[b]	PDBu binding to its receptor	EGF binding to its receptor	
12-O-tetradecanoylphorbol-13-acetate (TPA)	5.9	1.8	2.3×10^{-10}	1.8×10^{-9}	+++
Phorbol-12,13-dibutyrate (PDBu)	50.2	32.8	2.4×10^{-9}	3.9×10^{-8}	++
Phorbol-12,13-didecanoate (PDD)	83.5	53.8	3.2×10^{-9}	5.2×10^{-8}	++
Phorbol-12,13-dibenzoate (PDB)	104.0	105.0	4.4×10^{-9}	1.1×10^{-7}	+
4α-Phorbol-12,13-didecanoate (4-αPDD)	>100,000	>10,000	>1.6×10^{-4}	>9.6×10^{-6}	Nonpromoter
Phorbol-12,13-diacetate (PDA)	3,100	>10,000	>1.5×10^{-4}	>12.4×10^{-6}	Nonpromoter
4-O-Methyl-TPA (Me-TPA)	>100,000	>10,000	>1.7×10^{-4}	>9.5×10^{-6}	Nonpromoter
Phorbol	>100,000	>10,000	>2.7×10^{-4}	>16.5×10^{-6}	Nonpromoter
12-Deoxyphorbol-13-tetradecanoate (DPTD)	13.8	21.1	5.7×10^{-9}	2.3×10^{-8}	++
Mezerein (MZ)	42.5	9.8	1.7×10^{-9}	9.9×10^{-8}	?
Ingenol-13-hexadecanoate (IHD)	34.2	101	1.4×10^{-9}	10.3×10^{-8}	+
Ingenol-3,5,20-triacetate (ITA)	3,400	3,000	2.3×10^{-7}	3.6×10^{-6}	Nonpromoter
Ingenol	>100,000	>10,000	>2.8×10^{-4}	>17.2×10^{-6}	Nonpromoter

[a] Values for phorbol derivatives are taken from Shoyab et al. (33). The values for DPTD, MZ, and ingenol derivatives are from our unpublished results. 2 ng/ml of ^{125}I-EGF were used for binding.

[b] K_1 values were calculated according to the method of Cheng and Prusoff (5), using the equation K_1-$ID_{50} \times 1/(1 + L/K)$; where L and K denote concentration and affinity of labeled probe.

[c] Values derived from Fig. 3. 19.7 ng/ml of ^3H-PDBu was used for binding.

[d] See refs. 3, 14, 33, 36, 44.

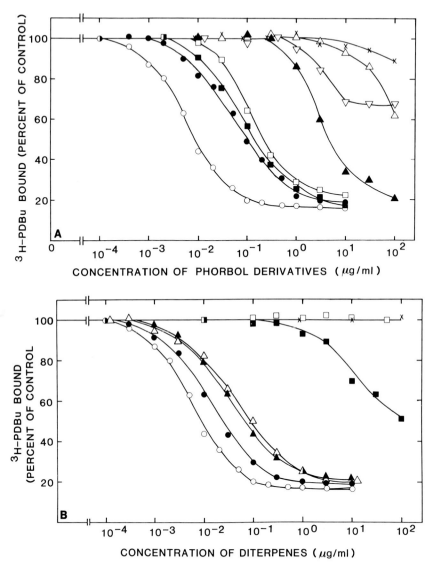

FIG. 3. A: Competition of the binding of ³H-PDBu to mink lung cells by various derivatives of phorbol. The binding assays were performed in the presence of ³H-PDBu (19.7 ng/ml) and the indicated concentrations of various derivatives of phorbol as described in the legend to Fig. 2. ○, TPA; ●, PDBu; □, PDB; ■, PDD; △, 4α-PDD; ▲, PDA; ▽, Me-TPA; x: phorbol. B: Competition of the binding of ³H-PDBu to mink lung cells by various derivatives of ingenol, mezerein, DPTD, and retinoic acid. Experiment was performed as in A. ○, TPA; ●, DPTD; △, MZ; ▲, IHD; □, ingenol; ■, ITA; x, retinoic acid.

TABLE 3. *Effect of tumor promoters and other compounds on the binding of* [3]H-
PDBu *to mink lung cells*

Compounds	Concentration (μg/ml)	Binding (cpm per 10^6 cells)[a]	Inhibition of binding (%)
None	—	2,049	0
TPA	10	62	97
Phorbol	10	2,039	0
Phenol	10	2,018	2
Iodoacetic acid	10	1,967	4
Lithocholic acid	10	2,070	−1
Na-Barbiturate	10	2,002	2
Na-Oleate	10	2,072	−1
Limonene	10	2,011	2
Anthradin	10	2,004	2
Anthralin	1	2,449	−20
Anthralin	5	3,133	−53
Anthralin	10	4,180	−104
Saccharin	10	2,041	0
Cyclamate	10	2,065	1
Vitamin K3	10	2,079	−1
Disulfiram	10	1,997	3
Retinoic acid	50	2,088	−2
EGF	10	2,075	−1
Dexamethasone	10	2,045	1
Insulin	50	2,155	−5
Prostaglandin E$_1$	50	2,106	−3
Prostaglandin F$_2$	50	1,905	−7

[a] The binding assays were performed and the nonspecific binding was corrected
as in Fig. 2.

phorbol or ingenol esters, EGF does not influence the interaction between PDBu
and its membrane receptors. These membrane receptors specifically bind biologically active phorbol and ingenol esters but not other nonditerpene ester tumor
promoters. Potent inhibitors of tumor promotion, such as retinoids, antiinflammatory steroids, prostaglandins, and cyclic nucleotides, do not interact with
these receptors. Interestingly, anthralin, a nonditerpene tumor promoter, increases the binding of PDBu to mink cells in a dose-dependent manner. We
do not know whether anthralin exhibits this effect by increasing the binding
capacity or the binding affinity or both, or acts by some other mechanism.
Whether anthralin enhances the tumor-promoting activity of PDBu and other
related compounds should be investigated.

Thus, why should mammalian cells have specific receptors for biologically
active phorbol and ingenol ester compounds of plant origin? TPA and certain
analogs may have some structural resemblance to the endogenous growth-promoting and/or differentiation-modulating substance(s) (agonists and/or antagonists) that have specific membrane receptors. The binding of PDBu to fixed
cells suggests that it interacts with the cellular components (receptors) located
on the plasma membrane of the cells. The isolation and further characterization

of PDBu receptors and a putative endogenous ligand(s) should help in understanding tumor promotion.

The general transformation model we are proposing has these features: Viruses and chemical carcinogens act by inducing cells to produce normally repressed or inactive growth-promoting factors. These factors, which may be endogenous or exogenous to given cells, could be important in embryonic development but, if inappropriately expressed later in life, could lead to transformation. Tumor viruses either provide transforming genes directly or activate cellular genes; chemical carcinogens do only the latter. These growth-promoting and transforming factors may be produced during early embryogenesis and then "switched off." The endogenous viruses, with their capacity to recombine with cellular genes, have the ability to transfer information between cells and presumably within a cell like bacterial insertion sequences. They may well be vehicles that allow expression of the endogenous growth promoter structural genes. In this model the promoters, be they endogenous (SGF) or exogenous (TPA), act as proximal effectors of transformation.

The virogene-oncogene hypothesis (17) points out the possibly erroneous assumption that virally induced tumors would have to arise through external infection by emphasizing that virus-coded or virus-associated genes are already present in several animal species. These genes, rather than the environmentally transmissible agents, are more likely to be involved in the origin of natural cancers. The tumor viruses, although unnatural in that they had often been selected for producing rapid disease, have provided extremely powerful tools to dissect out and understand the molecular mechanisms involved. Genetically transmitted viral genes and transforming genes are now accepted as being part of the normal genetic makeup of many organisms and of being activated by agents such as chemical carcinogens, hormones, and radiation (1,40). In parallel with this is the frequently made assertion that chemical carcinogenesis and environmental carcinogenesis, or even industrial carcinogenesis, are almost interchangeable with one another. The finding that SGF, produced by animal cells themselves, is an extremely potent promoter in cell culture systems suggests that endogenous growth promoters may be significant factors in naturally occurring cancers.

Since it was established that mouse sarcoma virus-transformed cells produced TGFs, we decided to screen human tumor cells for similar endogenous factors related to EGF and SGF (44). The human tumor cells tested for production of factors analogous to SGF were chosen for study because they had no apparent EGF receptors and readily form colonies in soft agar. Normal embryonal lung fibroblasts, unable to grow in soft agar, and A431 cells, which have a very high number of EGF receptors and grow poorly in soft agar, were used as controls.

Five human cultures were compared for their ability to form colonies in soft agar. The cells were grown in monolayer cultures, harvested, and seeded at varying densities into medium with 0.3% agar. Colonies were scored at 5 and 10 days. Colonies with more than 10 cells were counted as positive. The cell line 9812 (a bronchogenic carcinoma) formed progressively growing colonies even when relatively low numbers of cells were seeded. A431 (epidermoid carcinoma) cells only showed colony growth when high cell inocula were used. This suggests that a critical concentration of diffusible factors from these cells is required for anchorage-independent growth.

Cells that are potential producers of factors that stimulate growth in soft agar (e.g., human tumor cells) were seeded in one layer of agar at 1×10^6 cells per plate and overlaid with indicator cells (e.g., rat fibroblasts) at 1×10^4 cells per plate. The indicator cells formed colonies when certain human tumor cells were seeded in the other layer. A673 (human rhabdomyosarcoma), 9812, and A2058 (human metastatic melanoma) cells elicited the greatest response and released as much agar growth-stimulating activity as did a comparable number of MSV-transformed mouse 3T3 cells.

Figure 4 shows the results of experiments in which serum-free supernates from A673 cells were collected, concentrated, and run over a Bio-Gel P-100 column in 1 M acetic acid. Individual fractions were tested for protein concentration, ability to stimulate cells to form colonies in soft agar, and ability to compete with ^{125}I-labeled EGF (9). The majority of the protein is in the void volume of the column. A major peak of soft agar growth-stimulating activity was found in the included volume with maximal activity in fraction 54. When the same fractions were tested for competition with ^{125}I-EGF binding, one major peak was again found with maximal activity also in fraction 54. Aliquots were tested for stimulation of cell division in serum-depleted cultures of mouse 3T3 cells, rat NRK cells, and human skin fibroblasts; in all cases, the major growth-stimulating activity was found in fraction 54. Fractions 51 to 57 were pooled, concentrated by lyophilization, and used for further studies.

The identical procedure was used to test for growth-stimulating factors and EGF-competing peptides from the supernates of four other human cell cultures. The two highly transformed tumor cell lines, 9812 and A2058, release a growth-stimulating and EGF-competing factor with an apparent MW of 20,000 to 23,000 daltons. A2058 cells release a second factor with an apparent MW of 6,000 to 7,000 daltons. The supernate from normal human fibroblast cells did not release a detectable growth-stimulating factor and had no significant EGF-competing activity. A431 cells showed a smaller peak of growth-stimulating activity with an apparent MW of 21,000 daltons; no EGF-competing activity was found. When soft agar growth as a function of protein concentration was measured using a dose-response curve and the pooled, peak fractions from A673 cells were compared with those from normal human fibroblasts, there was a 50- to 100-fold difference in soft agar growth-stimulating activity.

The relative sensitivities of three different assays for growth-stimulating activity were compared and analyzed as the percentage of the maximal response. Induction of DNA synthesis as tested with serum-depleted rat fibroblast monolayer cultures was slightly more sensitive than the soft agar growth assay; EGF-

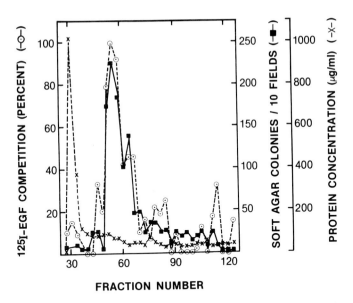

FIG. 4. Biological activity and protein determination of P-100 column fractions of concentrated conditioned media from A673 cells. EGF competition was performed as described in Todaro et al. (44). Nonspecific binding, determined by an addition of a 500-fold excess of unlabeled EGF, was approximately 200 cpm. Specific binding was approximately 1,200 cpm. Percent competition was determined after correcting for nonspecific binding. Soft agar assays were performed as described in Todaro et al. (44). Protein concentration was determined by the method of Lowry et al. (23).

competing ability was the least sensitive. The latter two assays were used in further studies since they have greater specificity. Each of the TGF activities was destroyed by trypsin or dithiothreitol but was stable at 100°C for 2 min and to repeated lyophilization from 1 M acetic acid.

Table 4 shows that the growth-stimulatory factor(s) released by the human tumor cells induces anchorage-independent growth of normal human fibroblasts. Two cell strains were tested; passage 8 of HEL 299 (a human embryonic lung cell line) and the 14th passage of HsF (a skin strain from a normal human adult). A673 cells were tested at 10 μg/ml and 1 μg/ml. 1 $\times$ 10^4 cells were seeded per plate and 1,000 single cells were followed for 2 weeks. Those that grew to colonies containing 10 cells were scored as positive. The percentages of HEL 299 and HsF single cells that gave rise to colonies were 4.2 and 3.1%, respectively, using 10 μg/ml of P-100 purified TGF. In contrast, 23.6% of the rat fibroblast cells showed a pronounced response even at 1 μg/ml. TGF also induced soft agar growth of a mouse epithelial cell line MMC-1 (19) (data not shown).

In order to test whether human tumor cell lines could also respond to TGFs, cells such as A431, which untreated could not form colonies in agar unless inoculated at high density, were used. Carcinoma cell growth in agar also depends

TABLE 4. *Stimulation of growth in agar of human diploid fibroblasts and human tumor cells by TGF*

| | | | Colonies >10 cells/1,000 cells | |
Cell	Type	Control	+TGF (10 μg/ml)	+TGF (1 μg/ml)
HEL 299	Embryonic lung fibroblast	1	42	3
HsF	Adult skin fibroblast	2	31	2
A431	Epidermoid carcinoma	3	31	8
TE85	Osteosarcoma	1	75	14
NRK (clone 49F)	Rat kidney fibroblasts	0	236	37

on "conditioning" factors, such as TGFs, which partially replace the requirement for high cell density. The results were more striking when the human osteosarcoma line TE85, which can be further transformed by MSV and certain chemical carcinogens (6), was used as an indicator cell. These results demonstrate that normal and tumor cells respond to TGFs in the same manner as rat fibroblasts. The results, then, are not dependent on an unusual property of a particular indicator cell.

The active fractions from P-100 columns of A673 and A431 cells were pooled, concentrated, and applied to carboxymethyl cellulose columns. Two peaks of agar growth-stimulating activity were obtained from A673 cells; only the major activity was associated with the peak of EGF-competing activity. Dose-response curves from each peak show an activity detectable when concentrations of 10 to 20 ng/ml are added to soft agar. The comparable fraction from supernates of cultures of the normal human fibroblasts showed no activity. Fractions derived from A431 cells (Fig. 5) showed only the less active, earlier eluting peak which is not associated with EGF-competing activity. We conclude that A431 cells which grow poorly in agar and have a high level of EGF receptors produce a factor capable of stimulating anchorage-independent growth of cells through a mechanism independent of the EGF receptor system. The highly transformed A673 cells, however, make at least two different factors. One interacts with the EGF receptor system and accounts for over 90% of the total activity in the fraction. The other is independent of the EGF receptor system and may be analogous to the factor produced by the A431 cells.

These results demonstrate that human tumor cells produce a growth factor(s) capable of inducing transformation in normal indicator cells. It has many properties in common with the factor from mouse and rat sarcoma virus-transformed cells. The major activity, although considerably larger than SGF, is closely associated with EGF-competing activity. We have found that a chemically transformed mouse 3T3 cell line produces growth-stimulating factor(s) active in the soft agar growth assay (G. Todaro et al., *unpublished data*). Production of these factors, then, is not restricted to RNA tumor virus-transformed cells,

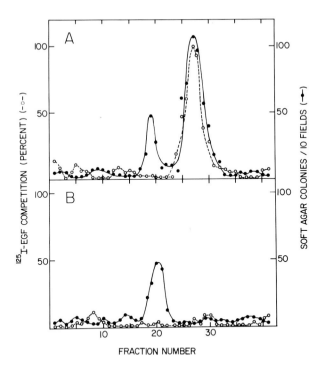

FIG. 5. Chromatography of biological activities in the peak region of Bio-Gel P-100 columns rechromatographed on a carboxymethyl cellulose column. **A:** A673. **B:** A431.

sarcoma cells, or rodent cells, but rather may be a more general expression of the transformed phenotype. In assays comparing growth stimulation of mouse, rat, and human fibroblasts in monolayer cultures, there is no evidence for species specificity of the factors produced by human cells. Conclusions as to whether the carcinoma, sarcoma, and melanoma cells are producing an identical factor(s) await further chemical purification. The present experiments show that anchorage-independent growth of tumor and normal cells is stimulated by these growth factors. Their production by transformed cells and the responses of their normal counterparts raise the possibility that cells "autostimulate" their growth by releasing factors that rebind at the cell surface (41). Experiments demonstrating that growth in soft agar of tumor cells depends on the number of cells seeded per unit area argue that diffusible substances released by cells stimulate neighboring cells. Those cells that grow best in soft agar are the most efficient producers of transforming peptides. Additional cell lines will have to be tested under different conditions before conclusions can be drawn as to the significance of this association.

Roberts et al. (30) described a procedure for purifying TGFs. The peptides are stable in acidic 70% alcohol. Intracellular growth factors have been extracted from cultured MSV-transformed mouse cells and from tumor cells in athymic mice. The major peptide with soft agar growth-stimulating activity has an apparent MW of 6,700 daltons. The peak of EGF-competing activity is in the same fraction. A transplantable, transitional cell, mouse bladder carcinoma had agar growth-stimulating activity for rat fibroblasts. Ozanne et al. (27) described a transforming factor from Kirsten sarcoma virus-transformed rat fibroblasts with properties like SGF and TGFs and report a similar activity in a spontaneously transformed rat cell line. The effect of the transforming factor on morphologic transformation can be blocked by actinomycin D early after treatment, suggesting that new RNA is produced prior to the change in phenotype of the indicator cells. Inhibitors of protein synthesis also produce a rapid reversion in the phenotype of the treated cells (27).

If release of the factor and rebinding to EGF receptors is essential for growth stimulation, tumor cell growth could be interrupted by exogenous agents, perhaps analogs that interact with the receptors but do not confer the ability to proliferate under anchorage-independent conditions (38). Anchorage-independent growth is a cell culture property closely associated with the transformed state *in vivo* (24,32). These peptides, then, are potent proximal effectors of cell transformation. Their continued production appears to play a role in maintaining the transformed phenotype. This can be directly demonstrated in temperature-sensitive mutant transformants of rodent cells (27,42), but has not yet been shown for factors produced by human tumor cells. The approach described here offers a sensitive assay for growth-stimulatory factors associated with maintaining the transformed state. Purification of such factors may lead to the development of specific immunologic assays for their production by tumor cells and their presence in body fluids. The factors may be analogous to peptide growth factors expressed early in normal embryonic development (42). This is supported by experiments by Nexo et al. (25). In the mouse embryo (days 11 to 18), there is 5 to 10 times more EGF-like material than mouse EGF. Why the factors produced by transformed cells are so potent in stimulating anchorage-independent growth while EGF is not effective is unclear but suggests the possibility that there may be more "transforming" variants of the normally expressed growth factors produced in adult life. We suggest that these factors, like SGFs, are EGF-related peptides, as insulin and somatomedins are related (29), and appear to have evolved from common ancestral proteins (26). Further purification of these and other growth factors from human tumor cells is needed to define their relationship to other biologically active peptides that cells produce. We are also testing the possibility that certain tumor cells may also produce factors related to the phorbol ester family of growth promoters.

ACKNOWLEDGMENTS

The authors gratefully acknowledge Patricia Ann Johnson for excellent technical information, support, and editorial assistance in the preparation of this manuscript.

REFERENCES

1. Aaronson, S. A., and Stephenson, J. R. (1976): Endogenous type-C RNA viruses of mammalian cells. *Biochim. Biophys. Acta,* 458:323–354.
2. Aaronson, S. A., and Todaro, G. J. (1968): Development of 3T3-like lines from Balb/c mouse embryo cultures: Transformation susceptibility to SV40. *J. Cell. Physiol.,* 72:141–148.
3. Boutwell, R. K. (1974): The function and mechanism of promoters of carcinogenesis. *Crit. Rev. Toxicol.,* 2:419–443.
4. Brown, K. D., Dicker, P., and Rozengurt, E. (1979): Inhibition of epidermal growth factor binding to surface receptors by tumor promoters. *Biochem. Biophys. Res. Commun.,* 86:1,037–1,043.
5. Cheng, C. Y., and Prusoff, W. H. (1973): Relationship between the inhibition constant (K_1) and the concentration of inhibitor which causes 50% inhibition (I_{50}) of an enzymatic reaction. *Biochem. Pharmacol.,* 22:3,099–3,108.
6. Cho, H. Y., and Rhim, J. S. (1979): Cycloheximide-dependent reversion of human cells transformed by MSV and chemical carcinogen. *Science,* 205:691–693.
7. Cifone, M. A., and Fidler, I. J. (1980): Correlation of patterns of anchorage-independent growth with *in vivo* behavior of cells from a murine fibrosarcoma. *Proc. Natl. Acad. Sci. USA,* 77:1,039–1,043.
8. Cohen, S., and Taylor, J. M. (1974): Part. I. Epidermal growth factor: Chemical and biological characterization. *Recent Prog. Horm. Res.,* 30:533–550.
9. De Larco, J. E., Reynolds, R., Carlberg, K., Engle, C., and Todaro, G. J. (1980): Sarcoma growth factor from mouse sarcoma virus-transformed cells: Purification by binding to and elution from epidermal growth factor receptor-rich cells. *J. Biol. Chem.,* 255:3,685–3,690.
10. De Larco, J. E., and Todaro, G. J. (1976): Membrane receptors for murine leukemia viruses: Characterization using the purified viral envelope glycoprotein, gp71. *Cell,* 8:365–371.
11. De Larco, J. E., and Todaro, G. J. (1978a): Growth factors from murine sarcoma virus-transformed cells. *Proc. Natl. Acad. Sci. USA,* 75:4,001–4,005.
12. De Larco, J. E., and Todaro, G. J. (1978b): Epithelioid and fibroblastic rat kidney cell clones: Epidermal growth factor (EGF) receptors and the effect of mouse sarcoma virus transformation. *J. Cell. Physiol.,* 94:335–342.
13. De Larco, J. E., and Todaro, G. J. (1980): Sarcoma growth factor: Specific binding to and elution from epidermal growth factor membrane receptors. *Symp. Quant. Biol.,* 44:643–649.
14. Dreidger, P. E., and Blumberg, P. M. (1980): Specific binding of phorbol ester tumor promoters. *Proc. Natl. Acad. Sci. USA,* 77:567–571.
15. Hecker, E. (1971): Isolation and characterization of the cocarcinogenic principles from croton oil. *Methods Cancer Res.,* 6:439–484.
16. Henderson, I. C., Lieber, M. M., and Todaro, G. J. (1974): Mink cell line Mv1Lu (CCL64): Focus formation and the generation of "nonproducer" transformed cell lines with murine and feline sarcoma viruses. *Virology,* 60:282–287.
17. Huebner, R. J., and Todaro, G. J. (1969): Oncogenes of RNA tumor viruses—as determinants of cancer. *Proc. Natl. Acad. Sci. USA,* 64:1,087–1,094.
18. Kahn, P., and Shin, S-I. (1979): Cellular tumorigenicity in nude mice: Test of associations among loss of cell surface fibronectin, anchorage independence, and tumor-forming ability. *J. Cell Biol.,* 82:1–16.
19. Keski-Oja, J., De Larco, J. E., Rapp, U. R., and Todaro, G. J. (1980): Murine sarcoma growth factors affect the growth and morphology of cultured mouse epithelial cells. *J. Cell. Physiol.,* 104:41–46.
20. Kubinyi, H. (1976): Quantitative structure-activity relationships. IV. Nonlinear dependence of biological activity on hydrophobic character: A new model. *Arzneim. Forest,* 26:1,991–1,997.
21. Lee, L. S., and Weinstein, I. B. (1978a): Tumor-promoting phorbol esters inhibit binding of epidermal growth factor to cellular receptors. *Science,* 202:313–315.
22. Lee, L. S., and Weinstein, I. B. (1978b): Uptake of the tumor-promoting agent 12-O-tetradecanoylphorbol-13-acetate by HeLa cells. *J. Environ. Pathol. Toxicol.,* 1:626–639.
23. Lowry, O. H., Rosebrough, N. J., Farr, A. L., and Randall, R. J. (1951): Protein measurement with the folin phenol reagent. *J. Biol. Chem.,* 193:265–275.
24. Montesano, R., Drevon, C., Kuroki, T., Saint Vincent, L., Handelman, S., Sanford, K. K., DeFeo, D., and Weinstein, I. B. (1977): Test for malignant transformation of rat liver cells in culture: Cytology, growth in soft agar, and production of plasminogen activator. *J. Natl. Cancer Inst.,* 59:1,651–1,658.

25. Nexo, E., Hollenberg, M. D., Figueroa, A., and Pratt, R. M. (1980): Detection of epidermal growth factor urogastrone and its receptor during fetal mouse development. *Proc. Natl. Acad. Sci. USA,* 77:2,782–2,785.

26. Niall, H. D. (1977): In: *Peptides: Proceedings of the Fifth American Peptide Symposium,* edited by G. Goodman and J. Meienhofer, pp. 127–135. Halsted Press, New York.

27. Ozanne, B., Fulton, J., and Kaplan, P. L. (1980): Kirsten murine sarcoma virus-transformed cell lines and a spontaneously transformed rat cell line produce transforming factors. *J. Cell Physiol.,* 105:163–180.

28. Pruss, R. W., and Herschman, H. R. (1977): Variants of 3T3 cells lacking mitogenic response to epidermal growth factor. *Proc. Natl. Acad. Sci. USA,* 74:3,918–3,921.

29. Rinderknecht, E., and Humbel, R. E. (1978): The amino acid sequence of human insulin-like growth factor I and its structural homology with proinsulin. *J. Biol. Chem.,* 253:2,769–2,776.

30. Roberts, A. B., Lamb, L. C., Newton, D. L., Sporn, M. B., De Larco, J. E., and Todaro, G. J. (1980): Transforming growth factors: Isolation of polypeptides from virally and chemically transformed cells by acid/ethanol extraction. *Proc. Natl. Acad. Sci. USA,* 77:3,494–3,498.

31. Rohrschneider, L. R., O'Brien, D. H., and Boutwell, R. K. (1972): The stimulation of phospholipid metabolism in mouse skin following phorbol ester treatment. *Biochim. Biophys. Acta,* 280:57–70.

32. Shin, S., Freedman, V. H., Risser, R., and Pollack, R. (1975): Tumorigenicity of virus-transformed cells in nude mice is correlated specifically with anchorage-independent growth *in vitro. Proc. Natl. Acad. Sci. USA,* 72:4,435–4,439.

33. Shoyab, M., De Larco, J. E., and Todaro, G. J. (1979): Biologically active phorbol esters specifically alter affinity of epidermal growth factor membrane receptors. *Nature,* 279:387–391.

34. Sivak, A. (1979): Cocarcinogenesis. *Biochim. Biophys. Acta,* 560:67–89.

35. Sivak, A., Mossman, B. F., and Van Duuren, B. L. (1972): Activation of cell membrane enzymes in the stimulation of cell division. *Biochem. Biophys. Res. Commun.,* 46:605–609.

36. Sivak, A., and Van Duuren, B. L. (1971): Cellular interactions of phorbol myristate acetate in tumor promotion. Chem. Biol. Interact., 3:401–411.

37. Slaga, T. J., Sivak, A., and Boutwell, R. K., editors (1978): *Mechanisms of Tumor Promotion and Carcinogenesis.* Raven Press, New York.

38. Sporn, M. B., Newton, D. L., Roberts, A. B., De Larco, J. E., and Todaro, G. J. (1981): Retinoids and the suppression of the effects of polypeptide-transforming factors—A new molecular approach to chemoprevention of cancer. In *Molecular Actions and Targets for Cancer Chemotherapeutic Agents,* edited by A. C. Sartorelli, J. R. Bertino, and J. S. Lazo. Academic Press, New York *(in press).*

39. Suss, R., Kinzel, V., and Kreibich, G. (1971): Cocarcinogenic croton oil factor A1 stimulates lipid synthesis in cell cultures. *Experientia,* 27:46–47.

40. Todaro, G. J., Callahan, R., Sherr, C. J., Benveniste, R. E., and De Larco, J. E. (1978): Genetically transmitted viral genes of rodents and primates. In: *Persistent Viruses, ICN-UCLA Symposia on Molecular Biology, Vol. 11,* edited by J. G. Stevens, G. J. Todaro, and C. F. Fox, pp. 133–145. Academic Press, New York.

41. Todaro, G. J., and De Larco, J. E. (1978): Growth factors produced by sarcoma virus-transformed cells. *Cancer Res.,* 38:4,147–4,154.

42. Todaro, G. J., and De Larco, J. E. (1980): Properties of sarcoma growth factors (SGFs) produced by mouse sarcoma virus-transformed cells in culture. In *Control Mechanisms in Animal Cells: Specific Growth Factors, Vol. 1,* edited by L. Jimenez de Asua, R. Levi-Montalcini, R. Shields, and S. Iacobelli, pp. 223–243. Raven Press, New York.

43. Todaro, G. J., De Larco, J. E., and Cohen, S. (1976): Transformation by murine and feline sarcoma viruses specifically blocks binding of epidermal growth factor (EGF) to cells. *Nature,* 264:26–31.

44. Todaro, G. J., Fryling, C., and De Larco, J. E. (1980): Transforming growth factors (TGFs) produced by certain human tumor cells: Polypeptides that interact with epidermal growth factor (EGF) receptors. *Proc. Natl. Acad. Sci. USA,* 77:5,258–5,262.

45. Van Duuren, B. L. (1969): Tumor-promoting agents in two-stage carcinogenesis. *Prog. Exp. Tumor Res.,* 11:31–68.

46. Weinstein, I. B., and Wigler, M. (1977): Cell culture studies provide new information on tumour promoters. *Nature,* 270:659–660.

47. Wenner, C., Hackney, J., Kimelberg, H., and Mayhew, E. (1974): Membrane effects of phorbol esters. *Cancer Res.,* 34:1,731–1,737.

Carcinogenesis, Vol. 7, edited by E. Hecker et al.
Raven Press, New York © 1982.

Interaction of Tumor Promoters and Growth Factors with Cultured Cells

*George T. Bowden, †Lynn M. Matrisian, †Jean M. Lockyer, and ‡Bruce E. Magun

*Department of Radiology (Division of Radiation Oncology), the University of Arizona Medical School, Arizona Health Sciences Center, Tucson, Arizona 85724; †Department of Anatomy, the University of Arizona Medical School, Arizona Health Sciences Center, Tucson, Arizona 85724; and ‡Departments of Radiology and Anatomy, the University of Arizona Medical School, Arizona Health Sciences Center, Tucson, Arizona 85724

An important aspect of tumor promotion in mouse skin is the stimulation of cell proliferation. In the mouse skin tumor model system, hyperplasia appears to be necessary but not sufficient for tumor promotion (12). Tumor promoters are also known to stimulate cell proliferation in primary cultures of mouse epidermal cells (10) and in cultured fibroblasts (7,13). Addition of tumor promoters to growing cell cultures does not increase the rate of cell growth and in fact causes a transient depression in deoxyribonucleic acid (DNA) synthesis. Only after cells have become confluent do tumor promoters cause an increase in cell numbers (9).

Phorbol ester tumor promoters and the mitogen epidermal growth factor (EGF) share a number of common biological effects (5). For this reason, Lee and Weinstein first examined the effects of tumor promoters on the binding of EGF to specific cell surface receptors (6). Using Scatchard analysis of ^{125}I-EGF receptor binding, Lee and Weinstein (5) showed that in HeLa cells, phorbol esters caused a decrease in the number of binding sites but not in receptor affinity, whereas others (2,11) concluded that phorbol esters induced a decrease in receptor affinity but not in the number of binding sites. Until recently no explanation had been given for the observation that despite the inhibited binding of EGF by phorbol esters, these compounds act synergistically to induce DNA synthesis in quiescent cells. The experiments which we conducted were designed to attempt to explain these paradoxical findings. We used both primary cultures of newborn mouse epidermal cells as well as Rat-1 fibroblasts (8) to examine the effects of the potent tumor promoter 12-O-tetradecanoylphorbol-13-acetate (TPA) on EGF binding and induction of DNA synthesis.

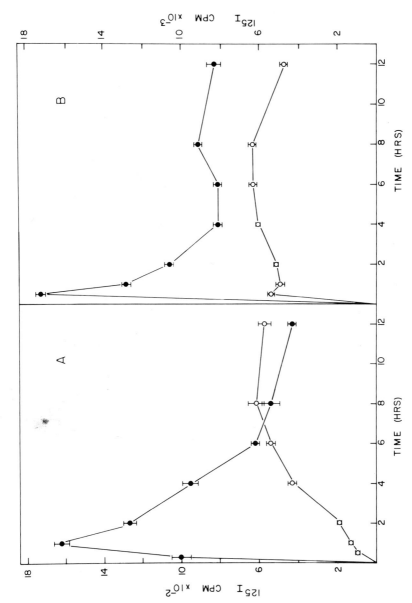

FIG. 1. Effect of TPA on time course of ^{125}I-EGF binding in Rat-1 cells. Rat-1 cells were incubated in binding medium containing 0.2 ng/ml (**A**) or 5 ng/ml (**B**) of ^{125}I-EGF at t = 0. The medium contained 0.1% DMSO (●) or 100 ng/ml TPA plus 0.1% DMSO (○). (From Magun et al., ref. 8.)

TPA-INDUCED ALTERATIONS OF EGF RECEPTOR NUMBER
AND AFFINITY

The time course of ^{125}I-EGF binding to Rat-1 cells was examined for 12 hr at 37° in the presence or absence of 100 ng/ml TPA (Fig. 1). In the absence of TPA at both high and low concentrations of EGF (0.20 and 5 ng/ml), maximum ^{125}I-EGF binding occurred within 1 hr, followed by a decrease in the amount of ^{125}I-EGF bound. With the lower concentration (Fig. 1A) of ^{125}I-EGF (0.2 ng/ml) in the presence of TPA (100 ng/ml), ^{125}I-EGF binding was decreased over the control (90% decrease at 1 hr) but by 12 hr the amount of ^{125}I-EGF bound was 30% greater than in the control. In the presence of the higher concentration of ^{125}I-EGF (5 ng/ml) plus TPA, ^{125}I-EGF binding was 30% of the control at 0.5 hr and stayed lower than the control thereafter (Fig. 1B). Similar results were found with primary newborn mouse epidermal cells grown under a low calcium concentration, except that the time course for TPA enhancement of EGF binding at a limiting EGF concentration was extended (enhanced binding was not seen until 18 hr after initial treatment; data not shown). The inhibitory effects of TPA on EGF binding were found to be reversible with time of incubation at 37° but not at 4° (8). The time course for reversibility showed a more delayed response in the primary epidermal cells as opposed to the Rat-1 cells (data not shown). The reversibility could not be explained by degradation of TPA in the medium in either cell type (8).

To relate the effects of TPA to receptor affinity and number, Scatchard analysis of EGF binding to its receptor was carried out in the presence and absence of TPA (Fig. 2). Using Scatchard analysis we observed for both cell types a decrease in EGF receptor number and affinity in the presence of TPA. The curvilinear Scatchard plots in the control cultures were explained by the presence of two classes of receptors with differing affinities. The effect of TPA was to eliminate binding to the class of high affinity receptors. Incubation with TPA at 37° for 8 to 12 hr, followed by Scatchard analysis at 4°, revealed that the initial decrease in affinity was overcome with time, such that the high affinity EGF receptors regained their ability to bind EGF (8). We found for both cell types that TPA did not alter the rate at which bound EGF was degraded (8). At low EGF concentrations, however, TPA reduced the amount of EGF that was metabolized over a 12- to 18-hr period, resulting in 50% more intact EGF in the medium of TPA-treated cells compared to controls (8). At a higher EGF concentration, TPA had a very small effect on EGF degradation (8). The ability of TPA to spare EGF from degradation at low EGF concentrations resulted from the initial TPA-induced reduction in EGF binding. The increased amounts of EGF remaining in the medium of cells exposed to a limiting concentration of EGF and TPA resulted in significantly more EGF binding in TPA-treated cells than in control cultures.

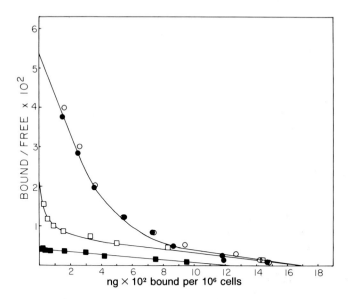

FIG. 2. Scatchard analysis of ^{125}I-EGF binding in the presence or absence of TPA in Rat-1 cells. Cells for Scatchard analysis were incubated with increasing concentrations of ^{125}I-EGF for 4 hr at 4° in the presence (□) or absence (○) of TPA (100 ng/ml). Another group of cells was first incubated in the binding medium containing DMSO (●) or TPA (100 ng/ml) (■) for 1 hr at 37° prior to Scatchard analysis. (From Magun et al, ref. 8.)

SYNERGISTIC INDUCTION OF DNA SYNTHESIS BY EGF AND TUMOR PROMOTERS

We have found EGF and phorbol ester tumor promoters to act synergistically at low (0.001 to 0.05 ng/ml) but not high (> 0.1 ng/ml) EGF concentrations to induce DNA synthesis in quiescent Rat-1 cells (Table 1). The degree of synergism was found to be correlated with the tumor-promoting ability of the phorbol ester. The phorbol esters decreased ^{125}I-EGF binding to cellular receptors in a dose-dependent manner that correlated with the tumor-promoting ability of the compound and thus resulted in a decrease in the amount of EGF degraded as compared to control cultures (Table 2). The ability of the phorbol ester compound to alter EGF degradation and to stimulate DNA synthesis synergistically with EGF correlated in both cases with the tumor-promoting ability of the compound and occurred only at low EGF concentrations.

HYPOTHESIS

Given the results presented above, we have proposed that the induction of DNA synthesis by TPA and related phorbol esters is related to the ability of the phorbol esters to transiently decrease binding of EGF or other growth factors to their receptors. This inhibition of binding would spare the degradation of

TABLE 1. *Effect of EGF and phorbol ester tumor promoters on DNA synthesis in rat-1 cells*[a]

EGF (ng/ml)	Percent replicated DNA			
	None	TPA	PDA	4-O-methyl-TPA
0	8	28	26	20
0.001	8	32	30	20
0.01	10	58	42	32
0.05	14	58	44	30
0.10	36	63	60	56
5.0	70	75	82	80

[a] Rat-1 cellular DNA was prelabeled with [^{14}C]thymidine and the cells were serum-deprived for 48 hr. At that time, fresh serum-free medium containing BrdUrd, FdUrd, 0.1% dimethylsulfoxide (DMSO), varying concentrations of EGF, and 100 ng/ml of the phorbol esters (TPA, phorbol 12, 13 diacetate (PDA), 4-O-methyl-TPA) were added to the plates. The cells were harvested 30 hr later and DNA was isolated and banded on CsCl gradients. Following centrifugation [^{14}C] activity recovered from the hybrid (newly synthesized DNA) peak divided by the [^{14}C] activity recovered from the entire gradient was taken as percent DNA replicated. Each value represents the result of a complete gradient.

TABLE 2. *Effect of phorbol esters on degradation of* ^{125}*I-EGF*[a]

Time of incubation (hr)	Percent immunoreactive ^{125}I-EGF				
	DMSO	TPA	PDB	PDA	4-O-methyl-TPA
1	78.9	85.1	84.2	81.3	79.8
2	64.8	83.1	83.2	73.0	70.8
4	45.9	77.7	75.5	58.2	55.5
8	24.3	54.4	52.4	35.5	36.0
12	17.8	32.5	31.5	21.4	17.0

[a] Rat-1 cells were exposed to 0.2 ng/ml immunoreactive ^{125}I-EGF in binding medium for times up to 12 hr. Binding medium also contained 0.1% DMSO and 100 ng/ml TPA, phorbol-12, 13-dibenzoate (PDB), PDA, or 4-O-methyl-TPA. At indicated times, the medium was removed and analyzed for the percent immunoreactive ^{125}I-EGF remaining in the medium. The standard error of the mean was always less than 5% of the mean.

the growth factor in the cellular milieu and would be more pronounced when the levels of growth factors were limiting. When the receptor affinity was restored, EGF concentrations would be greater in the cellular milieu of the phorbol ester-treated cells than in control cells. These higher growth factor concentrations would then be sufficient to induce a greater population of cells to enter DNA synthesis.

This model is consistent with the observation that phorbol esters decrease DNA synthesis shortly after addition to culture medium or application to the skin of mice (1,9) since its transient interference with EGF binding would be expected to prevent the entrance of cells into S phase. It has been observed that continuous exposure to growth factors must occur for a 12-hr period for cells to enter S phase (3). The reversibility of the TPA-induced inhibition of EGF binding which has been also reported by others (6) would explain the finding that TPA does not block mitogenic activity when cells have been exposed continuously to phorbol esters for several days. The observation that addition of phorbol esters to cell cultures results in an increased cell density would be explained by our observation that growth factor levels remain higher than in control cells, since the phorbol ester-induced inhibition of binding is coupled to decreased growth factor degradation. An additional piece of evidence that growth factor modulation may be an important aspect of phorbol ester action is that the phorbol esters are unable to induce hyperplasia in the absence of serum or serum factors (4,13).

Note added in proof: Results concerning the effects of phorbol esters on primary mouse epidermal cells in culture have been published by us (6a).

ACKNOWLEDGMENTS

This work was supported by United States Public Health Service Grant CA20913 and American Cancer Society Grant IN-110D. Lynn M. Matrisian was supported by Cellular and Molecular Biology Training Grant 5T32 GM07239.

REFERENCES

1. Baird, W. M., Sedgwick, J. A., and Boutwell, R. K. (1971): Effect of phorbol and four diesters of phorbol on the incorporation of tritiated precursors into DNA, RNA, and proteins in mouse epidermis. *Cancer Res.,* 31:1,434–1,439.
2. Brown, K. D., Dicker, P., and Rozengurt, E. (1979): Inhibition of epidermal growth factor binding to surface receptors by tumor promoters. *BBRC,* 86:1,037–1,043.
3. Carpenter, G., and Cohen, S. (1978): Epidermal growth factors. In: *Biochemical Actions of Hormones, Vol. V,* edited by G. Litwack, pp. 203–247. Academic Press, New York.
4. Dicker, P., and Rozengurt, E. (1978): Stimulation of DNA synthesis by tumor and pure mitogenic factors. *Nature,* 276:723–726.
5. Lee, L. S., and Weinstein, I. B. (1978): Tumor-promoting phorbol esters inhibit binding of epidermal growth factor to cellular receptors. *Science,* 202:313–315.
6. Lee, L. S., and Weinstein, I. B. (1979): Mechanism of tumor promoter inhibition of cellular binding of epidermal growth factor. *Proc. Natl. Acad. Sci. USA,* 76:5,168–5,172.
6a. Lockyer, J. M., Bowden, G. T., Matrisian, L. M., and Magun, B. E. (1981): Tumor promoter-induced inhibition to epidermal growth factor binding to cultured mouse primary epidermal cells. *Cancer Res.,* 41:2,308–2,314.
7. Magun, B. E., and Bowden, G. T. (1979): Effects of the tumor promoter TPA on the induction of DNA synthesis in normal and RSV-transformed rat fibroblasts. *J. Supramol. Struct.,* 12:63–72.
8. Magun, B. E., Matrisian, L. M., and Bowden, G. T. (1980): Epidermal growth factor: Ability of tumor promoter to alter its degradation, receptor affinity, and receptor number. *J. Biol. Chem.,* 255:6,373–6,381.
9. Peterson, A. R., Mondal, S., Brankow, D. W., Thon, W., and Heidelberger, C. (1977): Effect of promoters on DNA synthesis in C3H 10T ½ mouse fibroblasts. *Cancer Res.,* 37:3,223–3,227.

10. Samsel, W., Fischer, G., Kovar, R., and Fusenig, N. E. (1974): The effects of the tumor-promoting agent 12-O-tetradecanoylphorbol-13-acetate on proliferation and differentiation in primary cultures of mouse epidermal cells. *Physiol. Chem.*, 355:1,245–1,246.
11. Shoyab, M., DeLarco, J. E., and Todaro, G. J. (1979): Biologically active phorbol esters specifically alter affinity of epidermal growth factor membrane receptors. *Nature*, 279:387–391.
12. Slaga, T. J., Fischer, S. M., Nelson, K., and Gleason, G. L. (1980): Evidence for several stages in promotion. *Proc. Natl. Acad. Sci. USA*, 77:3,659–3,663.
13. Weinstein, I. B., Wigler, M., Fisher, P. B., Sisskin, E., and Pietropaolo, C. (1978): Cell culture studies on the biological effects of tumor promoters. In: *Mechanisms of Tumor Promotion and Cocarcinogenesis, Vol. 2,* edited by T. J. Slaga, A. Sivak, and R. K. Boutwell, pp. 313–334. Raven Press, New York.

Carcinogenesis, Vol. 7, edited by E. Hecker et al.
Raven Press, New York © 1982.

Inhibition of Epidermal Growth Factor Binding by Phorbol Esters, Saccharin, and Cyclamate and Its Implications in the Mechanism of Tumor Promotion

Lih-Syng Lee

*General Electric Corporate Research and Development Center,
Schenectady, New York 12301*

Tumor promotion in two-stage rodent tests has been demonstrated for phorbol esters, phenobarbital, saccharin, cyclamate, polycyclic aromatic hydrocarbons, butylated hydroxytoluene, and surfactants (13). In addition, substances such as cigarette tar, dietary fat, bile acids, and steroid hormones are known to increase cancer incidence despite lack of obvious tumor-initiating activity (13). Many of these are probably also promoters, although a few may instead derive their cocarcinogenic activity from the ability to stimulate the activation of procarcinogens. In any event, it is evident that tumor promotion can be effected by many different classes of substances which exhibit no structural similarity.

The most potent, known tumor promoters, the phorbol esters, especially 12-O-tetradecanoyl-β-phorbol-13-acetate (TPA), exert their effect at very low doses (about 1 μg on mouse skin), whereas most other suspect promoters exhibit their activity only upon lifetime feeding at maximal tolerable doses. Phorbol ester-induced carcinogenesis may therefore provide clues to a promotion pathway that is reachable only by other promoters at very high doses. On the other hand, there is evidence that not all the biological effects exerted by the pluripotent TPA are related to tumor promotion *(this volume).*

Since carcinogenesis involves loss of cellular regulation, we hypothesized that the TPA actions related to tumor promotion might interfere with the action systems of other growth regulators. This led to the discovery that TPA inhibits the binding of epidermal growth factor (EGF) to many types of cells (8,9).

EGF is a small peptide hormone (MW = 6,000). After it is bound to its receptor, the resulting receptor-EGF complexes undergo aggregation and internalization (1). At very high doses, EGF is tumor promoting (11), but at physiological levels, it is not tumor promoting, as shown by the feasibility of the classic two-stage rodent carcinogenesis assay.

EGF-BINDING INHIBITION BY PHORBOL ESTERS

Inhibition of EGF binding by phorbol esters is effected at very low concentrations (10^{-6} to 10^{-9} M), comparable to the levels required for tumor promotion (Table 1). Remarkable features of this system are: (a) Several of the biological effects exerted by EGF and TPA are similar (see ref. 8). (b) TPA potentiates the effects of EGF (3). (c) TPA binds to a receptor system that is distinct from the EGF-receptor system (9) since EGF does not inhibit phorbol ester binding (L. S. Lee, *unpublished results* and 2,5). (d) TPA cannot totally abolish all EGF binding (8,9). (e) TPA-induced inhibition of EGF binding occurs in all cells that have EGF receptors (9). (f) TPA has little effect on EGF binding at 4°C (9). (g) The kinetics of TPA and EGF "down-regulation" are different, indicating that the two receptor systems do not aggregate (L. S. Lee, *unpublished results*).

EGF-BINDING INHIBITION BY SACCHARIN AND CYCLAMATE

Saccharin and cyclamate exhibit tumor-promoting activity at relatively high doses (4). Such doses were also found to be required for inhibition of EGF binding (Fig. 1); at low doses (1 to 10 μg/ml) of saccharin and cyclamate, there was no inhibition. Other sweeteners and structural analogs were negative in EGF-binding inhibition: β-D(-)fructose (12 mg/ml), D-sorbitol (12 mg/ml), xylitol (13.3 mg/ml), 2-deoxy-D-glucose (13.3 mg/ml), L-glucose (13.3 mg/ml), β-D(+)glucose (13.3 mg/ml), α-D(+)glucose (13.3 mg/ml), sucrose (13.3 mg/ml), anthranilic acid (0.6%), and cyclohexylamine (0.03%). The inhibition by saccharin and cyclamate was observed with many types of cells in culture (Table

TABLE 1. *Inhibition of EGF binding to HeLa cells by phorbol esters and related compounds*

Test compounds (100 ng/ml)	^{125}I-EGF bound[a] (cpm)
None	6,149
TPA	255
β-Phorbol	5,792
4-O-Me-TPA	5,510
β-Phorbol-12,13-didecanoate (PDD)	1,349
β-Phorbol-12,13-dibenzoate	2,160
α-Phorbol-12,13-didecanoate (4αPDD)	5,956
Mezerein	620
Gnidipalmin	5,457
Gnidimacrin-20-palmitate	5,409
Gnilatimacrin	491
Gnidilatin	1,042

[a]Binding assays were done with HeLa cell cultures as described in ref. 8. The binding buffer contained 0.225 ng of ^{125}I-EGF in 1.5 ml. (Permission from L.S. Lee.)

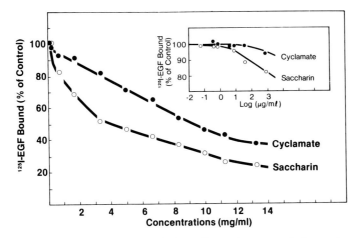

FIG. 1. Dependence of EGF binding to HeLa cells on the concentrations of saccharin or cyclamate. HeLa cells (3.65 × 10⁶) were assayed for EGF binding as described in ref. 8, except that various amounts of sodium cyclamate or sodium saccharin and 2 ng of ¹²⁵I-EGF were included in the binding buffer.

2 and ref. 6) and was temperature dependent. With HeLa cells, inhibition at 37°C was 73% for saccharin (13 mg/ml) and 70% for cyclamate (13 mg/ml), whereas the inhibition at 22°C was 54% for saccharin and 40% for cyclamate (13 mg/ml). We also observed that saccharin and cyclamate did not inhibit phorbol ester-binding to cellular receptors at the concentrations used, nor did they inhibit binding of concanavalin A.

EGF-BINDING INHIBITION BY PROMOTERS AND NONPROMOTERS

EGF-binding inhibition has now been observed for several phorbol esters (Table 1), derivatives of tricyclic diterpenes structurally related to phorbol (mezerein, gnidilatin, gnilatimacrin, Table 1; for structures of these compounds, see ref. 10), saccharin, cyclamate, human transforming growth factor (14), teleocidin (5), and melittin (5). All of these substances, except gnidilatin and gnilatimacrin, have been tested for tumor promotion. Activity has been observed for the phorbol esters, saccharin, cyclamate, and teleocidin *in vivo* and transforming growth factor *in vitro*. Promoting activity in initiated cells was not observed for melittin and mezerein at the levels tested. Mezerein, however, was found to have promoting activity in cells previously exposed to TPA (12).

THEORY OF THE HORMONE RESPONSE CONTROL UNIT

The observation that one substance with hormone-like activity (e.g. TPA) can inhibit the binding and modulate the activity of other hormones (e.g. EGF) having different receptors suggests that there exists in the cell some sort of

TABLE 2. *Effects of saccharin and cyclamate on EGF binding to animal cells in culture*

Cells	Control (ng EGF bound per ng added per 10^6 cells)	EGF bound (% control)[a]	
		Saccharin	Cyclamate
3T3 (mouse fibroblast)	0.011	70	56
3T3-BP (3T3-benzopyrene transformed)	0.001	63	37
K22 (rat liver)	0.0064	66	53
HTC (rat hepatoma)	0.00022	70	55
HeLa (cervical carcinoma)	0.068	20	38
XP1 (xeroderma pigmentosum skin, M)	0.042	63	48
XP11 (xeroderma pigmentosum skin, F)	0.043	23	41
WI38 (human lung)	0.036	18	17
WI38-VA13 (SV40 transformed WI38)	0.038	36	50

[a] The EGF binding assay was performed as described in Fig. 1. The cells were grown in monolayers and the assays were performed using about 1 to 2 ng of ^{125}I-EGF with or without 13.3 mg/ml of saccharin or cyclamate in the binding buffer.

hormone response control unit (HRCU) which can be stimulated by a group of hormone-receptor complexes, modulate the expression of their signals, and regulate the availability of the receptors (6). The observation that substances lacking in hormone-like structures or activities, and hence also lacking in hormone-like receptors (e.g. saccharin and cyclamate), can also affect EGF-binding inhibition suggests that such substances may be capable of directly stimulating the HRCU (6). The observation that diverse classes of substances that can stimulate the HRCU (as indicated by EGF-binding inhibition) are also tumor promoting suggests that HRCU stimulation in an initiated cell may be involved in tumor promotion. The observation that normal, HRCU-regulated growth can occur without tumor promotion suggests that the amount of stimulation of the HRCU needed for tumor promotion is greater than that required for normal growth and receptor regulation. The observation that normal growth hormones (e.g. EGF) can become tumor promoting at prolonged, high doses suggests that a threshold must be exceeded for promotion to occur. The observation that the threshold for tumorigenesis by a weak promoter (e.g. mezerein) can be lowered by prior treatment with a more potent one (e.g. TPA) suggests that the process of tumorigenesis may be simply one of progressive reduction in the promotional threshold of the HRCU, and hence a reduction in the required dose-threshold of the promoter (7).

In the ultimately resulting cancer cells, which are in a permanently "promoted" state, the promotional threshold has been lowered to a point that can be reached by stimulation by normal growth factors at or below their physiological levels. This reduction in the required level of extracellular growth factors for HRCU stimulation may be achieved, in some cases, by the internal generation of such factors (14). A lowered promotional threshold, however, does not imply a lowered threshold for receptor binding inhibition in cancer cells (6).

REFERENCES

1. Carpenter, G., and Cohen, S. (1979): Epidermal growth factor. In: *Annual Review of Biochemistry,* edited by E. F. Snell, P. D. Boyer, A. Meister, and C. C. Richardson, pp. 193–216. Annual Reviews Inc., California.
2. Delclos, K. B., Nagles, D. S., and Blumberg, P. M. (1980): Specific binding of phorbol ester tumor promoters to mouse skin. *Cell,* 19:1,025–1,032.
3. Dicker, P., and Rozengurt, E. (1978): Stimulation of DNA synthesis by tumor promoters and pure mitogenic factors. *Nature,* 276:723–726.
4. Hicks, R. M., Wakefield, J. St. J., and Chowaniec, J. (1975): Evaluation of a new model to detect bladder carcinogens or cocarcinogens: Results obtained with saccharin, cyclamate, and cyclophosphamide. *Chem. Biol. Interact.,* 11:225–233.
5. Horowitz, A. D., Greenebaum, E., and Weinstein, I. B. (1980): Identification and properties of phorbol ester receptor in rat embryo cells. *J. Cell Biol.,* 87:174a.
6. Lee, L. S. (1981*a*): Saccharin and cyclamate inhibit epidermal growth factor binding. *Proc. Natl. Acad. Sci. USA,* 78:1,042–1,046.
7. Lee, L. S. (1981*b*): Binding of phorbol esters to cells in culture: Its correlation with biological effects and implications in the mechanism of tumor promotion. *Biochem. Biophys. Res. Commun. (in press).*
8. Lee, L. S., and Weinstein, I. B. (1978): Tumor-promoting phorbol esters inhibit binding of epidermal growth factor to cellular receptors. *Science,* 202:313–315.
9. Lee, L. S., and Weinstein, I. B. (1979*a*): Mechanism of tumor promoter inhibition of cellular binding of epidermal growth factor. *Proc. Natl. Acad. Sci. USA,* 76:5,168–5,172.
10. Lee, L. S., and Weinstein, I. B. (1979*b*): Membrane effects of tumor promoters. Stimulation of sugar uptake in mammalian cell culture. *J. Cell Physiol.,* 99:451–460.
11. Rose, S. P., Stahn, R., Passovoy, D. S., and Hershman, H. (1976): Epidermal growth factor enhancement of skin tumor induction in mice. *Experientia,* 32:913–915.
12. Slaga, T. J., Fischer, S. M., Nelson, K., and Gleason, G. L. (1980): Studies on the mechanism of skin tumor promotion: Evidence for several stages in promotion. *Proc. Natl. Acad. Sci. USA,* 77:3,659–3,663.
13. Slaga, T. J., Sivak, A., and Boutwell, R. K. editors (1978): *Carcinogenesis, Vol. 2: Mechanisms of Tumor Promotion and Cocarcinogenesis.* Raven Press, New York.
14. Todaro, G. J., Fryling, C., and DeLarco, J. E. (1980): Transforming growth factors produced by certain human tumor cells: Polypeptides that interact with epidermal growth factor receptors. *Proc. Natl. Acad. Sci. USA,* 77:5,258–5,262.

Carcinogenesis, Vol. 7, edited by E. Hecker et al.
Raven Press, New York © 1982.

Effects of Tumor Promoters on Arachidonic Acid Metabolism by Cells in Culture

Lawrence Levine

Department of Biochemistry, Brandeis University, Waltham, Massachusetts 02254

The products of cellular arachidonic acid transformation that are secreted into culture media depend, quantitatively and qualitatively, on the relative activities of cellular enzymes such as acylhydrolases; CoA-acyltransferases; cyclooxygenases; prostacyclin, thromboxane, and the prostaglandin synthetases; lipoxygenases; glutathione S-transferases; γ-glutamyl transpeptidases; and the catabolizing enzymes, 15-hydroxydehydrogenases, and Δ13 reductases. Thus, it is not surprising that individual cell lines produce unique profiles of arachidonic acid metabolites (26). Stimulation of this metabolism by several compounds results in levels of products in the culture media in excess not only of that found free in the cells but also in excess of that synthesized from cellular nonesterified arachidonic acid. Unsaturated fatty acids do not exist free in cells. They are found in the form of phosphoglycerides and triglycerides, which must be deacylated to provide substrate for the lipoxygenases and cyclooxygenases (19,20,59). The tissue phospholipids are the richest source of these precursor polyunsaturated fatty acids, and it has been postulated that the phospholipases of the cell are part of the sequence of events involved in prostaglandin biosynthesis (19). In the scheme shown in Fig. 1, arachidonic acid, which is the unsaturated fatty acid found in highest concentration in membrane phospholipids, is shown as the fatty acid undergoing metabolism. Other unsaturated fatty acids, however, can serve as substrates for the cyclooxygenase. The endoperoxides are the immediate products of the cyclooxygenase (8,38). They then undergo enzymatic and nonenzymatic transformations to form the thromboxanes (TXA_2 and TXB_2) (10), the prostacyclins (PGI_2) (34), and the prostaglandins (PGE_2, $PGF_{2\alpha}$, and PGD_2). These endoperoxide metabolites can exist in classes depending on the degree of unsaturation in their precursor fatty acids; e.g., arachidonic acid is transformed to class-two (PGE_2, $PGF_{2\alpha}$, etc.) products, eicosatrienoic acid is transformed to class-one (PGE_1, $PGF_{1\alpha}$, etc.) products. The products formed from the endoperoxides, as well as the endoperoxides themselves, are potent pharmacologically and their activities qualitatively and quantitatively depend on the nature of the enzymatic (and nonenzymatic) transformations. Arachidonic acid also can be converted by lipoxygenase pathways to hydroperoxy-and hydroxyeicosatetraenoic acids and leukotrienes (9,36,37,42).

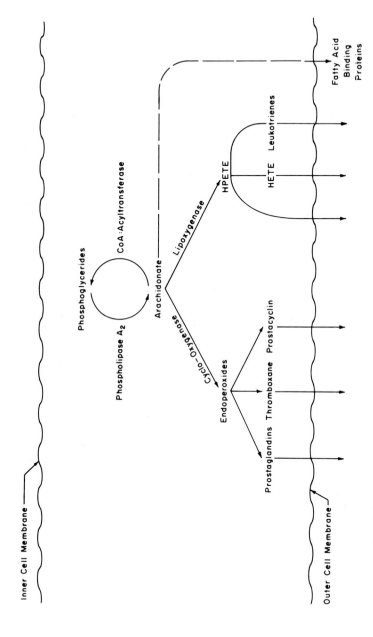

FIG. 1. Schematic representation of the components and characteristics of arachidonic acid utilization.

EFFECT OF 12-O-TETRADECANOYLPHORBOL-13-ACETATE ON BIOSYNTHESIS OF CYCLOOXYGENASE PRODUCTS BY CELLS IN CULTURE

12-O-Tetradecanoylphorbol-13-acetate (TPA), at 0.1 μg/ml or less, stimulates several types of cells to produce prostaglandins (Table 1). When stimulated by TPA, the profile of metabolites remains the same; i.e., the levels of each metabolite are increased to the same extent, suggesting that deacylation of cellular lipids is being stimulated followed by each cell's unique enzymatic utilization of the nonesterified substrate. Other cells probably are stimulated by TPA to deacylate cellular lipids, although the amount of TPA required may vary from cell to cell.

Most of the studies presented in this chapter were performed with cells cultured from dog kidney (MDCK). Two MDCK cell lines are available: one is being maintained in the American Type Culture Collection and a second is being studied extensively in Dr. Milton Saier's laboratories at the University of California, San Diego. These two cell lines have strikingly different arachidonic acid metabolic profiles and may respond differently to agonists (M. Lewis and A. A. Spector, *unpublished data*). Our studies were performed with the MDCK cell line obtained from Dr. Saier.

MDCK cells synthesize low but significant levels of PGE_2 and $PGF_{2\alpha}$ when incubated in nonserum-supplemented minimal essential medium. When incubated in the presence of TPA (1 and 10 ng/ml), the appearance in the medium of PGE_2 and $PGF_{2\alpha}$ is faster and their levels are higher. The rate of increase is greatest in the first 10 min (Fig. 2). Stimulation of PGE_2 production is seen even 5 min after addition of TPA (39). If the cells that are incubated with the TPA for these increments of time are washed several times with medium to remove all TPA not bound to the cells and reincubated with serum-supplemented medium for another 24 hr, they still produce increased levels of prostaglandins (39). In the presence of TPA (1 ng/ml) for 60 min, the stimulation was about threefold; but after a 24-hr incubation in serum-supplemented medium,

TABLE 1. *Cells in which arachidonic acid metabolism is stimulated by TPA[a]*

Cells	Cultured from
MDCK$_{S.D.}$	Dog kidney
WEHI-5	Mouse lymphoma
LC-540	Rat Leydig
Smooth muscle	Bovine aorta
WI-38	Human embryonic lung
D-550	Human foreskin
MC5-5	Transformed mouse fibroblast
Bone[b]	Mouse calvaria

[a] 0.1 μg/ml TPA, or less.
[b] Mixture of cell types.

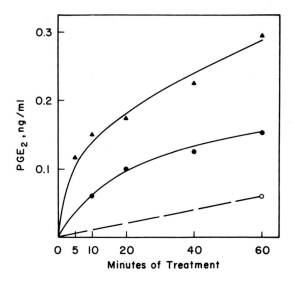

FIG. 2. Effect of time on stimulation of PGE₂ production by TPA. Cells (2 × 10⁵ cells/60-mm dish) were incubated with 4 ml of minimal essential medium containing 2mM 1-glutamate with or without TPA for indicated times. PGE₂ production during TPA treatment: Control, ○; TPA, 1 ng/ml, ●; TPA, 10 ng/ml, ▲. The values are the means of two dishes. Under the conditions of the radioimmunoassay used in these experiments, 0.05 ng of PGE₂/ml of culture fluid is the lower limit of sensitivity. Only in the 60-min control sample did we find PGE₂ at this lower limit of sensitivity. The differences in PGE₂ content obtained with TPA, 10 and 1 ng/ml, and the control culture fluids are significant. (From Ohuchi and Levine, ref. 39.)

14-fold more PGE₂ was found. This increased stimulation during the 24-hr incubation after removal of the TPA is more striking after incubation with TPA at 10 ng/ml. Stimulation of PGE₂ synthesis after the 10-min incubation was threefold, but after several washes of the cells and after incubation for another 24 hr in serum-supplemented medium, the stimulated PGE₂ synthesis was 50-fold. The levels of PGE₂ in the serum-supplemented medium, after treatment of the cells with TPA, phorbol-12, 13-didecanoate (PDD), and 4α-PDD for 60 min and after removal of the phorbol diesters, are shown in Fig. 3. PDD and TPA at 1 ng/ml are effective stimulators of prostaglandin production, but 4α-PDD even at 100 ng/ml is not. This stimulation of prostaglandin production during the 24 hr after removal of the phorbols is a slow process, and at low concentrations of promoters, the reaction(s) was not complete even after 24 hr. At all levels of the phorbol promoters, there is a pronounced lag time, the length of which depends on the amount of promoter used during the initial incubation.

Stimulation of prostaglandin production by cells was demonstrated not only by serologic analyses of the conditioned medium but also by release of radioactive compounds from the cells labeled with [³H] arachidonic acid (28). When the radioactively labeled cells are cultured for 14 hr in serum-supplemented medium

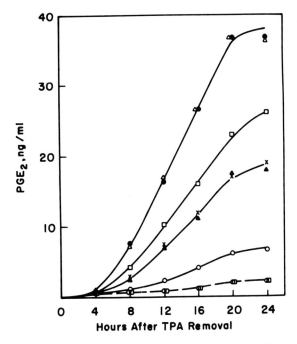

FIG. 3. Prostaglandin production as a function of time after phorbol diester treatment. Cells (2 × 10⁵ cells/60-mm dish) were incubated with 4 ml of minimal essential medium with and without the phorbol for 60 min. After three washes, cells were incubated with 4 ml of the medium containing 10% fetal bovine serum. At the times indicated, aliquots of 200 μl were withdrawn for assay of PGE_2. 200 μl of the fresh medium was added in the dish each time. TPA, 10 ng/ml, △; TPA, 5 ng/ml, ●; TPA, 1 ng/ml, □; TPA, 0.5 ng/ml, ▲; TPA, 0.1 ng/ml, ○; PDD, 1 ng/ml, X; 4α-PDD, 100 ng/ml, □---□; control, ○---○. Each value is the mean of duplicate dishes. The values agreed within 10% of these means. (From Ohuchi and Levine, ref. 39.)

in the presence of increments of TPA, increased quantities of radioactivity are found in the conditioned medium, even at a concentration of 125 pg/ml (2 × 10^{-10} M). Most of the identified radioactive materials released from MDCK cells growing in serum-supplemented medium alone corresponded to arachidonic acid, $PGF_{2\alpha}$, and PGE_2 (our chromatographic procedure did not separate 6-keto-$PGF_{1\alpha}$ from PGE_2). After 20 hr of incubation in the presence of TPA (250 pg/ml) or PDD (1.0 ng/ml), the radioactive compounds released were increased around fourfold, whereas that released by cells incubated in the presence of 4α-PDD (10 ng/ml) and the control serum-supplemented medium were equal (Table 2). The released radioactivity in the conditioned medium as a result of incubation with TPA and PDD is due mainly to increased PGE_2 and $PGF_{2\alpha}$ (14.5-fold with TPA and 10.6-fold with PDD); the arachidonic acid that had been made available by increased deacylation of the cellular phospholipids appears to have been efficiently converted to the prostaglandins by the cyclooxygenase and synthetase systems. MDCK cells, labeled with

TABLE 2. *Radioactive compounds in conditioned media of radioactively labeled MDCK cells and phorbol diesters*

Compound	Radioactivity (cpm)[a]			
	MEM (+)[b]	MEM (+) with TPA (0.25 ng/ml)	MEM (+) with PDD (1.0 ng/ml)	MEM (+) with 4α-PDD (10 ng/ml)
Phospholipids	281	718	457	144
Prostaglandin $F_{2\alpha}$	568	7,088	5,224	528
Prostaglandin E_2	300	5,507	3,996	302
Arachidonic acid	3,429	4,725	6,387	3,922
Triglycerides	122	214	241	33
Unidentified[c]	1,508	8,170	5,781	1,018
Total	6,208[d]	26,422[d]	22,086[d]	5,947[d]

[a] 1.6 ml radioactive medium (out of a total of 2 ml) was extracted and chromatographed. Incubation was for 20 hr.
[b] MEM (+) represents serum-supplemented medium.
[c] Scatter throughout thin-layer chromatography (TLC).
[d] Cell number initially was 0.64×10^6/60 mm dish, but cells were not counted after the 20-hr incubation.
From Levine and Hassid (28).

[14C]linoleic acid, are not stimulated by TPA to release radiolabeled compounds into the culture media; there appears to be specificity within the deacylation reaction (40).

EFFECT OF CYCLOHEXIMIDE ON TPA-STIMULATED PROSTAGLANDIN BIOSYNTHESIS

The effect of cycloheximide (0.5 μg/ml) on the prostaglandin synthesis expressed in the 24 hr after treatment of the cells with TPA (1.0 ng/ml) in nonserum-supplemented medium for 60 min is shown in Fig. 4 (39). Inhibition of prostaglandin synthesis was marked. Even with 0.05 μg/ml of cycloheximide, the TPA-stimulated prostaglandin biosynthesis was inhibited. The inhibition by cycloheximide is not observed when the cells are treated with cycloheximide for 1 hr during the TPA treatment or 2 hr before the TPA treatment if the cycloheximide is then removed with the residual TPA. The extent of inhibition of prostaglandin synthesis following TPA treatment depends on the time of addition of cycloheximide after the treatment with TPA and its removal (Fig. 4). When cycloheximide was added 8 hr after TPA treatment, it still inhibited: 30% inhibition with 0.05 μg/ml of cycloheximide and 58 and 55% inhibition of PGE_2 and $PGF_{2\alpha}$ synthesis, respectively, with 0.5 μg/ml of cycloheximide. Even when cycloheximide was added 16 hr after removal of residual TPA when the expression of increased prostaglandin synthesis was approaching completion as measured after the 24-hr incubation, inhibition was observed: 11% inhibition ($p < 0.025$) with 0.05 μg/ml and 22% (PGE_2) and 19% ($PGF_{2\alpha}$) with 0.5

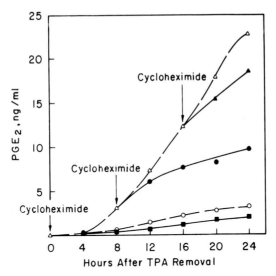

FIG. 4. Inhibition of PGE_2 production by cycloheximide. Cells (2 × 10^5/60-mm dish) were incubated for 60 min with 4 ml of the medium with or without TPA (1 ng/ml). After three washes, the cells were incubated for 24 hr, with 4 ml of the medium supplemented with 10% fetal bovine serum. At 0, 8, and 16 hr after the medium change, cycloheximide (0.5 μg/ml) was added *(arrows)*. Aliquots of the medium were withdrawn at the indicated times for assay of PGE_2. Each value is the mean of two dishes. The values agreed within 10% of these means. Cycloheximide added at: 0 time, ■; 8 hr, ●; 16 hr, ▲; no cycloheximide, △; control cells, ○. (From Ohuchi and Levine, ref. 39.)

μg/ml. Following a 2-hr pulse of cycloheximide treatment, inhibition of prostaglandin synthesis after 24-hr incubation was already 54% of that observed with cycloheximide present for the entire 24 hr (Fig. 5).

As shown above (Table 2), most of the extracted radioactive materials released from [³H]arachidonic acid-labeled cells incubated in serum-supplemented medium chromatographs as arachidonic acid, and only small amounts are converted to PGE_2 and $PGF_{2\alpha}$. The TPA-treated cells release more arachidonic acid, most of which is converted into PGE_2 and $PGF_{2\alpha}$. In the presence of indomethacin, the conversion of the released arachidonic acid into PGE_2 and $PGF_{2\alpha}$ was almost completely inhibited (Table 3). However, indomethacin, at 1.4 × 10^{-6} M, appears to be inhibiting a reaction in addition to the cyclooxygenase step, probably acylhydrolase activity, since the overall stimulation of released radioactivity was only 1.7-fold instead of 2.4-fold. Hydrocortisone, which inhibits prostaglandin production by many cells but not by MDCK cells, did not affect the stimulated release of radioactive compounds by TPA either qualitatively or quantitatively. Cycloheximide (0.5 μg/ml) inhibited both the release of radioactive materials stimulated by TPA and the conversion of the released arachidonic acid into prostaglandins.

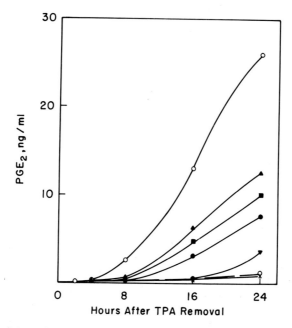

FIG. 5. Effect of time of cycloheximide treatment on PGE$_2$ production. Cells (2 × 10^5/60-mm dish) were incubated for 60 min with 4 ml of the medium with and without TPA (1 ng/ml). After three washes, the cells were incubated for increments of time with 4 ml of the medium supplemented with 10% fetal bovine serum containing cycloheximide (0.5 μg/ml). Time of treatment with cycloheximide: none, ○; 0 to 2 hr, ▲; 0 to 4 hr, ■; 0 to 8 hr, ●; 0 to 16 hr, ▲. After each time period, the cells were washed three times and incubated with cycloheximide-free medium. Cells treated with cycloheximide (0.5 μg/ml) just after TPA removal and incubated for 24 hr, X; control cells, no treatment with TPA or cycloheximide, ○---○. The values represent the means of two dishes. These values agreed within 10% of these means. (From Ohuchi and Levine, ref. 39.)

TABLE 3. *Radioactive PGE$_2$, PGF$_{2\alpha}$, and arachidonic acid released from TPA-treated MDCK cells, and the effect on this release of cycloheximide, hydrocortisone, and indomethacin*

	Radioactivity (cpm)			
Treatment	PGF$_{2\alpha}$ (% of total cpm)	PGE$_2$ (% of total cpm)	Arachidonic acid (% of total cpm)	Total[a]
TPA	16,561 (24.5)	14,129 (20.9)	27,520 (40.6)	67,721
TPA, cycloheximide	821 (2.2)	460 (1.2)	32,509 (86.0)	37,821
TPA, hydrocortisone	15,936 (26.4)	12,102 (20.2)	22,766 (37.7)	60,404
TPA, indomethacin	53 (0.1)	196 (0.4)	45,015 (95.9)	46,931
None	2,464 (8.8)	1,056 (3.8)	20,961 (75.1)	27,899

[a] Total radioactivity distributed on the thin layer plate.
From Ohuchi and Levine (40).

EFFECT OF RETINOIDS ON TPA-STIMULATED PROSTAGLANDIN BIOSYNTHESIS

Studies of the effects of vitamin A and its synthetic analogs (the retinoids) suggest that they may be useful in chemoprevention of cancer (50,51). Their biological properties, however, are manifold. They suppress *in vitro* malignant transformation induced chemically (33) or by radiation (11). They modify skin tumor promotion and prevent epithelial cancers (31). Topical applications of retinoids inhibit skin papilloma formation and TPA-induced ornithine decarboxylase activity (18,56,57). Retinoic acid inhibits the comitogenic action of TPA in bovine lymphocytes (17). Enhancement of the effects of the chemical carcinogens, similar to that of the tumor-promoting phorbol diesters, has also been described (22,23,43,49). Retinoids at low concentrations stimulate plasminogen activator synthesis in chick embryo fibroblasts, and at suboptimal levels of TPA, the effects of retinoic acid and TPA are synergistic (60). The retinoids, *cis*-retinoic acid, *trans*-retinoic acid, retinyl acetate, retinol, retinal, retinyl palmitate, and trimethylmethoxyphenyl retinoic acid, did not affect deacylation of phospholipids or prostaglandin production and, at relatively high concentrations, even enhanced them (30).

The retinoic acid analog, 4-hydroxyphenylretinamide is effective at preventing breast cancer in rats (35). In MDCK cells, 4-hydroxyphenylretinamide, at levels ranging from 0.025 to 3.1 μM, inhibited serum- and TPA-stimulated biosynthesis of $PGF_{2\alpha}$, 6-keto-$PGF_{1\alpha}$, and PGE_2 (Fig. 6). 4-Hydroxyphenylretinamide also was a potent inhibitor of PGE_2 and $PGF_{2\alpha}$ production by serum-stimulated, methylcholanthrene-transformed mouse fibroblasts, normal human fibroblasts, and the "spindle-shaped" smooth muscle cells present in the intima layer of rabbit aorta (25). In the presence of 10% fetal bovine serum, 4-hydroxyphenylretinamide inhibited prostaglandin production by MDCK cells four times less effectively than indomethacin and about 50 times more effectively than aspirin. 4-Hydroxyphenylretinamide did not affect the release of radiolabeled materials from TPA-stimulated labeled cells, however; cyclooxygenase activity appears to be inhibited, not acylhydrolases.

EFFECT OF α-TOCOPHEROL ON TPA-STIMULATED PROSTAGLANDIN BIOSYNTHESIS

Another inhibitor of TPA-stimulated prostaglandin production in MDCK cells is α-tocopherol (41). α-Tocopherol inhibited prostaglandin production in TPA-stimulated MDCK cells but not in control cells. This inhibitory effect was observed only if the cells were treated with TPA in the presence of α-tocopherol. Pretreatment or posttreatment with α-tocopherol was not effective (cycloheximide is inhibitory even after TPA treatment). α-Tocopherol inhibits TPA-stimulated prostaglandin production by inhibiting the binding of [^{3}H]TPA to the cells. Since a 10^2 to 10^3 mole excess of α-tocopherol to TPA was required

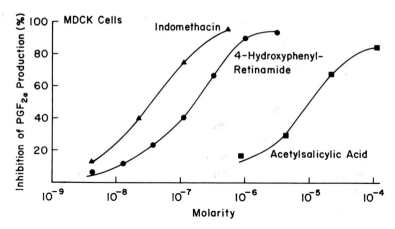

FIG. 6. Inhibition of serum-stimulated $PGF_{2\alpha}$ production by 4-hydroxyphenylretinamide, indomethacin, and aspirin (acetylsalicylic acid). Each point represents the mean value of two culture dishes. These values agreed within 20% of these means. (From Levine, ref. 25.)

to inhibit binding to the cells (Table 4), the mechanism is not clear. It is possible that TPA is more soluble in α-tocopherol bound in the MDCK cell membrane. It is also possible that a receptor site for TPA is being reversibly blocked by α-tocopherol. There appears to be some specificity for tumor promoters originating from *Croton tiglium* L. α-Tocopherol inhibited the effects of the tumor-promoting phorbol esters obtained from *Croton tiglium* L., but did not inhibit the stimulation of deacylation of phospholipids and prostaglandin production resulting from treatment of MDCK cells with diterpenoid esters isolated from the plant species *Daphne* or *Gnidia,* or with benzo(a)pyrene, adriamycin, or 17-β-estradiol. It has been difficult to demonstrate inhibition of TPA-stimulated prostaglandin production by α-tocopherol in cells other than MDCK cells. This may be related to the higher levels of TPA required to stimulate prostaglandin production in cells other than MDCK.

Inhibition of TPA-stimulated (a) deacylation of cellular lipids, (b) prostaglandin production, and (c) altered morphology in MDCK cells (altered morphology is not necessarily related to deacylation of phospholipids or prostaglandin production) by indomethacin, dexamethasone, retinoic acid, 4-hydroxyphenylretinamide, and cycloheximide is summarized in Table 5. Retinoic acid inhibits none of these responses, and at high concentrations it is synergistic with TPA (30). Indomethacin inhibits prostaglandin production very effectively, but it also inhibits the deacylation of cellular lipids (40). N-(4-hydroxyphenyl)retinamide inhibits TPA-stimulated prostaglandin production but does not affect deacylation of the lipids. α-Tocopherol inhibits all three effects, prostaglandin production, deacylation of cellular lipids, and altered morphology; it does this by blocking TPA binding to MDCK cells. Dexamethasone, not shown in Table 5, is ineffective; but dexamethasone, which inhibits prostaglandin production in several cells (14,16,52,53) by preventing the expression of acylhydrolase activ-

TABLE 4. *Effect of α-tocopherol on binding of*
³H-labeled TPA to MDCK cells

α-Tocopherol (μg/ml)	Radioactivity bound to cells (cpm/2 · 10⁵ cells) × 10⁻²
0	28.9 ± 0.9
0.1	20.4 ± 0.6[a]
1.0	7.5 ± 0.4[a]
10.0	3.9 ± 0.2[a]

[a] Statistically significant compared to control ($P < 0.001$). MDCK cells were incubated for 1 hr in 4 ml of the medium with 0.11 μCi of [³H]-labeled TPA containing increments of α-tocopherol. After a 1-hr incubation, the cells were washed five times with medium, the cell layer, dissolved in 0.1 N NaOH, was counted for radioactivity bound to the cells. The values are the mean $\pm$ SD of triplicate dishes.
From Ohuchi and Levine (41).

ity (14,52), does not do so in MDCK cells. Cycloheximide inhibits all three TPA-stimulated reactions in MDCK cells, most likely by inhibiting synthesis of a protein that stimulates prostaglandin production and acylhydrolase activity.

STIMULATION OF PROSTAGLANDIN PRODUCTION BY GROWTH FACTORS

Proteins stimulate acylhydrolase activity and prostaglandin production, e.g., epidermal growth factor and platelet-derived growth factor (4,29). Several growth factors recently have been described and characterized (5,6,32,45). All stimulate prostaglandin production; they probably do so by stimulating acylhydrolase activity. Some of these growth factors have been shown to confer transformed phenotypes on normal cells *in vitro* (6,45). A family of such growth factors probably exists in cells; their mitogenic effects and ability to transform phenotypes may be causally related to their capacity to stimulate acylhydrolase activities.

TABLE 5. *Inhibition of some TPA-stimulated effects on MDCK cells in culture*

Inhibitor	Morphology	Phospholipid deacylation	Prostaglandin production
Cycloheximide	+	+	+
Indomethacin	±[a]	±	+
Retinoic acid	−	−	−
4-Hydroxyphenylretinamide	−	−	+
α-Tocopherol	+	+	+

[a] +: 5×10^{-5} M; −: 1×10^{-6} M.

TUMOR PROMOTERS STIMULATE PROSTAGLANDIN PRODUCTION AND INDUCE SYNTHESIS OF GROWTH FACTORS: A MODEL FOR PROMOTION

Compounds of diverse biological activities are capable of stimulating acylhydrolase and prostaglandin biosynthesis in MDCK cells (24,27). Of those tested (eighteen), only stimulation by TPA and mezerein (both tumor promoters) is inhibited by cycloheximide (Table 6). As shown earlier, stimulation of prostaglandin production in MDCK cells by TPA occurs in two stages: an initial burst easily measurable 5 min after addition to TPA and lasting for about 60 min (Fig. 2), and a second much greater stimulation that is measurable after a lag of 4 to 8 hr and continuing for about 24 hr (Fig. 3). This secondary stimulation of prostaglandin production is inhibited by cycloheximide, an inhibitor of protein synthesis, and is not dependent on the presence of TPA, as it is not blocked by washing the TPA from the cells, even 5 min after the addition of TPA (39). Thus, stimulation of prostaglandin production in MDCK cells by TPA is biphasic: an initial burst of acylhydrolase activity and prostaglandin production which may or may not be causally related to a second burst of prostaglandin production mediated by an induced protein(s). The events leading to the induction probably include transport across the membrane, reaction with chromatin, translation, and protein synthesis. The inducing reaction is fast; it begins within 5 min of addition of TPA. That proteins can stimulate acylhydrolase activity and prostaglandin production has been demonstrated [thrombin and epidermal growth factors stimulate acylhydrolase activity and prostaglandin production (13,15,29)]; and, as shown in Table 7, proteins more relevant to mechanisms leading to transformation (6,45) also stimulate prostaglandin production. Some of these growth factors confer a transformed phenotype to untransformed cells.

Taken together, these results suggest a working model of a mechanism that leads to tumor promotion (Fig. 7). In this scheme, TPA induces synthesis of a protein(s) similar in function to growth factors. The induced protein(s) reacts

TABLE 6. *Stimulation of arachidonic acid transformation in MDCK cells and its inhibition by cycloheximide*

Stimulant	Inhibition by cycloheximide[a]	Stimulant	Inhibition by cycloheximide[a]
TPA	+	Norepinephrine	−
Mezerein	+	Dopamine	−
Sarcoma growth factor	−	Colchicine	−
Epidermal growth factor	−	Sodium vanadate	−
Platelet-derived growth factor	−	A-23187	−
Mononuclear growth factor	−	Thrombin	−
Benzo(a)pyrene	−	Bradykinin	−
7,12-Dimethylbenz(a)anthracine	−	17-β-Estradiol	−
Adriamycin	−	Iodoacetate	−

[a] 0.1 μg/ml. However, cycloheximide, at 2.0 μg/ml, inhibits serum- , thrombin- , and bradykinin-stimulated prostaglandin synthesis by MC5-5 cells.

TABLE 7. *Growth factors that stimulate arachidonic acid metabolism in MDCK cells*

Epidermal growth factor
Serum
Platelet-derived growth factor[a]
Sarcoma transforming growth factor[b]
"Kidney" transforming factor[b]
Bladder carcinoma transforming growth factor[b]
Rheumatoid stimulating factor[c]

[a] Coughlin et al. (4).
[b] Levine et al. *(unpublished data)*.
[c] Levine and Robinson *(unpublished data)*.

with a receptor on the cell membrane (the same or neighboring cells) to stimulate acylhydrolases. The resulting nonesterified fatty acids (probably arachidonic acid) are metabolized to prostaglandins, leukotrienes, and hydroxyfatty acids. As a result, the membrane contains additional lysophospholipids. Indomethacin (55,58) and corticosteroids (2,48) inhibit tumor formation by TPA. Since both indomethacin and corticosteroids inhibit prostaglandin production, indomethacin by inhibiting cyclooxygenase activity and, to a lesser extent, acylhydrolase activity, and dexamethasone by blocking expression of acylhydrolase activity in some, but not all, cells (7,14,52), the growth factor-stimulated arachidonic acid metabolic cascade may be causally related to promotion. If so, the transformation pathways must be unique to stimulation by growth factors. Multiple pathways within the overall acylhydrolase activity are just beginning to be recognized (1,3,12,21,40,44). It is probable that different acylhydrolases and substrates are utilized in different cells, or after stimulation by different agonists in the same cells. Arachidonic acid transformation may mediate promotion by altering the fluidity of the membrane. If so, such transformation initiated by growth factors after stimulation by tumor promoters catalyzes deacylation of phospholipids that have specific locations within the membrane. The arachidonic acid metabolism resulting from such stimulation, i.e. prostaglandins, leukotrienes, and hydroxyeicosatetraenoic acid production, with their potent chemotactic and chemokinetic properties, may either enhance or inhibit promotion. The direction of such modulation would depend on the arachidonic acid metabolizing enzymes present in the cells affected by the tumor promoter. Not all TPA-treated cells have the capacity to synthesize growth factor-like molecules; cells also may vary with respect to their content of specific growth factor receptors. In preliminary experiments we have observed such cell specificity, both for induction of TPA-induced growth factors and response to growth factors.

Among the pleiotypic effects of TPA is the induction of proteases. Several protease inhibitors, such as tosyl arginine methyl ester, N-α-tosyl-L-lysinechloromethylketone, and leupeptin, block tumor promotion by TPA in mouse skin (60). At relatively high levels (1.5×10^{-4} M) pepstatin, antipain, and leupeptin inhibit TPA-stimulated prostaglandin production in MDCK cells. These com-

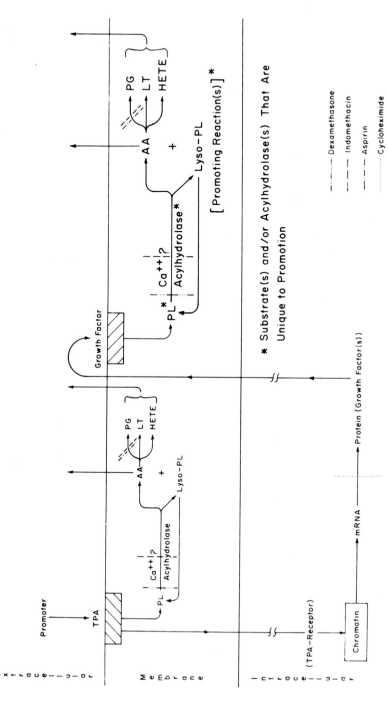

FIG. 7. TPA, arachidonic acid transformation, and tumor promotion. When TPA binds to MDCK cells, it stimulates acylhydrolases to deacylate phospholipids and consequently arachidonic acid metabolism, and induces synthesis of a protein(s). The protein "growth factor(s)" binds to receptors of the MDCK cells (or neighboring cells) and stimulates specific acylhydrolases to deacylate specific phospholipids (again followed by arachidonic acid metabolism) located in the membrane at sites that control membrane fluidity. The stability of this altered state is modulated by chemokinetic and chemotactic properties of the arachidonic acid metabolic products, the direction of modulation depending on the activities of the several metabolic enzymes unique to each cell. Cycloheximide inhibits synthesis of "growth factor(s)." Dexamethasone inhibits expression of acylhydrolase activity. Aspirin and indomethacin inhibit cyclooxygenase and, in addition, indomethacin inhibits acylhydrolase activity.

pounds may be acting at the chromatin level, a reaction leading to derepression, as suggested by Troll and his colleagues (54), or they may be blocking binding of the growth factor to its receptor.

Studies by Shier (46,47) show that several membrane phospholipases are activated by Ca^{2+}. Therefore, it is not unreasonable to suspect that altered Ca^{2+} transport within or across the cell membrane is one of the messengers leading to promotion.

ACKNOWLEDGMENTS

This work was supported by Grants GM 27256 and CA 17309 from the National Institutes of Health. This is Publication Number 1334 from the Department of Biochemistry, Brandeis University, Waltham, Massachusetts 02254. L. L. is a Research Professor of Biochemistry of the American Cancer Society (Award PRP-21).

Many tissue culture experiments and radioimmunoassays were performed to gather the data reported here. I would like to thank Mmes. Tamsin Shrubb and Nancy Worth, Mr. John Sullivan, and Misses Rhonda Gudewich, Adriana Uglesity, and Kathleen Sullivan for their assistance in performing these techniques. Some of the work reported here was taken from studies performed with my former colleague, Dr. Kazuo Ohuchi.

The expert typing of Mrs. Inez Zimmerman is gratefully acknowledged.

REFERENCES

1. Bell, R. L., Kennerly, D. A., Stanford, N., and Majerus, P. W. (1979): Diglyceride lipase: A pathway for arachidonate release from human platelets. *Proc. Natl. Acad. Sci. USA,* 76:3,238–3,241.
2. Belman, S., and Troll, W. (1972): The inhibition of croton oil-promoted mouse skin tumorigenesis by steroid hormones. *Cancer Res.,* 32:450–454.
3. Bills, T. K., Smith, J. B., and Silver, M. J. (1977): Platelet uptake, release, and oxidation of [^{14}C]arachidonic acid. *Prostaglandins Hematology Proc. Int. Symp.,* pp. 27–55.
4. Coughlin, S. R., Moskowitz, M. A., Zetter, B. R., Antoniades, H. N., and Levine, L. (1980): Platelet-dependent stimulation of prostacyclin synthesis by platelet-derived growth factor. *Nature,* 288:600–602.
5. Dayer, J., Robinson, D. R., and Krane, S. M. (1977): Prostaglandin production by rheumatoid synovial cells. *J. Exp. Med.,* 145:1,399–1,404.
6. De Larco, J. E., and Todaro, G. J. (1978): Growth factors from murine sarcoma virus-transformed cells. *Proc. Natl. Acad. Sci. USA,* 75:4,001–4,005.
7. Gryglewski, R. J., Panczenko, B., Korbut, R., Grodzinska, L., and Ocetkiewicz, A. (1975): Corticosteroids inhibit prostaglandin release from perfused mesenteric blood vessels of rabbit and from perfused lungs of sensitized guinea pig. *Prostaglandins,* 10:343–355.
8. Hamberg, M., and Samuelsson, B. (1973): Detection and isolation of an endoperoxide intermediate in prostaglandin biosynthesis. *Proc. Natl. Acad. Sci. USA,* 70:899–903.
9. Hamberg, M., and Samuelsson, B. (1974): Prostaglandin endoperoxides: Novel transformations of arachidonic acid in human platelets. *Proc. Natl. Acad. Sci. USA,* 71:3,400–3,404.
10. Hamberg, M., Svensson, J., and Samuelsson, B. (1975): Thromboxanes: A new group of biologically active compounds derived from prostaglandin endoperoxides. *Proc. Natl. Acad. Sci. USA,* 72:2,994–2,998.
11. Harisiadis, L., Miller, R. C., Hall, E. J., and Borek, C. (1978): A vitamin A analogue inhibits

radiation-induced oncogenic transformation. *Nature,* 274:486–487.

12. Hong, S. L., and Deykin, D. (1979): Specificity of phospholipases in methylcholanthrene-transformed mouse fibroblasts activated by bradykinin, thrombin, serum, and ionophore A23187. *J. Biol. Chem.,* 254:11,463–11,466.

13. Hong, S. L., and Levine, L. (1976a): Stimulation of prostaglandin synthesis by bradykinin and thrombin and their mechanisms of action on MC5-5 fibroblasts. *J. Biol. Chem.,* 251:5,814–5,816.

14. Hong, S. L., and Levine, L. (1976b): Inhibition of arachidonic acid release from cells as the biochemical action of antiinflammatory corticosteroids. *Proc. Natl. Acad. Sci. USA,* 73:1,730–1,734.

15. Hong, S. L., Polsky-Cynkin, R., and Levine, L. (1976): Stimulation of prostaglandin production by vasoactive substances in methylcholanthrene-transformed mouse BALB/3T3. *J. Biol. Chem.,* 251:776–780.

16. Kantrowitz, F., Robinson, D. R., McGuire, M. B., and Levine, L. (1975): Corticosteroids inhibit prostaglandin production by rheumatoid synovia. *Nature,* 258:737–739.

17. Kenzler, T. W., and Mueller, G. C. (1978): Retinoic acid inhibition of the comitogenic action of mezerein and phorbol esters in bovine lymphocytes. *Cancer Res.,* 38:771–775.

18. Kenzler, T. W., Verma, A. K., Boutwell, R. K., and Mueller, G. C. (1978): Effects of retinoic acid and juvenile hormone on the induction of ornithine decarboxylase activity by 12-O-tetradecanoylphorbol-13-acetate. *Cancer Res.,* 38:2,896–2,899.

19. Kunze, H., and Vogt, W. (1971): Significance of phospholipase A for prostaglandin formation. *Ann. N.Y. Acad. Sci.,* 180:123–125.

20. Lands, W. E. M., and Samuelsson, B. (1968): Phospholipid precursor of prostaglandins. *Biochim. Biophys. Acta,* 164:426–429.

21. Lapetina, E. G., Schmitges, C. J., Chandrabose, K., and Cuatrecasas, P. (1978): Regulation of phospholipase activity in platelets. *Adv. Prostagland. Thrombox. Res.,* 3:127–135.

22. Levij, I. S., and Polliack, A. (1968): Potentiating effect of vitamin A on 9, 10-dimethyl-1,2-benzanthracene carcinogenesis in the hamster cheek pouch. *Cancer,* 22:300–306.

23. Levij, I. S., Rwomushana, J. W., and Polliack, A. (1979): Enhancement of chemical carcinogenesis in the hamster cheek pouch by prior topical application of vitamin A palmitate. *J. Invest. Dermatol.,* 53:228–231.

24. Levine, L. (1979): Deacylation of cellular lipids and arachidonic acid metabolism in cultured cells. In: *Hormones and Cell Culture. Cold Spring Harbor Conferences on Cell Proliferation, Vol. 6,* edited by G. Sato and R. Ross, pp. 623–640. Cold Spring Harbor Laboratory, New York.

25. Levine, L. (1980): N-(4-hydroxyphenyl)retinamide: A synthetic analog of vitamin A that is a potent inhibitor of prostaglandin biosynthesis. *Prostaglan. Med.,* 4:285–296.

26. Levine, L., and Alam, I. (1979): Arachidonic acid metabolism by cells in culture: Analyses of culture fluids for cyclooxygenase products by radioimmunoassay before and after separation by high pressure liquid chromatography. *Prostaglan. Med.,* 3:295–304.

27. Levine, L., and Alam, I. (1981): Deacylation of cellular lipids and arachidonic acid metabolism. *Progr. Lipid Res. (in press).*

28. Levine, L., and Hassid, A. (1977a): Effects of phorbol-12,13-diesters on prostaglandin production and phospholipase activity in canine kidney (MDCK) cells. *Biochem. Biophys. Res. Commun.,* 79:477–484.

29. Levine, L., and Hassid, A. (1977b): Epidermal growth factor stimulates prostaglandin biosynthesis by canine kidney (MDCK) cells. *Biochem. Biophys. Res. Commun.,* 76:1,181–1,187.

30. Levine, L., and Ohuchi, K. (1978): Retinoids as well as tumour promoters enhance deacylation of cellular lipids and prostaglandin production in MDCK cells. *Nature,* 276:274–275.

31. Mayer, H., Bollag, W., Hänni, R., and Rüegg, R. (1978): Retinoids, a new class of compounds with prophylactic and therapeutic activities in oncology and dermatology. *Experientia,* 34:1,105–1,119.

32. Meats, J. E., McGuire, M. B., and Russell, R. G. G. (1980): Human synovium releases a factor which stimulates chondrocyte production of PGE and plasminogen activator. *Nature,* 286:891–892.

33. Merriman, R. L., and Bertram, J. S. (1979): Reversible inhibition by retinoids of 3-methylcholanthrene-induced neoplastic transformation in C3H/10T½ CL8 cells. *Cancer Res.,* 39:1,661–1,666.

34. Moncada, S., and Vane, J. R. (1977): The discovery of prostacyclin—A fresh insight into

arachidonic acid metabolism. In: *Biochemical Aspects of Prostaglandins and Thromboxanes,* edited by N. Kharasch and J. Fried, pp. 155–177. Academic Press, New York.

35. Moon, R. C., Thompson, H. J., Becci, P. J., Grubbs, C. J., Gander, R. J., Newton, D. L., Smith, J. M., Phillips, S. L., Henderson, W. R., Mullen, L. T., Brown, C. C., and Sporn, M. B. (1979): N-(4-hydroxyphenyl)retinamide, a new retinoid for prevention of breast cancer in the rat. *Cancer Res.,* 39:1,339–1,346.

36. Morris, H. R., Taylor, G. W., Piper, P. J., Samhoun, M. N., and Tippins, J. R. (1980): Slow reacting substances (SRSs): The structure identification of SRSs from rat basophil leukaemia (RBL-1) cells. *Prostaglandins,* 19:185–201.

37. Murphy, R. C., Hammarstrom, S., and Samuelsson, B. (1979): Leukotriene C: A slow reacting substance from murine mastacytoma cells. *Proc. Natl. Acad. Sci. USA,* 76:4,275–4,279.

38. Nugteren, D. H., and Hazelhof, E. (1973): Isolation and properties of intermediates in prostaglandin biosynthesis. *Biochim. Biophys. Acta,* 326:448–461.

39. Ohuchi, K., and Levine, L. (1978a): Stimulation of prostaglandin synthesis by tumor-promoting phorbol-12,13-diesters in canine kidney (MDCK) cells: Cycloheximide inhibits the stimulated prostaglandin synthesis, deacylation of lipids, and morphological changes. *J. Biol. Chem.,* 253:4,783–4,790.

40. Ohuchi, K., and Levine, L. (1978b): Tumor-promoting phorbol diesters stimulate release of radioactivity from [³H]arachidonic acid-labeled but not [¹⁴C]linoleic acid-labeled cells. Indomethacin inhibits the stimulated release from [³H]arachidonate-labeled cells. *Prostagland. Med.,* 1:421–431.

41. Ohuchi, K., and Levine, L. (1980): α-Tocopherol inhibits 12-O-tetradecanoylphorbol-13-acetate-stimulated deacylation of cellular lipids, prostaglandin production, and changes in cell morphology of Madin-Darby canine kidney cells. *Biochim. Biophys. Acta,* 619:11–19.

42. Parker, C. W., Stenson, W. F., Huber, M. G., and Kelly, J. P. (1979): Formation of thromboxane B₂ and hydroxyarachidonic acids in purified human lymphocytes in the presence and absence of PHA. *J. Immunol.,* 122:1,572–1,577.

43. Prutkin, L. (1968): The effect of vitamin A acid on tumorigenesis and protein production. *Cancer Res.,* 28:1,021–1,030.

44. Rittenhouse-Simmons, S. (1979): Production of diglyceride from phosphatidylinositol in activated human platelets. *J. Clin. Invest.,* 63:580–587.

45. Roberts, A. B., Lamb, L. C., Newton, D. L., Sporn, M. B., De Larco, J. E., and Todaro, G. J. (1980): Transforming growth factors: Isolation of polypeptides from virally and chemically transformed cells by acid/ethanol extraction. *Proc. Natl. Acad. Sci. USA,* 77:3,494–3,498.

46. Shier, W. T. (1979): Activation of high levels of endogenous phospholipase A₂ in cultured cells. *Proc. Natl. Acad. Sci. USA,* 76:195–199.

47. Shier, W. T. (1980): Serum stimulation of phospholipase A₂ and prostaglandin release in 3T3 cells is associated with platelet-derived growth-promoting activity. *Proc. Natl. Acad. Sci. USA,* 77:137–141.

48. Slaga, T. J., Fischer, S. M., Viaje, A., Berry, D. L., Bracken, W. M., LeClerc, S., and Miller, D. R. (1978): Inhibition of tumor promotion by antiinflammatory agents: An approach to the biochemical mechanism of promotion. In: *Carcinogenesis, Vol. 2: Mechanisms of Tumor Promotion and Cocarcinogenesis,* edited by T. J. Slaga, A. Sivak, and R. K. Boutwell, pp. 173–195. Raven Press, New York.

49. Smith, D. M., Rogers, A. E., Herndon, B. J., and Newberne, P. M. (1975): Vitamin A (retinyl acetate) and benzo(a)pyrene-induced respiratory tract carcinogenesis in hamsters fed a commercial diet. *Cancer Res.,* 35:11–16.

50. Sporn, M. B., Dunlop, N. M., Newton, D. L., and Smith, J. M. (1976): Prevention of chemical carcinogenesis by vitamin A and its synthetic analogs. *Fed. Proc.,* 35:1,332–1,338.

51. Sporn, M. B., and Newton, D. L. (1979): Chemoprevention of cancer with retinoids. *Fed. Proc.,* 38:2,528–2,534.

52. Tam, S., Hong, S. L., and Levine, L. (1977): Relationships, among the steroids, of antiinflammatory properties and inhibition of prostaglandin production and arachidonic acid release by transformed mouse fibroblasts. *J. Pharmacol. Exp. Ther.,* 203:162–168.

53. Tashjian, A. H., Jr., Voelkel, E. F., McDonough, J., and Levine, L. (1975): Hydrocortisone inhibits prostaglandin production by mouse fibrosarcoma cells. *Nature,* 258:739–741.

54. Troll, W., Meyn, M. S., and Rossman, T. G. (1978): Mechanisms of protease action in carcinogenesis. In: *Carcinogenesis, Vol. 2: Mechanisms of Tumor Promotion and Cocarcinogenesis,* edited

by T. J. Slaga, A. Sivak, and R. K. Boutwell, pp. 301–312. Raven Press, New York.

55. Verma, A. K., Ashendel, C. L., and Boutwell, R. K. (1980): Inhibition by prostaglandin synthesis inhibitors of the induction of epidermal ornithine decarboxylase activity, the accumulation of prostaglandins, and tumor promotion caused by 12-O-tetradecanoylphorbol-13-acetate. *Cancer Res.,* 40:308–315.

56. Verma, A. K., and Boutwell, R. K. (1977): Vitamin A acid (retinoic acid), a potent inhibitor of 12-O-tetradecanoylphorbol-13-acetate-induced ornithine decarboxylase activity in mouse epidermis. *Cancer Res.,* 37:2,196–2,201.

57. Verma, A. K., Rice, H. M., Shapas, B. G., and Boutwell, R. K. (1978): Inhibition of 12-O-tetradecanoylphorbol-13-acetate-induced ornithine decarboxylase activity in mouse epidermis by vitamin A analogs (retinoids). *Cancer Res.,* 38:793–801.

58. Viaje, A., Slaga, T. J., Wigler, M., and Weinstein, I. B. (1977): Effects of antiinflammatory agents on mouse skin tumor promotion, epidermal DNA synthesis, phorbol ester-induced cellular proliferation, and production of plasminogen activator. *Cancer Res.,* 37:1,530–1,536.

59. Vonkeman, H., and Van Dorp, D. A. (1968): The action of prostaglandin synthetase on 2-arachidonyllecithin. *Biochim. Biophys. Acta,* 164:430–432.

60. Wilson, E. L., and Reich, E. (1978): Plasminogen activator in chick fibroblasts: Induction of synthesis by retinoic acid; synergism with viral transformation and phorbol ester. *Cell,* 15:385–392.

Carcinogenesis, Vol. 7, edited by E. Hecker et al.
Raven Press, New York © 1982.

Tumour-Promoter-Induced Proliferation of 3T3 Cells Is Independent of Prostaglandin Release and Ornithine Decarboxylase Induction

René Lanz and Kay Brune

Department of Pharmacology, Biozentrum, University of Basel, CH-4056 Basel, Switzerland

Among other effects, tumour-promoting phorbol esters elicit inflammatory reactions (3) along with prostaglandin (PG) release, induction of ornithine decarboxylase (ODC), and cell proliferation (4). The importance of inflammation-related cell proliferation for tumour promotion has been studied extensively but remains unclear. Recent studies suggest that prostaglandins released by inflammagens may initiate cell proliferation by allowing for the expression of malignant cell transformation (1,8). We have now investigated if 12-O-tetradecanoylphorbol-13-acetate (TPA)-induced prostaglandin release causes cell proliferation in cultures of Swiss mouse 3T3 fibroblasts, and if ODC induction is an obligatory event in TPA-stimulated deoxyribonucleic acid (DNA) synthesis.

MATERIALS AND METHODS

The chemicals were from the following sources: TPA from Prof. Dr. E. Hecker, German Cancer Research Centre, Heidelberg, F.R.G.; indomethacin from Sigma Chemical Co., St. Louis, MO, USA; 1, 3-diaminopropane from Merck-Schuchardt, München, F.R.G. The labeled compounds were all from the Radiochemical Centre Amersham, Bucks., U.K. Other chemicals were from commercial sources and of analytical or reagent grade.

Swiss mouse 3T3 cells (nontransformed) were cultured in Dulbecco's modified Eagle's medium containing 10% (v/v) newborn calf serum and 1% (v/v) penicillin-streptomycin solution (10,000 units/ml) from Gibco Bio-Cult., Glasgow, Scotland, U.K. Cells were seeded at a density of about 5×10^3 cells per cm^2 in Falcon plastic culture dishes. Cultures were incubated at 37°C in a humidified atmosphere containing 10% CO_2. Experiments were performed 4 to 5 days after plating when the cells just reached confluency.

PGE_2 release was measured as described by Glatt et al. (2), ODC as published (4), and DNA synthesis as described by Puzas and Goodman (7).

For determination of cell proliferation, cells were treated with trypsin and portions of the cell suspension were counted in a Coulter counter.

RESULTS

Effects of TPA on Prostaglandin Release, ODC Induction, and Cell Proliferation

TPA caused the release of PGE_2 (Fig. 1) and PGI_2 (4), which reached a maximum 2 hr after TPA treatment. This effect was dose-dependent, the maximum being at 10^{-7} M. TPA also markedly increased ODC activity at the same concentrations at which PG release occurred (Fig. 1). The ODC-inducing potency of TPA was most pronounced at day 4 after plating, at which stage the cells had just reached confluency (4). Peak activity of ODC was found 4 hr after TPA treatment (Fig. 1). Incorporation of ^{3}H-thymidine into DNA was

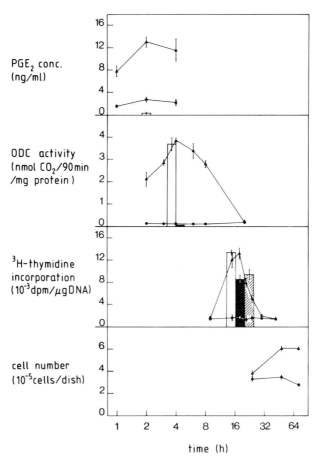

FIG. 1. Drug effects *(bars)* were measured at the time of maximal TPA stimulation. Values given comprise means ± SD of each time five experiments. ●, control; ▲, TPA 10^{-7} M; ▫, TPA 10^{-7} M + indomethacin 10^{-6} M; ■, TPA 10^{-7} M + 1,3-diaminopropane 10^{-2} M; ▨, TPA 10^{-7} M + indomethacin 10^{-6} M + 1,3-diaminopropane 10^{-2} M. (Figure from Lanz and Brune, ref. 5, with kind permission.)

also stimulated by 10^{-7} M TPA, the maximum being at 18 hr after TPA addition (Fig. 1). Also, addition of 10^{-7} M TPA increased the cell number per culture significantly within 2 days after treatment (Fig. 1), i.e., TPA consecutively stimulated PG release, ODC activation, and cell proliferation.

Effects of Inhibitors of Prostaglandin Release on TPA-Induced ODC Activity and Cell Proliferation

Pretreatment (1 hr) of cultures of 3T3 cells with 10^{-6} M indomethacin caused a complete inhibition of TPA-induced release of PGE_2, (Fig. 1) and PGI_2. The TPA effect on ODC and cell proliferation, however, was not affected by this drug, whereas pretreatment (24 hr) of the cells with 10^{-6} M dexamethasone, which reduced PG release to control values, even enhanced the proliferative effect of TPA (4). PGE_2 even at high concentrations of 10^{-5} M did not mimic the effects of TPA in unstimulated cells (4). No correlation was found between PG release, ODC induction, and cell proliferation when inhibitors of PG synthesis were applied.

Effects of Inhibitors of Polyamine Synthesis on TPA-Induced Cell Proliferation

ODC induction by 10^{-7} M TPA was depressed by 80% after pretreatment (2 hr) of the cells with 10^{-3} M 1,3-diaminopropane (DAP) which inhibits the synthesis of the enzyme. At this concentration, TPA-stimulated thymidine incorporation into DNA was not affected (4). Complete suppression of ODC activity by 10^{-2} M DAP resulted in a significant decrease of TPA-stimulated thymidine incorporation (Fig. 1). Nevertheless, TPA induced DNA synthesis in the total absence of measurable ODC activity and PG production (Fig. 1). Similar results were obtained with a competitive inhibitor of ODC activity, α-methylornithine (5×10^{-3} M). No correlation was found between TPA-induced ODC activity and thymidine incorporation into DNA when the synthesis or activity of ODC was blocked by inhibitors.

DISCUSSION

We have shown that the tumour promoter TPA is unlikely to exert its cell proliferative effect in 3T3 cells via PG production and ODC activation. Thymidine incorporation proceeded almost uninhibited after exposure of these cells to TPA, although both biochemical events were totally blocked. The question remains of which messengers, if any, trigger cell proliferation subsequent to TPA administration. Two possibilities are worth mentioning. Recently, evidence was produced that the cytoskeleton might be involved in mediating cell proliferation induced by growth factors (6). This suggestion appears attractive since TPA enters the cell interior almost instantaneously and changes the morphology of macrophages within minutes and of 3T3 cells within hours. On the other hand, TPA is known to initiate the release of the serine proteinase, plasminogen activator. This enzyme appears to be involved in the malignant transformation of cells in culture subsequent to TPA exposure (9). It may also be a factor that leads to enhanced cell proliferation as shown for other proteinases and hence deserves further investigation.

ACKNOWLEDGMENTS

This work was supported by a grant from the Swiss National Science Foundation (3.588-0.75). We thank Dr. B. A. Peskar for generous gifts of PG-antibodies and Prof. Dr. E. Hecker and Dr. R. Schmidt for supplying TPA and ³H-TPA.

REFERENCES

1. Fürstenberger, G., and Marks, F. (1978): Indomethacin inhibition of cell proliferation induced by the phorbol ester TPA is reversed by prostaglandin E_2 in mouse epidermis in vivo. Biochem. Biophys. Res. Commun., 84:1,103–1,111.
2. Glatt, M., Peskar, B., and Brune, K. (1974): Leukocytes and prostaglandins in acute inflammation. Experientia, 30:1,257–1,259.
3. Hecker, E. (1971): Isolation and characterization of the cocarcinogenic principles from croton oil. Methods Cancer Res., 6:439–484.
4. Lanz, R., and Brune, K. (1981): Dissociation of tumour promoter-induced effects on prostaglandin release, polyamine synthesis, and cell proliferation of 3T3 cells. Biochem. J., 194:975–982.
5. Lanz, R., and Brune, K. (1981): Tumor promoter-induced proliferation of 3T3 cells: The role of prostaglandin release and polyamine synthesis. In: Cellular Interactions, edited by J. T. Dingle and J. L. Gordon. Elsevier/North Holland.
6. Otto, A. M., Zumbé, A., Gibson, L., Kubler, A. M., and Jimenez de Asua, L. (1979): Cytoskeleton-disrupting drugs enhance effect of growth factors and hormones on initiation of DNA synthesis. Proc. Natl. Acad. Sci. USA, 76:6,435–6,438.
7. Puzas, J. E., and Goodman, D. B. P. (1978): A rapid assay for cellular deoxyribonucleic acid. Anal. Biochem., 86:50–55.
8. Verma, A. K., Rice, H. M., and Boutwell, R. K. (1977): Prostaglandins and skin tumor promotion: Inhibition of tumor promoter-induced ornithine decarboxylase activity in epidermis by inhibitors of prostaglandin synthesis. Biochem. Biophys. Res. Commun., 79:1,160–1,166.
9. Wigler, M., and Weinstein, I. B. (1976): Tumour promotor induces plasminogen activator. Nature, 259:232–233.

Carcinogenesis, Vol. 7, edited by E. Hecker et al.
Raven Press, New York © 1982.

A Possible Role of Protein Alkylation in Phorbol Ester Action

Gerald C. Mueller and Philip W. Wertz

*McArdle Laboratory for Cancer Research, University of Wisconsin,
Madison, Wisconsin 53706*

A SEARCH FOR A TUMOR-PROMOTING PROCESS

Certain phorbol esters, such as 12-O-tetradecanoylphorbol-13-acetate (TPA), promote the development of skin tumors in mice that have been treated with an initiating dose of a chemical carcinogen (2). A remarkable aspect of the cocarcinogenic action of this family of agents is that their action can be prevented by retinoic acid and a variety of related retinoids (1). This antagonism between phorbol esters and retinoids is especially interesting since it now provides a basis for identifying, among the pleiotropic effects of phorbol esters, those reactions and metabolic events that are involved in cocarcinogenesis. The reactions of interest presumably lie on the pathways that lead to the hyperproliferation or aberrant differentiation of cells and involve processes that are opposed or counteracted by retinoids. It is proposed that the identification of such processes will provide clues to the mechanism and control of certain types of carcinogenesis, even though the actual oncogenic event takes place in single cells of a population and is relatively infrequent.

The present studies have been carried out in normal lymphocytes from bovine lymph nodes. These cells are highly sensitive to low levels of TPA, and a number of the responses are selectively antagonized by retinoic acid. While it remains to be shown that these cells can exhibit a two-stage carcinogenesis process analogous to that most frequently studied in mouse skin, their responsiveness to the above agents and their ease in handling prompts their use for study of the metabolic interactions of phorbol esters and retinoids. This chapter presents evidence that TPA activates certain preexisting enzymatic processes and induces gene expression for others through an oxygen-mediated mechanism. In one instance, this has been shown to involve the formation of a highly reactive intermediate of arachidonic acid which then binds covalently to proteins. Our evidence supports the view that protein alkylation is an important process in enzyme activity and gene regulation in general, and that such an event specifically brings about the activation of cytidyl transferase, the rate-limiting enzyme in phosphatidyl choline synthesis. This process is of special interest as a mediator of cocarcinogenesis since it is also inhibited by retinoic acid.

THE LYMPHOCYTE RESPONSE TO PHORBOL ESTERS AND RETINOIDS

Extending our very early studies in human lymphocytes (11), TPA has also been found to be a powerful comitogen in bovine lymphocytes when combined with a low dose of phytohemagglutinin (PHA). The chronology of the phorbol ester response in bovine lymphocyte cultures is depicted in Fig. 1. Analogous to the situation in human lymphocytes, mitogenic activation involves an initial stimulation of preexisting membrane processes which lead in turn, during the ensuing 36 hr, to a cascading increase in gene expression and a resultant cell hypertrophy. Cells that have been made competent by these early events then engage in nuclear and cellular replication. For optimal comitogenesis, however, it is necessary to treat the lymphocytes simultaneously with these two agents using a limiting dose of PHA (6). For example, delaying the TPA as little as 2 hr dramatically decreases the mitogenic response when measured 48 hr after PHA treatment. En route to the mitogenic response, the two agents appear to act synergistically during a very short time interval to facilitate the expression of the many genes that underlie the synthesis of the proteins involved in the dramatic cell hypertrophy. An important example of this cooperation in an induced response appears to be ornithine decarboxylase (ODC) (12), the synthesis of which peaks at 18 hr (8). The induction of mitogenesis, as well as the induction of ODC, can be blocked completely by retinoic acid and certain related retinoids (6,8,17) which are also antagonists of tumor promotion. It is of considerable interest, however, that the induced gene expression leading to the synthesis of many other proteins during the cell hypertrophy is not blocked by the retinoids (6). This observation suggests that whereas phorbol esters may activate many gene expressions, only a few of such genes are actually under the control of the retinoids. This observation also implies that retinoids are not likely to directly oppose the primary action of the phorbol esters, but rather to interfere with some process that is set in motion by the phorbol esters and is required for amplification of the phorbol ester action. This separability of the triggering action of phorbol esters and the retinoid-sensitive amplification events provides a basis for the identification of the type of metabolic processes that might play a role in tumor promotion.

A ROLE FOR OXYGEN IN CERTAIN EARLY PHORBOL ESTER RESPONSES

As shown in Fig. 1, phorbol esters have several acute effects on lymphocytes which appear to arise through the interaction of this class of agents with the cell surface. Within 3 min, TPA promotes the capping reaction in lymphocytes as measured with fluorescein-labeled concanavalin A (Con A) (10). In this same time frame, TPA accelerates glucose transport (Wrighton and Mueller, *unpublished observations*). Neither of these two responses is inhibited by retinoids or

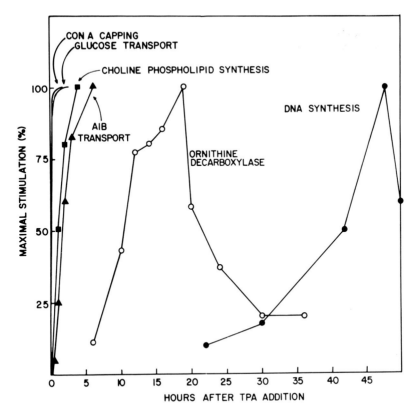

FIG. 1. The time course of the early and late TPA responses in the bovine lymphocyte system. The activation of Con A capping (10), glucose transport, α-aminoisobutyric acid (AIB) transport (9), and phosphatidyl choline synthesis (18,19), following treatment of lymphocytes with 10 nM TPA are shown. In addition, the kinetics of ODC (8), and DNA synthesis (6) are plotted after a combination treatment of the cells with 10 nM TPA and PHA at 0 time. The data are expressed as the percent of maximal stimulation.

TABLE 1. *Oxygen requirement for TPA response[a]*

Atmosphere	Phosphatidyl choline synthesis (19) TPA effect (percent of control)
Air	235
Nitrogen	83

[a] Lymphocytes were preequilibrated with an atmosphere of air or nitrogen at 37°C. At 0 time, 10 nM TPA plus [³H]choline was added to replicate cultures. The incorporation of [³H]choline into the phospholipid fraction was measured over a 1-hr period. Data are presented as the percent of the activity of untreated control cells in the respective atmosphere.

requires the presence of oxygen. In addition, neither process depends on the synthesis of new ribonucleic acid (RNA) or protein.

Although oxygen is not required for the above early responses, it is of considerable interest that TPA activates other processes that do require oxygen. For example, TPA is remarkably effective as an activator of superoxide anion production in polymorphonuclear cells and macrophages (3). This response can even be elicited in membrane vesicle preparations. The rapid response is clearly independent of protein synthesis and reflects the dramatic release of a DPNH-flavoprotein oxidoreductase system from some inhibited state in association with other membrane components. Recently, Kensler and Trush (7) have shown that TPA can trigger a chemoluminescence response in small lymphocytes, which appears to involve the generation of the singlet oxygen state.

Thus it appears that TPA causes acute alterations in the association of membrane macromolecules, which are reflected in the increased capping reaction, the accelerated glucose transport, and activation of certain aspects of oxygen metabolism. Since these reactions take place in the presence of retinoic acid, it appears that they may be more closely tied to the triggering action of phorbol esters than to the amplification or extension of the initial phorbol ester effects.

Although it is evident that the TPA action sets in motion a number of membrane-related systems, there still remains the problem of identifying the pathways and metabolic processes involved in its tumor-promoting action. To this end, we have searched for retinoic acid-sensitive processes ensuing from the initial triggering actions of TPA. The theme of this search was prompted by the earlier demonstrations by Boutwell and associates (2) and others (14,16) that a retinoid-sensitive process is involved in tumor promotion and ODC induction by TPA.

As shown in Fig. 1, TPA causes an early and rapid acceleration of phosphatidyl choline synthesis. Very importantly, retinoic acid blocks this response selectively when administered simultaneously (18); however, when it is added during the acceleration interval, further acceleration is prevented without depressing the rate of choline phospholipid synthesis that has already been achieved. The observation that 5,6-epoxyretinoic acid was even more effective than retinoic acid (Fig. 2; 17) prompted an inquiry into the possibility that retinoic acid might have to be oxidatively activated in order to be effective. Accordingly, the TPA acceleration of phosphatidyl choline synthesis was studied under anaerobic conditions. Instead of demonstrating that oxygen is required for the retinoic acid effect, we found, to our surprise, that oxygen is required for the TPA acceleration of phosphatidyl choline synthesis (Table 1). While this observation precluded our inquiry into the possible activation of retinoic acid for its effects, it provided the first clues to the role of an oxygen-requiring process in the extension or amplification of the TPA triggering action.

To investigate this subject further, a variety of inhibitors of oxygen-dependent pathways were tested for their possible influence on the TPA acceleration of phosphatidyl choline synthesis. Indomethacin, an inhibitor of cyclooxygenase, inhibited the response, but high levels were required and the action appeared

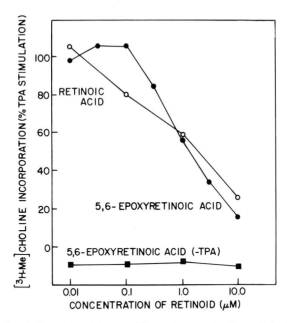

FIG. 2. Effect of retinoic acid and its epoxide on the acceleration of choline incorporation into the phospholipid fraction of bovine lymphocytes by TPA (17). Lymphocytes (15×10^6) were incubated for 15 min at 37°C in the presence of retinoic acid or 5,6-epoxyretinoic acid. [^{3}H]Choline (2 μCi/culture) and TPA (10 nM) were then added and the incubation continued for 1 hr. Following the incubation, the cells were harvested, the phospholipids extracted, and the radioactivity determined as described (19). ○: TPA + retinoic acid; ●: TPA + 5,6-epoxyretinoic acid; ■: 5,6-epoxyretinoic acid without TPA.

nonspecific. This view was further substantiated by the failure of prostaglandin, thromboxane, and prostacyclin analogs to influence the TPA acceleration of phosphatidyl choline synthesis. Similarly, the limited inhibition with tocopherol and related antioxidants appeared unselective. In contrast, 5,8,11,14-eicosatetray-noic acid (ETYA), which is also a lipoxidase inhibitor, was highly effective and very selective towards the TPA action (19). As shown in Fig. 3, this analog of arachidonic acid acted like retinoic acid in that it prevented the acceleration of phosphatidyl choline synthesis when it was added simultaneously with TPA, but blocked the further acceleration without depressing the established rate when it was added midway in the acceleration interval (Fig. 4). In contrast to the situation with retinoic acid, the simultaneous addition of arachidonic acid counteracted the effects of ETYA; however, the delayed addition of arachidonic acid (i.e., once the ETYA inhibition had been established) failed to counteract the ETYA. Accordingly, it was concluded that arachidonic acid protected the ETYA-sensitive system; however, the possibility remained that an oxidation product of arachidonic acid might also be involved in the TPA-mediated accelera-tion of phosphatidyl choline synthesis.

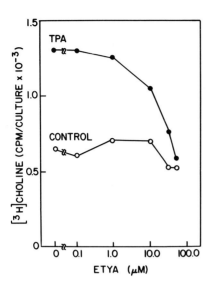

FIG. 3. The effect of ETYA on the acceleration of choline incorporation into the phospholipid fraction (19). Lymphocytes (15 × 10⁶) were incubated for 1 hr at 37°C in the presence of [³H]choline (2 μCi/culture) ± 10 nM TPA and the indicated concentration of ETYA. All agents were added in dimethylsulfoxide (DMSO). After the incubation, the cells were harvested, the lipid fraction extracted, and the radioactivity in the samples determined as described (19). ○: DMSO control; ●: TPA.

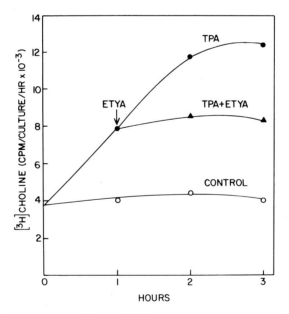

FIG. 4. Effect of the delayed addition of ETYA on the acceleration of choline incorporation in lymphocytes by TPA (19). Lymphocytes (15 × 10⁶) were treated ± TPA (10 nM) for 1 hr at 37°C prior to the addition of 100 μM ETYA to the indicated cultures. All agents were added in DMSO. The incorporation of [³H]choline (2 μCi/culture) was measured over a 1-hr interval. At the end of the labeling period, the cells were harvested, and the radioactivity in the lipid fraction was determined as described (19).○: DMSO control; ▲: TPA + ETYA; ●: TPA.

ROLE OF OXYGEN IN THE ACTIVATION OF CYTIDYL TRANSFERASE

To explore the above situation in more detail, we attempted to account for the TPA acceleration in terms of an altered enzyme activity in the pathway for choline phospholipid synthesis. Since cycloheximide experiments showed that this response does not require the synthesis of new proteins (18), an activation of an enzyme that is common to the synthesis of all three choline phospholipid products was indicated. Previous investigators (5,13,15) had clearly shown that the rate-limiting step in phosphatidyl choline synthesis is the formation of CDP-choline. Accordingly, the rate-limiting enzyme, cytidyl transferase, which catalyzes the formation of CDP-choline from cytosine triphosphate (CTP) and phosphocholine, was assayed during the TPA response (P. W. Wertz and G. C. Mueller, *unpublished observations*). It was found that this enzyme increased in activity in a manner that paralleled the acceleration of phosphatidyl choline synthesis during TPA treatment of the cells (Fig. 5). In accord with our expectations, both ETYA and retinoic acid treatment of the cells prevented this response (Fig. 6); whereas, neither inhibitor affected the activity of the enzyme when added directly to the assay.

The nature of this enzyme activation process was revealed in experiments in which arachidonic acid was added directly to sonicated preparations of TPA-treated lymphocytes. As shown in Fig. 7, the synthesis of CDP-choline in such

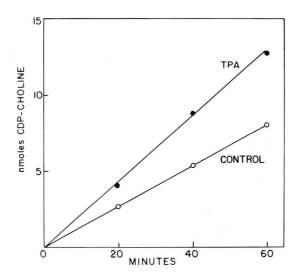

FIG. 5. Activation of cytidyl transferase in lymphocytes by TPA. Lymphocyte cultures were incubated for 2 hr at 37°C in the presence or absence of 10 nM TPA. Following incubation, the cells were harvested, disrupted by sonication, and the level of cytidyl transferase activity in the sonicates was determined using [^{14}C]choline phosphate and the charcoal procedure of Fiscus and Schneider (4). Results are expressed as nmole CDP-choline formed per 15 $\times$ 10^6 cells. ○: DMSO control; ●: TPA.

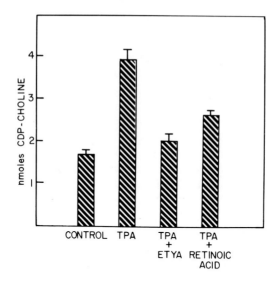

FIG. 6. The effect of ETYA and retinoic acid on the activation of cytidyl transferase. TPA (10 nM), ETYA (50 μM), and retinoic acid (30 μM) were added as indicated to replicate cultures of lymphocytes. After 2 hr of incubation at 37°C, the cells were harvested, disrupted by sonication, and centrifuged at 100,000 × g for 1 hr to yield a particulate fraction. The activity of cytidyl transferase in the particulate fraction was measured using [¹⁴C]choline phosphate and the charcoal procedure of Fiscus and Schneider (4). The results are expressed as nmole CDP-choline formed by 16 × 10⁶ cell equivalents in 20 min.

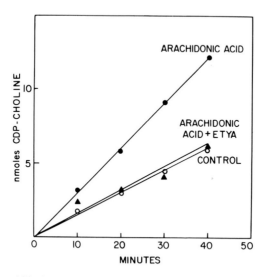

FIG. 7. Effect of arachidonic acid and ETYA on the cytidyl transferase activity in lymphocyte sonicates. Lymphocytes were disrupted by sonication and the level of cytidyl transferase activity in the sonicates was determined. Arachidonic acid (0.1 mg/ml) and ETYA (0.2 mg/ml) were added as indicated. Results are expressed as nmole CDP-choline formed by 15 × 10⁶ cell equivalents. ○: control; ●: arachidonic acid; ▲: arachidonic acid + ETYA.

sonicates was increased by the addition of arachidonic acid. This effect was prevented by ETYA, suggesting either a direct competition or the interference with an essential oxygenase-mediated process under the influence of TPA.

When the distribution of the enzyme in the subcellular fractions was studied, it was found that the changes in the activity of cytidyl transferase in the intact cell experiments correlated with a shift of the enzyme from the soluble protein fraction of the sonicate to the membrane/particulate fraction. Thus it appeared that the activation of phospholipid synthesis must result from some change in the cytidyl transferase or a membrane receptor that causes the enzyme to translocate to the membrane where it has close communication with the other enzymes involved in choline phospholipid synthesis. Furthermore, the data suggested that some oxidized metabolite of arachidonic acid might mediate this change in cytidyl transferase or receptor properties.

To explore this possibility, the soluble protein fraction of control lymphocytes was prepared and exposed to arachidonic acid. In contrast to the situation in the whole cell sonicates, the addition of arachidonic acid to such preparations was somewhat inhibitory (Fig. 8). If the arachidonic acid was oxidized briefly with crystalline soybean lipoxidase, however, the arachidonic acid preparation, at a level of 0.03 mg/ml, resulted in a striking activation of the soluble cytidyl transferase; higher levels of the oxidized arachidonic acid became inhibitory—

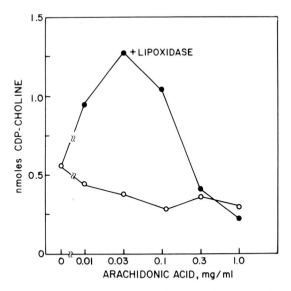

FIG. 8. Activation of soluble cytidyl transferase by lipoxidase-treated arachidonic acid. Control lymphocytes were disrupted by sonication, and the sonicate was centrifuged at 100,000 × g for 1 hr. Cytidyl transferase in the resulting supernatant fraction was assayed after the addition of the individual level of arachidonic acid or arachidonic acid preoxidized with soybean lipoxidase (100 μg/ml). Results are expressed as nmole CDP-choline formed by 18 × 10⁶ cell equivalents in 20 min in the presence of the indicated level of arachidonic acid preparation.

suggesting that the enzyme might have been inactivated by multiple attacks of a reactive intermediate in the oxidized arachidonic acid preparation. The lack of a positive effect on, and even inhibition of, cytidyl transferase activity by pure arachidonic acid in cytosol preparations, as contrasted to the results with whole cell sonicates, is best explained by the localization of a TPA-activated oxygenase system in the membranes or cell particulates.

Taken together, these results support the concept that phorbol esters, in the course of acutely mobilizing oxygen metabolism in the cell membrane, provide a system that can oxidatively convert arachidonic acid to a metabolite which in turn activates cytidyl transferase. The mechanism of this activation is not fully established, but it appears most likely to involve the initial formation of a hydroperoxide or an epoxide of arachidonic acid; this entity then either alkylates or oxidizes a specific site in the enzyme or another protein required for transferase activity. The data obtained using the soybean lipoxidase suggest that this enzyme can be used to bypass the TPA-activated lipoxidase in making the active metabolite directly.

With respect to the above two possibilities, recent studies on the metabolism of arachidonic acid in TPA-stimulated bovine lymphocytes support the view that the retinoic acid/ETYA-sensitive activation process involves an alkylation of target proteins. As shown in Fig. 9, TPA treatment of lymphocytes strikingly increases the amount of [³H]arachidonic acid that is covalently bound to the acid insoluble macromolecular fraction of these cells (P. W. Wertz and G. C.

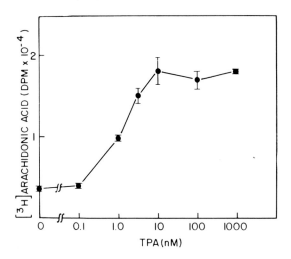

FIG. 9. Effect of TPA on the covalent linking of arachidonic acid to lymphocyte proteins. Lymphocytes (10⁸/culture) were incubated at 37°C for 2 hr in the presence of the indicated concentration of TPA and [³H]arachidonic acid (5 μCi/culture). The cells were sedimented, acid-precipitated, and lipid-extracted in a Soxhlet apparatus to remove free arachidonic acid and small MW metabolites. Radioactivity that remained covalently attached to the protein in the macromolecular residue was measured. Results are expressed as DPM [³H]arachidonic acid per culture.

Mueller, *unpublished observations*). Fractionation studies show that a radioactive metabolite of arachidonic acid is bound largely to cell proteins without significant labeling of the RNA or deoxyribonucleic acid (DNA) fractions. Proteolytic digestion of the proteins liberates peptides with the radioactivity still bound covalently. Treatment of the latter, however, with cyanogen bromide or silver nitrate and acetic acid liberates the radioactivity as an ether-soluble form, which is currently the subject of characterization studies. Since the cyanogen bromide and silver nitrate are effective reagents for cleaving thio-ether bridges, it is anticipated that the arachidonic acid metabolite may be bound to its target protein through such a bond. Test of this hypothesis is also a topic of current investigation.

POSSIBLE ROLE OF PROTEIN ALKYLATION IN PHORBOL ESTER RESPONSES RELATED TO TUMOR PROMOTION

In summary, our experiments on the interacting effects of phorbol esters and retinoids have provided evidence that the two types of agents act quite separately. The phorbol esters, acting presumably through a receptor-like mechanism, acutely activate the cell membrane for membrane movement, acceleration of glucose transport, and the generation of active oxygen species (Fig. 10). The latter process appears in some way to be involved in the generation of reactive lipid intermediates which, in the one case studied so far, can be deriva-

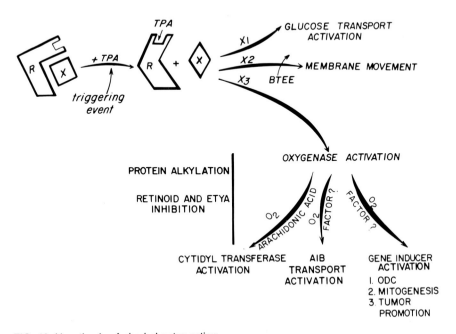

FIG. 10. Hypothesis of phorbol ester action.

tives of arachidonic acid. This active metabolite, in turn, appears to alkylate proteins in the model system, with the result that cytidyl transferase becomes more active as an enzyme and translocates to the cell membrane. Retinoic acid and ETYA block this process—possibly by interfering at the level of the oxygenase, but more likely by competitively alkylating the target proteins in a manner that redirects their role in the biological response. In support of this view, we have found that TPA treatment, in a manner quite analogous to that observed for arachidonic acid, also increases the covalent binding of [^{3}H]retinoic acid to cell proteins.

On the basis of these findings, we propose that other retinoid-sensitive processes that ensue from the TPA activation event, including tumor promotion in mouse skin, may operate in a very similar manner. It is suggested that whereas a single oxygenase system may be common to all such responses, the range of lipid mediators that can be activated might be quite diverse. In such a case, the nature of the biological response that ensues would be directed by the specificity exhibited in the interaction of the different lipid mediators with specific target proteins. The responses that take place would then depend on whether that protein is involved in a catalytic or a genetic process. This view of phorbol ester/retinoic acid interaction not only provides an explanation for the pleiotropic effects of phorbol esters, but provides a strategy for identifying the processes leading more specifically to tumor promotion.

REFERENCES

1. Bollag, W. (1972): Prophylaxis of chemically induced benign and malignant epithelial tumors by vitamin A acid (retinoic acid). *Eur. J. Cancer,* 8:689–693.
2. Boutwell, R. K. (1974): The function and mechanism of promoters of carcinogenesis. *CRC Crit. Rev. Toxicol.,* 2:419–443.
3. DeChatelet, L. R., Shirley, P. S., and Johnson, R. B., Jr. (1976): Effect of phorbol myristate acetate on the oxidative metabolism of human polymorphonuclear leukocytes. *Blood,* 47:545–554.
4. Fiscus, W. G., and Schneider, W. C. (1966): The role of phospholipids in stimulating phosphorylcholine cytidyl transferase activity. *J. Biol. Chem.,* 241:3,324–3,330.
5. Kennedy, E. P. (1962): The metabolism and function of complex lipids. *The Harvey Lectures,* 57:143–171.
6. Kensler, T. W., and Mueller, G. C. (1978): Retinoic acid inhibition of the comitogenic action of mezerein and phorbol esters in bovine lymphocytes. *Cancer Res.,* 38:771–775.
7. Kensler, T. W., and Trush, M. A. (1980): Inhibition of phorbol ester-stimulated chemiluminescence in human polymorphonuclear leukocytes by retinoic acid and 5,6-epoxyretinoic acid. *Cancer Res.,* 41:216–222.
8. Kensler, T. W., Verma, A. K., Boutwell, R. K., and Mueller, G. C. (1978): Effects of retinoic acid and juvenile hormone on the induction of ornithine decarboxylase activity by 12-O-tetradecanoylphorbol-13-acetate. *Cancer Res.,* 38:2,896–2,899.
9. Kensler, T. W., Wertz, P. W., and Mueller, G. C. (1979): Inhibition of phorbol ester-accelerated amino acid transport in bovine lymphocytes. *Biochim. Biophys. Acta,* 585:43–52.
10. Kwong, C. H., and Mueller, G. C. (1979): Effects of hexachlorocyclohexane isomers on concanavalin A capping in bovine lymphocytes. *Biochim. Biophys. Acta,* 586:501–511.
11. Mueller, G. C., and Kajiwara, K. (1966): Regulatory steps in the replication of mammalian cell nuclei. In: *Developmental and Metabolic Control Mechanisms and Neoplasia,* edited by D. N. Ward, pp. 452–474. The Williams and Wilkins Company, Baltimore.

12. O'Brien, T. G., Simsiman, R. C., and Boutwell, R. K. (1975): Induction of the polyamine biosynthetic enzymes in mouse epidermis and their specificity for tumor promotion. *Cancer Res.*, 35:1,662–1,670.

13. Schneider, W. J., and Vance, D. E. (1978): Effect of choline deficiency on the enzymes that synthesize phosphatidylethanolamine in rat liver. *Eur. J. Biochem.*, 85:181–187.

14. Sporn, M. B. (1977): Retinoids and carcinogenesis. *Nutr. Rev.*, 35:65–69.

15. Vance, D. E., and Choy, P. C. (1979): How is phosphatidylcholine biosynthesis regulated? *Trends Biol. Sci.*, 4:145–148.

16. Verma, A. K., Shapas, B. G., Rice, H. M., and Boutwell, R. K. (1979): Correlation of the inhibition by retinoids of tumor promoter-induced mouse epidermal ornithine decarboxylase activity and of skin tumor promotion. *Cancer Res.*, 39:419–425.

17. Wertz, P. W., Kensler, T. W., Mueller, G. G., Verma, A. K., and Boutwell, R. K. (1979): 5,6-Epoxyretinoic acid opposes the effects of 12-O-tetradecanoylphorbol-13-acetate in bovine lymphocytes. *Nature*, 277:227–229.

18. Wertz, P. W., and Mueller, G. C. (1978): Rapid stimulation of phospholipid metabolism in bovine lymphocytes by tumor-promoting phorbol esters. *Cancer Res.*, 38:2,900–2,904.

19. Wertz, P. W., and Mueller, G. C. (1980): Inhibition of 12-O-tetradecanoylphorbol-13-acetate-accelerated phospholipid metabolism by 5,8,11,14-eicosatetraynoic acid. *Cancer Res.*, 40:776–781.

Carcinogenesis, Vol. 7, edited by E. Hecker et al.
Raven Press, New York © 1982.

Studies on Antagonistic Actions of TPA and Retinoic Acid

Anton M. Jetten and Luigi M. De Luca

Differentiation Control Section, Laboratory of Experimental Pathology, National Cancer Institute, National Institutes of Health, Bethesda, Maryland 20205

A conceptual approach for studying the biochemical mechanism by which 12-O-tetradecanoylphorbol-13-acetate (TPA) promotes neoplasia is furnished by the consideration that retinoids are powerful antipromoting agents (2,3,10,11). Thus, one expects that in the simplest case, TPA should interfere with biochemical processes sustained by vitamin A and its active analogs in normal tissues. The expressions and modalities of this process will depend on the specific commital pathways of the cell.

Initital work in our laboratory has centered on attempts to find key biological processes that are affected in opposite ways by TPA and retinoic acid (RA).

ANTAGONISTIC EFFECTS OF RA AND TPA ON ADHESION, SATURATION DENSITY, AND BINDING OF EPIDERMAL GROWTH FACTOR

Table 1 summarizes results on the effects of RA and/or TPA treatment on adhesiveness, saturation density, and binding of epidermal growth factor (EGF) in mouse fibroblast cells Balb/c 3T6 and Balb/c 3T3 A31-1-BP-2 (the latter obtained from Dr. T. Kakunaga, NCI, Bethesda, Maryland). Untreated 3T6 cells showed no contact inhibition and grew to a high density; addition of TPA had little effect on both adhesiveness and density of these cells. Treatment of 3T6 cells with RA restored contact inhibition, resulting in a reduction in saturation density and an increase in adhesion. Contact inhibition could be overcome when RA-treated cells were exposed to TPA. Moreover, adhesiveness of RA-treated cells was reduced by addition of TPA. The binding of EGF to 3T6 cells was drastically reduced within 5 hr of TPA treatment (Table 1). Cells grown for several days in the presence of RA exhibited a fivefold enhancement of EGF binding (4,5); subsequent treatment of these cells with TPA strongly reduced EGF binding. Although TPA and RA caused opposite effects on 3T6 cells, it seems that RA did not prevent the action of TPA on saturation density, EGF binding, and adhesiveness. This is in contrast to the action of RA and TPA on 3T3 A31-1-BP-2 cells: addition of TPA to RA-treated cells did not significantly alter adhesiveness or saturation density.

TABLE 1. *Action of RA and TPA on saturation density, cell substratum adhesiveness, and EGF binding*

Cell line	Treatment	Saturation density[a] (10^5 cells/cm²)	Adhesiveness[b] (min)	^{125}I-EGF binding[c] (pg per 10^6 cells)
3T6	Untreated	2.54	2.5	87.0
	+ RA	0.88	12.0	443.9
	+ TPA	2.62	2.0	4.8
	+ RA + TPA	2.20	8.0	77.7
3T3 A31-1-BP-2	Untreated	2.27	8.0	2.9
	+ RA	0.76	15.0	3.3
	+ TPA	3.43	1.5	N.D.[d]
	+ RA + TPA	0.93	15.0	N.D.

[a] For measurement of saturation density, cells were grown in the presence or absence of 2.10^{-6} M RA for 4 days. Then to some dishes TPA (50 ng/ml) was added, and 5 days later the total number of cells was determined in a Coulter counter.

[b] For measurement of adhesiveness, cells were grown for 4 days in the presence or absence of RA (10^{-6} M) and/or with TPA (30 ng/ml) for 18 hr. Adhesion was determined by treatment with trypsin (100 g/ml). Numbers indicate time at which 50% of the cells were released.

[c] EGF binding was determined as described previously (4). Cells were treated with 10^{-5} M RA for 5 days and with TPA (50 ng/ml) for 5 hr.

[d] N.D. = Not done.

ANTAGONISTIC EFFECTS OF RETINOIDS AND PHORBOL ESTERS ON THE FORMATION OF TRANSFORMED FOCI AND COLONIES IN SOFT AGAR

Mouse fibroblast Balb/c 3T3 A31-1-BP-2 cells appeared to be contact inhibited when grown in tissue culture dishes and remained so for some time when reaching confluence. Upon further incubation, and only in certain spots, contact inhibition was abolished and foci were formed consisting of piled-up, noncontact inhibited cells (Fig. 1). Approximately 65% of the foci were of type II, whereas 15% were of type III. The total number of foci was independent of the initial plating density but was dependent on the serum concentration: the number of foci increased with higher concentrations of serum. When 3T3 A31-1-BP-2 cells were grown in the presence of RA, the formation of foci was inhibited at low concentrations and was prevented at concentrations higher than 10^{-7}M (Fig. 2). The pyrimidyl analog for RA (pyrRA), which has been shown to be biologically inactive in other systems (1,6,7), had no major inhibitory effect. TPA treatment enhanced focus formation by almost twofold and increased the number of type III foci to approximately 60% of the total number of foci. RA also inhibited drastically the formation of foci in the presence of TPA, indicating the antagonistic nature of the effects of these two compounds.

Although not an absolute criterion, colony formation in soft agar correlates in many instances with the malignant behavior of cells. As shown in Table 2, untreated 3T3 A31-1-BP-2 cells exhibited a low frequency of colony formation in agar. TPA increased colony formation by almost sevenfold, whereas phorbol-

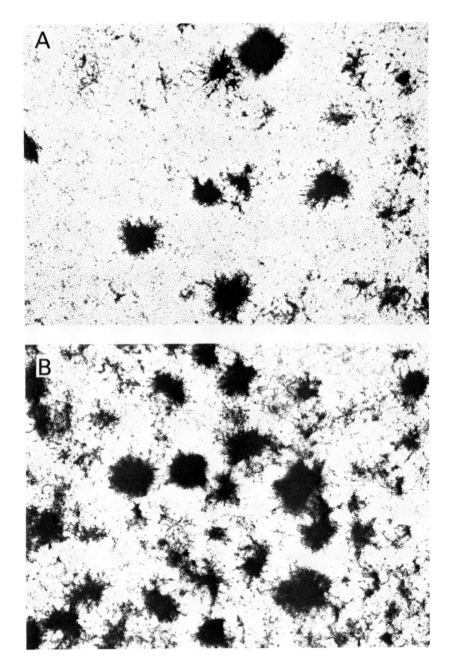

FIG. 1. Focus formation by Balb/c 3T3 A31-1-BP-2 cells. Confluent cells were grown in the presence **(B)** or absence **(A)** of TPA (30 ng/ml) in Dulbecco's modified Eagle's/Ham's F12 (1:1) medium containing 1% calf serum. After 1-week incubation, cells were fixed and stained with Giemsa. × 6.

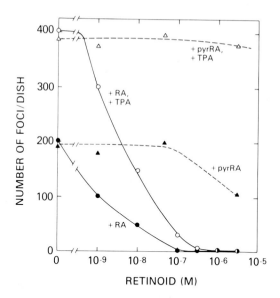

FIG. 2. Antagonistic action of RA and TPA on the formation of type I, II, and III foci by mouse fibroblast 3T3 A31-1-BP-2 cells. Cells were grown in 10-cm tissue culture dishes in Dulbecco's modified Eagle's/Ham's F12 (1:1) medium containing 1% calf serum in the presence and absence of various concentrations of RA or pyrRA. After 1 day of incubation, TPA (30 ng/ml) was added to half of the dishes. One week after reaching confluence, cells were stained with Giemsa and the number of foci greater than 1 mm were scored as described by Kakunaga (8). Total number of foci of RA-treated cells, ●; RA plus TPA-treated cells, ○; pyrRA-treated cells, ▲; and pyrRA plus TPA-treated cells, △.

13,20-diacetate (PDA), a biologically inactive phorbol ester, did not enhance colony formation significantly. Both retinol and RA, in the presence or absence of TPA, prevented colony formation in soft agar, whereas pyrRA was inactive.

DISCUSSION

In contrast to TPA treatment, RA treatment of mouse fibroblasts caused an increase in adhesiveness and EGF binding and a reduction in saturation density. Furthermore, in 3T3 A31-1-BP-2 cells RA inhibited, whereas TPA enhanced, focus and colony formation. When cells were treated simultaneously with RA and TPA, the action of either compound could prevail, dependent on the cell line: RA prevailed in 3T3 A31-1-BP-2 cells, whereas in 3T6 cells, TPA could overcome the action of the retinoid. It can be concluded from these results that RA can inhibit the expression of the transformed phenotype by preventing progression from the preneoplastic to the neoplastic state of the cell, whereas TPA promotes this process. The increase in adhesiveness produced by retinoids may be associated with the restoration of contact inhibition and reduction in saturation density, resulting in inhibition of focus formation and reduction of colony formation in soft agar.

TABLE 2. *Effect of various retinoids and phorbol esters on colony formation of mouse fibroblast 3T3 A31-1-BP-2 cells plated in soft agar*

Treatment		Colonies per dish[a]
Control		6.3
+ RA	(10^{-7} M)	0.0
+ Retinol	(10^{-7} M)	0.0
+ Pyrimidyl RA	(10^{-7} M)	7.0
+ TPA	(30 ng/ml)	43.5
+ PDA	(30 ng/ml)	6.5
+ RA + TPA	$(10^{-7} \text{ M},$ 30 ng/ml)	0.0
+ Retinol + TPA	$(10^{-7} \text{ M},$ 30 ng/ml)	0.0

[a] Cells were grown in DMEM/F12 medium containing 10% calf serum in the presence and absence of the indicated retinoid (10^7 M) for 3 days. Then cells were trypsinized and seeded at 10^4 cells per 6-cm plate in soft agar containing the additions indicated. After 2 weeks of incubation, colonies larger than 20 cells were scored.

The appearance of foci after the 3T3 A31-1-BP-2 cells reached confluence resembles the behavior of the X-irradiated CH3 10T ½ cells described by Kennedy et al. (9). One interpretation of this phenomenon is that incubation of these cells at confluence alters their physiological state and thereby promotes the expression of certain transformed characteristics, such as the release of cells from contact inhibition. This phenomenon is not unique to these cells, since embryonal carcinoma cells are endowed with an enhanced probability to differentiate when maintained at confluence.

These studies suggest that further insight into the problem of promotion by TPA may be gained by an investigation of cell surface molecules involved in maintenance of contact inhibition, adhesiveness, and reception of growth factors.

REFERENCES

1. Adamo, S., De Luca, L. M., Akalovsky, I., and Bhat, P. V. (1979): Retinoid-induced adhesion in cultured transformed mouse fibroblasts. *J. Natl. Cancer Inst.,* 62:1,473–1,477.
2. Colburn, N. (1979): The use of tumor promoter-responsive epidermal cell lines to study preneoplastic progression. In: *Neoplastic Transformation in Differentiated Epithelial Cell Systems in vitro,* edited by L. M. Franks and C. B. Wigley, p. 113–134. Academic Press, New York.
3. Diamond, L., O'Brien, T. G., and Baird, W. M. (1980): Tumor promoters and the mechanism of tumor promotion. *Adv. Cancer Res.,* 32:1–74.
4. Jetten, A. M. (1980a): Retinoids specifically enhance the number of epidermal growth factor receptors. *Nature,* 284:626–629.
5. Jetten, A. M. (1981b): Action of retinoids and phorbol esters on cell growth and the binding of epidermal growth factor. *Ann. N.Y. Acad. Sci.,* 359:200–217.

6. Jetten, A. M., and Jetten, M. E. R. (1979): Possible role of retinoic acid-binding protein in retinoid stimulation of embryonal carcinoma cell differentiation. *Nature,* 278:180–182.
7. Jetten, A. M., Jetten, M. E. R., Shapiro, S., and Poon, J. (1979): Characterization of the action of retinoids on mouse fibroblast cell lines. *Exp. Cell Res.,* 119:289–299.
8. Kakunaga, T. (1973): A quantitative system for assay of malignant transformation by chemical carcinogens using a clone derived from Balb/c 3T3. *Int. J. Cancer,* 12:463–473.
9. Kennedy, A. R., Fox, M., Murphy, G., and Little, J. (1980): On the relationship between X-ray exposure and malignant transformation in C3H 10T ½ cells. PNAS 77:7,262–7,266.
10. Lotan, R. (1980): Effects of vitamin A and its analogs (retinoids) on normal and neoplastic cells. *Biochim. Biophys. Acta,* 605:33–91.
11. Merriman, R. L., and Bertram, J. S. (1979): Reversible inhibition by retinoids of 3-methylcholan-threne-induced neoplastic transformation in C3H 10T ½ Clone 8 cells. *Cancer Res.,* 39:1,661–1,666.

Carcinogenesis, Vol. 7, edited by E. Hecker et al.
Raven Press, New York © 1982.

Specific Binding of Phorbol Ester Tumor Promoters to Mouse Tissues and Cultured Cells

Peter M. Blumberg, K. Barry Delclos, William G. Dunphy, and
Susan Jaken

Department of Pharmacology, Harvard Medical School, Boston, Massachusetts 02115

The phorbol ester tumor promoters induce a large number of cellular and biochemical changes, both in mouse skin *in vivo* and in cultured cells *in vitro* (3,8,39). As described in this volume, a major focus of effort has been to trace the pathway of these biological cascades and to identify which of the many alterations either are directly responsible for causing papilloma outgrowth or are essential intermediates in the critical pathways that lead to papilloma outgrowth.

In contrast to the multiplicity of biological responses, the similarity in structure-activity relations for induction of these responses strongly suggested that the various responses are triggered by interaction of the phorbol esters at no more than a few classes of targets. The high potency of the phorbol esters, which are active in the nanomolar concentration range, and the marked differences in activity associated with small structural modifications in the molecule, indicated that the phorbol esters probably acted through receptor binding rather than through a nonspecific interaction with the cell membrane. On the other hand, initial attempts to demonstrate such specific binding by using [³H]phorbol 12-myristate 13-acetate (PMA) and [³H]phorbol 12,13-didecanoate had been unsuccessful (19,27,29,41), probably on account of the substantial lipophilicity of these derivatives (24).

Recently, the use of a less lipophilic derivative, [³H]phorbol 12,13-dibutyrate (PDBu), has permitted the demonstration of specific phorbol ester binding to cultured cells (12) and to tissues (6,13,31). The structure-activity relations for binding are consistent with this binding activity mediating both tumor promotion in skin and biological responses *in vitro*. The ongoing characterization of this binding activity provides insights into the nature of the receptor, and demonstration of receptor modulation both by phorbol esters and by other factors indicates that it may be subject to regulatory control. This chapter summarizes the current state of knowledge concerning the phorbol ester receptor.

MATERIALS AND METHODS

Centrifugation Binding Assay

Binding was carried out in 400-μl microcentrifuge tubes containing, in a total volume of 250 μl, 0.01 to 0.5 mg of particulate protein preparation, 0.05 M Tris-Cl (pH 7.4), 4 mg/ml bovine serum albumin, 0.8% dimethylsulfoxide (DMSO), [^{3}H]PDBu, and other ligands as specified in the figure and table legends. The tubes were maintained at 0°C while additions were made. They were then mixed thoroughly and incubated for 30 min (unless otherwise specified) at 37°C. After incubation, the tubes were immediately centrifuged for 45 min at 4°C and 17,500 × g (12,500 rpm in the HB-4 rotor of a Sorvall RC-5 centrifuge equipped with custom-made adapters giving the rotor a total capacity of 24 tubes). A 100-μl aliquot of the supernatant was withdrawn for scintillation counting to determine the actual concentration of free [^{3}H]PDBu. The remaining supernatant was removed and discarded. The tip of the centrifuge tube containing the pellet was cut off and transferred to a counting vial. Radioactivity was quantitated by counting in Scintiverse (Fisher Scientific). Specific binding represents the difference between total and nonspecific binding. Nonspecific binding was determined as follows: The partitioning of [^{3}H]PDBu into the pellet under the conditions of the particular experiment was determined in the presence of 30 μM nonradioactive PDBu. Nonspecific binding for each tube was then calculated from this partition coefficient, and the actual amount of [^{3}H]PDBu was measured in the supernatant of that tube.

Filtration Binding Assay

Brain particulate protein, [^{3}H]PDBu, and, in some cases, excess nonradioactive PDBu (30 μM) were incubated in 50 mM Tris-Cl (pH 7.4) containing 4 mg/ml bovine serum albumin (incubation buffer). At the end of the incubation, 1-ml aliquots were removed from the incubation mixture and rapidly filtered on Whatman GF/F filters presoaked in incubation buffer. After sample filtration, each filter was immediately washed once with 5 ml of ice-cold incubation buffer, dried, and radioactivity was determined. In each assay, 0.1-ml aliquots were removed from the incubation mixture and counted for determination of total [^{3}H]PDBu. Free [^{3}H]PDBu represents the difference between total and bound [^{3}H]PDBu. Nonspecific [^{3}H]PDBu binding was determined in the presence of 30 μM nonradioactive PDBu as before.

Whole Cell Binding Assay

Cells were grown in 16-mm multiwell dishes (Falcon) in 0.5 ml of serum-containing medium. For assay, cell monolayers were incubated in binding medium consisting of 200 μl of serum-containing medium, 50 μl of 0.75% DMSO in serum-containing medium, and other compounds as indicated. [^{3}H]PDBu was added to each well in a volume of 50 μl of serum-containing medium. The dishes were returned to the incubator (37°C in a 5% CO_2, 95% air atmosphere) for 30 min. They were then removed and placed in an ice bucket, and aliquots of the medium were removed to measure directly the concentration of free [³H]PDBu. The remaining medium was aspirated off, and the cell monolayers were rinsed quickly three times with 0.2 ml of ice-cold serum-containing medium. Cell lysates were collected in 0.6 ml of 0.1 N NaOH, and aliquots were prepared for scintillation counting in Aquasol (New England Nuclear). Specific binding was calculated from the difference in radioactivity in the absence or presence of excess PDBu. Nonspecific binding was measured in the presence of 20 μM PDBu.

RESULTS

[³H]PDBu was chosen as the radioactive ligand for binding studies because it appeared to maximize biological potency relative to lipophilicity (28). Mouse skin was of greatest interest for analysis of binding since the biological phenomenon of phorbol ester tumor promotion has been best characterized in that system. The studies of binding to mouse skin are described in ref. 6.

[³H]PDBu bound to particulate preparations from mouse skin in a saturable fashion with high affinity (Fig. 1A). Specific binding ranged from 72% of total binding at the lowest ligand concentration to 16% at the highest concentration. Nonspecific binding was defined as that binding occurring in the presence of 30 μM nonradioactive PDBu. Over the range of concentrations examined, nonspecific binding was linear with the concentration of free [³H]PDBu present.

When the equilibrium binding data were analyzed by the Scatchard method (Fig. 1B) and fitted by linear regression analysis to the model of a single binding site, the following parameters were derived: binding at saturation, 3.9 ± 0.3 pmole/mg; $K_D = 24 \pm 6$ nM. It is clear, however, that the Scatchard plot has a slight upward concavity. This shape could indicate more than one class of phorbol ester receptors. Alternatively, it might reflect partial association of a single receptor class with a factor modulating binding affinity, it might indicate negative cooperativity, or it might represent an assay artifact. Because the points accounting for the concave shape largely were determined in a concentration range in which errors were relatively large due to the low ratio of specific to total binding (16 to 18%), meaningful quantitation of the binding in terms of two binding sites did not appear practical.

The most critical feature in evaluation of a binding activity is that of specificity. Binding affinities of derivatives were measured by inhibition of [³H]PDBu binding as described (6). Both for mouse skin and brain preparations, the structure-activity requirements for binding corresponded to the promoting activity of the phorbol esters (Table 1). Although binding activity was measured with [³H]PDBu, the phorbol ester of highest affinity for the PDBu target was in fact PMA, the most potent tumor promoter.

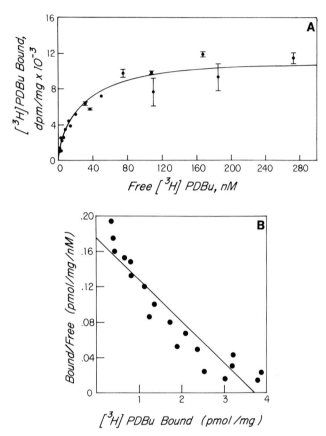

FIG. 1. Specific binding of [³H] PDBu to particulate preparations from whole mouse skin as a function of ligand concentration. **A:** Saturation curve. The particulate fraction (300 μg/tube) prepared from whole mouse skin as described (6) was incubated with increasing concentrations of [³H]PDBu for 30 min at 39°C (see "Materials and Methods"). Nonspecific binding was determined in the presence of 30 μM nonradioactive PDBu at each concentration of [³H]PDBu used. The curve was calculated using values for the dissociation constant and the amount of binding at saturation estimated from the Scatchard plot. **B:** Scatchard plot.

Several phorbol-related diterpene esters have been identified that, although highly inflammatory, are only weak or nonpromoters. 12-Deoxyphorbol 13-isobutyrate 20-acetate is 1.5-fold less potent than PMA in the mouse ear inflammation assay (20). Resiniferatoxin is at least 100-fold more inflammatory than is PMA (17,36). Neither is active as a tumor promoter (20,47). Resiniferatoxin at a concentration of 160 nM caused no inhibition of [³H]PDBu binding to skin preparations, 12-deoxyphorbol 13-isobutyrate 20-acetate was 19,000-fold less potent than PMA as an inhibitor of [³H]PDBu binding. These findings provide strong evidence that the [³H]PDBu target is that involved in phorbol ester tumor promotion and is not instead a secondary target associated only with inflammation.

TABLE 1. *Comparison of the tumor-promoting and binding activities of the phorbol-related diterpene esters in the mouse*

Derivative	Relative tumor-promoting activity	Ref.	Potency in binding assay (K_i relative to PMA)	
			Skin[a]	Brain[b]
PMA	1		1	1
Phorbol 12,13-didecanoate	1.5	(43)	<7[c]	<4[c]
Mezerein	49	(30)	132	20
PDBu	180–72	(38,43)	32	112
Phorbol 12,13-dibenzoate	20–100	(1)	100	98
Phorbol 12,13-diacetate	>50	(35)	4,000	8,500
Phorbol 12,13,20-triacetate	>200	(18)	7,600	440,000
Phorbol 13-acetate	NT[d]		86,000	240,000

[a] Data from Delclos et al., (6); K_i for PMA = 0.74 nM.
[b] Data from Dunphy et al., (13); K_i for PMA = 0.066 nM.
[c] Upper limits determined by assuming that phorbol-12,13-didecanoate and PMA nonspecifically partition into the particulate preparations to an equal extent.
[d] NT, not tested.

The data obtained with the resiniferonol derivative mezerein support this same conclusion. Mezerein has a potency within a factor of two of PMA as an inflammatory agent (17) and is more potent than, or nearly as potent as, PMA in several *in vitro* assays (26,45). On the other hand, mezerein is approximately 50-fold less potent than PMA as a promoter in CD-1 mice (30). We find that mezerein is 20- to 132-fold less active than PMA as an inhibitor of [³H]PDBu binding.

The binding results from mouse skin allow several predictions. Separate high affinity receptors for resiniferatoxin and 12-deoxyphorbol 13-isobutyrate 20-acetate should exist. In addition, the weakly inflammatory phorbol esters phorbol 12,13-diacetate, phorbol 12,13,20-triacetate, and phorbol 13-acetate should be promoting, provided that sufficiently high concentrations are used and corrections are made for differences in rates of absorption and degradation. Although phorbol 12,13-diacetate and phorbol 12,13,20-triacetate were reported to be non-promoting or only weakly promoting, they were only tested in amounts 200- and 50-fold greater than for PMA. In contrast, amounts at least 4,000- and 7,600-fold greater than for PMA would be predicted from the binding data to be required.

[³H]PDBu was not inhibited by the nonphorbol-related tumor promoters anthralin (1 μM), cantharidin (300 μM), iodoacetic acid (1.7 μM), or phenol (1mM) (6). This finding suggests that these compounds act via a mechanism different from that of the phorbol esters. The dissimilarity of biological effects *in vitro* of these compounds and of the phorbol esters (9 and references cited therein) had earlier suggested the same conclusion. Likewise, since dexamethasone acetate (2 μM), retinoic acid (10 μM), epidermal growth factor (100 ng/ml), and melittin

(25 μg/ml) did not block [³H]PDBu binding (6), these putative antagonists or analogs must interact at a different target.

Although the mouse skin system may be biologically the most relevant to tumor promotion, *in vitro* systems possess the advantage of greater experimental manipulability. [³H]PDBu binding to chick embryo fibroblasts (12), the GH_4C_1 cell line (25), human lymphocytes (34), and rat embryo cells (21) has been reported. [³H]PMA binding to human lymphocytes (14) and MDCK cells (32) has also been found. Binding can be measured to particulate preparations, as was done in the early studies on chick embryo fibroblasts (12). Measurement of binding to whole cells has proved to be easier, however (see "Materials and Methods" for details of the whole cell binding assay used with GH_4C_1 cells).

Total binding at saturation was 75,000 molecules/cell for chick embryo fibroblasts (12), 200,000 molecules/cell for GH_4C_1 (25) and rat embryo cells (21), and 200,000 to 600,000 molecules/cell for human lymphocytes (14,34). Detailed structure-activity analysis was carried out for the chick embryo fibroblasts (12). For derivatives varying over a range of 1.5×10^5 in binding affinity, the binding affinity and the ED_{50} for the biological response of fibronectin loss were the same within a factor of 3.5 (Table 2). Such quantitative agreement provides strong evidence that the specific PDBu binding mediates the biological response.

The tissue distribution of specific [³H]PDBu binding was examined. With three exceptions, specific binding was found for all tissues examined. Human red blood cells bound -0.1 ± 0.2 pmole/mg; degradation of PDBu interfered with measurement in the cases of mouse liver and kidney. The two tissues showing highest [³H]PDBu binding were spleen and brain. The widespread tissue distribution of phorbol ester receptors supports recent *in vivo* studies which report phorbol ester tumor promotion in a variety of tissues including forestomach, lung, and ovary (37).

This laboratory has recently begun analysis of the phylogenetic distribution of phorbol ester receptors. Bresch and Arendt had earlier reported activity of PMA at nM concentrations on the sea urchin *Sphaerechinus granularis* (4). In collaboration with Dr. Kenneth Lew (Children's Hospital, Boston, Massachusetts), we have found biological responsiveness and specific binding of [³H]PDBu with the nematode *Caenorhabditis elegans* (K. Lew et al., *in preparation*). No binding was seen with *Bacillus subtilis,* however (12). These results suggest that PDBu receptors were highly conserved during evolution. They raise the possibility, moreover, that the unique advantages of certain nonmammalian systems may be available for studying aspects of phorbol ester receptor structure and function.

At saturation, mouse brain showed a very high level of specific [³H]PDBu binding, 28.4 pmole/mg protein—7.5-fold that of skin (13). This finding has two important consequences. Conceptually, the result implies that the phorbol ester receptor is a major brain constituent. Were it to have a MW of 100,000, the phorbol ester receptor would comprise 0.3% of the total particulate protein

TABLE 2. *Comparison in chick embryo fibroblasts of binding affinity and biological activity of phorbol esters*

Compound	Binding assay K_i, nM[a]	Biological activity ED$_{50}$ for fibronectin loss, nM[b]
PMA	1.9	6.5
Phorbol 12,13-didecanoate	<9	7
PDBu	25	50
Mezerein	180	56
Phorbol 12,13-dibenzoate	180	84
Phorbol 12,13-diacetate	1,700	1,200
Phorbol 12,13,20-triacetate	39,000	12,900
Phorbol 13-acetate	120,000	85,000

[a] From Driedger and Blumberg (12).
[b] From Driedger and Blumberg (10,11).

(0.2% of the total cellular protein). Receptors for neurotransmitters, in contrast, are present at 1/20 to 1/1,000 of this level. It therefore seems likely that the phorbol ester receptor serves a functional, rather than an exclusively information-transducing, role in the cell. The receptor may thus be more analogous to the Na^+, K^+-ATPase than to the opiate receptor.

Technically, the high level of specific binding by brain, coupled with somewhat lower K_D's in this system for all derivatives (see Table 1), has greatly facilitated the assay of binding. At the K_D for PDBu, for example, specific binding by brain was 96% of total binding, as compared to only 54% for mouse skin. We have therefore used the brain system extensively to characterize phorbol ester binding (13,31).

Using brain preparations, we were able to measure [^{3}H]PMA binding directly (see ref. 13 for experimental details). This assay permitted analysis of a critical issue. We had previously shown that PMA had higher affinity for the PDBu receptor than did PDBu itself and that it blocked [^{3}H]PDBu binding > 95%. These results implied that [^{3}H]PDBu binding in fact measured the PMA receptor. Nevertheless, could PMA possess in addition a second class of receptors with which PDBu did not interact? We find no evidence for this possibility. Nonradioactive PDBu inhibited [^{3}H]PMA binding at least 95% (Fig. 2). Moreover, the competition curves for inhibition of [^{3}H]PMA binding by nonradioactive PMA or PDBu showed quantitative agreement with those obtained for inhibition of [^{3}H]PDBu binding.

The centrifugation assay that we used in the initial studies to measure specific [^{3}H]PDBu binding was unsuitable for rapid kinetic measurements. A filtration assay was therefore developed that permits measurements on a time scale of seconds (see "Material and Methods") (13a). Under equilibrium conditions, the filtration and centrifugation assays yielded the same values for K_D and specific binding activity of particulate brain preparations.

At 23°C, the association rate constant k_1 for PDBu was $3.75 \pm 0.17 \times 10^7$

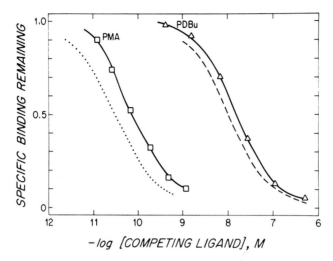

FIG. 2. Inhibition of specific [³H]PMA binding by nonradioactive phorbol esters. Specific binding of [³H]PMA to brain particulate fraction (40 μg protein) was measured in a 1.0-ml reaction volume using a modification (see ref. 13) of the usual centrifugation binding assay described in "Materials and Methods." In each experiment, specific binding of [³H]PMA in the presence of nonradioactive phorbol esters was expressed as a fraction of the total specific binding in the absence of competing ligand. The nominal concentrations of the nonradioactive phorbol esters were corrected for the decrease in concentrations due to binding to the particulate fraction and for competition with [³H] PDBu (see ref. 13). Concentrations of PMA were also corrected for nonspecific partitioning into the particulate fraction. The nonradioactive ligands were PMA (K_1, 70 pM) and PDBu (K_1, 14 nM). Curves showing inhibition of specific [³H]PDBu binding by PMA (.....) and by PDBu (----) are presented for comparison.

$M^{-1} min^{-1}$. The dissociation rate constant k_2 was 0.209 ± .006 min⁻¹. From these kinetic values, a K_D of 5.6 nM was calculated, in good agreement with the value of 7.4 ± 0.5 nM determined from equilibrium measurements (13). The dissociation rate constant showed marked temperature dependence (Fig. 3). The half-time for release decreased from 62 min at 4°C to 1.75 min at 30°C. The rate of release at 37°C was too fast for convenient measurement; the half-time for release obtained by extrapolation was 0.69 min. The association rate constant showed a similar dependence on temperature.

The second-order association rate constant for PDBu predicts a half-time for binding at 23°C of 10 sec at a PDBu concentration of 100 nM. At 37°C the extrapolated half-time would be < 2 sec. The rate of binding is therefore potentially fast enough to account for the most rapid biological responses observed (15,44).

The marked temperature dependence of the binding kinetics is of considerable experimental utility. Because of the slow half-time of release at 4°C, preparations can be rinsed in the cold to remove unbound ligand after equilibration has been achieved. It is thus possible to quickly and efficiently remove specifically bound PDBu from cells in biological experiments when desired.

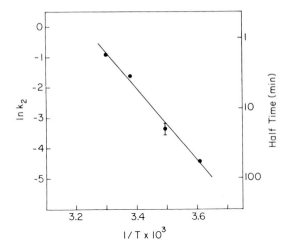

FIG. 3. Temperature dependence of the dissociation rate constant K_2 for [³H]PDBu binding to brain. [³H]PDBu was bound to brain particulate preparations. After binding had reached equilibrium, excess nonradioactive PDBu (30 μM) was added to the incubation mixture. The rate of dissociation of specific [³H]PDBu binding was then measured by the filtration assay as described in "Materials and Methods."

The thermodynamics of PDBu binding were determined from the temperature dependence of the K_D. Binding to the brain receptor occurred with a small, unfavorable increase in enthalpy ($\Delta H = +0.4$ kcal/mole) and a large, favorable increase in entropy ($\Delta S = 38.4$ e.u.). Such values are typical for hydrophobic interactions, which result in the displacement of water molecules ordered around a ligand and its binding site. This finding supports the conclusions from *in vivo* structure-activity studies, which emphasized the important role of the hydrophobic side chains in determining phorbol ester activity (16,28).

The binding activity of the mouse brain particulate preparation was destroyed by boiling for 5 min (13). Binding was likewise sensitive to papain, provided that high concentrations of the protease were used. Although vesicles prepared from total lipid extract of calf brain did not bind [³H]PDBu specifically, and purified sulfatides, cerebrosides, and gangliosides had no effect on [³H]PDBu binding, binding was inhibited by phospholipase A_2. Lipids or the proper lipid environment may therefore be necessary for the phorbol esters to bind to their target.

To examine the subcellular distribution of specific [³H]PDBu binding activity (13a), mouse brain was homogenized and fractionated by a combination of differential and sucrose gradient centrifugation as described by DeRobertis et al. (7; Fig. 4). Specific binding to cytosol, assayed by the gel filtration technique of Hummel and Dreyer (22), accounted for < 1% of the total specific binding

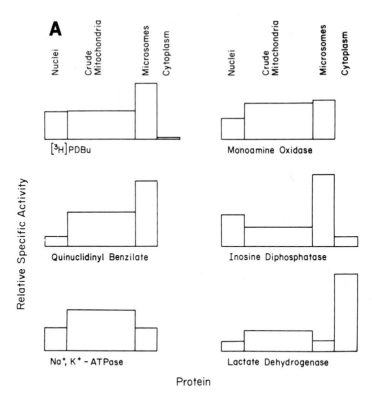

FIG. 4. Subcellular localization of [³H]PDBu binding from mouse brain. Mouse brain was homogenized and fractionated as described by DeRobertis et al. (7). **A:** Differential centrifugation. Nuclei, crude mitochondria, and microsomes were the pellets obtained by centrifugation for 10 min at 900 × g, 20 min at 17,500 × g, and 60 min at 100,000 × g, respectively. **B:** Sucrose density centrifugation. The crude mitochondrial fraction from **A** was osmotically lysed according to the procedure of Cotman and Matthews (5) and then centrifuged at 10,000 × g for 20 min. The pellet was resuspended in 0.32 M sucrose and subfractionated on discontinuous sucrose gradients centrifuged for 2 hr at 25,000 rpm in an SW 27 rotor (Beckman Instruments, Irvine, California).

activity. Binding clearly did not cofractionate with nuclei, which contained 100% of the recovered deoxyribonucleic acid (DNA), or with the mitochondrial marker monoamine oxidase. On the other hand, [³H]PDBu binding was more diffusely distributed throughout the density gradient than either the Na⁺, K⁺-ATPase activity or the binding activity for quinuclidinyl benzilate (an antagonist that binds to the muscarinic acetylcholine receptor). [³H]PDBu may therefore bind specifically to cell membranes in addition to the plasma membrane. Alternatively, the pattern of [³H]PDBu binding may simply reflect the heterogeneity of the plasma membranes of the numerous cell types in the brain. For example, differential centrifugation caused enrichment of quinuclidinyl benzilate binding in the microsomal fraction relative to Na⁺, K⁺-ATPase.

Within the brain, specific [³H]PDBu binding showed marked regional localiza-

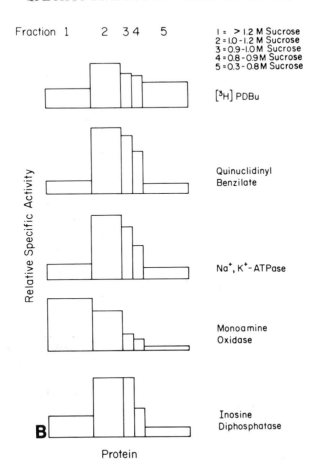

FIG. 4B. See legend on facing page.

tion (31). Upon assay of dissected bovine brain, specific binding to frontal cortex was 38.1 pmole/mg protein (Fig. 5). On contrast, specific binding to medulla was only 4.6 pmole/mg, just slightly greater than that found for mouse skin (6).

Specific binding also changed substantially during development (31). Binding of chicken brain preparations was assayed because of the ease in obtaining embryos. Binding rose linearly with time between 7 and 18 days of development, reflecting a sixfold increase in specific activity (Fig. 6). A further small increase in activity was found in brains from chicks 2-days posthatching or from the adult. Binding affinities for brain preparations from 10- and 11-day-old embryos were compared with that from the adult. No difference was observed.

Comparison of the pattern of increase of specific [³H]PDBu binding in chicken brain during development resembles that for markers of synaptogenesis and for membrane markers (42). In contrast, structural proteins, (2,33) and metabolic

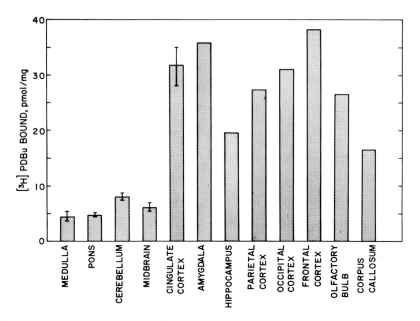

FIG. 5. Regional localization in calf's brain of specific [³H]PDBu-binding activity. Portions of calf's brain were excised (46) and specific [³H]PDBu binding activity was determined by the centrifugation binding assay as described in "Materials and Methods." The concentration of free [³H]PDBu was 112 ± 9 nM (± SD). Each point is the average of four or more determinations per membrane preparation. Two preparations were made for medulla, pons, cerebellum, midbrain, and cingulate cortex. One preparation was analyzed for each of the other regions. Under the conditions of these experiments, nonspecific binding was 6.5 ± 1.3 (± SD) pmole/mg.

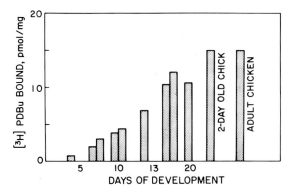

FIG. 6. Specific binding activity of embryonic chicken brain as a function of development. Brains from developing chicken embryos of the indicated ages were removed, pooled, and homogenized. Specific [³H]PDBu binding to the particulate fractions was determined as described in "Materials and Methods." The concentration of free [³H]PDBu was 38 ± 4 nM (± SD). Each point is the average of three or more determinations on a single batch of embryonic brain. Under the conditions of these experiments, nonspecific binding was 2.7 ± .3 (± SD) pmole/mg.

enzymes show little developmental change (42), whereas those involved in DNA synthesis decrease markedly (23). The inverse relationship between phorbol ester binding activity and DNA synthesis in brain provides no support for a normal role of the receptor in cell division. Likewise, the occurrence of maximal binding in mature brain does not support the concept that the phorbol ester receptor functions as the target for an embryonic inducer of development.

Accumulating evidence indicates that phorbol ester binding is sensitive to multiple modulating factors. A number of the effects of the phorbol esters are interrelated with those of Ca^{2+}. Addition of ethylene glycol-bis-β-aminoethyl ether-N,N'-tetraacetic acid (EGTA) to mouse brain preparations caused a 2.4 ± 0.4- (mean $\pm$ S.E.M., four experiments) fold increase in the K_D for PDBu with no change in binding at saturation (13a). The inhibition by EGTA can be reversed by addition of an excess of calcium.

Preliminary results from this laboratory reveal inhibition of specific PDBu binding to brain preparations by a low MW inhibitor from the supernatant of either acidified or boiled bovine brain. Brain was examined for the presence of inhibitors because of the high level of phorbol ester receptors. The receptors in the preparation of inhibitor were denatured both to prevent interference with the binding assay and to allow release of inhibitor potentially bound to the receptors. For intact rat embryo cells, inhibition of PDBu binding by serum has been reported in an abstract (21).

The response of phorbol ester receptors in intact cells to incubation in the presence of phorbol ester was examined in the GH_4C_1 rat pituitary cell line (25). This cell line was chosen because of the presence of well-characterized functional receptors for several growth factors and hormones, including thyrotropin-releasing hormone (TRH), epidermal growth factor, and somatostatin. Incubation of the cells in the presence of PDBu caused a dose-dependent down-modulation of [^{3}H]PDBu receptor levels (Fig. 7), measured using an intact cell assay. Down-modulation reflected a reduction in receptor number with no change in receptor affinity. The decrease in specific binding occurred slowly. Binding was reduced to 20% of control by 24 hr and, in the continued presence of PDBu, remained at that level for an additional 5 days. Upon removal of PDBu from the medium, PDBu receptor levels had returned to 75% of the control level within 24 hr and to the control level within 48 hr.

For the GH_4C_1 cells, PDBu receptors were also subject to heterologous down-modulation by TRH, once again associated with a decrease in receptor number. The dose-response curves for TRH were the same for down-modulation of either the PDBu receptor or its own receptor. The kinetics of down-modulation of PDBu receptors by TRH and their recovery upon removal of TRH were similar to those obtained for down-modulation by PDBu. The ability to independently regulate PDBu receptor levels with TRH may be of substantial utility for analyzing the biological significance of PDBu receptor modulation.

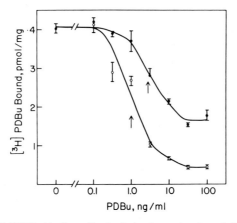

FIG. 7. Decrease in [³H]PDBu binding with phorbol ester pretreatment. GH₄C₁ cells were grown to plateau density in Ham's F10 medium supplemented with 15% horse serum and 2.5% fetal bovine serum. The cultures were incubated with PDBu for 6 or 24 hr. The PDBu was then removed by two washes with serum-containing medium each followed by a 10-min incubation at 37°C in serum-containing medium. Specific [³H]PDBu binding was then determined as described in "Materials and Methods." Dose-response curve: ●, 6-hr incubation; ○, 24-hr incubation. Each point represents the mean ± range of triplicate determinations. Similar results were obtained in two additional experiments.

DISCUSSION

The findings summarized in this chapter strongly argue that at least some of the biological responses to the phorbol esters, probably including that of tumor promotion, are mediated through binding to the receptor detected with [³H]PDBu. Confirmation by genetic techniques of this conclusion, which is derived from pharmacological and kinetic evidence, would be desirable. Distinct objectives are the demonstration that a subclass of phorbol ester unresponsive cell variants are lacking receptors and that receptor-minus mutants of mice are resistant to promotion. If the receptor plays an important role in cell functioning, as its conservation in evolution may imply, then variants altered in the receptor may be a relatively minor subclass of the total unresponsive variants obtained.

The relative inactivity of mezerein, the short-chain substituted 12-deoxyphorbol derivatives, and resiniferatoxin at the PDBu receptor suggests the likelihood that distinct receptors for these classes of compounds may also exist, at least in certain cell types. Identification of these receptors should facilitate dissection of the biochemical cascades induced by the phorbol-related diterpenes. Such studies, moreover, should provide the biochemical analysis to complement the emerging *in vivo* results that subdivide tumor promotion into multiple stages (40).

Perhaps the two most critical questions related to the phorbol ester receptor are the following. What is the single biochemical response that is directly coupled to phorbol ester binding to its receptor, i.e., what is the second messenger for the phorbol esters? Secondly, what endogenous compounds normally interact at this receptor, and are there "endogenous phorboids"? Humans possess a receptor, the homolog of which in the mouse mediates tumor promotion. The biochemical process directly coupled to this receptor and modulation of this process by endogenous or exogenous factors are therefore important candidates for determinants of human cancer development.

SUMMARY

Phorbol esters bind to mouse tissues and chick embryo fibroblasts in a specific, saturable, and reversible fashion. The binding site, located in the membrane fraction, is heat and protease sensitive. Binding can be measured most readily with [^{3}H]PDBu. Binding of [^{3}H]PDBu is of high affinity and is inhibited competitively by nonradioactive phorbol esters; the dissociation constants of the phorbol esters correspond quantitatively to their respective biological and tumor-promoting activities. Of particular significance, highly inflammatory but weakly promoting or nonpromoting diterpene esters are much less potent than PMA. Binding of [^{3}H]PMA has been measured directly. The results confirm that PMA and PDBu interact at the same major high-affinity binding site. [^{3}H]PDBu binding is entropy driven. The equilibrium dissociation constant is independent of temperature, whereas the off-rate is highly temperature dependent.

In vivo, specific binding activity increases during embryonic development. It also shows considerable variation among tissues. In the mouse, highest binding activity, 28 pmole/mg, is in the brain (skin, for example, binds 3.9 pmole/mg). Between regions of the brain, 10-fold differences in binding activity are found. The high level of phorbol ester binding in brain suggests that the phorbol ester receptor plays a functional rather than an exclusively information-transducing role in the cell.

Growth of cells in the presence of PDBu causes marked down-modulation of phorbol ester receptors. In the GH_4C_1 rat pituitary cell line, receptor number is decreased by 80% in 24 hr. In membrane preparations, the phorbol ester binding affinity is calcium sensitive. It has been speculated that endogenous ligands interacting at the phorbol ester receptor may exist. The finding that the supernatant fraction from boiled or acidified brain inhibits [^{3}H]PDBu binding is therefore exciting.

ACKNOWLEDGMENTS

This research was supported by grant CA 22895 from the National Cancer Institute and by grant BC-345 from the American Cancer Society. P.M.B. is a recipient of a Research Career Development Award from the National Institutes of Health. K.B.D. is a predoctoral trainee for the N.I.H. S. J. is a fellow of the Interdisciplinary Programs in Health, Harvard School of Public Health.

REFERENCES

1. Baird, W. M., and Boutwell, R. K. (1971): Tumor-promoting activity of phorbol and four diesters of phorbol in mouse skin. *Cancer Res.,* 31:1,074–1,079.
2. Bamburg, J. R., Shooter, E. M., and Wilson, L. (1973): Developmental changes in microtubule protein of chick brain. *Biochemistry,* 12:1,476–1,482.
3. Blumberg, P. M. (1980): *In vitro* studies on the mode of action of the phorbol esters, potent tumor promoters. *Crit. Rev. Toxicol.,* 8:153–234.
4. Bresch, H., and Arendt, U. (1978): Disturbances of early sea urchin development by the tumor promoter TPA (phorbol ester). *Naturwissenschaften,* 65:660–662.
5. Cotman, C. W., and Matthews, D. A. (1971): Synaptic plasma membranes from rat brain synaptosomes: Isolation and partial characterization. *Biochim. Biophys. Acta,* 249:380–394.
6. Delclos, K. B., Nagle, D. S., and Blumberg, P. M. (1980): Specific binding of phorbol ester tumor promoters to mouse skin. *Cell,* 19:1,025–1,032.
7. DeRobertis, E., Rodriguez de Lores Arnaiz, G., Alberici, M., Butcher, R. W., and Sutherland, E. W. (1967): Subcellular distribution of adenyl cyclase and cyclic phosphodiesterase in rat brain cortex. *J. Biol. Chem.,* 242:3,487–3,493.
8. Diamond, L., O'Brien, T. G., and Baird, W. M. (1980): Tumor promoters and the mechanism of tumor promotion. *Adv. Cancer Res.,* 32:1–74.
9. Driedger, P. E., and Blumberg, P. M. (1978): Nonphorbol mouse skin tumor promoters do not mimic phorbol myristate acetate in its effects on chick embryo fibroblasts. *Int. J. Cancer,* 22:63–69.
10. Driedger, P. E., and Blumberg, P. M. (1979): Quantitative correlation between *in vitro* and *in vivo* activities of phorbol esters. *Cancer Res.,* 39:714–719.
11. Driedger, P. E., and Blumberg, P. M. (1980*a*): Structure-activity relationships in chick embryo fibroblasts for phorbol-related diterpene esters showing anomalous activities *in vivo*. *Cancer Res.,* 40:339–346.
12. Driedger, P. E., and Blumberg, P. M. (1980*b*): Specific binding of phorbol ester tumor promoters. *Proc. Natl. Acad. Sci. USA,* 77:567–571.
13. Dunphy, W. G., Delclos, K. B., and Blumberg, P. M. (1980): Characterization of specific binding of [³H]phorbol 12,13-dibutyrate and [³H]phorbol 12-myristate 13-acetate to mouse brain. *Cancer Res.,* 40:3,635–3,641.
13a. Dunphy, W. G., Kochenburger, R. J., Castagna, M., and Blumberg, P. M. (1981): Kinetics and subcellular localization of specific [³H]phorbol 12,13-dibutyrate binding by mouse brain. *Cancer Res.,* 41:2,640–2,647.
14. Estensen, R. D., DeHoogh, D. K., and Cole, C. F. (1980): Binding of [³H]12-O-tetradecanoyl-phorbol-13-acetate to intact human peripheral blood lymphocytes. *Cancer Res.,* 40:1,119–1,124.
15. Estensen, R. D., and White, J. G. (1974): Ultrastructural features of the platelet response to phorbol myristate acetate. *Am. J. Pathol.,* 74:441–448.
16. Hecker, E. (1968): Cocarcinogenic principles from the seed oil of *Croton tiglium* and from other *Euphorbiaceae. Cancer Res.,* 28:2,338–2,348.
17. Hecker, E. (1978): Structure-activity relationships in diterpene esters irritant and cocarcinogenic to mouse skin. In: *Mechanisms of Tumor Promotion and Cocarcinogenesis,* edited by T. J. Slaga, A. Sivak, and R. K. Boutwell, pp. 11–48. Raven Press, New York.
18. Hecker, E., and Schmidt, R. (1974): Phorbol esters—the irritants and cocarcinogens of *Croton tiglium L. Fortschr. Chem. Org. Naturst.,* 31:377–467.
19. Helmes, C. T., Hillesund, T., and Boutwell, R. K. (1974): The binding of tritium-labeled phorbol esters to the macromolecular constituents of mouse epidermis. *Cancer Res.,* 34:1,360–1,365.
20. Hergenhahn, M., Kusumoto, S., and Hecker, E. (1974): Diterpene esters from *Euphorbium* and their irritant and cocarcinogenic activity. *Experientia,* 30:1,438–1,440.
21. Horowitz, A. D., Greenebaum, E., and Weinstein, I. B. (1980): Identification and properties of phorbol ester receptors in rat embryo cells. *J. Cell Biol.,* 87:174a.
22. Hummel, J. P., and Dreyer, W. J. (1962): Measurement of protein binding phenomena by gel filtration. *Biochim. Biophys. Acta,* 63:530–532.
23. Hyndman, A. G., and Zamenhof, S. (1978): Thymidine phosphorylase, thymidine kinase, and thymidylate synthetase activities in cerebral hemispheres of developing chick embryos. *J. Neurochem.,* 31:577–580.
24. Jacobson, K., Wenner, C. E., Kemp, G., and Papahadjopoulos, D. (1975): Surface properties of phorbol esters and their interaction with lipid monolayers and bilayers. *Cancer Res.,* 35:2,991–2,995.

25. Jaken, S., Tashjian, A. H., Jr., and Blumberg, P. M. (1981): Characterization of phorbol ester receptors and their down-modulation in GH$_4$C$_1$ rat pituitary cells. *Cancer Res.*, 41:2,175–2,181.
26. Kensler, T. W., and Mueller, G. C. (1978): Retinoic acid inhibition of the comitogenic action of mezerein and phorbol esters in bovine lymphocytes. *Cancer Res.*, 38:771–775
27. Kubinski, H., Strangstalien, M. A., Baird, W. M., and Boutwell, R. K. (1973): Interactions of phorbol esters with cellular membranes *in vitro*. *Cancer Res.*, 33:3,103–3,107.
28. Kubinyi, H. (1976): Quantitative structure-activity relationships. IV. Nonlinear dependence of biological activity on hydrophobic character. A new model. *Arzneim.-Forsch.*, 26:1,991–1,997.
29. Lee, L.-S., and Weinstein, I. B. (1978): Uptake of the tumor-promoting agent 12-O-tetradecanoyl-phorbol-13-acetate by Hela cells. *J. Environ. Pathol. Toxicol.*, 1:627–639.
30. Mufson, R. A., Fischer, S. M., Verma, A. K., Gleason, G. L., Slaga, T. J., and Boutwell, R. K. (1979): Effects of 12-O-tetradecanoylphorbol-13-acetate and mezerein on epidermal ornithine decarboxylase activity, isoproterenol-stimulated levels of cyclic adenosine 3′:5′-monophosphate, and induction of mouse skin tumors *in vivo*. *Cancer Res.*, 39:4,791–4,795.
31. Nagle, D. S., Jaken, S., Castagna, M., and Blumberg, P. M. (1981): Variation with embryonic development and regional localization of specific [^{3}H]phorbol 12,13-dibutyrate binding to brain. *Cancer Res.*, 41:89–93.
32. Ohuchi, K., and Levine, L. (1980): α-Tocopherol inhibits 12-O-tetradecanoylphorbol-13-acetate-stimulated deacylation of cellular lipids, prostaglandin production, and changes in cell morphology of Madin-Darby canine kidney cells. *Biochim. Biophys. Acta.*, 619:11–19.
33. Pardee, J. D., and Bamburg, J. R. (1976): Quantitation of actin in developing brain. *J. Neurochem.*, 26:1,093–1,098.
34. Sando, J. J., Hilfiker, M. L., Salomon, D. S., and Farrar, J. J. (1981): Evidence that specific receptors mediate phorbol ester-enhanced production of T cell growth factor. *Proc. Natl. Acad. Sci. USA*, 78:1,189–1,193.
35. Schmidt, R., and Hecker, E. (1971): Untersuchungen über die Beziehungen zwischen Strucktur und Wirkung von Phorbolestern. In: *Aktuelle Probleme aus dem Gebiet der Cancerologie III*, edited by H. Lettré and G. Wagner, pp. 98–108. Springer Verlag, Berlin.
36. Schmidt, R. J., and Evans, F. J. (1979): Investigations into the skin-irritant properties of resiniferonol orthoesters. *Inflammation*, 3:273–280.
37. Schweizer, J., Loehrke, H., and Goerttler, K. (1978): Transmaternal modification of the Berenblum/Mottram experiment in mice. *Bull. Cancer (Paris)*, 65:265–270.
38. Scribner, J. D., and Boutwell, R. K. (1972): Inflammation and tumor promotion: Selective protein induction in mouse skin by tumor promoters. *Eur. J. Cancer*, 8:617–621.
39. Scribner, J. D., and Süss, R. (1978): Tumor initiation and promotion. *Int. Rev. Exp. Pathol.*, 18:137–198.
40. Slaga, T. J., Fischer, S. M., Nelson, K., and Gleason, G. L. (1980): Studies on the mechanism of skin tumor promotion: Evidence for several stages in promotion. *Proc. Natl. Acad. Sci. USA*, 77:3,659–3,663.
41. Slaga, T. J., Scribner, J. D., Rice, J. M., Das, S. B., and Thompson, S. (1974): Inhibition by dexamethasone of intracellular binding of phorbol esters to mouse skin. *J. Natl. Cancer Inst.*, 52:1,611–1,618.
42. Szutowicz, A., Frazier, W. A., and Bradshaw, R. A. (1976): Subcellular localization of nerve growth factor receptors. Developmental correlations in chick embryo brain. *J. Biol. Chem.*, 251:1,524–1,528.
43. Thielmann, H.-W., and Hecker, E. (1969): Beziehungen zwischen der Struktur von Phorbolderivaten und ihren entzündlichen und tumorpromovierenden Eigenschaften. *Forschr. Krebsforsch*, 7:171–179.
44. Whitin, J. C., Chapman, C. E., Simons, E. R., Chobaniec, M. E., and Cohen, H. J. (1980): Correlation between membrane potential changes and superoxide production in human granulocytes stimulated by phorbol myristate acetate. Evidence for defective activation in chronic granulomatous disease. *J. Biol. Chem.*, 255:1,874–1,878.
45. Yamasaki, H., Fibach, E., Nudel, U., Weinstein, I. B., Rifkind, R. A., and Marks, P. A. (1977): Tumor promoters inhibit spontaneous and induced differentiation of murine erythroleukemia cells in culture. *Proc. Natl. Acad. Sci. USA*, 74:3,451–3,455.
46. Yoshikawa, T. (1968): *Atlas of the Brains of Domestic Animals*. University of Tokyo Press, Tokyo.
47. Zur Hausen, H., Bornkamm, G. W., Schmidt, R., and Hecker, E. (1979): Tumor initiators and promoters in the induction of Epstein-Barr virus. *Proc. Natl. Acad. Sci. USA*, 76:782–785.

Carcinogenesis, Vol. 7, edited by E. Hecker et al.
Raven Press, New York © 1982.

Possible Molecular Mechanisms of Action of Tumor Promoters

J. R. Smythies

The Department of Psychiatry and The Neurosciences Program, The University of Alabama in Birmingham, Birmingham, Alabama 35294

The enzyme phospholipase A_2 (PLA_2) plays an important role in prostaglandin synthesis and tumor production. 12-O-Tetradecanoylphorbol-13-acetate (TPA) is known to activate powerfully this enzyme (5), but whether it does this indirectly, e.g. by action on a receptor on the membrane surface, or directly, by acting as a cofactor on the enzyme, is unknown. Recently, the X-ray structure of bovine pancreatic PLA_2 has been reported (2,7). The reported amino acid sequence of a number of phospholipases from different sources allows us to identify the invariant residues presumably located on functionally important parts of the enzyme. Examination of a CPK molecular model of this enzyme reveals three lipophilic grooves identified by a group of invariant residues radiating from the active hydrolytic center [aspartate (asp) (49) and histidine (his) (48)] in trifoliate fashion (Fig. 1). Experiments with molecular models reveal that groove A is highly complementary to the molecules of the potent tumor promoters, TPA and teleocidin. In the case of TPA, the pattern of complementarity is 4 OH to asp (99); 2 CH_3 to leucine (leu) (2); 3 O from NT; OH to tyrosine (tyr) (28); 20 OH to substrate; and multiple lipophilic and van der Waals' interactions with phenylalanine (phe) (5), isoleucine (ile) (9), leu (or equivalent) (20), phe (106), alanine (ala) (102), and ala (103). For teleocidin the pattern is OH to asp (99), O from tyr (28), and multiple lipophilic and van der Waals' interactions with phe (5), ile (9), ala (103), ala (104), phe (106), and tyr (28). This complementarity is shared by inflammatory, but nontumor-promoting, relatives of TPA, such as mezerein and TPA analogs with largely double-bonded side chains. This suggests, but of course does not prove, that such an interaction is both necessary and sufficient for the inflammatogenic action of these drugs, but is only necessary, but not sufficient, for their tumor-promoting activity for which action at another site is also necessary. Alternatively, TPA may bind to pro-PLA_2 and may relate to activation of PLA_2 by pronase.

The fact that the mere replacement of the flexible hydrocarbon chain of TPA by a stiff, largely double-bonded chain abolishes promoting activity, suggests that this second factor may be some biophysical effect on the membrane itself, such as a change in membrane fluidity.

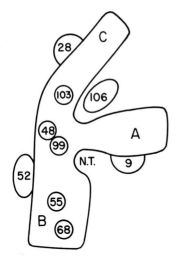

FIG. 1. Trifoliate lipophilic area on the molecule of PLA_2—invariant amino acids or conservative substitutions only.

TPA and teleocidin may mimic some endogenous factor normally stimulatory to PLA_2. This might be a phospholipid (see e.g. ref. 1); however, the structure of teleocidin suggests that this factor might be a polypeptide with a sequence akin to ile–valine (val)–val–ala, with a β-turn conformation.

Prostaglandin E_1 (PGE_1) has been reported to have antitumor effects and to inhibit PLA_2 (3,4). Molecular modeling shows that PGE_1 is highly complementary to groove B on the enzyme (for details, see ref. 6). It seems likely that the substrate itself may bind to groove C with its arachidonic acid side chain and to groove B with its saturated chains. If so, PGE_1 bound to groove B would competitively inhibit this binding. This hypothesis suggests the following experiments to test it:

(a) Binding experiments between TPA, teleocidin, PGE_1, PLA_2, and pro-PLA_2. The binding of TPA may be cooperative with substrate. Furthermore, normal binding, if it occurs, would take place in the structured environment of the lipid bilayer rather than in water.

(b) Co-crystallization experiments with these agents and PLA_2 for X-ray analysis.

(c) Experiments to test the comparative effect of the biophysical properties (such as fluidity) of the membrane of TPA and its closely allied nonpromoting analogs described above.

(d) The testing of polypeptides related to teleocidin (such as ile–val–val–ala, or variants) for inflammatogenic and promoting properties.

NOTE ADDED IN PROOF

Another candidate for the "endogenous ligand" at the TPA receptor is some relative of the chemotactic factor for leukocytes. Molecular models indicate that the peptide N-formyl–methionine (met)–leu–phe–OH, when forming a β-turn, is quite similar to teleocidin in its molecular structure. This peptide is known to induce PLA_2 as part of its effect. Possible such candidates are N-formyl–leu–val–ala–OH (particularly with methylation of the first two peptide NHs), and (N-formyl)–val–ile–val–serine (ser)–OH. Such peptides may play important roles in the modulation of cell growth, growth of axons, etc.

REFERENCES

1. Adamich, L. M., Roberts, M. F., and Dennis, E. A. (1980): Phospholipid activation of cobra venom phospholipase A_2. 2. Characterization of the phospholipid enzyme interaction. *Biochemistry,* 18:3,308–3,314.
2. Dijkstra, B. U., Drenth, J., Kalk, D. H., and Vandermallen, P. G. (1978): Three-dimensional structure and disulfide bond connections in bovine pancreatic phospholipase A_2. *J. Mol. Biol.,* 124:53.
3. Fischer, S. M., Mills, G. D. and Slaga, T. J. (1980): *Abstract,* International Symposium on Cocarcinogenesis and Biological Effects of Tumor Promoters, Elmau, Bavaria. p. 88.
4. Horrobin, D. F. (1978): *Prostaglandins.* Eden Press, Montreal, p. 22.
5. Levine, L., and Hassid, A. (1977): Effects of phorbol-12, 13-diesters on prostaglandin production and phospholipase activity in canine kidney (MDCK) cells. *Biochem. Biophys. Res. Commun.,* 79:477.
6. Smythies, J. R. (1979): On the molecular structure of some prostaglandin receptors. *Prostagland. Med.,* 2:393–400.
7. Verheij, H. M., Volwerk, J. J., Jansen, E. H. J. M., Puyk, W. C., Dijkstra, B. W., Drenth, J., and de Haas, G. H. (1980): Methylation of histidine-48 in pancreatic phospholipase A_2. Role of histidine and calcium ion in the catalytic mechanism. *Biochemistry,* 19:3,308–3,314.

Carcinogenesis, Vol. 7, edited by E. Hecker et al.
Raven Press, New York © 1982.

Spin-Labeled Phorbol Esters and Their Interaction with Cellular Membranes

*,†S. Pečar, †M. Šentjurc, †M. Schara, †M. Nemeč, ‡B. Sorg, and ‡E. Hecker

Department of Pharmacy and †J. Stefan Institute, E. Kardelj University of Ljubljana, 61000 Ljubljana, Yugoslavia; and ‡Institute of Biochemistry, German Cancer Research Center, D-6900 Heidelberg 1, Federal Republic of Germany

SUMMARY

A series of homologous spin-labeled fatty acid analogs of the type 12-O-FASL *(n,m)*-phorbol-13-acetate [*(n,m)*PA] of 12-O-tetradecanoylphorbol-13-acetate (TPA) with variable chain length N of the fatty acid moiety and various positions of the nitroxide group were synthesized. Their irritant doses 50 (ID_{50}) on the ear and their initiation-promoting activities on the back skin of NMRI mice were determined. The irritancy $1/ID_{50}$ of the *(n,m)*PA follows the simple linear relation $ln(1/ID_{50}) = \alpha N + \beta$. In an "equilibrium" approach, the electron paramagnetic resonance (EPR) spectra measured in absence and in presence of erythrocytes (E) were used to determine the partition coefficients $K_{M,o}$ between the erythrocyte membrane (M) and the extracellular solution (o). The $K_{M,o}$ depend on the chain length N of the fatty acid moieties following the equation $ln\ K_{M,o} = aN + b$ and show that the *(n,m)*PA are accumulated preferentially in the *erythrocyte membrane*. In a "kinetic" approach, the decay rate $J(t)/J(o)$ of the EPR signal intensity of *(n,m)*PA molecules in absence and in presence of equilibrated E was measured during oxidation with ferricyanide and reduction with ascorbate, respectively. From the data obtained by the "kinetic" approach, a "two-compartment model" is shown to be the most simple approximation to describe the system, in which finite concentrations of the *(n,m)* PA are postulated for the extracellular and the membrane compartment only. EPR data indicate that generally the *(n,m)*PA are buried with their acyl chain in the E membrane with the phorbol moiety close to the outer membrane surface. Apparently only in case of (1,12)PA is the acyl chain long enough to be anchored in the lipid layer of the membrane in a way similar to the tetradecanoyl residue of TPA. A possible relationship with biological activities is discussed.

INTRODUCTION

Certain diterpene esters with tigliane, ingenane, or daphnane structures were established as the first molecularly defined and most active cocarcinogens of the initiation (or tumor) promoter-type (6–9). As a prototype promoter, TPA with tigliane structure (see Fig. 1) is widely used experimentally. It was originally isolated from croton oil (7,9) and exhibits its effects in doses similar to those of hormones (6,8). TPA was shown to induce at the cell level a surprisingly large number of biochemical events (for a recent review, see loc.cit. ref. 1). There are several indications that the primary sites of interaction of TPA and other diterpene ester-type promoters with cells are membrane structures (e.g., 8,13). It may be speculated that they carry specific "receptors" that trigger preformed biochemical events or even cascades of events in a similar manner as, for example, receptors of hormones. Therefore, the hypothesis was put forward that instead of with putative physiologic agonists, TPA interacts with their "receptors" to induce the biochemical events observed (13). To develop a new and possibly informative means of study of the microenvironment of putative TPA "receptors," a series of certain spin-labeled analogs of TPA was prepared and tested for their irritant and promoting activities. Simultaneously, their EPR spectra were investigated in the presence of E as a first model for interaction with biological membranes. For other approaches to the study of receptor/agonist interaction of diterpene ester-type promoters see also Schmidt and Hecker *(this volume)* and Adolf et al. *(this volume)*.

MATERIALS AND METHODS

General

Spin-labeled fatty acids "HO-FASL *(n,m)*" of the doxyl (4,4-dimethyloxazolidine-N-oxyl)-type derived from keto acids of the general structure $CH_3(CH_2)_m$-$CO(CH_2)_nCOOH$ were prepared (Pecar et al., *in preparation*) according to known general procedures (5). They were used to synthesize spin-labeled TPA analogs of the type *(n,m)*PA with (a) different lengths $N = m + n + 3$ of the 12-O-acyl residue and (b) with various positions of the nitroxide group within the

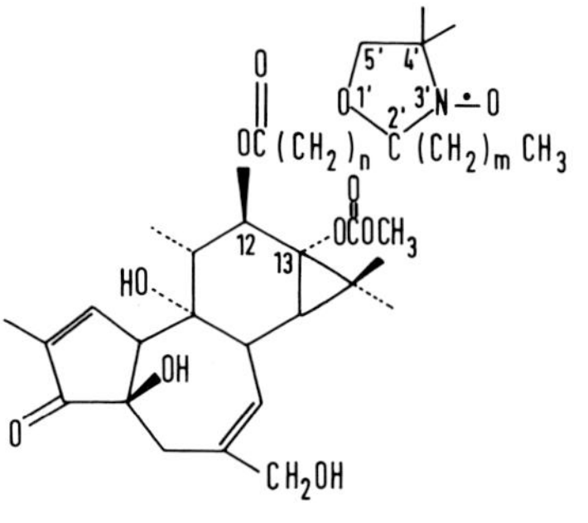

(n,m) PA	n	m	N
(4,2) PA	4	2	9
(5,2) PA	5	2	10
(5,4) PA	5	4	12
(1,12) PA	1	12	16

FIG. 1. Chemical structure of some spin-labeled analogs of TPA of the type *(n,m)*PA. The length of the alkyl chain of the 12-O-acyl group, which includes C-2' of the spin label, is $N = n + m + 3$. For a "spin-labeled-TPA," the alkyl chain would be $N = 14$.

acyl residue (see Fig. 1). Because of lack of adequate precursors for spin-labeled analogs of tetradecanoic acid, corresponding *(n,m)*PA with $N = 14$ (i.e., "spin-labeled TPA") were not prepared. For biological testing of irritant and promoting activities, the standard procedures on NMRI mice were used (7,9). For determinations of the phospholipid (PL) content of E preparations, the lipids were extracted with chloroform/methanol 2:1 (v/v), the dry residue of the extracts was oxidized with perchloric acid, and, after evaporation, phosphate was determined according to ref. 4. To prepare aqueous solutions of *(n,m)*PA, the esters were dissolved in 2 μl of ethanol and mixed with 2 ml of isotonic (0.166 mole/1) Tris-HCl buffer, pH 7.4. E were isolated from freshly drawn citrated bovine blood (11). Standard amounts of E were added to solutions of *(n,m)*PA in Tris-HCl buffer. The final concentrations of *(n,m)*PA in the samples used were between 2.0×10^{-6} to 2.3×10^{-5} M. EPR spectroscopy shows that the lower end of this range safely avoids molecular aggregation of *(n,m)*PA molecules with chain lengths of $N \geq 10$. Before EPR measurements, the *(n,m)*PA/E preparations were incubated for 1 hr at 20°C, placed in 1-mm inner diameter glass capillaries, and scanned in a Varian E-9 X band EPR spectrometer with dual sample cavity. To measure the EPR intensity decay, Varian strong pitch was used as a standard.

EPR Measurements

The EPR characteristics of *(n,m)*PA molecules were evaluated by EPR for two situations: *(n,m)*PA equilibrated with E ("equilibrium" approach) and *(n,m)*PA equilibrated as before and reacted with ferricyanide or ascorbate (final concentration between 2.0×10^{-4} to 2.3×10^{-3} M, respectively), to oxidize or reduce the spin label ("kinetic" approach).

Equilibrium Approach

EPR spectra measured without and with added E may be used to separate the free and the bound portion of the composite spectrum and hence to determine the partition coefficient $K_{M,o}$ of individual, immobilized, and free *(n,m)*PA

$$K_{M,o} = \frac{c_M}{c_o} \tag{1}$$

where c_M is the concentration of *(n,m)*PA associated with membranes, expressed as mole *(n,m)*PA/mole PL, and c_o is the concentration of free *(n,m)*PA in the extracellular solution.

Kinetic Approach

In the chemical reactions with ferricyanide or ascorbate, respectively, the nitroxide free radical of the *(n,m)*PA disappears through conversion to a nonparamagnetic group. Such reactions may be followed by the decay of intensities of EPR spectra expressed as the function $J(t)/J(o)$. Usually this was measured over at least 30 min. By defining the parameters characteristic for the system (n,m)PA/cell, e.g., in compartment models involving certain partition coefficients of (n,m)PA (see Chart 1), the decay role of EPR intensities may be calculated by the expression.

$$J(t)/J(O) = \frac{c_x(t)V_x + c_o(t)V_o + c_M(t)V_M}{c_x(O)V_x + c_o(O)V_o + K_{M,o}c_o(O)V_M} \tag{2}$$

Thus, for a three-compartment model (see Chart 1), it may be postulated that in an equilibrated (n,m)PA/cell preparation, finite concentrations of (n,m)PA may occur in the extra (c_o)- and the intracellular (c_x) compartments as well as in the membrane (c_M) compartment, with the corresponding volumes V_o, V_x, and V_M. For this model it is assumed that an exchange of (n,m)PA molecules between the membrane and the extra- and intracellular compartments is possible and, further, that the partition coefficients $K_{M,o}$ and $K_{M,x}$ are equal. For pseudo first-order kinetics of oxidation or reduction reactions in the extracellular compartment, the following system of differential equations may describe the reaction rates in the various compartments:

$$\frac{dc_o}{dt} = - kc_o + \frac{P_1 S}{V_o}(c_x - c_o) + \frac{P_3 S}{V_o}\left(\frac{c_M}{K_{M,o}} - c_o\right); \tag{3}$$

$$\frac{dc_x}{dt} = - \frac{P_1 S}{V_x}(c_x - c_o) - \frac{P_2 S}{V_x}\left(c_x - \frac{c_M}{K_{M,o}}\right); \tag{4}$$

$$\frac{dc_M}{dt} = - \frac{P_3 S}{V_M}\left(\frac{c_M}{K_{M,o}} - c_o\right) + \frac{P_2 S}{V_M}\left(c_x - \frac{c_M}{K_{M,o}}\right); \tag{5}$$

CHART 1. *Hypothetical three-compartment model of* (n,m)*PA/cell/reactant preparations*

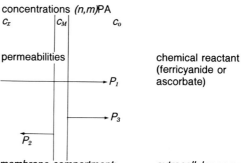

intracellular compartment:

volume V_x

$K_{M,x} = \dfrac{c_M}{c_x}$

membrane compartment:

volume V_M

surface area: S

extracellular compartment:

volume V_o

$K_{M,o} = \dfrac{c_M}{c_o}$

k is the pseudo first-order rate constant of the chemical reaction, which may be determined independently using *(n,m)*PA buffer solution with the reactant only (without E). S is the membrane surface area. P_j are permeabilities: P_1—intra- to extracellular compartment; P_3—membrane to extracellular compartment; and P_2—intracellular to membrane compartment (see Chart 1). Assuming that $P_2 = P_3$, and with the initial conditions $c_x(O) = c_0(O)$ and $c_M(O) = K_{M,o} c_0(O)$, the reaction rates $dc_j(t)/dt$ may be calculated with a computer from Eqs. 3 to 5 for certain values of $K_{M,o}$, V_j, P_j, and S. By inserting in Eq. 2 these $C_j(t)$ and the other parameters required (see also Table 4), $J(t)/J(o)$ may be varied by computer to fit the experimental EPR decay curves. Those partition coefficients $K_{M,o}$ giving an optimally fitting decay may be compared with the partition coefficients obtained by the equilibrium approach (Eq. 1). A corresponding two-compartment model assumes that finite concentrations of *(n,m)*PA are present only in the membrane and in the extracellular compartment. Thus in Eq. (3 to 5) $c_x(O) = 0$, and $P_1 = P_2 = 0$ have to be inserted.

The polarity of the nitroxide microenvironment was obtained from the EPR spectra by measuring the contact hyperfine splitting (15). For distinguishing the portion of free *(n,m)*PA molecules in the intra- from those in extracellular solution, the paramagnetic ion ferricyanide, which does not penetrate the membrane, was used. Due to the close encounters between the ferricyanide ions and the nitroxide group in the extracellular solution, the EPR lines of the *(n,m)*PA molecules were broadened (12).

RESULTS

The TPA analogs prepared and their irritant and promoting activities as determined in the standardized assays in NMRI mice are summarized in Table 1. It may be seen that in the dose tested, (1,12)PA, i.e., that TPA analog with the nitroxide group closest to the phorbol moiety (see Fig. 1), exhibits similar activities to TPA. The rest of the *(n,m)*PA, although tested in higher doses than (1,12)PA, exerted little [(5,4)PA] or no promoting activities at all (Table 1). As may be seen from Fig. 2, the irritancy of the *(n,m)*PA expressed as *ln (1/ID₅₀)* follows a linear relationship with respect to the total length N of the alkyl chain, governed by

$$ln(1/ID_{50}) = \alpha N + \beta \tag{6}$$

The irritancy of TPA as calculated from the ID_{50} (Table 1) fits reasonably with Eq. 6 (see Fig. 2).

Typical EPR spectra of *(n,m)*PA in Tris-buffer solutions without and with added E are shown in Fig. 3. It should be noted that in *(n,m)*PA/E preparations, the spectrum pertaining to the portion of free *(n,m)*PA does not differ significantly from the spectra of *(n,m)*PA in buffer alone. This is a prerequisite for using the spectra to measure partition coefficients. The spectra of (1,12)PA without and with E were found to be practically identical (not shown). For partition coefficients obtained in the equilibrium approach, see Table 5. They

TABLE 1. *Irritant and initiation-promoting activities of the (n,m)PA synthesized*[a]

| | Irritant activity[b] | | Initiation-promoting activity[c] | | |
Compound	ID_{50}^{24} (nmole)	$1/ID_{50}^{24}$ (nmole^{-1})	single dose p (nmole/appl.)	tumor rate[d] (% survivors with tumor)	tumor yield[d] (tumors/ survivor)
(4,2)PA	0.34	2.9	20	0	0
(5,2)PA	0.19	5.3	20	0	0
(5,4)PA	0.058	17	20	15	0.6
(1,12)PA	0.001	1,000	5	88	8.4
TPA	0.016[e]	63	5	78	4.9

[a] Irritation: Standard procedure, mouse ear, NMRI mice (7,9). Initiation promotion: Standard procedure, NMRI mice (7,9).
[b] Read 24 hr after administration (ID_{50}^{24}), standard deviation $\sigma = 1.3$; significance level $\alpha = 0.05$.
[c] Initiator dose $i = 100$ nmole DMBA.
[d] After 24 weeks = 48 single doses p.
[e] See, for example, loc. cit. ref. 6; Table 5.

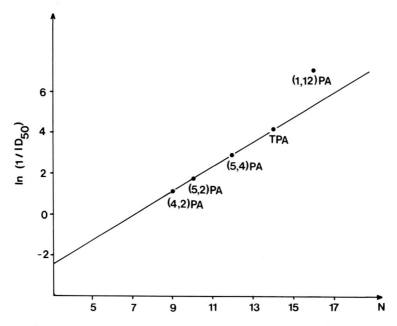

FIG. 2. Irritancy of the *(n,m)PA* expressed as *In (1/ID$_{50}$)* as a function of their acyl chain length *N*. ID$_{50}$ is expressed in nmole/ear; $N = n + m + 3$.

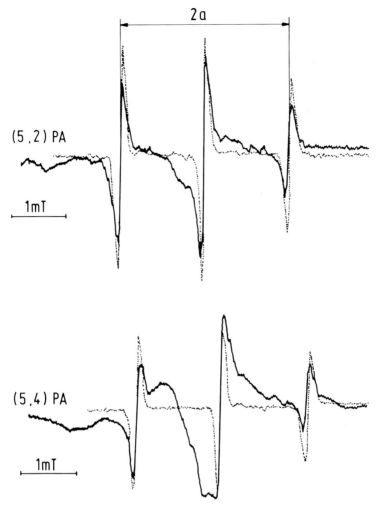

FIG. 3. EPR spectra of typical *(n,m)*PA in Tris-HCl buffer without E (.......) and equilibrated with E (———). The latter represent composite spectra provided by the free, mobile portion *(narrow)* and the membrane-bound, immobilized portion *(broad)* of the *(n,m)*PA molecules.

show that the *(n,m)*PA are associated preferentially with the E membrane.

Some typical data taken from EPR spectra used in the equilibrium and/or the kinetic approaches are collected in Table 2. In solutions of *(n,m)*PA in buffer without E, it is typical and indeed expected that the hyperfine splittings *(a)*, the linewidths ΔH, and the reaction rate constants k' of, for example, ascorbate reduction, vary with respect to the length of the alkyl chain and the position of the nitroxide therein. Thus, (1,12)PA shows the largest hyperfine splitting, reflecting for its nitroxide group in buffer solution the highest polarity.

TABLE 2. *Some typical data taken from EPR spectra of* (n,m)*PA dissolved in Tris-HCl buffer, without E*[a]

(n,m)PA	hyperfine splitting a[mT]	line width ΔH[mT] buffer	line width ΔH[mT] buffer/KFC[b]	k' I mole^{-1}sec^{-1}
(4,2)PA	1.52	0.10 (0.12)	0.12 (0.16)	1.05
(5,2)PA	1.52	0.11 (0.12)	0.12 (0.14)	0.68
(5,4)PA	1.52	0.11 (0.12)	0.12 (0.14)	0.23
(1.12)PA	1.65	0.12 (0.12)	0.16 (0.17)	22.8

[a] For ΔH, the values with added E are given in brackets. $k' = k/c_{ASC}$.
[b] 7.5×10^{-3} mole/l KFC.

In presence of paramagnetic ions, potassium ferricyanide (KFC), the line widths are slightly increased for both the buffer solution and buffer E suspension. (1, 12)PA shows the largest increase of ΔH. Pseudo first-order sodium ascorbate (ASC) reduction rate constants, determined without E, are also largest for (1, 12)PA.

The relative signal intensities *J(t)/J(o)* taken from EPR spectra of *(n,m)*PA/ E preparations after 10 min of ascorbate reduction are increased as compared to *(n,m)*PA alone (Table 3), indicating that by binding to the E the rate of reduction of *(n,m)*PA is diminished.

In Table 4 the parameters P_j, k, and $K_{M,o}$ for the "best fit" are presented for the three- and the two-compartment models. In the fit, the rest of the parameters (V_j, S, $P_2 = P_3$, c_x) were used as a "fixed set" (see Table 4). Whereas satisfactory $K_{M,o}$ for (4,2)PA and (5,2)PA were obtained, with KFC no oxidations took place in case of (1,12)PA and (5,4)PA in presence of E. Therefore, for the latter, no $K_{M,o}$ values were obtained. Without E, however, at least (5,4)PA reacted with KFC, whereas (1,12)PA again did not react. As may be seen from Table 4, the $K_{M,o}$ obtained in KFC oxidation for (4,2)PA and (5,2)PA are about one order of magnitude higher than those obtained for the same compounds in ascorbate reduction.

TABLE 3. Relative EPR signal intensities J(t)/J(o) *of the* (n,m)*PA nitroxide group at 10 min after start of ASC reduction in buffer without and with E*

(n,m)PA	100 [J(t)/J(o)] t = 10 min buffer %	100 [J(t)/J(o)] t = 10 min buffer + E (%)
(4.2)PA	24.5	62.7
(5.2)PA	39.0	80.3
(5,4)PA	71.6	100.0
(1,12)PA	11.8	12.7

TABLE 4. *Fitting the EPR decay function calculated according to Eq. 2 with the decay function observed during the reactions of* (n,m)*PA for the hypothetical three- and two-compartment models[a]*

Sample	Three-compartment model (A)			
	P_1(cm/sec)	P_3(cm/sec)	k (sec^{-1})	$K_{M,o}^b$
(4,2)PA + E + KFC	8×10^{-9}	8×10^{-9}	8×10^{-3}	2,100
(4,2)PA + E + ASC	6×10^{-8}	8×10^{-9}	1.57×10^{-3}	210
(5,2)PA + E + KFC	7×10^{-9}	8×10^{-9}	7.0×10^{-3}	4,500
(5,2)PA + E + ASC	8×10^{-7}	8×10^{-9}	6.8×10^{-4}	215
	Two-compartment model (B)			
(4,2)PA + E + KFC	0	8.2×10^{-9}	5.85×10^{-3}	2,100
(4,2)PA + E + ASC	0	5.8×10^{-9}	1.18×10^{-3}	233
(5,2)PA + E + KFC	0	1.4×10^{-8}	6.4×10^{-4}	4,800
(5,2)PA + E + ASC	0	3.0×10^{-7}	5.3×10^{-4}	210

[a] The columns of the table show the parameters adjusted to obtain optimal fit. The set of fixed parameters was as follows:
(A) $V_M = 10^{-3}$ ml, $S = 5 \times 10^3$ cm^2, $V_o = 0.66$ ml, $P_2 = P_3$, $V_x = 0.34$ ml, $c_x(o) = c_o(o)$
(B) $V_M = 10^{-3}$ ml, $S = 5 \times 10^3$ cm^2, $V_o = 0.6$ ml, $c_x = 0$, $V_x = 0$

[b] $K_{M,o} = \dfrac{[\text{mole} (n,m)\text{PA/l}]_{\text{membrane}}}{[\text{mole} (n,m)\text{PA/l}]_{\text{extracellular solution}}}.$

In the reaction with ascorbate, for (5,4)PA without and with E, a decrease in the EPR intensity was observed only for the free molecules (nonbound to E), indicating no significant reduction of the membrane-bound entity. In case of (1,12)PA, there was no difference in the ascorbate reduction rates without and with membranes. Hence, in both cases, again it was impossible to obtain a $K_{M,o}$ value by ascorbate reduction. Where $K_{M,o}$ values were determined by best fit (Table 4), no significant difference was seen between the $K_{M,o}$ obtained for the three- and two-compartment models. Therefore, the two-compartment model, with which also a better fit of the experimental curves were obtained, may be considered the most simple description of the system.

The partition coefficients obtained by the equilibrium (see Eq. 1) and by the kinetic (see Eq. 2) approaches are collected and compared in Table 5. The $K_{M,o}^{KFC}$ values in Table 5 determined by the kinetic approach correspond reasonably well with the $K_{M,o}$ values obtained by the equilibrium approach. Although $K_{M,o}$ values obtained by the kinetic approach are lacking for (5,4)PA and (1,12)PA, the observations made from their EPR spectra during oxidation and reduction, respectively, may contribute appreciably in the development of a model for the molecular environment of *(n,m)*PA bound to the E membrane (see Discussion).

The partition coefficients from the equilibrium approach (Table 5) increase with the overall length N of the acyl chain. For (1,12)PA, $K_{M,o}$ cannot be determined directly. Yet the $K_{M,o}$ of the rest of the *(n,m)*PA obtained fit the general equation

TABLE 5. *Typical partition coefficients in (n,m)PA/E preparations as obtained by the equilibrium and by the kinetic approaches*

	equilibrium approach $K_{M,o}^a$	kinetic approach	
		ferricyanide	ascorbate
(n,m)PA		$K_{M,o}^{KFCa}$	$K_{M,o}^{ASCa}$
(4,2)PA	2,845	2,188	241
(5,2)PA	4,411	5,000	217
(5,4)PA	31,309	—	—
(1,12)PA	~730,000 [b]	—	—

^{a} $K_{M,o} = \dfrac{\text{mole}(n,m)\text{PA/l}_{membrane}}{\text{mole}(n,m)\text{PA/l})_{extracellular\ solution}}$.

^{b} Extrapolated from Eq. 7.

$$ln\ K_{M,o} = aN + b \qquad (7)$$

as shown in Fig. 4, indicating a linear relationship with respect to the length N of the alkyl chain in the *(n,m)*PA measured. Therefore, for the partition coefficients, at least of this (small) set of *(n,m)*PA, the relative position of the nitroxide group within the chain does not appear critical. With this assumption in mind, by extrapolation an estimate of $K_{M,o}$ of (1,12)PA (Table 5) may be obtained. Also Eq. 7 may be used to determine the $K_{M,o}$ value of a hypothetical "spin-labeled TPA" with $N = 14$, assuming a position of the spin label comparable with that in the *(n,m)*PA described.

DISCUSSION

It has been shown previously (17) for a series of phorbol-12,13-diesters of the phorbol-12,13-didecanoate (PDD)-type that both the logarithms of their irritancies and the logarithms of their partition coefficients—the latter measured in the system carbon tetrachloride/methanol/water (2/1/0.15)—exhibit linear relationships with respect to the number of C-atoms in the acyl residues of the ester groups. Starting with phorbol-12,13-diacetate, the irritancies and the partition coefficients were shown to increase linearly with increasing chain length and—only in case of the irritancies—reach a maximum located between phorbol-12,13-dioctanoate and -didecanoate. A similar linear relationship was demonstrated also for the initiation-promoting activities of some 12-O-acylphorbol-13-acetates of the TPA-type (6).

As shown here, comparable relationships hold true for the irritancies of the *(n,m)*PA synthesized, without reaching the maximum to be expected (10) (see Fig. 2), as well as for the partition coefficients $K_{M,o}$ determined by ESR techniques (see Fig. 4) in the *(n,m)*PA/E system.

It should be stressed that the partition coefficients $K_{M,o}$ were determined by two independent EPR approaches (Table 5). There is a fairly good agreement between the $K_{M,o}^{KFC}$ values determined by the kinetic and by the equilibrium approaches. On the other hand, $K_{M,o}^{ASC}$ by the kinetic approach is by an order of

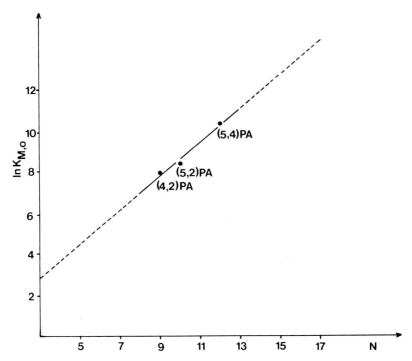

FIG. 4. Partition coefficients $K_{M,o} = c_M/c_o$ of the *(n,m)*PA molecules as a function of their acyl chain length N $(N = n + m + 3)$ $K_{M,o} = \dfrac{[\text{mole}(n,m)\text{PA}/\text{mole PL}]_{\text{membrane}}}{[\text{mole}(n,m)\text{PA}/\text{l}]_{\text{extracellular solution}}}$.

magnitude smaller than the corresponding values mentioned above. This is probably due to partial penetration of the ascorbate ion into the E membrane (16).

EPR techniques in both the equilibrium and the kinetic approach allow the development of a detailed proposition for the interaction of *(n,m)*PA with E membranes. From the $K_{M,o}$ values (Table 5) and the reduction kinetic measurements (Table 3), it may be concluded that the molecules, especially the short chain length esters, do exchange between the membrane and the buffer solution. The portion associated with membranes increases with the chain length. The permeability coefficients P_3 describing the rate of release of *(n,m)*PA molecules from the membrane are less sensitive to the chain length than the partition coefficient $K_{M,o}$ (Table 4). This conclusion is based only on the differences between (4,2)PA and (5,2)PA.

Besides the role of the fatty acid chain length N on the strength of *(n,m)*PA binding to the membrane, there is other relevant information available due to the position of the nitroxide group in the acyl chain in various *(n,m)*PA. EPR spectra reflect the microenvironment of the nitroxide group because the reaction kinetics depend on the accessibility of this group to the reactants. For example, membrane-bound (5,4)PA molecules, with the nitroxide group located approximately in the middle of the chain, are very stable against the reactants, as compared to the buffer-dissolved ones. On the other hand, (1,12)PA does not show any significant changes between the reaction rates in bound and unbound states (Table 3). For the (1,12)PA molecules with the nitroxide group close to the phorbol moiety, it should be emphasized that, as compared to *(n,m)*PA molecules with nitroxide group at least four C-atoms from the phorbol moiety, different EPR results might be expected. Though the (1,12)PA molecules are associated strongly with the membrane (they cannot be removed by repeated washing of the labeled cells), their EPR spectra indicate free mobility of the nitroxide group in a hydrophilic environment. The motional freedom is only partly diminished as the rotational correlation time increases from 4.5×10^{-11} sec in the buffer solution to 1.5×10^{-10} sec for the membrane-bound molecules. There is no significant difference in ΔH between the buffer-dissolved and membrane-bound (1,12)PA molecules in presence of KFC (Table 2). This indicates that there are no barriers for close encounters between the nitroxide group of (1,12)PA and the ferricyanide ions. Since ferricyanide ions do not penetrate the E membranes, it can be concluded that these molecules bind only to the external surfaces of the membrane. This observation is strongly supported by the reduction rate with ASC shown in Table 3, where no significant differences between the reduction rates in buffer solution and the E buffer suspension can be observed for (1,12)PA molecules.

Binding of the *(n,m)*PA molecules to the external surface of the membrane is also supported by results of the kinetic approach. The evaluation of the two- and three-compartment models gave a better fit for the two-compartment model which provides exchange of molecules only between the extracellular solution and the membrane. Therefore it can be assumed that the esters bind only to the external surface of the E membrane, most likely with the acyl chain burying itself in hydrophobic regions of the membrane. At least for (1,12)PA, the phorbol moiety and the adjacent CH_2 groups remain in the hydrophilic region, i.e., they are exposed to the buffer solution.

The partition coefficient as well as the irritancy are both proportional to the free-energy changes caused by the transfer of the *(n,m)*PA molecules from the buffer solution to the membrane. Assuming that only the fatty acid chain is buried in hydrophobic regions and with the free-energy change as an additive quantity, a value of about -2.0 kJ/mole for the transfer of each CH_2 group from the buffer to the E membrane was estimated. This value is in good accordance with similar evaluations for the hydrocarbon/water system (3).

We believe that this is the first direct spectroscopic evaluation of the binding of TPA analogs to membranes. In our experiments, about 10^5 to 10^6 of the biologically active *(n,m)*PA molecules are bound per cell. Though their binding in E without specific receptors (14) is expected to be nonspecific in this concentration range, we demonstrated that anchoring of the phorbol ester molecules in the membrane is accomplished most likely by burying of the acyl chain in the PL bilayer. In target cells, firm anchoring might be a condition for maintaining concentrations high and long enough for interference of the phorbol moiety with receptor groups. Therefore, the length of the fatty acid chain contributes directly to the biological activities of the TPA analogs, although it was shown independently (8) that also the specific structure of the phorbol moiety is determining the biological activity of these molecules. It might be speculated, therefore, that the appropriate chain length of the phorbol ester molecule ensures firm binding close to the receptor site(s) of membranes. Thus the specific structure of the phorbol moiety can interact optimally with the receptor to release biochemical events.

REFERENCES

1. Blumberg, P. (1980): *In vitro* studies on the mode of action of the phorbol esters, potent tumor promoters. Part 1. *CRC Crit. Rev. Toxicol.*, 8:153–197.
2. Blumberg, P. (1981): *In vitro* studies on the mode of action of the phorbol esters, potent tumor promoters. Part 2. *CRC Crit. Rev. Toxicol.*, 8:199–234.
3. Diamond, J. M., and Katz, Y. (1974): Interpretation of nonelectrolyte partition coefficients between dimyristoyl lecithin and water. *J. Membr. Biol.*, 17:121–154.
4. Eible, H., and Lands, W. E. M. (1969): A new, sensitive determination of phosphates. *Anal. Biochem.*, 30:51–57.
5. Gaffney, B. J. (1976): The chemistry of spin labels. In: *Spin Labeling. I.*, edited by L. J. Berliner, pp. 183–238. Academic Press, New York.
6. Hecker, E. (1968): Cocarcinogenic principles from the seed oil of croton tiglium and from other Euphorbiaceae. *Cancer Res.*, 28:2,338–2,349.
7. Hecker, E. (1971): Isolation and characterization of the cocarcinogenic principles from croton oil. In: *Methods in Cancer Research, Vol. 6*, edited by H. Busch, pp. 439–484. Academic Press, New York.
8. Hecker, E. (1978): Structure-activity relationships in diterpene esters irritant and cocarcinogenic to mouse skin. In: *Carcinogenesis, Vol. 2: Mechanisms of Tumor Promotion and Cocarcinogenesis*, edited by T. J. Slaga, A. Sivak, and R. K. Boutwell, pp. 11–48. Raven Press, New York.
9. Hecker, E., and Schmidt, R. (1974): Phorbol esters—The irritants and cocarcinogens of *Croton tiglium L. Chem. Org. Natur. Prod.*, 31:377–467.
10. Kubinyi, H. (1976): Quantitative structure-activity relationships. *Drug Res.*, 26:1,991–1,997.
11. Passow, H. (1969): Ion permeability of erythrocyte ghosts. In: *Laboratory Techniques in Membrane Biophysics*, edited by H. Passow, pp. 21–27. Springer Verlag, Berlin.
12. Salikhov, K. M., Doctorov, A. B., Molin, Yu. N., and Zamaraev, K. I. (1971): Exchange broadening of ESR lines for solutions of free radicals and transition metal complexes. *J. Magnetic Res.*, 5:189–205.
13. Shoyab, M., De Larco, J. E., and Todaro, G. J. (1979): Biologically active phorbol esters specifically alter affinity of epidermal growth factor membrane receptors. *Nature*, 279:387–391.
14. Shoyab, M., and Todaro, G. J. (1980): Specific high affinity cell membrane receptors for biologically active phorbol and ingenol esters. *Nature*, 288:451–455.
15. Smith, I. C. P. (1972): The spin label method. In: *Biological Application of Electron Spin Resonance*, edited by H. Swartz, J. R. Bolton, and D. C. Borg, pp. 483–539. Wiley–Interscience, New York.
16. Smith, I. C. P., Schreier-Muccillo, S., and Marsh, D. (1976): Spin-labeling. In: *Free Radicals in Biology*, edited by W. A. Pryor, pp. 149–197. Academic Press, New York.
17. Thielmann, H. W. (1968): Ph.D. thesis, University of Heidelberg.

Carcinogenesis, Vol. 7, edited by E. Hecker et al.
Raven Press, New York © 1982.

Ionophoretic Effect of Tumor Promoter Phorbol Diester: A Clue to Its Insulinotropic Action?

*M. Castagna, †M. Deleers, and †W. J. Malaisse

*Institute for Scientific Research in Cancer, Villejuif, France; and †Laboratory of
Experimental Medicine, Brussels University, Brussels, Belgium*

The tumor promoter 12-O-tetradecanoylphorbol-13-acetate (TPA) affects functional events in several target cells, but its primary site of action is not fully elucidated. This chapter deals with the capacity of TPA to stimulate insulin release from the pancreatic B-cell, with emphasis on the possible interference of TPA with Ca^{2+} translocation. Preliminary data on the effect of TPA on ionophoresis in liposomes are also presented.

INSULINOTROPIC CAPACITY OF TPA

Virji and his colleagues (4) were the first to report on the insulinotropic capacity of TPA, these authors being unable to detect any significant effect of TPA on insulin release in the absence of extracellular glucose. At variance with the latter observation, we found that TPA stimulates insulin release from isolated pancreatic rat islets both in the absence and presence of glucose. The insulinotropic action of TPA was related to its concentration in the 2.10^{-9} to 2.10^{-7} M range. Both the magnitude of the drug-induced increment in insulin output and the sensitivity of the B-cell to increasing concentrations of TPA were positively related to the ambiant concentration of glucose. In perifused islets, the TPA-induced increment in insulin output was significant within 8 min of exposure to the drug, progressively increased during administration of TPA, and was not rapidly reversible upon removal of TPA from the perifusion medium (Fig. 1).

The release of insulin evoked by TPA in the absence of glucose was abolished by antimycin A, epinephrine, and at low temperature, inhibited in the absence of extracellular Ca^{2+}, unaffected by indomethacin, and potentiated by theophylline.

The non-tumor-promoting TPA analog, 4-methylphorbol-12-13-didecanoate, failed to stimulate insulin release in the absence of glucose (2).

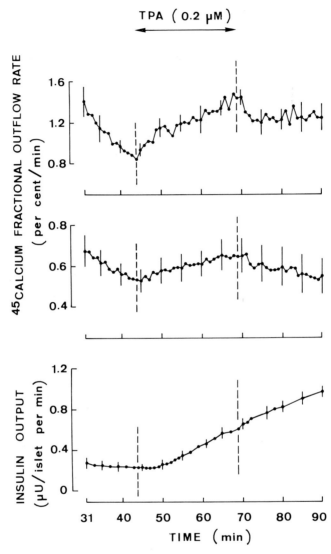

FIG. 1. Effect of TPA (0.2 μM) administered from the 45th to 69th min *(vertical dotted lines)* on ⁴⁵Ca²⁺ FOR and insulin release in islets perifused for 90 min with glucose-free media either deprived of Ca²⁺ and containing ethylene glycol-bis-β-aminoethyl ether-N, N¹=-tetraacetic acid (EGTA) 0.5 mM **(upper panel)** or containing Ca²⁺ 1.0 mM **(middle and lower panels).**

EFFECTS OF TPA ON METABOLIC AND IONIC VARIABLES IN THE ISLETS

TPA failed to affect significantly glucose oxidation, ⁸⁶Rb or ³²P fractional outflow rate, and ⁴⁵Ca²⁺ net uptake by the islets. However, TPA caused a progressive increase in ⁴⁵Ca²⁺ fractional outflow rate from perifused islets. The latter effect, which was reversed in part when TPA was removed from the perifusate, was observed both in the absence or presence of extracellular Ca^{2+} (Fig. 1). TPA also caused a slowly induced rise in the cyclic AMP content of the islets and their surrounding medium (2).

POSSIBLE MODE OF ACTION OF TPA IN THE B-CELL

The findings so far outlined suggest that the process of TPA-induced insulin release, although representing an energy-dependent phenomenon, cannot be attributed to any facilitation of the metabolism of glucose or endogenous nutrients in the islet cells.

An alternative hypothesis would be that TPA exerts a primary effect on Ca^{2+} fluxes across membrane systems in the islet cells. An effect of TPA to facilitate Ca translocation from the extracellular fluid and/or intracellular organelles into the cytosolic compartment was considered to be compatible with both the effect of the drug on $^{45}Ca^{2+}$ outflow from the islets (Fig. 1) and the influence of Ca^{2+}-deprivation, epinephrine, and theophylline on TPA-stimulated insulin output. Moreover, the TPA-induced accumulation of cyclic AMP may well be secondary to the increase in cytosolic Ca^{2+} concentration since, in the islets, adenylate cyclase activity is stimulated by endogenous calmodulin in a Ca^{2+}-dependent fashion (3).

EFFECT OF TPA ON CALCIUM IONOPHORESIS

The postulated effect of TPA to affect Ca^{2+} fluxes across membrane systems in the B-cell led us to investigate the influence of TPA on Ca^{2+} ionophoresis in artificial systems.

Preliminary observations that TPA facilitates, under suitable conditions and to a limited extent, the translocation of Ca^{2+} from an aqueous into an organic phase as mediated by either the ionophore A23187 or native ionophoretic material extracted from the islets were not conclusive, as they could reflect a tensioactive artifact.

The results illustrated in Fig. 2 indicate that in multilamellar liposomes formed of dipalmitoylphosphatidylcholine and maintained at 37°C, TPA (10 mole of TPA/100 mole of lipid) failed to facilitate $^{45}Ca^{2+}$ outflow. Likewise, the ionophore A23187 (1 mole of ionophore/100 mole of lipid) was unable to display its ionophoretic capacity in these relatively rigid liposomes. In the simultaneous presence of TPA and A23187, however, a dramatic increase in the rate of $^{45}Ca^{2+}$ outflow was observed. The latter effect coincided with a dose-related effect of TPA to decrease fluorescence polarization when the dipalmitoylphosphatidylcholine liposomes were labeled with 1,6-diphenyl-1,3,5-hexatriene (data not shown), the latter decrease being obvious in the 35 to 40°C range of temperature. These findings are compatible with the view that TPA, by increasing the fluidity of liposomes, facilitates the process of A23187-mediated

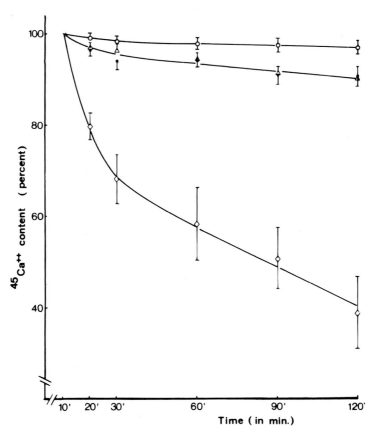

FIG. 2. Time-related changes in $^{45}Ca^{2+}$ content of dipalmitoylphosphatidylcholine liposomes (after a preliminary 10-min washing) maintained at 37°C. Control liposomes are shown as closed circles. Other liposomes contained TPA *(open circles)*, A23187 *(closed triangles)* or both drugs *(open diamonds)*. See text for drug concentrations and reference for methodological considerations.

Ca^{2+} transport across the lipid bilayer. Indeed, we have recently demonstrated that the fluidity of the liposomes exerts a major influence on the efficiency of ionophore-mediated Ca^{2+} transport (1).

CONCLUSION

The present observations call for a more extensive study on the effects of both active and inactive analogs of TPA on insulin release, membrane fluidity, and ionophore-mediated Ca^{2+} transport. Such a study is presently in progress. Within given limits, the data so far obtained are compatible with the view that the interference of TPA and its analogs on ionophore-mediated Ca^{2+} transport is indeed relevant to their insulinotropic action, which itself appears to correlate tightly with their tumor-promoting capacity. Therefore, the present study affords further support to the idea that the biological properties of TPA are somehow related to the effect of the drug on Ca^{2+} handling by target cells.

ACKNOWLEDGMENTS

This work was supported in part by grants from the Belgian Foundation for Scientific Medical Research (grant 3.4528.79) and the French General Delegation for Scientific and Technical Research (grant 79.7.0795).

REFERENCES

1. Deleers, M., and Malaisse, W. J. (1980): Ionophore-mediated calcium exchange diffusion in liposomes. *Biochem. Biophys. Res. Commun.,* 95:650–667.
2. Malaisse, W. J., Sener, A., Herchuelz, A., Carpinelli, A. R., Poloczek, P., Winand, J., and Castagna, M. (1980): Insulinotropic effect of the tumor promoter 12-O-tetradecanoylphorbol-13-acetate in rat pancreatic islets. *Cancer Res.,* 40:3,827–3,831.
3. Valverde, I., Vandermeers, A., Anjaneyulu, R., and Malaisse, W. J. (1979): Calmodulin activation of adenylate cyclase in pancreatic islets. *Science,* 206:225–227.
4. Virji, M. A. G., Steffes, M. W., and Estensen, R. D. (1978): Phorbol myristate acetate: Effect of a tumor promoter on insulin release from isolated islets of Langerhans. *Endocrinology,* 102:706–711.

Carcinogenesis, Vol. 7, edited by E. Hecker et al.
Raven Press, New York © 1982.

Phorbol Myristate Acetate Uncouples the Relationship Between β-Adrenergic Receptors and Adenyl Cyclase in Mouse Epidermis: A Phenotypic Trait in Papillomas

Sidney Belman and Seymour J. Garte

*Institute of Environmental Medicine, New York University Medical Center,
New York, New York 10016*

Reactions of phorbol myristate acetate (PMA) with cell membranes are manifold and undefined. A clear understanding of how PMA reacts with cell membranes to produce a particular biochemical effect would be useful in the elucidation of its mechanism of action in tumor production and cell differentiation.

The effect of PMA on β-adrenergic hormone stimulation of mouse epidermal adenyl cyclase is a suitable model system for such studies. The hormone-regulated adenyl cyclase reaction appears to be part of a series of events that is responsible for membrane transmission of external signals to the cell. Other components of the membrane transmission complex include phospholipids and phospholipase A_2, which are altered in mouse epidermis and other cells by PMA. Recently developed methods, which are helping to clarify the biochemical events involved, can be used to define the effects of PMA on this system.

Mouse epidermal adenyl cyclase was shown (5) to be stimulated *in vivo* and *in vitro* by the β-adrenergic hormone isoproterenol. This stimulation was prevented by β-adrenergic, but not by α-adrenergic, blockers (5). The receptor in mouse epidermis appears to be β_2 in nature (2). The isoproterenol-stimulated adenyl cyclase was inhibited, in a dose-dependent fashion, by prior application of PMA (5). Grimm and Marks (5) also obtained a good correlation between promoting activity and inhibition by phorbol esters and anthralin.

Direct evidence for the presence of β-adrenergic receptors in mouse epidermis was demonstrated by binding experiments using the specific β-antagonist L-dihydroalprenolol (DHA) (1). The stereospecific nature of the β-receptor was indicated by competition experiments with D-propanolol. The application of PMA *in vivo* had no subsequent effect on DHA binding *in vitro*. Further experiments *in vitro* (4) showed that the PMA inhibition of isoproterenol-stimulated adenyl cyclase is due to an uncoupling of the relationship between the β-adrenergic hormone receptor and adenyl cyclase, and not on the binding of the β-hormone to its receptor. This was established by criteria that distinguished coupled from uncoupled systems.

The ratio (K_D/K_{act}) of the dissociation constant, K_D, for agonist binding to the activation constant, K_{act}, for agonist activation of adenyl cyclase was lower (0.60) for PMA-treated mouse epidermis than for controls (4.33). This means that more agonist is required in PMA-treated epidermis to activate the enzyme. In addition, guanine triphosphate (GTP), which is involved in the coupling of receptor to enzyme, decreased agonist binding in untreated but not in PMA-treated tissue. The PMA uncoupling effect is a direct one which is reversed when PMA treatment is stopped. The loss of sensitivity to β-adrenergic hormones, however, becomes manifest in papillomas obtained during initiation-promotion (3). Mice initiated with dimethylbenzanthracene (DMBA) and promoted with PMA for 17 weeks were allowed to rest without treatment for 3 additional weeks to permit the direct effects of PMA to subside. Normal-looking epidermis in mice bearing papillomas had a β-response (isoproterenol-stimulated/basal levels of cyclic AMP) of 3.85, which was similar to the untreated value of 3.36. The papillomas, however, had a β-response of 1.63. This decreased response appears to be due to a phenotypic alteration in papilloma cells and may serve as a marker for such cells.

Recently developed methods for studying the relationships between the various factors involved in β-adrenergic stimulation of adenyl cyclase (7) can be used to determine whether PMA reacts directly with one of these, such as the GTP-binding coupling factor (7), or whether the uncoupling is an indirect consequence of binding to other membrane receptors.

POSSIBLE MECHANISM FOR PMA PROMOTION

The various biochemical effects of PMA in mouse epidermis and other cells suggest a sequence of events outlined in Fig. 1. Two consequences of this are a decreased β-hormone responsiveness of adenyl cyclase and increased cyclic GMP levels. This hypothetical scheme would account for the ability of protease inhibitors and glucocorticoid hormones to act as promotion inhibitors. We are currently studying the involvement of the depicted factors in PMA-treated epidermis to provide evidence for or against this scheme.

Hirata and Axelrod (6) have recently proposed a scheme for transmission of biochemical signals through membranes. PMA affects many components of this scheme (Fig. 2), which suggests that it acts to alter the normal process of membrane transmission of external (e.g. hormonal) signals.

ACKNOWLEDGMENT

This work was supported by Grant No. CA18536, awarded by the National Cancer Institute, DHEW, and is part of center programs supported by Grant

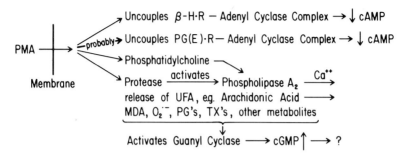

FIG. 1. Partial paradigm for PMA promotion. Abbreviations used are: H, hormone; R, receptor; UFA, unsaturated fatty acids; MDA, malondialdehyde; TX, thromboxane.

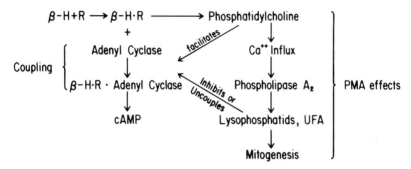

FIG. 2. Scheme of Hirata and Axelrod, ref. 6. Abbreviations as for Fig. 1.

No. ES00260 from the National Institute of Environmental Health Science, and Grant No. CA13343 from the National Cancer Institute, DHEW.

REFERENCES

1. Belman, S., and Garte, S. J. (1980): Antagonism between phorbol myristate acetate and butyric acid on isoproterenol elevation of cyclic adenosine 3',5'-monophosphate and their effects on β-adrenergic receptors in mouse epidermis. *Cancer Res.,* 40:240–244.
2. Duell, E. A. (1980): Identification of a beta₂-adrenergic receptor in mammalian epidermis. *Biochem. Pharmacol.,* 29:97–101.
3. Garte, S. J., and Belman, S. (1980a): Decreased β-adrenergic responsiveness in mouse epidermal papillomas during tumor promotion with phorbol myristate acetate. *Cancer Letters,* 9:245–249.
4. Garte, S. J., and Belman, S. (1980b): Tumour promoter uncouples β-adrenergic receptor from adenyl cyclase in mouse epidermis. *Nature,* 284:171–173.
5. Grimm, W., and Marks, F. (1974): Effect of tumor-promoting phorbol esters on the normal and the isoproterenol-elevated level of adenosine-3',5'-cyclic monophosphate in mouse epidermis *in vivo. Cancer Res.,* 34:3,128–3,134.
6. Hirata, F., and Axelrod, J. (1980): Phospholipid methylation and biological signal transmission. *Science,* 209:1,082–1,090.
7. Limbird, L. E., Gill, D. M., and Lefkowitz, R. J. (1980): Agonist-promoted coupling of the β-adrenergic receptor with the guanine nucleotide regulatory protein of the adenylate cyclase system. *Proc. Natl. Acad. Sci.,* 77:775–779.

Carcinogenesis, Vol. 7, edited by E. Hecker et al.
Raven Press, New York © 1982.

Inhibition of Cell-Cell Communication by Tumor Promoters

James E. Trosko, Larry P. Yotti, Stephen T. Warren,
Gen Tsushimoto, and Chia-cheng Chang

*Department of Pediatrics and Human Development, Michigan State University,
East Lansing, Michigan 48824*

The genesis of a metastasizing tumor has been characterized as a progressive and complex process (19,41,42,89,90,96). During the process, an evolution of a series of phenotypic changes occurs from the normal to the premalignant and malignant stages. The biological phenotypes of "selective growth advantage," "loss of growth control," and metastasis are among those most described. *In vitro* transformation studies have also shown a similar evolutionary progression before a "transformed" cell can have tumorigenic properties when placed in an appropriate *in vivo* host (5). Loss of contact inhibition, growth in soft agar, low Ca^{2+} dependence, and anchorage independence are characteristic phenotypes demonstrated by cells *in vitro* during the evolution from normal to the "transformed" state (25,131).

The multistage concept of carcinogenesis, first described by Rous and Kidd (105), Berenblum (6), Mottram (85), and Boutwell (13) in mouse and rabbit skin, has been an operational means to place some order in the complex carcinogenic process. Although this initiation and promotion model of carcinogenesis was first postulated to explain skin tumorigenesis, many *in vivo,* as well as *in vitro,* transformation models have been used to illustrate its wide-spread applicability to tumorigenesis in several organs of many species (for reviews, see refs. 26,32,94,95,117). In addition, interpretation of several examples of cancers in human beings is consistent with the initiation/promotion model being applicable to human carcinogenesis (23,33,101,147,149).

Although the molecular and biological bases for the initiation and promotion phases are not yet unequivocally delineated, there are several distinguishing characteristics of initiators and promoters that might provide clues to their mechanisms of action (4). Initiation can be brought about by agents, given with a single exposure, that seem to induce a permanent genetic effect and are additive with increasing doses. Furthermore, initiators are known to induce deoxyribonucleic acid (DNA) damage and cause mutations. All kinds of *in*

Dr. Yotti's present address is Biology Division, Oak Ridge National Laboratory, Oak Ridge, Tennessee.

vivo and *in vitro* evidence exist that implicate the need for DNA replication to occur after DNA has been damaged in order for the lesion to act as a substrate for mutation fixation, *in vitro* transformation, and *in vivo* tumorigenesis (for reviews, see refs. 134,135). Consequently, the induction of DNA damage and the error-prone replication of unrepaired DNA lesions causing mutations seem to be a reasonable explanation for the initiation phase. Assuming this to be the case, initiation itself is seen as a complex process, involving many genetic, physiological, and environmental factors that can modify either the amount of DNA damage and its error-prone repair/replication (134,135).

Promotion caused by chemical agents, although brought about by several different means (i.e., repeated wounding, surgery, cytotoxicity of initiating agents, "growth factors" during normal development, and exogenous chemicals; 43) (Fig. 1), requires multiple exposures that are not additive, are reversible to some extent (121), and appear to act only above a certain threshold (14). Promoters at biological dose levels do not seem to induce DNA damage, inhibit the repair of DNA damaged by mutagens (139), nor are they mutagenic in bacterial (79) or mammalian cells (136). Although there have been some reports of observations leading some to interpret the results as indicating that some tumor promoters are "recombinogenic" (64), others have either not repeated those results (132,75) or have questioned its universal applicability (67).

The pleiotropic biochemical and biological responses in different species, organs, or developmental stages to various chemical promoters appear, at first glance, to lead to no unifying mechanism by which tumor promoters might act. Alteration of phenotypes of certain cells, blockage or induction of terminal differentiation in various cell types, stimulation of protein, ribonucleic acid (RNA), DNA, phospholipid, and prostaglandin synthesis under certain conditions in certain cells, alteration of cell surface glycoproteins, modified membrane transport of 2-deoxyglucose, phosphorylation of histones, induction of plasminogen activator, ornithine decarboxylase, and induction of latent viruses are among the many reports of 12-O-tetradecanoylphorbol-13-acetate (TPA) effects (see refs. 32,148). In general, these responses to tumor promoters can be classified, in our opinion, as hormone-like effects. Indeed, some hormones appear to behave like promoters (51,123). Thus, conceptually, chemical and physical promoters would seem to us to be viewed as "gene modulators," not as gene mutagens. Promoters appear to act epigenetically to modulate the expression of genes

FIG. 1. A diagrammatic heuristic scheme to depict the postulated mechanisms of the initiation and promotion phase of carcinogenesis. DNA lesions, induced by physical or chemical mutagens, are substrates that can be fixed if they are not removed in an error-free manner prior to DNA replication. Promotion includes those conditions (i.e., wounding, cytotoxicity, exogenous promoters) in which a pluripotent, but surviving, initiated cell can escape the nonproliferative state. The buildup of initiated cells allows them to "resist" the antimitotic influence of neighboring noninitiated cells. This, together with a second mutation, might allow a given cell to have autonomous, invasive properties of a malignant cell. Reprinted, with permission from Springer-Verlag, from Trosko et al. (140).

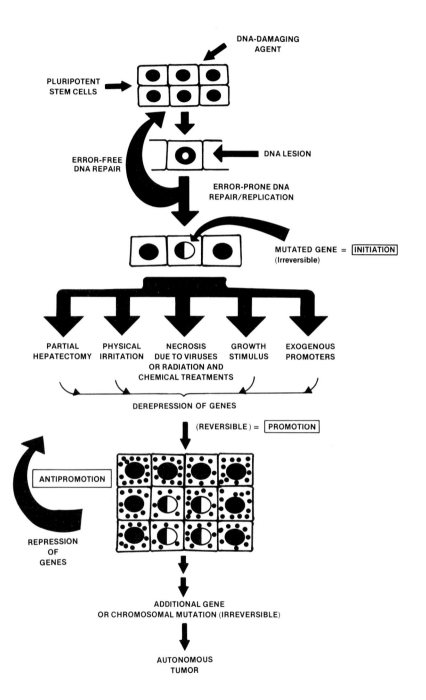

via some as yet to be delineated mechanism(s).

A plethora of evidence suggests that, among the many pleiotropic effects of promoters on cells, the primary or initial effect occurs at the membrane (10, 12,21,30,56,68,84,87,111,115,118,120,150,153,159). Using the model that transmits signals from the cell membrane to the nuclear genes for the regulation of their expression (16,52,54), promoters might be conceived as agents that perturb membranes (possibly by many different mechanisms; e.g., specific membrane receptors to modifiers of critical membrane macromolecules), which then transmit the perturbation via a complex concatenation of biochemical reactions to derepress or repress certain genes (133).

DEVELOPMENT OF AN *IN VITRO* ASSAY TO DETECT TUMOR PROMOTERS

Based on the previous discussion, it should be obvious that the study of the mechanism(s) of tumor promotion and the detection of environmental promoters will be as important as the study and detection of tumor initiators. The strategy to design an *in vitro* assay for such purposes can be based either on fundamental assumptions concerning the mechanisms of promotion or on some empirical generalizations about the properties of promoters. Since it is not known what might be the unifying molecular basis (if there is one) for promotion, the design of any *in vitro* assay system for promoters is going to be as difficult a problem, if not more so, as the design of mutation or transformation screening systems. Intrinsic limitations, such as species, tissue, and developmental specificity of promoters, must be attended to in such an assay. In addition, assuming promotion to include more than just cell problems (i.e., immune surveillance mechanisms), an *in vitro* assay could, at best, give only limited information for understanding the total mechanism of promotion (which would be an *in vivo* process). In addition, one has to recognize that the initiation and promotion concepts are artificial constructs. In reality, these two processes are not clearly demarcated. Many "carcinogens" seem to have the properties of both initiation and promotion (i.e., "complete carcinogens") when applied at certain concentrations. "Incomplete" carcinogens need promoters. Although the idea of a "pure" promoter does exist, the reality is that these promoters always seem to "induce" some cancers without a known pretreatment of an initiator (60). Since all organisms are exposed to initiators ("spontaneous" mutations), however, most, if not all, nonmutagenic promoters ("pure") would be associated with a higher than background amount of tumors (see Potter, ref. 97 for discussion on this point).

The historical roots of this assay are found in a hypothesis provided by Gaudin et al. (46). The tests of the direct predictions of this hypothesis did not support the hypothesis. Instead, they led to an interesting observation, namely that the tumor promoter TPA enhanced the recovery of ultraviolet (UV) and chemical carcinogen-induced 6-thioguanine [hypoxanthine guanine phosphoribosyltransferase$^-$ (HG-PRT$^-$)]- and ouabain (defective NA$^+$/K$^+$ATPase)-resistant mutant

Chinese hamster cells (136), under conditions where it did not inhibit DNA repair or induce mutations by itself. It is now clear that the survival of some induced ouabain-resistant mutants is TPA dependent (Chang and Trosko, *unpublished data*) and that the enhancement of the recovery of 6-thioguanine-resistant mutants is due to the elimination of metabolic cooperation (159). Based on this observation that TPA could block metabolic cooperation between cells, Trosko et al. (140,141) developed an *in vitro* assay.

The details (141), as well as applications (137,138,142), of the procedure have been reported. Independently, observations based on the use of a similar principle have been published by Murray and Fitzgerald (86) and Fitzgerald and Murray (39). In addition, verification of the principle and modification to rat liver cells have been reported by Williams (152).

The principle of the assay is based on the phenomenon of "metabolic cooperation" between cells. Metabolic cooperation is known to play an important role in the recovery of mutant HG-PRT⁻ cells in the 6-thioguanine or 8-azaguanine selection system (129,144). In brief, when an HG-PRT⁻ cell is cocultivated in a population of wild-type HG-PRT⁺ cells, the wild-type cells can transport the toxic metabolite (phosphorylated 6-thioguanine) formed in the presence of the HG-PRT⁺ enzyme and 6-thioguanine to the HG-PRT⁻ cells only if they are in physical contact (Fig. 2). Consequently, the transfer of the phosphorylated 6-thioguanine (presumably) will kill the mutant HG-PRT⁻ cell. We have now demonstrated that many known tumor promotors have this property of blocking metabolic cooperation (138,140,141,142,159). They all do so at noncytotoxic levels, many in a dose-dependent fashion, and each with its own "potency";

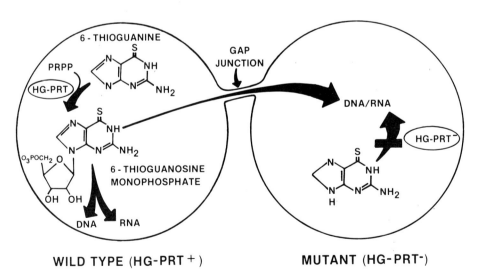

WILD TYPE (HG-PRT⁺)   **MUTANT (HG-PRT⁻)**

FIG. 2. Diagram illustrating the postulated mechanism by which metabolic cooperation occurs in V79 cells at the HG-PRT locus. 6-Thioguanine-resistant cells will die in the presence of 6-thioguanine if they are in physical contact with 6-thioguanine-sensitive cells.

those tested seem to demonstrate a "threshold" level, above which the blockage occurs (137,138,142). One of the most interesting observations to date is that several known "carcinogens" in several animal tumor systems, which have not been shown to be mutagenic (with or without metabolic activating systems) in the Ames assay (79,99), are positive in this metabolic cooperation assay (i.e., TPA, saccharin, 2,2-di(p-chlorophenyl)-1,1,1-trichloroethane (DDT), kepone, polybromobiphenyl (PBB), mirex, phenobarbital, and butylated hydroxytoluene).

Based on the assumption that the property of inhibition of metabolic cooperation is common to many or most TPA-like promoters, and recognizing the aforementioned limitations of the *in vitro* assay, we feel the assay has the potential of screening for tumor promoters and for the study of the mechanisms of tumor promotion (Fig. 3). To date, a number of chemicals, chosen because they have been reported to have, or not to have, promoting activity are listed in Table 1. Obviously, the assay can discriminate between chemicals (i.e., not all chemicals have this property). Most importantly, we feel it might have the potential of predicting what chemicals could be promoters in animal systems. For example, we have recently shown (Trosko et al., *unpublished results*) that two similar congeners of PBB, 2,4,5,2',4',5'-hexabromobiphenyl and 3,4,5,3',4',5'-hexabromobiphenyl, have very distinctively different effects in our *in vitro* assay (Fig. 4). It remains to be shown how each behaves *in vivo*.

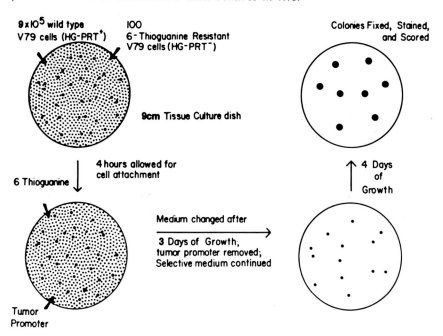

FIG. 3. Protocol to test for chemicals that can block metabolic cooperation. Reprinted, with permission from Springer-Verlag, from Trosko et al. (140).

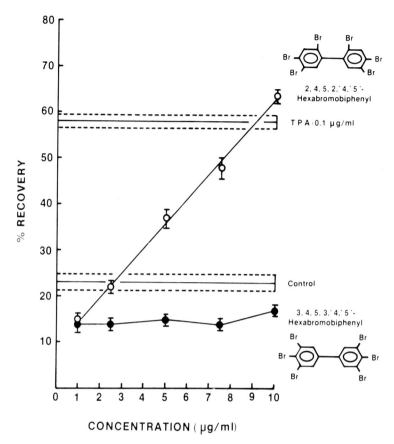

FIG. 4. Dose-response curve for the effect of two congeners of PBB on the inhibition of metabolic cooperation between 6-thioguanine-sensitive and resistant Chinese hamster V79 cells. The shaded areas correspond to the mean recovery of 6-thioguanine-resistant cells for the control and TPA-treated groups ± S.E.M. The data are expressed as the percentage of the plated 6-thioguanine cells that formed colonies in the presence of 9×10^5 6-thioguanine-sensitive cells in a 9-cm Petri dish. From G. Tsushimoto et al. *(in preparation)*.

SPECULATED ROLE OF THE INHIBITION OF CELL-CELL COMMUNICATION IN TUMOR PROMOTION

During the development, differentiation, and maintenance of complex specialized functions of a multicellular organism, a variety of cell-cell communication mechanisms (i.e., systemic, portal, local, long and short half-life-types ref. 97) is used to integrate and "orchestrate" all the organ and tissue systems needed for homeostatic balance. They appear to play fundamental roles in developmental processes (36,47,72,114,130), as well as in the control of cellular proliferation and differentiation in multicellular organisms (24,61,70). Communication appears to involve molecular movement over a distance (i.e., hormone to target cells) or from contact between like or unlike cells (97). One means of allowing

TABLE 1. *Chemicals tested for their ability to inhibit metabolic cooperation in Chinese hamster V79 cells* in vitro

Chemical	Maximum concentration used (noncytotoxic)	Relative effect
Phorbol	1 μg/ml	−
4-α-Phorbol-12,13-didecanoate	1 μg/ml	−
Phorbol-12,13-diacetate	1 μg/ml	+
4-o-Methylphorbol-12-myristate-13-acetate	1 μg/ml	+
Phorbol-12,13-dibutyrate	1 μg/ml	++
Phorbol-12,13-didecanoate	1 μg/ml	+++
Phorbol-12-myristate-13-acetate	1 μg/ml	++++
Phenobarbital	200 μg/ml	++
Butylated hydroxytoluene	40 μM	++
Mezerein	.1 μg/ml	+++
DDT	5 μg/ml	++
Lindane	15 μg/ml	++
Chlordane	1 μg/ml	−
Kepone	3 μg/ml	+++
Mirex	10 μg/ml	++
Antralin	.05 μg/ml	++
Saccharin (pure)	5 mg/ml	+
Saccharin (impure)	6 mg/ml	+
Tween 60	.002% V/V	++
Tween 80	.002% V/V	+
Deoxycholic Acid	10 μg/ml	++
Lithocholic Acid	10 μg/ml	++
Cholesterol	50 μg/ml	−
Taurodeoxycholic acid	100 μg/ml	−
Cytocalasin B	0.1 μg/ml	++
Cytocalasin D	0.01 μg/ml	−
Dinitrofluorobenzene	0.1 μg/ml	++
Polybromobiphenyl (Firemasters)	10 μg/ml	++
3'4'5',3,4,5-Hexabromobiphenyl	2.5 μg/ml	−
2',4',5',2,4,5-Hexabromobiphenyl	7.5 μg/ml	++
3'4'5',2,4,5-Hexabromobiphenyl	7.5 μg/ml	+
3',4',2,4,5-Pentabromobiphenyl	5 μg/ml	+
2',4',5',2,3,4,5-Heptabromobiphenyl	10 μg/ml	++
2',3',4',5',2,3,4,5-Octobromobiphenyl	10 μg/ml	++
Heptochlor epoxide	8 μg/ml	++
Melittin	1 μg/ml	++
Hydroquinone	1.0 μg/ml	++
Benzyl peroxide	1.0 μg/ml	++
Valium	1.25 μg/ml	+
Methyl clofenopate	0.5 μg/ml	−
Nafenopin	2.5 μg/ml	++
[4-chloro-6-(2,3-xylidino)-2-pyrimidinylthio]acetic acid (Wy-14,643)	10 μg/ml	++
[4-chloro-6-(2,3-xylidino)-2-pyrimidinylthio (N-B-hydroxyethyl)-acetamide] (BR 931)	1 μg/ml	−
Thalidomide	1 μg/ml	−
Diphenylhydantoin	100. μg/ml	++
9-Methylpteroylglutamic acid	50 μg/ml	+
Formaldehyde	0.3 μg/ml	−

TABLE 1. *(Continued)*

Chemical	Maximum concentration used (noncytotoxic)	Relative effect
Mestranol	2.5×10^{-6}M	++
Ethinyl estradiol	2.5×10^{-6}M	++
Norethynodrel	2.5×10^{-6}M	++
Ethyl alcohol	1 mg/ml	−
Retionic acid	1 μM	−
Dibutyryl cAMP	0.05 μM	−
Dimethylsulfoxide	0.5% V/V	−
Epidermal growth factor	0.05 μg/ml	−
Fibroblast-derived growth factor	0.01 μg/ml	−

intercellular communication involves junctional complexes between cells, which are mediated by membrane proteins (48,124). A subclass of these junctional complexes includes the "gap junction," which facilitates the direct transfer of ions, metabolites, nucleotides, interferon, and other small regulatory molecules from cytoplasm to cytoplasm (40,72).

Regulation of the various complex cellular functions (i.e., growth control, differentiation, immune responses, and gene modulation) appears to be affected by the modulation of cell surface components by various intracellular structural elements (124). The transfer of the signal received by the cellular membrane to the genome in the nucleus appears to be facilitated, in part, by an elaborate array of microtubules, microfilaments, and contractile and membrane proteins, and the disruption of the information flow can lead to cellular dysfunction (34,35,71,88,92,98,116). By means of carefully coordinated series of feedback mechanisms between molecular signals, receptors, effectors, gene targets, and products, the delicately balanced communication mechanisms can control proliferation and differentiation. Chalones (17,31,91,127,145) and control of uptake of essential nutrients (9,55) are only some of several postulated means by which cell proliferation is regulated.

In principle, either genetic (i.e., "receptor disease," ref. 104) or environmental factors could interfere with this regulatory control of proliferation and differentiated functions. The results obtained with our *in vitro* assay, which is based on the principle of cell-cell communication, clearly demonstrate that many of the known tumor promoters have the ability to inhibit one important form of cell-cell communication, that is, "metabolic cooperation." This has led to our working hypothesis that tumor promoters allow initiated cells (containing a single mutated gene at some critical locus) to be "amplified" into a large clone of like-type cells. During this amplification process, the probability of having one cell with a second mutation at this locus is enhanced (133). Potter has recently elaborated on the details of this postulated mechanism occurring during rat liver hepatocarcinogenesis (97).

Membranes obviously play a key role in cell-cell communication processes that regulate proliferation and differentiation. It is now becoming very apparent that one of the primary effects of promoters is on membrane structure and function (10,12,20,21,56,68,84,87,111,115,118,120,150,153,159), as well as on the related cytoskeleton (102). The fact that tumor promoters can either induce (59,62,83,100,106,128,156) or block terminal differentiation (37,57,58,73, 107,108,109) in various cell types presumably depends on differences in the promoter-membrane interface on the membrane-genome connection (146).

The regulation of the normal balance between the proliferative capacity of a cell and the specific differentiated function of that cell appears to depend on the cell's ability, through specific membrane receptors, to respond to various cell-cell signals (i.e., hormones, chalones, and growth factors).

Contact inhibition (69) is one example whereby physical contact of cells, mediated by gap junctions, prevents uncontrolled cell division. One major criterion of whether a cell has been transformed is the loss of contact inhibition (1,27), indicating that during the transformation process, the genetic control of contact inhibition has been altered (possibly by mutations). The postulation of chalones (17,91) as cell-specific inhibitors of proliferation affords another example of a cell-cell communication device. The recent demonstration of "chalone-like" molecules affecting various cell functions has recently been reported (127,145). Assuming that "immune surveillance" plays some role in the suppression of the progression and development of tumors, the communication mechanisms in the immune system would depend on specific membrane states of each component of the system.

Tumor promoters appear to (a) inhibit contact inhibition or metabolic cooperation between cells (39,86,152,159); (b) alter the receptor sites of growth factors (21,115); (c) affect the immune system (29,63,110); and (d) block chalones (66). Consequently, it appears that one of the primary effects of the tumor promoter on the cell is the modulation of membrane structure/function in such a way as to mimic the transformed state (i.e., loss of contact inhibition).

Observations *in vivo* (14) lead one to conclude that both normal and initiated tissues respond to tumor promoters. If after prolonged application the promoter exposure is stopped, however, normal tissue appears to restore itself to its original prepromoted state. Some cells in the initiated tissue, after prolonged promoter exposure, seem to lose this ability (18). One could surmise that this ultimate change might reside in an alteration in the membrane, or in the ability of the membrane to transmit a signal to the nucleus. One explanation for such a stable change would be a mutation in the gene(s) coding for specific membrane components, which could cause a cell to respond abnormally to the external control of cell proliferation and differentiation. For example, an initiated cell, because it might fail to produce enough negative feedback factors, would proliferate when a promoter inhibits local communication from the normal surrounding cells (97).

On the biochemical level, observations have been made that relate tumor promoter effects on membranes to the role of Ca^{2+} in cell proliferation and differentiation. The role of Ca^{2+} on the growth or differentiation of normal epithelial cells appears to mimic (2) that of a tumor promoter on the inhibition of terminal differentiation of normal rat tracheal cells (128), as well as the induction of latent viruses (3,38,49,78,155,160). In addition, it is well known that transformed cells have a low Ca^{2+} requirement for growth (131). The role of calcium in membrane structure and function (50), as well as in cytoskeleton structure (77) and regulation of cell division, has been noted (7,15,53,80,81, 143,151). Gap junction function is influenced by modulating Ca^{2+} fluxes (103). Tumor promoters have been shown to induce rapid alteration in both calcium content and transport in cultured differentiated chick myoblasts (112). A calcium antagonist has been reported to inhibit a tumor promoter-induced release of granule enzymes for human neutrophils (122). There is a possibility that all tumor promoters, independent of their specific membrane interactions (i.e., promoter-receptors, alteration of the redox state of important membrane components), affect cell membranes in a way so as to alter the flux of Ca^{2+}, which could then trigger a series of Ca^{2+}-dependent protein functions (151) through the Ca^{2+} binding protein calmodulin (22).

Included in these Ca^{2+}-dependent enzyme functions (i.e, gap junction function, assembly of microtubules, ornithine decarboxylase induction) might be the modulation of cyclic nucleotides (28,45,80). Although reports of promoter modulation of cyclic nucleotides have been conflicting, there is recently more evidence favoring a promoter alteration of cyclic nucleotide levels (93). Bertram (8) showed that the mechanism by which nontransformed 10T½ cells inhibit the growth of cocultivated malignant cells seems to involve the modulation of cyclic nucleotides in mediating intercellular communication between normal and transformed cells.

A prediction from the hypothesis that tumor promoters block intercellular communication or metabolic cooperation between contacting cells by altering gap junction function is that labeled nucleotides could not be transferred from cell to cell in the presence of a promoter. This prediction was tested in the experiment reported in Fig. 5. By cocultivation of ^{3}H-uridine-labeled cells with unlabeled cells, in the presence or absence of a tumor promoter, and analysis through autoradiography, this prediction is supported.

In preliminary experiments using freeze fracture techniques (157), we have shown that under identical conditions when TPA inhibits metabolic cooperations, TPA also significantly reduces the number of gap junctions/unit surface area of Chinese hamster V79 cells (Yancey and Trosko, *in preparation*). The disappearance of gap junctions in regenerating rat liver (158) and the lack of gap junctions in the myometrium of immature hypophysectomized rats, but their appearance after administration of estrogen (82), obviously do not constitute direct proof of the role gap junctions might play in regulating hyperplasia and cell differentiation. In light of a recent observation that showed a human breast cancer cell line to be responsive to estrogen in the nude mouse, but unresponsive in culture medium (113), however, the authors suggested an "indirect" mecha-

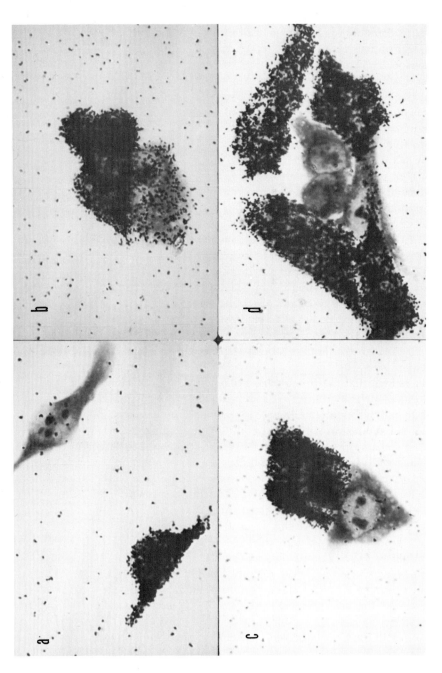

FIG. 5. Autoradiograms of ³H-uridine-labeled V79 cells in the absence (**a** and **b**) or presence (**c** and **d**) of the tumor promoter (TPA; 0.1 µg/ml). Autoradiograms illustrate that the transference of the labeled material is blocked in TPA-treated cells even though there is physical contact between the cells. From S. T. Warren, et al. *(in preparation)*.

nism of action of the hormones on tumor growth *in vivo.* They inferred that mammary carcinoma cell growth *in vivo* is subject to inhibition that can be overcome by estrogen. In light of our results and discussion, the inhibition of growth *in vivo* might be the result of gap junction formation between normal and tumor cells. *In vitro,* this would not occur, unless cocultivated with normal cells. *In vivo,* estrogens could facilitate their disappearance for this tissue mix, allowing the tumor cell to escape the antiproliferative influence of the normal tissue.

One might speculate that the cell has a very tightly coordinated control over permeability and gap junction transfer of different classes of molecules for either its proliferative or differentiated functions (154). When a cell is triggered to divide, it might need to facilitate the influx of certain molecules needed for rapid synthesis of most of the cellular macromolecules. At the same time, it might shut off the transference of important molecules (i.e., nucleotides, small peptides, etc.) through the gap junctions. When a cell is in a nonproliferative or quasidifferentiated state, however, the plasma membrane restricts certain molecules from entering, while the gap junctions allow certain "differentiation-type" or antiproliferative molecules (i.e, interferon, chalones, cyclic nucleotide, etc.) to pass throughout a network of such cells. It seems logical to us that chemical disruption of cell-cell communication plays not only an important role in tumor promotion, but also in teratogenesis. One would predict that many teratogens could be promoters and vice-versa. A classic example, illustrating the ability to be both a teratogen and a liver tumor promoter without being a mutagen, is phenobarbital (76).

On the genetic level, a mechanism must be postulated to explain how tumor promoters appear to give a selective growth advantage to an initiated cell. If we assume initiation involves a mutation in one of a few number of genetic loci affecting cell growth, and if we further assume that for nonviral transformation, the mutation that occurs is recessive to the normal gene (i.e., somatic hybrid cells, fused from normal and transformed cells, retain the normal, not the transformed, phenotype; refs. (20,65,74,125,126), then we must postulate that the initiated cell has only one normal allele at this critical locus. The concept of gene dosage refers to the phenomenon whereby the phenotype of a cell is dependent on a critical level of gene products from the number of functioning alleles.

Now if we further assume that both the quality and quantity of specific membrane components on a cell is necessary to maintain a nonproliferative state (i.e., receptors for cell division repressors), then mechanisms to reduce either the number and the function of these specific membrane receptors (permanently—mutation, or reversibly—epigenetic mechanism) could induce the proliferative state. For example, if cells producing cell division repressors are destroyed (e.g. cytotoxic doses of radiations, chemicals, or viruses, surgery, or wounding); if the ability of repressors to bind to cell receptors is inhibited; or if the receptor type or numbers have been altered by mutational or epigenetic repression of the genes controlling these receptors, then cell proliferation can occur. If these mechanisms do not irreversibly affect the cell's ability to restore the original number and state of these "receptors," then the cell has a feedback mechanism to control proliferation/differentiation.

If, on the other hand, a mutation has occurred in one gene controlling the number of functional membrane "receptors," then when the initial number of those receptors falls below a given number, regulation of proliferation will be weakened (i.e., the cell has a slight growth advantage). This would give some initiated cells a slight growth advantage for forming a clone of such cells. Even if a mutation affecting this specific membrane "receptor" occurs in one gene of a cell, the close physical exchange of these "receptors" from the normal to initiated cells restores the number of functional receptors to the initiated cell. This would have the effect of repressing the initiated cell's tendency to proliferate, as in the case of cocultivation experiments (11,119). It has been observed that membrane antigens of one cell can be transferred to other cells (44).

If, by cell death, cell removal, tumor promoters, or growth factors, cell-cell communication is reduced, then preferential growth of initiated cells could occur. After a large enough number of these initiated cells have been produced, those cells in the interior of the clone would be resistant to the contact of the normal cells. In addition, each time a cell divides, there is a finite probability that any gene can mutate either spontaneously or via replication of an unrepaired lesion in the DNA. Obviously, increasing the number of cells with a single mutation in the critical locus enhances the chance that one of these cells will have a second mutation occur during this proliferative amplification stage. After this second mutation occurs in one cell, the chances of a normal homozygous or heterozygous cell being able to transfer enough of the needed receptors by direct contact to the double mutated cell will be small.

Although highly speculative, if one of those potential critical genetic loci controlling cell proliferation codes for a protein on the gap junction, then all those cellular functions and structures related to the gap junction will be grossly altered. Since cytoskeletal structures (i.e., microtubules and microfilaments needed for chromosome organization and movement) are related in some way to normal gap junctions (124), it is conceivable that the high aneuploid situation in neoplastic cells might be related to this kind of defect. Tumor promotors might mimic this phenotype in cells having normal genes controlling gap junction-microtubule function. When genetic mutations occur that cause this dysfunction, tumor promoters are no longer needed.

In conclusion, we have developed an *in vitro* assay, using Chinese hamster cells, that has the potential of detecting chemicals that inhibit cell-cell communication, presumably by blocking gap junction function/structures. Many tumor promoters, but not nontumor promoters, appear to inhibit metabolic cooperation. We speculate that tumor promoters, give initiated cells a selective growth advantage, increasing the likelihood of a second mutational event to occur at a genetic locus affecting gap junction function and structure. Once this occurs, the cell has the means to incur additional genetic changes (i.e., loss of chromosomes due to faulty microtubules, etc.) in order to gain the metastatic phenotype.

ACKNOWLEDGMENTS

This work was supported by grants from the National Cancer Institute (CA21104), MSU-All University Grant (80–37), MSU-Agriculture Experiment Station, MSU-Toxicology Center, and the College of Human Medicine. We wish to thank Ms. Olivia Reid and Mrs. Judy Copeman for their excellent typing assistance.

REFERENCES

1. Abercrombie, M. (1979): Contact inhibition and malignancy. *Nature,* 281:259–262.
2. Andreis, P. G., Draghi, E., Mengato, L., and Armato, U. (1979): Calcium and cyclic AMP interplay in the positive control of *in vitro* hepatocyte growth. (Abstr.). *30th Annual Tissue Culture Assoc. Meeting.* Seattle, Washington.
3. Arya, S. K. (1980): Phorbol ester-mediated stimulation of the synthesis of mouse mammary tumor virus. *Nature,* 284:71–72.
4. Barrett J. C., and Sisskin, E. E. (1980): Studies on why 12-0-tetradecanoyl-phorbol-13-acetate does not promote epidermal carcinogenesis of hamsters. In: *Carcinogenesis: Vol. 13, Fundamental Mechanisms and Environmental Effects,* edited by B. Pullman, P. O. P. Ts'o and H. Gelboini, pp. 427–439. D. Reidel, The Netherlands.
5. Barrett, J. C., and Ts'o, P. O. P. (1978): Evidence for the progressive nature of neoplastic transformation *in vitro. Proc. Natl. Acad. Sci. USA,* 75:3,761–3,765.
6. Berenblum, I. (1941): The cocarcinogenic actions of croton resin. *Cancer Res.,* 1:44–48.
7. Berridge, M. J. (1975): Control of cell division: A unifying hypothesis. *J. Cycl. Nucl. Res.,* 1:305–320.
8. Bertram, J. S. (1979): Modulation of cell/cell interactions *in vitro* by agents that modify cAMP metabolism. *Proc. Am. Assoc. Cancer Res.* (abstract), 20:212.
9. Bhargava, P. M., Dwarakanath, V. N., and Prasad, K. S. N. (1979): Regulation of cell division and malignant transformation through control of uptake of essential nutrients. *Cell. Mol. Biol.,* 25:85–94.
10. Blumberg, P. M., Driedger, P. E., and Rossow, P. W. (1976): Effect of a phorbol ester on a transformation-sensitive surface protein of chick fibroblasts. *Nature,* 264:446–447.
11. Borek, C., and Sachs, L. (1966): The difference in contact inhibition of cell replication between normal cells and cells tranformed by different carcinogens. *Proc. Natl. Acad. Sci. USA,* 56:1705–1711.
12. Bos. C. J., and Emmelot, P. (1974): Studies on plasma membranes. XXI. Inhibition of liver plasma membrane enzymes by tumor-promoting phorbol ester, mitotic inhibitors, and cytochalasin B. *Chem. Biol. Interact.,* 8:249–261.
13. Boutwell, R. K. (1964): Some biological aspects of skin carcinogenesis. *Prog. Exp. Tumor Res.,* 4:207–250.
14. Boutwell, R. K. (1974): The function and mechanism of promoters of carcinogenesis. *Crit. Rev. Toxicol.,* 2:419–443.
15. Boynton, A. L., Whitfield, J. F., and Isaacs, R. J. (1975): Calcium-dependent stimulation of BALB/c 3T3 mouse cell DNA synthesis by a tumor-promoting phorbol ester. *J. Cell. Physiol.,* 87:25–32.
16. Brunner, G. (1977): Membrane impression and gene expression. *Differentiation,* 8:123–132.
17. Bullough, W. S. (1965): Mitotic and functional homeostasis: A speculative review. *Cancer Res.,* 25:1,683–1,727.
18. Burns, F. J., Van der Laan, M., Sivak, A., and Albert, R. E. (1976): Regression kinetics of mouse skin papillomas. *Cancer Res.,* 36:1,422–1,427.
19. Cairns, J. (1975): Mutation, selection, and natural history of cancer. *Nature,* 225:197–200.

20. Carney, D., Edgell, C. A., Gazdos, A., and Minna, V. (1979): Suppression of malignancy in human lung cancer (A54918) × mouse fibroblast (3T3-4E) somatic cell hybrids, *J. Natl. Cancer Inst.,* 62:411–415.
21. Castagna, M., Rochette-Egly, C., Rosenfeld, C., and Mishal, Z. (1979): Altered lipid microviscosity in lymphoblastoid cells treated with 12-O-tetradecanoylphorbol-13-acetate, a tumor promoter. *FEBS Letters,* 100:62–66.
22. Cheung, W. Y. (1980): Calmodulin plays a pivotal role in cellular regulation. *Science,* 207:19–27.
23. Christopherson, W. M., and Mays, E. T. (1977): Liver tumors and contraceptive steroids: Experience with the first hundred registry patients. *J. Natl. Cancer Inst.,* 58:167–171.
24. Cline, M. J., and Golde, D. W. (1979): Cellular interactions in haematopoiesis. *Nature,* 227:177–181.
25. Colburn, N. H. (1978): *In Vitro* Carcinogenesis. *NCI Technical Report,* 44:57–64.
26. Colburn, N. H. (1980): Tumor promotion and preneoplastic progression. In: *Carcinogenesis, Vol. 5: Modifiers of Chemical Carcinogenesis,* edited by T. J. Slaga, pp. 33–56. Raven Press, New York.
27. Corsaro, C. M., and Migeon, B. R. (1977): Comparison of contact-mediated communication in normal and transformed human cells in culture. *Proc. Natl. Acad. Sci. USA,* 74:4,476–4,480.
28. Costa, M., and Nye, J. S. (1978): Calcium, asparagine, and c-AMP are required for ornithine decarboxylase activation in intact Chinese hamster ovary cells. *Biochem. Biophys. Res. Commun.,* 85:1,156–1,164.
29. Curtis, G. L., Stenback, R., and Ryan, W. L. (1975): Initiation-promotion skin carcinogenesis and immunological competence. *Proc. Soc. Exp. Biol. Med.,* 150:61–64.
30. Delclos, K. G., Nagle, D. S., and Blumberg, P. M. (1980): Specific binding of phorbol ester tumor promoters to mouse skin. *Cell,* 19:1,025–1,032.
31. DePaermentier, F., Barbason, H., and Bassleer, R. (1979): Controle de la differenciation et de la proliferation par une "chalone hepatique" dans des cellules d'un hepatome de rat cultiveés *in vitro. Bio. Cell.,* 34:205–212.
32. Diamond, L., O'Brien, T. G., and Rovera, G. (1978): Tumor promoters: Effects on proliferation and differentiation of cells in culture. *Life Sci.,* 23:1,979–1,988.
33. Domellof, L. (1979): Gastric carcinoma promoted by alkaline reflex gastritis—with special reference to bile and other surfactants as promoters of postoperative gastric cancer. *Med. Hypoth.,* 5:463–476.
34. Edelman, G. M. (1976): Surface modulations in cell recognition and cell growth. *Science,* 192:218–226.
35. Evans, R., and Alexander, P. (1970): Cooperation of immune lymphoid cells with macrophages in tumor immunity. *Nature,* 228:620–622.
36. Evans, W. H. (1980): Communication between cells. *Nature,* 283:521–522.
37. Fibach, E. Gambari, R., Shaw, P. A., Maniatis, G., Reuben, R. C., Sassa, S., Rifkind, R. A., and Marks, P. A. (1979): Tumor promoter-mediated inhibition of cell differentiation: Suppression of the expression of erythroid functions in murine erythroleukemia cells. *Proc. Natl. Acad. Sci. USA,* 76:1,906–1,910.
38. Fisher, P. B., Weinstein, I. B., Eisenberg, D., and Ginsberg, H. S. (1978): Interactions between adenovirus, a tumor promoter, and chemical carcinogens in transformation of rat embryo cell culture. *Proc. Natl. Acad. Sci. USA,* 75:2,311–2,314.
39. Fitzgerald, D. J., and Murray, A. W. (1979): Inhibition of intercellular communication by tumor-promoting phorbol esters. *Cancer Res.,* 40:2,935–2,937.
40. Flagg-Newton, J., Simpson, I., and Loewenstein, W. R. (1979): Permeability of the cell to cell membrane channels in mammalian cell junction. *Science,* 205:404–407.
41. Foulds, L. (1969): *Neoplastic Development, Vol. 1.* Academic Press, London.
42. Foulds, L. (1975): *Neoplastic Development, Vol. 2.* Academic Press, London.
43. Frei, J. V. (1976): Some mechanisms operative in carcinogenesis: A review. *Chem. Biol. Interact.,* 12:1–25.
44. Frye, L. D., and Edidin, M. (1970): The rapid intermixing of cell surface antigens after formation of mouse-human heterokaryons. *J. Cell Sci.,* 7:319–335.
45. Garland, D. L. (1979): c-AMP inhibits the *in vitro* assembly of microtubules. *Arch. Biochem. Biophys.,* 198:335–337.

46. Gaudin, D., Gregg, R., and Yielding, K. (1972): Inhibition of DNA repair by cocarcinogens. *Biochem. Biophys. Res. Commun.,* 48:945–959.
47. Gilula, N. B. (1980): Cell to cell communication and development. In: *Cell Surface: Mediator of Developmental Processes,* edited by S. Subtelny and N. K. Wessells, pp. 23–42. Academic Press, New York.
48. Goodenough, D. A. (1980): Intercellular Junctions. In: *Membrane-Membrane Interactions,* edited by N. B. Gilula, pp. 167–178. Raven Press, New York.
49. Gottesman, M. M., and Sobel, M. E. (1980): Tumor promoters and Kirsten Sarcoma virus increase synthesis of a secreted glycoprotein by regulating levels of translatable RNA. *Cell,* 19:449–455.
50. Gupta, K. C., Turner, F. R., and Taylor, M. W. (1979): Calcium-mediated cell surface changes in Chinese hamster cells. *Exp. Cell Res.,* 120:39–46.
51. Hall, W. H. (1948): The role of initiating and promoting factors in the pathogenesis of tumors of the thyroid. *Br. J. Cancer,* 2:273–280.
52. Harris, P. (1978): Triggers, trigger waves, and mitosis: A new model. In: *Cell Cycle Regulation,* edited by J. R. Jeter, I. L. Cameron, and G. M. Padilla, pp. 75–104. Academic Press, New York.
53. Hennings, H., Michael, D., Chang, C., Steinert, P., Holbrook, K., and Yuspa, S. H. (1980): Calcium regulation of growth and differentiation of mouse epidermal cells in culture. *Cell,* 19:245–254.
54. Hirata, F., and Axelrod, J. (1980): Phospholipid methylation and biological signal transmission. *Science,* 209:1,082–1,090.
55. Holley, R. W. (1972): A unifying hypothesis concerning the nature of malignant growth. *Proc. Natl. Acad. Sci. USA,* 69:2,840–2,841.
56. Horton, A. W., Eshleman, D. N., Schuff, A. R., and Perman, W. H. (1976): Correlation of cocarcinogenic activity among *n*-alkanes with their physical effects on phospholipid micelles. *J. Natl. Cancer Inst.,* 56:387–391.
57. Huberman, E., and Callahan, M. F. (1979): Induction of terminal differentiation in human promyelocytic leukemic cells by tumor-promoting agents. *Proc. Natl. Acad. Sci. USA,* 76:1,293–1,297.
58. Huberman, E., Heckman, C., and Langenbach, R. (1979): Stimulation of differentiated functions in human melanoma cells by tumor-promoting agents and dimethyl sulfoxide. *Cancer Res.,* 39:2,618–2,624.
59. Ishii, D. N., Fibach, E., Yamasaki, H., and Weinstein, I. B. (1978): Tumor promoters inhibit morphological differentiation in cultured mouse neuroblastoma cells. *Science,* 200:556–559.
60. Iverson, U. M., and Iverson, O. H. (1979): The carcinogenic effect of TPA (12-O-tetradecanoyl-phorbol-13-acetate) when applied to the skin of hairless mice. *Virchows Arch. (zellpath.),* 30:33–42.
61. Jacob, F. (1978): The Leeuwenhoek Lecture 1977: Mouse teratocarcinoma and mouse embryo. *Proc. R. Soc. London Ser. B.,* 201:249–270.
62. Kasukabe, T., Honma, Y., and Hozumi, M. (1979): Inhibition of functional and morphological differentiation of cultured mouse myeloid leukemia cells by tumor promoters. *Gann,* 70:119–123.
63. Keller, R. (1979): Suppression of natural antitumor defense mechanisms by phorbol esters. *Nature,* 282:729–730.
64. Kinsella, A., and Radman, M. (1978): Tumor promoter induces sister chromatid exchanges: Relevance to mechanisms of carcinogenesis. *Proc. Natl. Acad. Sci. USA,* 75:6,149–6,153.
65. Klein, G., Bregula, V., Wiener, F., and Harris, H. (1971): The analysis of malignancy by cell fusion: Hybrid between tumor cells and L-cell derivatives. *J. Cell Sci.,* 8:659–672.
66. Krieg, L., Kuhlmann, I., and Marks, F. (1974): Effect of tumor-promoting phorbol esters and of acetic acid on mechanisms controlling DNA synthesis and mitosis (chalones) and on the biosynthesis of histidine-rich protein in mouse epidermis. *Cancer Res.,* 34:3,135–3,146.
67. Kunz, B. A., Hannan, M. A., and Haynes, B. H. (1980): Effect of tumor promoters on ultraviolet light-induced mutation and mitotic recombination in *Saccharomyces cerevisiae. Cancer Res.,* 40:2,323–2,329.
68. Lee, L., and Weinstein, I. B. (1978): Tumor-promoting phorbol esters inhibit binding of epidermal growth factor to cellular receptors. *Science,* 202:313–315.
69. Levine, E. M., Beck, Y., Boone, C. W., and Eagle, H. (1965): Contact inhibition, macromolecu-

lar synthesis, and polyribosomes in cultured human diploid fibroblasts. *Proc. Natl. Acad. Sci. USA,* 53:350–356.

70. Lipton, J. H. (1979): The relationship of cell surface receptor interactions to the differentiation potential of myeloid leukemic cells. *Cell Differ.,* 8:353–363.

71. Lloyd, C. (1979): Fibronectin: A function at the junction. *Nature,* 279:473–474.

72. Loewenstein, W. R. (1979): Junctional intercellular communication and the control of growth. *Biochim. Biophys. Acta,* 560:1–65.

73. Lotem, J., and Sachs, L. (1979): Regulation of normal differentiation in mouse and human myeloid leukemic cells by phorbol esters and the mechanism of tumor promotion. *Proc. Natl. Acad. Sci. USA,* 76:5,158–5,162.

74. Louis, C. J., and Rose, G. B. (1978): Suppression of malignancy in mouse-man hybrid cells. *Pathologica,* 10:343–350.

75. Loveday, K. S., and Latt, S. A. (1979): The effect of a tumor promoter, 12-O-tetradecanoylphorbol-13-acetate on sister chromatid exchange formation in cultured Chinese hamster cells. *Mutat. Res.,* 67:343–348.

76. Majewski, F., Raff, W., Fisher, P., Huenges, R., and Petruch, F. (1980): Zur teratogenitat von antikonvulsiva. *Deutsche Medizinishe Wochenschrift,* 105:719–723.

77. Marcum, J. M., Dedman, J. R., Brinkley, B. R., and Means, A. R. (1978): Control of microtubule assembly-disassembly by calcium-dependent regulation protein. *Proc. Natl. Acad. Sci. USA,* 75:3,771–3,775.

78. Matsumura, T., and Yamshita, H. (1978): Effects of Ca^{++} ion on the liberation of Dengue virus from BHK-21 cells in culture. *Microbiol. Immunol.,* 22:803–807.

79. McCann, J., Choi, E., Yamasuki, E., and Ames, B. N. (1975): Detection of carcinogens as mutagens in the Salmonella/Microsome test: Assay of 300 chemicals. *Proc. Natl. Acad. Sci. USA,* 72:5,135–5,139.

80. McKeehan, W. L., and McKeehan, K. A. (1979): Epidermal growth factor modulates extracellular Ca^{++} requirement for multiplication of normal human skin fibroblasts. *Exp. Cell Res.,* 123:397–400.

81. McKeehan, W. L., and McKeehan, K. A. (1980): Calcium, magnesium, and serum factors in multiplication of normal and transformed human lung fibroblasts. *In Vitro,* 16:475–485.

82. Merk, F. B., Kwan, P. W. L., and Lean, I. (1980): Gap junctions in the myometrium of hypophysectomized, estrogen-treated rats. *Cell Biol. Intern. Reports,* 4:287–293.

83. Miao, R. M., Fieldsteel, A. H., and Fodge, D. W. (1978): Opposing effects of tumor promoters on erythroid differentiation. *Nature,* 274:271–272.

84. Moroney, J., Smith, A., Tomei, L. D., and Wenner, L. E. (1978): Stimulation of ^{86}Rb and [32]P_i movements in 3T3 cells by prostaglandins and phorbol esters. *J. Cell. Physiol.,* 95:287–294.

85. Mottram, J. C. (1944): A developing factor in experimental blastogenesis. *J. Pathol. Bacteriol.,* 56:181–187.

86. Murray, A. W., and Fitzgerald, D. J. (1979): Tumor promoters inhibit metabolic cooperation in cocultures of epidermal and 3T3 cells. *Biochem. Biophys. Res. Commun.,* 91:395–401.

87. Murray, A. W., and Fusenig, N. E. (1979): Binding of epidermal growth factor to primary and permanent cultures of mouse epidermal cells: Inhibition by tumor-promoting phorbol esters. *Cancer Letters,* 7:71–77.

88. Nicolson, G. L. (1976): Transmembrane control of the receptors on normal and tumor cells. *Biochim. Biophys. Acta,* 458:1–71.

89. Nicolson, G. L. (1979): Cancer metastasis. *Sci. Am.,* 240:66–67.

90. Nowell, P. C. (1976): The clonal evolution of tumor cell populations. *Science,* 194:23–28.

91. Onda, H. (1979): A new hypothesis on mitotic control mechanism in eukaryotic cells: Cell-specific mitosis-inhibiting protein excretion hypothesis. *J. Theor. Biol.,* 77:367–377.

92. Otto, A. M., Zumbe, A., Gilson, L., Kubler, A., and deAsua, L. J. (1979): Cytoskeleton-disrupting drugs enhance effect of growth factors and hormones on initiation of DNA synthesis. *Proc. Natl. Acad. Sci. USA,* 76:6,435–6,438.

93. Perchellet, J. P., and Boutwell, R. K. (1980): Enhancement by 3-isobutyl-l-methylxanthine and cholera toxin of 12-O-tetradecanoylphorbol-13-acetate-stimulated cyclic nucleotide levels and ornithine decarboxylase activity in isolated epidermal cells. *Cancer Res.,* 40:2,653–2,660.

94. Pitot, H. C. (1979): Biological and enzymatic events in chemical carcinogenesis. *Ann. Rev. Med.,* 30:25–39.

95. Pitot, H. C., and Sirica, A. E. (1980): The stages of initiation and promotion in hepatocarcinogenesis. *Biochim. Biophys. Acta*, 605:191–215.
96. Poste, G., and Fidler, I. M. (1980): The pathogenesis of cancer metastasis. *Nature*, 283:139–146.
97. Potter, V. R. (1980): Initiation and promotion in cancer formation: The importance of studies on intercellular communication. *Yale J. Biol. Med.*, 53:367–384.
98. Puck, T. T. (1977): Cyclic AMP, the microtubule-microfilament system and cancer. *Proc. Natl. Acad. Sci.*, 74:4,491–4,495.
99. Purchase, I. F. H., Longstaff, E., Ashby, J., Styles, J. A., Anderson, D., Lefevre, P. A., and Westwood, F. R. (1978): An evaluation of 6 short-term tests for detecting organic chemical carcinogens. *Br. J. Cancer*, 37:873–902.
100. Raick, A. N. (1974): Cell differentiation and tumor-promoting action in skin carcinogenesis. *Cancer Res.*, 34:2,915–2,925.
101. Reddy, B. S., Weisburger, J. H., and Wynder, E. L. (1978): Colon cancer: Bile salts as tumor promoters. In: *Carcinogenesis, Vol. 2: Mechanisms of Tumor Promotion and Cocarcinogenesis*, edited by T. J. Slaga, A. Sivak, and R. K. Boutwell, pp. 453–464. Raven Press, New York.
102. Rifkin, D. B., Crowe, R. M., and Pollack, R. (1979): Tumor promoters induce changes in the chick embryo fibroblast cytoskeleton. *Cell*, 18:361–368.
103. Rose, B., and Loewenstein, W. R. (1975): Permeability of cell junction depends on local cytoplasmic calcium activity. *Nature*, 254:250–254.
104. Roth, J., Lesniak, M. A., Bar, R. S., Muggeo, M., Megyesi, K., Harrison, L. C., Flier, J. S., Wachslicht-Rodbard, H., and Gorden, P. (1979): An introduction to receptor and receptor disorders. *Proc. Soc. Exp. Biol. Med.*, 162:3–12.
105. Rous, P., and Kidd, J. G. (1941): Conditional neoplasms and subthreshold neoplastic states. A study of the tar tumors of rabbits. *J. Exp. Med.*, 73:365–390.
106. Rovera, G., O'Brien, T., and Diamond, L. (1977): Tumor promoters inhibit spontaneous differentiation of Friend erythroleukemia cells in culture. *Proc. Natl. Acad. Sci. USA*, 74:2,894–2,898.
107. Rovera, G., O'Brien, T. G., and Diamond, L. (1979): Induction of differentiation in human promyelocytic leukemia cells by tumor promoters. *Science*, 204:868–870.
108. Rovera, G., Olashaw, N., and Meo, P. (1980): Terminal differentiation in human promyelocytic leukaemic cells in the absence of DNA synthesis. *Nature*, 284:69–70.
109. Rovera, G., Santolik, D., and Damsky, C. (1979): Human promyelocytic leukemic cells in culture differentiate into macrophage-like cells when treated with a phorbol diester. *Proc. Natl. Acad. Sci. USA*, 76:2,779–2,783.
110. Ryan, W. L., Curtis, G. L., Heidrick, M. L., and Stenback, F. (1980): Autoantibody and tumor promotion. *Proc. Soc. Exp. Biol. Med.*, 163:212–215.
111. Schimmel, S. D., Grotendorst, G. R., and Grove, R. I. (1980): Binding of phorbol-12-myristate-13-acetate to cultured myoblasts. *Cancer Letters*, 9:229–236.
112. Schimmel, S. D., and Hallam, T. (1980): Rapid alteration in Ca^{++} content and fluxes in phorbol-12-myristate-13-acetate-treated myoblasts. *Biochem. Biophys, Res. Commun.*, 92:624–630.
113. Shafie, S. M. (1980): Estrogen and the growth of breast cancer: New evidence suggests indirect action. *Science*, 209:701–702.
114. Sheridan, J. D. (1976): *The Cell Surface in Animal Embryogenesis and Development*, pp. 409–447. Elsevier-North Holland, New York.
115. Shoyab, M., DeLarco, J. E., and Todaro, G. (1979): Biologically active phorbol esters specifically alter affinity of epidermal growth factor membrane receptors. *Nature*, 279:387–391.
116. Singer, S. J. (1974): The molecular organization of membranes. *Annu. Rev. Biochem.*, 43:805–833.
117. Sivak, A. (1979): Cocarcinogenesis. *Biochim. Biophys. Acta*, 560:67–89.
118. Sivak, A., Mossman, B. T., and Van Duuren, B. L. (1972): Activation of cell membrane enzymes in the stimulation of cell division. *Biochem. Biophys. Res. Commun.*, 46:605–609.
119. Sivak, A., and Van Duuren, B. L. (1967): Phenotypic expression of transformation: Induction in cell culture by a phorbol ester. *Science*, 157:1,443–1,444.
120. Sivak, A., and Van Duuren, B. L. (1971): Cellular interactions of phorbol myristate acetate in tumor promotion. *Chem. Biol. Interact.*, 3:401–411.
121. Slaga, T. J., Fischer, S. M., Nelson, K., and Gleason, G. L. (1980): Studies on the mechanism

of skin tumor promotion—Evidence for several stages of promotion. *Proc. Natl. Acad. Sci.,* 77:3,659–3,663.

122. Smith, R. J., and Iden, S. S. (1979): Phorbol myristate acetate-induced release of granule enzymes from human neutrophils: Inhibition by the calcium antagonist 8-(N,N-diethylamino)-octyl-3,4,5-trimethoxybenzoate hydrochloride. *Biochem. Biophys. Res. Commun.,* 91:263–271.

123. Sonnenschein, C., and Soto, A. M. (1980): But . . . are estrogens *per se* growth-promoting hormones? *J. Natl. Cancer Inst.,* 64:211–215.

124. Staehelin, A. L., and Hull, B. E. (1978): Junctions between living cells. *Sci. Am.,* 338:141–152.

125. Stanbridge, E. M. (1976): Suppression of malignancy in human cells. *Nature,* 260:17–20.

126. Stanbridge, E. M., and Wilkinson, J. (1978): Analysis of malignancy in human cells: Malignant and transformed phenotypes are under separate genetic control. *Proc. Natl. Acad. Sci. USA,* 75:1,465–1,469.

127. Steck, P. A., Voss, P. G., and Wang, J. L. (1979): Growth control in cultured 3T3 fibroblasts. *J. Cell Biol.,* 83:562–575.

128. Steele, V. E., Marchok, A. C., and Nettesheim, P. (1978): Establishment of epithelial cell lines following exposure of cultured tracheal epithelium to 12-O-tetradecanoylphorbol-13-acetate. *Cancer Res.,* 32:3,563–3,565.

129. Subak-Sharpe, J. H., Burk, R. R., and Pitts, J. D. (1969): Metabolic cooperation between biochemically marked mammalian cells in tissue culture. *Cell Sci.,* 4:353–367.

130. Subtelny, S., and Wessells, N. K. (1980): *Cell Surface: Mediator of Developmental Processes.* Academic Press, New York.

131. Swierenga, S. H., Whitefield, J. F., and Karasaki, S. (1978): Loss of proliferative calcium dependence: Simple *in vitro* indication of tumorigenicity. *Proc. Natl. Acad. Sci. USA,* 75:6,069–6,072.

132. Thompson, L. H., Baker, R. M., Carrano, A. V., and Brookman, K. W. (1980): Failure of the phorbol ester 12-O-tetradecanoylphorbol-13-acetate to enhance sister chromatid exchange, mitotic segregation, or expression of mutations in Chinese hamster cells. *Cancer Res.,* 40:3,245–3,451.

133. Trosko, J. E., and Chang, C. C. (1980): An integrative hypothesis linking cancer, diabetes, and atherosclerosis: The role of mutations and epigenetic changes. *Med. Hypoth.,* 6:455–468.

134. Trosko, J. E., and Chang, C. C. (1981): The role of DNA repair capacity and somatic mutations in carcinogenesis and aging. In: *Handbook of the Diseases of Aging: A Pathogenic Perspective,* edited by H. T. Blumenthal. Van Nostrand Reinhold Company, New York *(in press).*

135. Trosko, J. E., and Chang, C. C. (1981): The role of radiation and chemicals in the induction of mutations and epigenetic changes during carcinogenesis. In: *Advances in Radiation Biology, Vol. 9,* edited by J. Lett and H. Adler, pp. 1–36. Academic Press, New York.

136. Trosko, J. E., Chang, C. C., Yotti, L. P., and Chu, E. H. Y. (1977): Effect of phorbol myristate acetate on the recovery of spontaneous and ultraviolet light-induced 6-thioguanine and ouabain-resistant Chinese hamster cells. *Cancer Res.,* 37:188–193.

137. Trosko, J. E., Dawson, B., and Chang, C. C. (1981): PBB inhibits metabolic cooperation in Chinese hamster cells *in vitro:* Its potential as a tumor promoter. *Environ. Health Perspect.,* 37:179–182.

138. Trosko, J. E., Dawson, B., Yotti, L. P., and Chang, C. C. (1980): Saccharin may act as a tumor promoter by inhibiting metabolic cooperation between cells. *Nature,* 285:109–110.

139. Trosko, J. E., Yager, J. D. Bowden, G. T., and Butcher, F. R. (1975): The effect of several croton oil constituents on two types of DNA repair and cyclic nucleotide levels in mammalian cells *in vitro. Chem. Biol. Interact.,* 11:191–205.

140. Trosko, J. E., Yotti, L. P., Dawson, B., and Chang, C. C. (1981): *In vitro* assay for tumor promoters. In: *Short Term Tests for Chemical Carcinogens,* edited by H. Stich and R. H. C. San, pp. 420–427. Springer-Verlag, New York.

141. Trosko, J. E., Yotti, L. P., Warren, S. T., and Chang, C. C. (1979): *In vitro* detection of potential tumor promoters. In: *Short Term Tests for Prescreening of Potential Carcinogens,* edited by L. Santi and S. Parodi, pp. 45–53. Istituto Scientifico per lo Studio e la Cura dei Tumori, Genova.

142. Tsushimoto, G., Chang, C. C., Trosko, J. E., and Matsumura, F. (1981): Cytotoxic, mutagenic, and tumor-promoting properties of DDT, lindane, and chlordane on Chinese hamster cells *in vitro. J. Environ. Pathol. Toxicol. (in press).*

143. Tupper, J. T., and Zorgniotti, F. (1977): Calcium content and distribution as a function of growth and transformation in the mouse 3T3 cell. *J. Cell Biol.*, 75:12–22.

144. Van Zeeland, A. A., Van Diggelen, M. C. E., and Simons, J. W. I. M. (1972): The role of metabolic cooperation in selection of hypoxanthine-guanine-phosphoribosyl (HG-PRT)-deficient mutants from diploid mammalian cell strains. *Mutat. Res.*, 14:355–363.

145. Wang, J. L., McClain, D. A., and Edelman, G. M. (1975): Modulation of lymphocytic mitogenesis. *Proc. Natl. Acad. Sci. USA*, 72:1,917–1,921.

146. Warren, S. T., Yotti, L. P., Moskal, J. R., Chang, C. C., and Trosko, J. E. (1981): Metabolic cooperation in CHO and V79 cells following treatment with a tumor promoter. *Exp. Cell Res.*, 131:427–430.

147. Weber, J., and Hecker, E. (1978): Cocarcinogen of the diterpene ester-type from *Croton Flavens L.* and esophageal cancer in Curacao. *Experientia*, 34:679–682.

148. Weinstein, I. B., Yamasaki, H., Wigler, M., Lee, L., Fisher, P. B., Jeffrey, A., and Grunberger, D. (1979): Molecular and cellular events associated with the action of initiating carcinogens and tumor promoters. In: *Carcinogens: Identification and Mechanisms of Action*, edited by A. C. Griffen and C. R. Shaw, pp. 399–418. Raven Press, New York.

149. Weiss, W. (1979): Changing incidence of thyroid cancer. *J. Natl. Cancer Inst.*, 62:1,137–1,142.

150. Wenner, C. E., Hackney, J., Kimelberg, H. K., and Mayhew, E. (1974): Membrane effects of phorbol esters. *Cancer Res.*, 34:1,731–1,736.

151. Whitfield, J. F., Boynton, A. L., MacManus, J. P., Sikorska, M., and Tsang, B. K. (1979): The regulation of cell proliferation by calcium and cyclic AMP. *Mol. Cell. Biochem.*, 27:155–179.

152. Williams, G. M. (1980): Classification of genotoxic and epigenetic hepatocarcinogens using liver culture assays. *Annu. N.Y. Acad. Sci.*, 349:273–282.

153. Witz, G., and Banerjee, S. (1979): Divalent cation effects in the interaction of the tumor promoter phorbol myristate acetate with rat liver plasma membranes. *Chem. Biol. Interact.*, 28:127–131.

154. Yabrov, A. (1980): Adequate function of the cell: Interactions between the needs of the cell and the needs of the organism. *Med. Hypoth.*, 6:337–374.

155. Yamamoto, N., and Zur Hausen, H. (1980): Tumor promoter TPA enhances transformation of human leukocytes by Epstein-Barr virus. *Nature*, 280:244–245.

156. Yamasaki, H., Fibach, E., Nudel, U., Weinstein, I. B., Rifkind, R. A., and Marks, P. A. (1977): Tumor promoters inhibit spontaneous and induced differentiation of murine erythroleukemia cells in culture. *Proc. Natl. Acad. Sci. USA*, 74:3,451–3,455.

157. Yancey, S. B., Easter, D., and Revel, J. P. (1979): Cytological changes in gap junctions during liver regeneration. *J. Ultrastruct. Res.*, 67:229–249.

158. Yee, A. G., and Revel, J. P. (1978): Loss and reappearance of gap junctions in regenerating liver. *J. Cell Biol.*, 78:554–563.

159. Yotti, L. P., Chang, C. C., and Trosko, J. E. (1979): Elimination of metabolic cooperation in Chinese hamster cells by a tumor promoter. *Science*, 206:1,089–1,091.

160. Zur Hausen, H., O'Neill, F. J., and Freese, U. K. (1978): Persisting oncogenic herpes virus induced by the tumor promoter TPA. *Nature*, 272:373–375.

Carcinogenesis, Vol. 7, edited by F. Hecker et al.
Raven Press, New York © 1982.

Inhibition of Intercellular Communication by Tumor Promoters

Andrew W. Murray, D. James Fitzgerald, and Graeme R. Guy

School of Biological Sciences, Flinders University, Bedford Park, South Australia 5042

Recent results from our own (2,4) and Trosko's (7,8) laboratories have established that many tumor-promoting compounds inhibit the transfer of low MW molecules between contacting cultured mammalian cells. This transfer is believed to occur via gap junctions. A promoter-induced breakdown in communication may metabolically isolate initiated cells from any restraining influence of their neighbours, enabling them to proliferate into clones of transformed cells (4,8).

In this chapter we summarize data obtained using an autoradiographic procedure (2) and a cell "rescue" method (5) to determine intercellular communication.

MATERIALS AND METHODS

Materials

Mouse epidermal cells (HEL/37) and PG-19 cells were maintained as described before (2,4). PG-19 cells lack the enzyme hypoxanthine-guanine phosphoribosyltransferase (HPRT).

12-O-Tetradecanoylphorbol-13-acetate (TPA), 4-O-methyl TPA, phorbol-12,13-didecanoate (PDD), and 4α-PDD were obtained from P-L Biochemicals, Milwaukee, USA. Phorbol-12,13-dibutyrate (PDBu), phorbol-12,13-diacetate (PDAc), phorbol-12,13-dibenzoate (PDBe), phorbol-13-acetate, phorbol, and mezerein were from Life Systems, Newton, Massachusetts, USA.

[Methyl-³H]thymidine (sp. act. 24 Ci/mmole) was obtained from the Radiochemical Centre, Amersham, England. Eagles minimal essential medium (MEM) was from Commonwealth Serum Laboratories, Melbourne, and medium containing hypoxanthine, aminopterin, and thymidine (HAT) was from Flow Laboratories, Stanmore, N.S.W., Australia.

Methods

Autoradiography

The technique for detection of metabolic cooperation between cocultured HEL/37 and PG-19 cells has been described (2).

Detection of intercellular communication by incubation in HAT medium

The method used has been described (5). PG-19 cells were prelabeled with 10 μCi of [^{3}H]thymidine/10^6 cells (20 hr). Labeled PG-19 cells (2 $\times$ 10^5) and HEL/37 cells (2 $\times$ 10^5) were cocultured for 5 hr in 35-mm plastic dishes in 2 ml MEM. The cells were washed and incubated in HAT medium containing the test compound. All compounds were added in 2 μl dimethylsulfoxide (Me$_2$SO); Me$_2$SO alone was added to controls. In HAT medium, PG-19 cells (HPRT$^-$) die unless "rescued" by metabolic cooperation with HEL/37 cells (HPRT$^+$). The extent of PG-19 cell death in cultures was measured by determining radioactivity released into the medium over a 48-hr period, and expressed as the lytic index essentially as described (5). The proportion of released radioactivity was calculated from the means of four replicate dishes.

RESULTS

As summarized in Table 1, a range of phorbol esters and mezerein inhibit metabolic cooperation as detected by autoradiography. Although detailed dose-

TABLE 1. *Effects of phorbol esters and mezerein on intercellular communication between HEL/37 and PG-19 cells detected by autoradiography*

Compound	Relative proportion of labeled contacting PG-19 cells[a]	Estimate of relative activity as a complete *in vivo* promoter (3)
Me$_2$SO Control	100	
10^{-7} M TPA	42[b]	
10^{-8} M TPA	38[b]	++++
10^{-9} M TPA	99	
10^{-7} M 4-O-methyl TPA	99	
10^{-7} M PDD	46[b]	+++
10^{-7} M 4α-PDD	101	−
10^{-7} M Mezerein	71[b]	++
10^{-7} M PDBu	52[b]	+
10^{-7} M PDBe	56[b]	+
10^{-7} M PDAc	96	±
10^{-7} M Phorbol-13-acetate	105	
10^{-7} M Phorbol	104	−

[a] A minimum of three replicate slides were scored for each treatment. In control cocultures, between 84 and 95% of contacting PG–19 cells were labeled.
[b] Significantly different from control (χ^2 test).

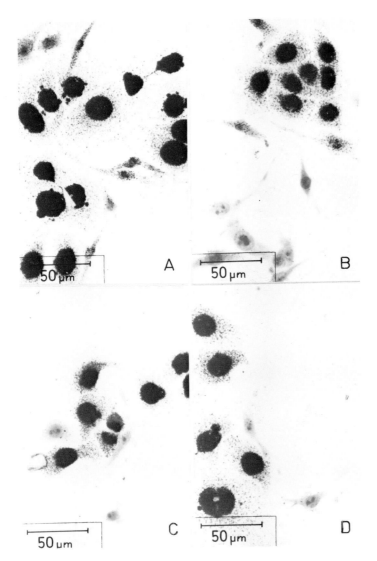

FIG. 1. Autoradiographs demonstrating the transfer of label between HEL/37 cells and PG-19 cells. **A,B:** Cocultures contained Me₂SO. **C,D:** Cocultures contained 10⁻⁷ M TPA. From Fitzgerald and Murray, ref. 2.

response studies have not been done, there is a reasonable correlation between the extent of communication inhibition and potency as a complete *in vivo* promoter. Representative autoradiographs of coculture experiments are shown in Fig. 1. HEL/37 cells can be clearly identified by the heavily grained nuclei resulting from the [³H]thymidine prelabeling. Contacting PG-19 cells in control cocultures (plates A and B) are heavily labeled; noncontacting PG-19 cells are unlabeled (plate B). Examples of contacting but unlabeled PG-19 cells in cocultures treated with 10^{-7} M TPA are shown in plates C and D. As a routine, contacting PG-19 cells are scored only as labeled or unlabeled (2); this has tended to underestimate the effect of promoters. Thus, on average, contacting PG-19 cells labeled in the presence of TPA contain fewer grains than in controls (data not shown).

The effect of TPA on the lysis of cocultured PG-19 cells in HAT medium is shown in Table 2. In the controls the lytic index (5) is low, indicating almost complete "rescue" of the PG-19 cells by contacting HEL/37 cells. Control experiments were done to confirm that the low lytic index did not result from reutilization of released radioactivity by the HEL/37 cells (5). The index is significantly increased by 10^{-7} M TPA or by 10^{-7} M PDD, indicating that the promoters partially abolish the protective effect of HEL/37 cells. The most likely explanation for this effect is an inhibition of the transfer of purine nucleotides from HEL/37 cells to PG-19 cells via gap junctions. Because cocultures were established 5 hr before the test substances were added, the promoter effect is on already established communication links (2).

CONCLUSIONS

Promoters can inhibit the passage of nucleotides between cocultured mammalian cells. There is evidence that normal cells can limit the growth of transformed cells in culture (1) and that this effect can be overcome by promoters (6). It has not, however, been established that the effect of normal cells on transformed cell growth is mediated via intercellular communication. Demonstration that this was the case, together with evidence that promoters interfere with intercellular communication *in vivo,* would strengthen proposals for a link between such communication and promotion.

ACKNOWLEDGMENTS

This work was supported by grants from the Australian Research Grants Committee, the University of Adelaide Anti-Cancer Foundation, and the Na-

TABLE 2. *Detection of intercellular communication between HEL/37 and PG-19 cells by growth in HAT medium (5)*

Treatment	Lytic index
Me$_2$SO control	0.056
10^{-7} M TPA	0.39
10^{-7} M 4-O-methyl TPA	0.024
10^{-7} M PDD	0.38
10^{-7} M 4α-PDD	0.032
10^{-7} M PDBu	0.20

tional Health and Medical Research Council. Mrs. Anne Rogers provided excellent technical assistance.

REFERENCES

1. Bertram, J. S. (1978): Effects of serum concentration on the expression of carcinogen-induced transformation in the C3H/10T½ CL8 cell line. *Cancer Res.,* 37:514–523.
2. Fitzgerald, D. J., and Murray, A. W. (1980): Inhibition of intercellular communication by tumor-promoting phorbol esters. *Cancer Res.,* 40:2,935–2,937.
3. Kinzel, V., Kreibich, G., Hecker, E., and Suss, R. (1979): Stimulation of choline incorporation in cell cultures by phorbol derivatives and its correlation with their irritant and tumor-promoting activity. *Cancer Res.,* 39:2,743–2,750.
4. Murray, A. W., and Fitzgerald, D J. (1979): Tumor promoters inhibit metabolic cooperation in cocultures of epidermal and 3T3 cells. *Biochem. Biophys. Res. Commun.,* 91:395–401.
5. Nicolas, J. F., Jakob, H., and Jacob, F. (1978): Metabolic cooperation between mouse embryonal carcinoma cells and their differentiated derivatives. *Proc. Natl. Acad. Sci. USA,* 75:3,292–3,296.
6. Sivak, A., and Van Duuren, B. L. (1967): Phenotypic expression of transformation: Induction in cell culture by a phorbol ester. *Science,* 157:1,443–1,444.
7. Trosko, J. E., Dawson, B., Yotti, L. P., and Chang, C. C. (1980): Saccharin may act as tumor promoter by inhibiting metabolic cooperation between cells. *Nature,* 285:109–110.
8. Yotti, L. P., Chang, C. C., and Trosko, J. E. (1979): Elimination of metabolic cooperation in Chinese hamster cells by a tumor promoter. *Science,* 206:1,089–1,091.

Carcinogenesis, Vol. 7, edited by E. Hecker et al.
Raven Press, New York © 1982.

The Role of Free Oxygen Radicals in Tumor Promotion and Carcinogenesis

*Walter Troll, †Gisela Witz, †Bernard Goldstein, *Donna Stone, and ‡Takashi Sugimura

Department of Environmental Medicine, New York University Medical Center, New York, New York 10016; †Department of Environmental and Community Medicine, Rutgers Medical School, Piscataway, New Jersey 08854; and ‡National Cancer Center Research Institute, Chuo-ku, Tokyo, Japan

Promoting agents can be defined as damaging materials capable of causing tumorigenesis only to cells that have been modified genetically by a carcinogen. This chapter proposes that the damage caused by two chemically different promoters, phorbol-12-myristate-13-acetate (PMA) and the alkylated indole teleocidin (TEL), is in part due to formation of free oxygen radicals by the cell membrane. These promoters are hormone-like materials combining with receptors on the cell membrane, causing a multitude of tissue reactions (Blumberg and Weinstein, *this volume*). A prompt consequence of the interaction of the tumor promoter with human polymorphonuclear leukocytes (PMN) is oxygen uptake resulting in formation of superoxide anions ($O_2^- \cdot$) and hydrogen peroxide (H_2O_2) (5). Two types of inhibitors of tumor promotion, protease inhibitors and retinoids, block the oxygen response in these cells. This correlation between the action of tumor promoters and the action of inhibitors in PMNs and in tumor promotion in mouse skin led us to the hypothesis that one of the damaging actions in tumor promotion may be due to free oxygen radicals. This mechanism of tumor promotion brings together earlier observations by Kennedy and Little of inhibition by protease inhibitors of transformation by X-ray and PMA in C_3H 10T½ cells (7), and of inhibition by antioxidants of croton oil promotion in mouse skin, as reported by Shamberger (11).

Dr. Slaga has reported *(this volume)* that benzoyl peroxide acts as a tumor promoter in Sencar mice and that antioxidants are inhibitors of tumor promotion by PMA. Edgar Pick reported that the main biochemical event induced by PMA in macrophages was the release of $O_2^- \cdot$ and H_2O_2. He concluded that PMA is an active inducer of "macrophage activation" which is responsible for the expression of the tissue-damaging potential of macrophages.

The role of free oxygen radicals in promotion offers new opportunities for studying the mechanism of tumor promotion and its inhibition.

METHODS AND RESULTS

PMA and other membrane-disturbing materials (e.g., zymosan and Concanavalin A) cause rapid uptake of oxygen, and formation of $O_2^- \cdot$ and H_2O_2. The measurement of these materials depends on the specific enzymes, superoxide dismutase (SOD) and horseradish peroxidase (HRP). Superoxide is measured by the quantity of cytochrome C reduction sensitive to SOD, and hydrogen peroxide by oxidation of a fluorescent compound catalyzed by HRP (5).

In PMNs, the tumor promoters PMA, mezerein, and TEL cause superoxide anion formation (Fig. 1). On the other hand, analogs of PMA (4-me-phorbol-12-myristate-13-acetate and phorbol-12,13-diacetate) that are inactive as tumor promoters do not cause $O_2^- \cdot$ formation (Table 1). Protease inhibitors, retinoids (Tables 2 and 3), and dexamethasone, which block tumor promotion by PMA in skin, also block $O_2^- \cdot$ formation in PMNs (4,17). When retinol and antipain are used together to counteract the effect of PMA on PMNs, their blocking effect on $O_2^- \cdot$ is amplified (Fig. 2). Soybean trypsin inhibitor plus retinol, and phosphoramidon plus retinol show additive effects. Thus, the action of protease inhibitors plus retinol on blocking $O_2^- \cdot$ formation may be due to separate mechanisms. The action of the antiinflammatory hormone dexamethasone in this system may also be distinct. It may act by preventing the influx of phagocytic cells. The application of using several types of blocking agents of promotion together may be a promising technique for preventing cancer. The toxicity resulting from using retinoids might be avoided because lower concentrations of this agent could be used.

Vegetarian populations have a relatively low occurrence of breast and colon cancers (2,9). We assume that these populations consume a greater quantity of retinoids and protease inhibitors. The prevention of experimental breast cancer

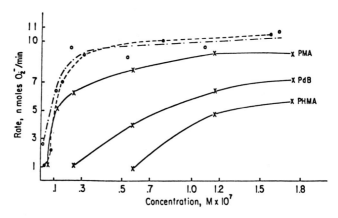

FIG. 1. Dose response for $O_2^- \cdot$ production by PMNs stimulated with tumor promoters: phorbol esters phorbolol myristate acetate (PHMA), phorbol dibutyrate (PdB), and PMA, X—; mezerein, O·-·; teleocidin B, O---.

TABLE 1. *Stimulation of human PMN $O_2^-\cdot$ production by phorbol esters*

Compound[a]	$O_2^-\cdot$ Produced,[b] n mole/min
PMA	7.9
PdB	4.0
PHMA	0.9
4-O-Me-phorbol myristate acetate	0
Phorbol diacetate	0

[a] 5.8×10^{-8} M.
[b] 0.71×10^{-6} cell/ml; 0.55 mg cytochrome cell/ml.

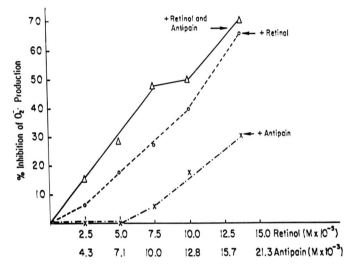

FIG. 2. Combined effect of retinol and antipain on $O_2^-\cdot$ production in polymorphonuclear leukocytes stimulated with phorbol myristate acetate. Cells were stimulated with PMA (71 ng/ml) in the absence or presence of either retinol, antipain, or both. The percent inhibition of $O_2^-\cdot$ production refers to the reduction in the rate of $O_2^-\cdot$ formation in the presence of inhibitors relative to that of cells stimulated in the absence of inhibitors. Data are average of two experiments.

by protease inhibitors or retinyl acetate has been shown in rats (8,15). The combined action remains to be tested.

The response of producing H_2O_2 by cell membranes has unexpected useful applications as well. For example, in sea urchins the production of H_2O_2 during fertilization prevents polyspermic fertilization by inactivating excess sperms. Removal of H_2O_2 by catalase causes polyspermy (3). Protease inhibitors and retinol prevent the production of H_2O_2, also resulting in polyspermy (10,12). This inhibition is analogous to the inhibition of superoxide anion formation observed in PMNs.

TABLE 2. *Inhibition of $O_2^-\cdot$ production in PMA-stimulated PMNs by protease inhibitors[a]*

Protease inhibitor	Concentration	Percent inhibition
Soybean trypsin inhibitor	80 μM	47
Lima bean trypsin inhibitor	430 μM	50
Phosphoramidon	20 mM	95
Benzamidine	67 mM	55
Antipain	60 mM	56
Elastatinal	40 mM	63
Chymostatin	2.8 mM	38

[a] 1.75 $\times$ 10^6 cell/ml; 44 μM cytochrome C; 1.7 μg PMA/ml.

TABLE 3. *Inhibition of $O_2^-\cdot$ production in PMA-stimulated PMNs by retinoids[a]*

Retinoid (μM)	$O_2^-\cdot$ Produced (nmole/min)	% Reduction in rate of $O_2^-\cdot$ formation
Retinol		
0	5.55	—
50	4.50	18
150	3.18	43
250	1.66	70
Retinyl acetate		
0	3.93	—
44	4.41	0
130	3.32	16
270	1.28	67
Retinoic acid		
0	3.55	—
48	2.37	33
240	1.90	47

[a] 71.4 ng PMA/ml; 0.71 $\times$ 10^6 cell/ml; 0.57 mg cytochrome c/ml.

CONCLUSION

Tumor promoters are responsible for many tissue reactions and it has remained difficult to identify those responsible for promotion. The first response to tumor promoters as reported in mouse skin was the induction of proteases (14). The action of PMA was inhibited by a variety of protease inhibitors (6,13,15). Two other inhibitors of tumor promotion were described—dexamethasone and retinoids (1,16). Inhibition of promotion may be explained in a number of ways. (a) Proteases may remove a protein repressor, permitting expression of the tumorigenic potential of the inhibited cell. (b) Inflammation that can be blocked by antiinflammatory hormones may be an essential part of promotion (1). (c) Because mezerein, a poor tumor promoter when compared with PMA, gives more $O_2^-\cdot$, it might be that oxygen radicals are a necessary but insufficient part of promotion.

The free oxygen radicals may be considered to be the agents responsible for the damage caused by the promoting agents.

ACKNOWLEDGMENTS

This work was supported by NIH grants ES-00606 and ES-006737, and by the National Cancer Institute, Tokyo, Japan.

REFERENCES

1. Belman, S., and Troll, W. (1972): The inhibition of croton oil-promoted mouse skin tumorigenesis by steroid hormones. *Cancer Res.,* 32:450–454.
2. Carroll, K. K. (1975): Experimental evidence of dietary factors and hormone-dependent cancers. *Cancer Res.,* 35:3,374–3,383.
3. Coburn, M., Schuel, H., and Troll, W. (1981): A hydrogen peroxide block to polyspermy in the sea urchin *Arbacia punctulata. Dev. Biol.,* 84:235–238.
4. Goldstein, B. D., Witz, G., Amoruso, M., Stone, D. S., and Troll, W. (1981): Stimulation of human polymorphonuclear leukocyte superoxide anion radical production by tumor promoters. *Cancer Letters* 11:257–262.
5. Goldstein, B. D., Witz, G., Amoruso, M., and Troll, W. (1979): Protease inhibitors antagonize the activation of polymorphonuclear leukocyte oxygen consumption. *Biochem. Biophys. Res. Commun.,* 88:854–860.
6. Hozumi, M., Ogawa, M., Sugimura, T., Takeuchi, T., and Umezawa, H. (1972): Inhibition of tumorigenesis in mouse skin by leupeptin, a protease inhibitor from actinomycetes. *Cancer Res.,* 32:1,725.
7. Kennedy, A. R., and Little, J. B. (1978): Protease inhibitors suppress radiation-induced malignant transformation *in vitro. Nature,* 276:825–826.
8. Moon, R. C., Thompson, H. J., Becci, P. J., Grubbs, C. J., Gander, R. J., Newton, D. L., Smith, J. M., Phillips, S. L., Henderson, W. R., Mullen, L. T., Brown, C. C., and Sporn, M. B. (1979): *N*-(4-hydroxyphenyl)retinamide, a new retinoid for prevention of breast cancer in the rat. *Cancer Res.,* 39:1,339–1,346.
9. Philips, R. L. (1975): Role of life style and dietary habits in risk of cancer among Seventh-Day Adventists. *Cancer Res.,* 35:3,513–3,522.
10. Schuel, H., Longo, F. J., Wilson, W. L., and Troll, W. (1976): Polyspermic fertilization of sea urchin eggs treated with protease inhibitors: Localization of sperm receptor sites at the egg surface. *Dev. Biol.,* 49:178–184.
11. Shamberger, R. J. (1972): Increase of peroxidation in carcinogenesis. *J. Natl. Cancer Inst.,* 48:1,491.
12. Sinsheimer, P., Coburn, M., and Troll, W. (1980): The toxic effects of vitamin A on sea urchin gametes. *Biol. Bull.,* 159:469.
13. Troll, W., Belman, S., Wiesner, R., and Shellabarger, C. J. (1979): Protease action in carcinogenesis. In: *Biological Functions of Proteinases,* edited by H. Holzer and H. Tschesche, pp. 165–170. Springer-Verlag, Berlin/Heidelberg.
14. Troll, W., Klassen, A., and Janoff, A. (1970): Tumorigenesis in mouse skin: Inhibition by synthetic inhibitors of proteases. *Science,* 169:1,211–1,213.
15. Troll, W., Wiesner, R., Shellabarger, C. J., Holtzman, S., and Stone, J. P. (1980): Soybean diet lowers breast tumor incidence in irradiated rats. *Carcinogenesis,* 1:469–472.
16. Verma, A. K., and Boutwell, R. K. (1977): Vitamin A acid (retinoid acid), a potent inhibitor of 12-O-tetradecanoylphorbol-13-acetate-induced ornithine decarboxylase activity in mouse epidermis. *Cancer Res.,* 37:2,196–2,201.
17. Witz, G., Goldstein, B. D., Amoruso, M., Stone, D. S., and Troll, W. (1980): Retinoid inhibition of superoxide anion radical production by human polymorphonuclear leukocytes stimulated with tumor promoters. *Biochem. Biophys. Res. Commun. (in press).*

Carcinogenesis, Vol. 7, edited by E. Hecker et al.
Raven Press, New York © 1982.

Results and Speculations Related to Recent Studies on Mechanisms of Tumor Promotion

I. Bernard Weinstein, Ann D. Horowitz, R. Alan Mufson, Paul B. Fisher, Vesna Ivanovic, and Ellen Greenebaum

Division of Environmental Sciences and Cancer Center/Institute of Cancer Research and Departments of Medicine, Microbiology and Pathology, Columbia University, College of Physicians and Surgeons, New York, New York 10036

The importance of the covalent binding of certain initiating chemical carcinogens or their metabolites to cellular deoxyribonucleic acid (DNA) and other macromolecules has provided a unifying concept in terms of understanding their mechanisms of action (20,39). Until recently, relatively little was known in terms of the cellular targets and mechanisms of action of tumor promoters. Within the past few years, however, studies on the action of 12-O-tetradecanoyl-phorbol-13-acetate (TPA) and related phorbol ester tumor promoters in cell culture systems have provided a virtual plethora of biologic effects (11,54,58,59). We have previously emphasized that these effects can be grouped into three categories, all of which coveniently begin with the letter "M" (57,58). These are: (a) *m*imicry of cell transformation in normal cells and enhancement of expression of markers of transformation in cells transformed by chemical carcinogens or oncogenic viruses; (b) *m*odulation of differentiation, which can take the form of either induction or inhibition of differentiation, depending on the particular target cells; and (c) *m*embrane changes, which appear to reflect the primary site of action of these compounds. These aspects have been reviewed in detail elsewhere (11,57,58).

In this chapter, we will review recent results and speculations related to certain topics that we believe are emerging as major themes in understanding tumor promotion and multistage carcinogenesis. These topics include the following: (a) the phorbol ester tumor promoters apparently exert their primary effects by binding to specific receptors on the cell surface membrane; (b) this receptor binding results in rapid alterations in membrane phospholipid metabolism, membrane structure, and membrane function; (c) the subsequent cytoplasmic and nuclear effects of the phorbol esters may relate, at least in part, to alterations in Ca^{2+} flux; (d) the highly pleiotropic effects of these compounds are best understood within the context of hormone action; and (e) the processes of initiation and promotion in two-stage carcinogenesis involve distortions of the normal processes of cell commitment and differentiation, respectively.

At the present time, we have only fragmentary knowledge of the normal mechanisms responsible for membrane structure and function, the molecular basis of action of growth factors and hormones, and the molecular details of development and differentiation. Thus, hypotheses related to the fundamental mechanisms of tumor initiation and promotion must be highly speculative. It is apparent, however, that the phorbol ester tumor promoters are providing powerful tools for obtaining insights into these processes in normal cells and during the process of carcinogenesis.

INTACT CELLS CONTAIN HIGH-AFFINITY RECEPTORS FOR PHORBOL ESTER TUMOR PROMOTERS

A few years ago, we postulated that the phorbol ester tumor promoters act by binding to and usurping the function of membrane-associated receptors that are normally utilized by an endogenous growth factor (30,59). Indirect evidence for this hypothesis includes: (a) the fact that these compounds act in a concentration range similar to that of several hormones and growth factors (i.e., $\sim 10^{-8}$ to 10^{-10} M); (b) the fact that these compounds display very similar structure-function requirements on cells from diverse species and tissues; and (c) the fact that, like known hormones, they induce highly pleiotropic effects that vary considerably depending on the target cell (30,58,59). Since the earliest cellular responses to these agents occur at the cell surface membrane (57), we suggested that the putative receptors were associated with the plasma membrane (57,58).

Utilizing ^{3}H-TPA, however, we were not able to demonstrate the existence of a specific saturable receptor in intact HeLa cells, but we were concerned that the detection of these receptors might have been masked by the nonspecific partitioning of the highly hydrophobic TPA into the lipid phases of the cell (31). Recently, Blumberg and his colleagues have utilized ^{3}H-phorbol dibutyrate (PDBu), which is much less hydrophobic, to overcome this problem and have obtained direct evidence for specific high-affinity, saturable receptors in crude membrane preparations of chick embryo fibroblasts (13) and mouse epidermis (9). In an extension of these important results, we have utilized ^{3}H-PDBu to demonstrate cell surface receptors for this class of compounds in intact cell monolayers of rat embryo (RE) fibroblast cultures and have characterized several properties of these receptors (23,58).

When subconfluent monolayer cultures of a cloned subline of a Fischer RE cell line, designated CREF, were incubated with 3 nM ^{3}H-PDBu at 37°C, we found that specific binding occurred rapidly and reached a maximum within 10 min (Fig. 1A). Specific binding decreased slightly (24%) by 20 min, but remained constant thereafter for at least 3 hr at 37°C. The decrease between 10 and 20 min was observed repeatedly but its significance is not known. At 4°C, specific ^{3}H-PDBu binding required 3 hr to reach a maximum but the plateau value was similar to that at 37°C. Nonspecific binding, i.e. binding in the presence of an excess of unlabeled PDBu (50 μM), was measured in parallel

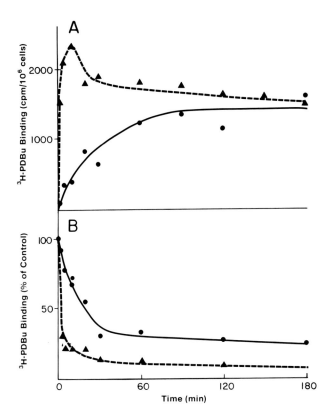

FIG. 1. A: Time course of specific binding of ^{3}H-PDBu to monolayers of intact CREF cells. ^{3}H-PDBu binding was conducted at: ▲, 37°C; or ●, 4°C. Each point is the average of duplicate plates. Duplicates agreed within 10%. All values have been corrected for nonspecific binding, which was determined in parallel assays. For additional details, see ref. 23. **B:** Dissociation of ^{3}H-PDBu from CREF cells. ^{3}H-PDBu was allowed to bind to monolayers of CREF cells (2 × 10⁶ cell/dish) at 37°C for 30 min, as in **A.** The assay buffer was then rapidly replaced with fresh assay buffer lacking ^{3}H-PDBu, and the monolayers were incubated for varying time intervals at: ▲, 37°C; or ●, 4°C. Binding of ^{3}H-PDBu is plotted as percent of the initial binding. All values have been corrected for nonspecific binding.

with total binding and the former value was subtracted from the total binding to obtain the specific binding. We found that nonspecific ^{3}H-PDBu binding was complete within 30 min, at either 37°C or 4°C. At equilibrium binding of 3 nM ^{3}H-PDBu, it accounted for less than one-third of the total cell-associated radioactivity.

When binding of ^{3}H-PDBu at 37°C was allowed to reach a plateau and the cell monolayer then transferred to buffer lacking ^{3}H-PDBu, the bound radioactivity was rapidly released from the cells. At 37°C most of the specifically bound ^{3}H-PDBu was released within 10 min. At 4°C, 70% of the specifically bound ^{3}H-PDBu was released within 30 min, and a slow release of the remaining radioactivity occurred thereafter (Fig. 1B). Since in intact cell monolayers [3]H-

PDBu binding at 37°C rapidly reaches a plateau and is also rapidly reversible, it appears that these receptors are on the cell surface, presumably associated with the plasma membrane (see also Shoyab and Todaro, *this volume*).

Several types of compounds were tested at 37°C for inhibition of specific binding of ^{3}H-PDBu to CREF cells. Phorbol and 4-α-phorbol-12,13-didecanoate (4-αPDD), which lack tumor-promoting activity in mouse skin and also lack activity in various cell culture assays (3,54,57), were inactive, even when tested at 1,000 ng/ml. TPA was a potent inhibitor and had an ID_{50} of 30 ng/ml (i.e., concentration required to inhibit specific ^{3}H-PDBu binding 50%). In collaboration with Umezawa et al. (55), we found that teleocidin B is also a potent inhibitor of ^{3}H-PDBu binding with an ID_{50} of 3 ng/ml. Mezerein, which has many of the same effects as TPA in cell culture (54,57) and is quite potent when used during the second phase of tumor promotion on mouse skin (53 and Slaga, *this volume*) had an ID_{50} of 20 ng/ml. Although in monolayer cultures, epidermal growth factor (EGF)-receptor binding is inhibited by TPA and PDBu (7,30,32,33,52), EGF did not inhibit ^{3}H-PDBu binding. These results are consistent with evidence that the phorbol ester inhibition of EGF binding is exerted via an indirect mechanism, rather than by direct competition for binding to the same set of receptors (7,32,33,52). Platelet-derived growth factor and fibroblast growth factor also failed to inhibit ^{3}H-PDBu binding. Arginine and lysine vasopressins, luteinizing hormone releasing hormone (LHRH), diazepam, concanavalin A, wheat germ agglutinin, and 4-α-methyl glucoside were also negative. The vasopressins were of interest since they share certain effects in cell culture with TPA (12). Diazepam was tested since it binds to high-affinity receptors, can modulate differentiation in cell culture (36), and, like TPA, inhibits metabolic cooperation (Trosko et al., *this volume*). The negative results obtained with concanavalin A, wheat germ agglutinin, and 4-α-methyl-glucoside suggest that the related polysaccharide residues are not part of the phorbol ester binding sites.

The fact that the abilities of a series of TPA analogs to compete with ^{3}H-PDBu for binding to cell surface receptors correlates with their known potencies in cell culture and, with the exception of mezerein, with their activities as tumor promoters on mouse skin provides evidence that these receptors mediate the biologic action of these compounds. Similar structure-activity correlations have been seen in the phorbol ester-receptor binding studies of Blumberg et al. (9,13) and of Shoyab and Todaro *(this volume)*. Our finding that teleocidin B is a potent inhibitor of ^{3}H-PDBu binding is of particular interest since, although this compound is structurally unrelated to the phorbol esters, it shares with these compounds a number of biologic effects in cell culture (18) and is also as potent as TPA as a tumor promoter on mouse skin (19). In separate collaborative studies (55), we have found that like TPA, nanomolar concentrations of teleocidin B and dihydroteleocidin induce a rapid increase in 2-deoxyglucose uptake, induce arachidonic acid release and prostaglandin synthesis, and inhibit EGF-receptor binding. The results obtained with the teleocidins greatly strengthen the conclusion that the ^{3}H-PDBu receptors play a role in mediating the action of these tumor promoters. Further studies are, of course, required to determine if all of the biologic effects of the phorbol esters and teleocidins are mediated via these receptors and whether or not cellular internalization of the occupied receptors plays a role in mediating the pleiotropic cytoplasmic and nuclear events induced by these tumor promoters.

A Scatchard analysis of ^{3}H-PDBu binding to intact CREF cells indicated that the binding was nonlinear (Fig. 2). Although other interpretations have not been excluded, the results suggest that there are at least two classes of binding sites, a high-affinity class with a K_D of about 8 nM and 1.6 × 10^5 sites per cell, and a low-affinity class with a K_D of 710 nM and about 3 × 10^6 sites per cell. The large number of the latter sites suggests that they are not specific phorbol ester receptors, but structural elements in the cell to which these compounds also happen to bind. Our values for the K_D and total number of high-affinity ^{3}H-PDBu receptors in intact rat fibroblasts are in good agreement with the values obtained with crude membrane preparations from avian fibro-

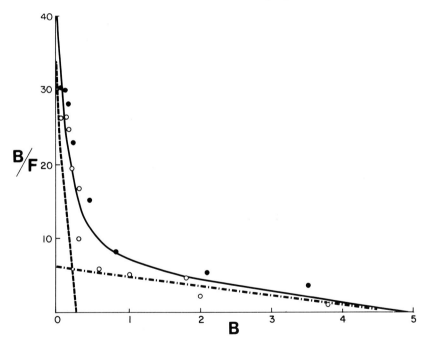

FIG. 2. Scatchard plot of specific binding of ^{3}H-PDBu to CREF cells. Each point is the average of duplicate plates. The results from two separate experiments are shown (● and ○). Binding assays were performed on approximately 2 × 10^6 cell/dish at 37°C for 30 min. Bound ^{3}H-PDBu (B) is expressed as pmole per 10^6 cells, and is corrected for nonspecific binding. The concentration of ^{3}H-PDBu in the binding solution (F) is in μmole/l. The data are consistent with two binding sites, with K_{D_1} = 7.6 nM, at 1.6 × 10^5 sites/cell; and K_{D_2} = 710 nM, at 2.8 × 10^6 sites/cell. Binding to the first site is shown by -----; and to the second, by ...... For additional details, see ref. 23.

blasts or mouse epidermis (9,13).

Using our intact cell assay, we have also detected similar ^{3}H-PDBu receptors in a variety of cell types including Friend erythroleukemia cells, the mouse embryo fibroblast cell line 10T½, the rat liver epithelial cell line K22, and an adenovirus-transformed RE cell line. The intact cell assay for phorbol ester receptors should facilitate further studies on the physiology of this unusual receptor-ligand system.

A curious finding is that after prolonged exposure, cells in culture can become refractory to TPA-induced inhibition of EGF-receptor binding (32,33). This is consistent with evidence that following prolonged exposure, cell cultures can escape from TPA inhibition of differentiation (10,43). Although other mechanisms have not been excluded, this could reflect down-regulation of the phorbol ester receptors. This phenomenon could play an important role in tissue-specific and dose-scheduling effects of TPA.

INHIBITION OF ^{3}H-PDBu BINDING BY SERUM AND TISSUE EXTRACTS

During the course of our studies, we found that preincubation of cultures in the absence of serum at 37°C for 30 min prior to the addition of ^{3}H-PDBu led to a twofold increase in specific ^{3}H-PDBu binding. This suggested that serum might contain a substance that inhibits ^{3}H-PDBu binding. Indeed, we found that sera from several species caused a concentration-dependent inhibition of ^{3}H-PDBu binding to CREF cells (23). The human serum produced 50% inhibition of ^{3}H-PDBu binding at a concentration of about 4 mg/ml. Human serum from platelet-depleted plasma was also active, suggesting that the inhibitory activity is not derived from platelets. Lipoprotein-depleted human serum was also active, suggesting that the effect did not reflect nonspecific trapping of the ^{3}H-PDBu in serum lipids. Significant activity was also detected in rhesus monkey serum, rat serum, human amniotic fluid, and extracts from RE or rat liver. Although purified serum albumin did inhibit ^{3}H-PDBu binding, this occurred only with concentrations that were 10-fold greater than that required with an equivalent amount of serum. Presumably, the inhibition obtained with these high concentrations of albumin reflects its capacity to bind phorbol esters nonspecifically (31).

When CREF cells were incubated in serum, the inhibition of ^{3}H-PDBu binding was immediate and sustained. If cells were preincubated in the presence of 50% serum for 60 min and binding of ^{3}H-PDBu was then measured, after replacing the medium with serum-free medium, a gradual recovery of ^{3}H-PDBu binding was seen, which reached a maximum after about 2 hr. This indicates that inhibition of ^{3}H-PDBu binding by serum is reversible. The effect of human serum on ^{3}H-PDBu binding did not require cellular metabolic functions or intact cells, since we found that serum and amniotic fluid inhibited ^{3}H-PDBu binding in a crude membrane preparation to a similar extent as with intact cells. In addition, human serum was able to inhibit ^{3}H-PDBu binding at both 4° and 37°C. The latter findings are in contrast to the inhibition by tumor-promoting phorbol esters of EGF-receptor binding, which appears to be due to an indirect effect rather than direct competition for EGF receptors (32,33).

Human serum was fractionated by affinity chromatography, ion exchange, and gel filtration to partially purify the above factor. This yielded material that was enriched about 135-fold, with an ID_{50} of 0.04 mg/ml compared to 5.4 mg/ml for the unfractionated serum. The partially purified serum factor was free of albumin, was active after precipitation with cold 80% ethanol, was inactivated by heating at 70°C for 10 min, and had a MW of approximately 60,000 (23). Studies are in progress to determine whether this factor inhibits ^{3}H-PDBu binding to cells by binding ^{3}H-PDBu itself, by indirectly inhibiting cellular binding of ^{3}H-PDBu, or by actually occupying the cellular phorbol ester receptors. It will also be of interest to determine whether this factor inhibits the biologic effects of the phorbol ester tumor promoters or actually produces effects on cells similar to those of tumor promoters.

ASSOCIATED CHANGES IN PHOSPHOLIPID METABOLISM

It is of interest that the high-affinity binding sites for phorbol ester tumor promoters appear to be located, at least in part, in the plasma membrane, since there is considerable evidence that the earliest responses of cells to these compounds involve alterations in membrane structure and function (57). These aspects also apply to teleocidin B (55). Several of these membrane-related effects occur within minutes after exposing cell cultures to TPA and are not blocked by inhibitors of protein or ribonucleic acid (RNA) synthesis, suggesting that they result from a direct action of TPA on cell membranes. This is true for the enhancement of 2-deoxyglucose uptake, altered membrane "fluidity," altered cell adhesion, the induction of phospholipid turnover, and the inhibition of EGF-receptor binding (57). The facts that TPA can induce morphologic changes in enucleated chick embryo fibroblasts and induce aggregation of platelets (that lack a nucleus) provide further evidence that the primary effects of TPA do not occur at the nuclear level. On the other hand, several later effects, for example, plasminogen activator synthesis (59), do require RNA and protein synthesis.

The effects of TPA on phospholipid metabolism may be of particular importance, since alterations in the lipid matrix of cell membranes might play a role in mediating some of the membrane-related effects of TPA. Previous studies have shown that TPA induces an increase in the incorporation of P^{32} or choline into membrane phospholipids (27,50,61). It also induces deacylation of phospholipids with release of arachidonic acid and an increase in prostaglandin synthesis (34,42,63).

Recently, we have discovered that TPA induces the release of choline from the phospholipids of C3H10T½ cells prelabeled with ^{3}H-choline (45,58). Within

5 min of exposure to TPA, the release of radioactivity was enhanced twofold, and by 60 to 120 min the release was four to five times that of vehicle controls. Choline metabolite release was concentration-dependent between 10 and 100 ng TPA/ml. PDD was also active, but 4-αPDD, which is not a tumor promoter, was inactive. The radioactivity released by TPA appears to be derived from phosphatidyl choline, since changes in the acid-soluble pool of choline metabolites or in labeled sphingomyelin were insufficient to account for the amount of material released. The released material was identified by chromatography as choline and phosphoryl choline. Neither cycloheximide (4 to 40 μg/ml) nor cordycepin (4 to 40 μg/ml) blocked the TPA-induced release. The release was, however, temperature sensitive and did not occur at 4°C. Although previous studies indicate that certain mitogens and other agonists induce the release of inositol from phosphatidyl inositol (38), we found that this was not the case with TPA. The calcium ionophore A23187 and EGF enhanced ^{3}H-arachidonic acid and ^{3}H-prostaglandin release, but neither of these compounds induced choline release. This difference between the effects of A23187 and TPA is of interest since although A23187 is not a complete tumor promoter on mouse skin (Marks, *this volume,* and Slaga, *this volume*), it can induce epidermal hyperplasia (Marks, *this volume*), it enhances the first stage of tumor promotion, and induces an increase in dark cells (Slaga, *this volume*). It is possible, therefore, that the TPA-induced release of choline from phosphatidyl choline is a necessary event during tumor promotion.

The major pathways of phosphatidyl choline turnover and a hypothetical scheme for the effects of TPA on these pathways is given in Fig. 3. Our studies suggest that TPA-induced choline release is due to activation of an endogenous membrane-associated phospholipase C or D, although other mechanisms have not been excluded. TPA-induced arachidonic acid release and prostaglandin synthesis could be due to the subsequent action of a diacylglycerol lipase. Alternatively, TPA could have an independent effect on phospholipase A_2. To our knowledge, the phorbol ester tumor promoters are the only known agonists that specifically induce choline release from cellular phospholipids. Since other investigators have found that TPA also specifically induces the incorporation of P^{32} or choline into phosphatidyl choline (27,50,61), it appears that the action of TPA is intimately involved in the turnover of phosphatidyl choline. The studies of Wertz and Mueller (61), indicating that TPA enhances the activity of CDP-choline transferase in bovine lymphocytes, is consistent with this conclusion and might reflect compensatory resynthesis of phosphatidyl choline. Presumably, the occupancy of different cell surface receptors by their respective agonists induces different types of alterations in membrane phospholipids. As mentioned above, certain mitogens and cholinergic agonists affect phosphatidyl inositol metabolism (38). Hirata and Axelrod (22) have demonstrated that certain ligands enhance the methylation of phosphatidyl ethanolamine, but this effect is not seen with TPA (Mufson and Weinstein, *unpublished studies*).

It is not known how these membrane effects of TPA might induce signals

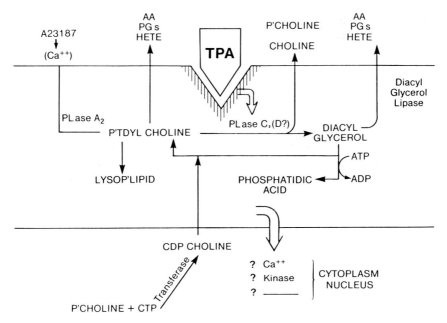

FIG. 3. Schematic diagram of effects of TPA and related compounds on phosphatidylcholine turnover. We postulate that the binding of TPA to specific cell membrane receptors activates phospholipase (PLase) C and/or D, resulting in the conversion of phosphatidylcholine (P'TDYL Choline) to diacylglycerol plus choline. Arachidonic acid (AA) is then released by diacylglycerol lipase; prostaglandins (PGs) and other AA metabolites are also formed. AA also may be released by the direct action of PLase A₂ on P'TDYL Choline. The calcium ionophore A23187 and melittin may induce AA release via the latter mechanism. P'TDYL Choline may be resynthesized via CDP choline, as shown. Presumably, during these biochemical transformations, a transmembrane signal to the cytoplasm and/or nucleus is generated, i.e., increased Ca^{2+} uptake or redistribution, activation of a protein kinase, or some other mediator. For additional details see text and refs. 45 and 58.

or second messengers that mediate the subsequent cytoplasmic and nuclear events. An increase in intracellular Ca^{2+} concentration, enhanced protein kinase activity, or release of yet unidentified mediators remain to be explored as potential candidates for these effects. Studies related to the effects of TPA on Ca^{2+} metabolism are discussed below. Elsewhere, we have postulated that the apparent role of dietary lipid in enhancing colon and breast cancer may be mediated by changes in membrane lipids similar to those produced by TPA (56).

PHORBOL ESTERS AND CALCIUM METABOLISM

Several findings suggest that alterations in Ca^{2+} uptake and/or intracellular distribution may play a role in mediating the cytoplasmic and nuclear events induced by TPA. As mentioned above, the calcium ionophore A23187 mimics some but not all of the actions of TPA. Michell et al. (38) have proposed that the effects of certain agonists on phosphatidyl inositol turnover might be coupled to alterations in membrane Ca^{2+} flux. The above described effects of TPA on phosphatidyl choline turnover might, therefore, also alter Ca^{2+} flux. In chick embryo myoblasts, TPA induced inhibition of Ca^{2+} influx within 90 sec after its addition, whereas TPA increased Ca^{2+} uptake in multinucleated myotubes (51). TPA is mitogenic to lymphocytes but only in the presence of Ca^{2+}, and this mitogenic effect is synergistic with the calcium ionophore A23187 (62).

There is considerable evidence that Ca^{2+} plays an important role in modulating the growth of normal fibroblast and epithelial cells. In general, normal cells exhibit negligible or limited growth in media containing a low Ca^{2+} concentration (0.001 to 0.01 mM rather than 1.25 mM), and transformation by chemical carcinogens or viruses enhances the ability of cells to grow in low Ca^{2+} media (for review, see refs. 4,16,17). Since TPA induces a number of phenotypic effects that mimic properties of transformed cells (57), and since EGF and TPA share a number of similar phenotypic effects (30), it is of interest that both TPA (4,5,16,17) and EGF (17,29,37) can enhance the growth of either normal or transformed cells in media containing low Ca^{2+}. Our recent studies (17) on the effects of TPA on Ca^{2+} requirements for growth of normal RE and adenovirus-transformed RE cells at various stages of progression of the transformed phenotype are summarized below.

We found that several early passage normal RE cultures grew two- to sixfold better during a 5-day period in standard Ca^{2+} (1.25 mM) medium than in low Ca^{2+} (0.01 mM) medium. The addition of TPA enhanced growth two- to threefold in the low Ca^{2+} medium, but produced less than a 1.25-fold enhancement in standard medium. An early passage clone (A18-E) of RE cells transformed by the H5ts125 mutant of adenovirus type 5, which shows morphologic transformation but is still anchorage-dependent for growth (14,15), grew 3.5-fold better in 1.25 mM than in 0.01 mM Ca^{2+} medium. With a late passage of the same clone (A18-L), which had acquired anchorage independence (14,15), this difference in Ca^{2+} requirement disappeared. TPA caused about a twofold enhancement of the growth of A18-E and A18-L cells in low Ca^{2+} medium, but produced less than a 1.25-fold stimulation in standard medium.

Dose-response studies with A18-E cells indicated that concentrations of TPA as low as 0.1 ng/ml enhanced growth in low Ca^{2+} medium and that 10 ng/ml gave the maximum stimulation. The tumor-promoting phorbol esters, phorbol-12,13-dibenzoate (PDB) and PDD, as well as the antileukemic compounds, mezerein and ingenol-3,20-dibenzoate, also stimulated the growth of A18-E cells in both the standard and low Ca^{2+} media. With these compounds, as with TPA, the stimulation in low Ca^{2+} was greater than in standard Ca^{2+} medium. The compounds, phorbol, 4-αPDD, and 4-O-MeTPA, which are inactive as tumor promoters on mouse skin, did not enhance growth in either of these media. EGF and melittin (44) also stimulated the growth of A18-E cells, particularly in low Ca^{2+} medium. When 10 ng of TPA was combined with 10 ng of EGF, the growth-enhancing effect was greater than that obtained with either agent alone in low Ca^{2+} medium.

We also examined the uptake and accumulation of ^{45}Ca by normal and adeno-virus-transformed RE cells in the absence and presence of TPA (17). In the absence of TPA, there was a rapid uptake of cell-associated and membrane-associated ^{45}Ca during the first minute of exposure to ^{45}Ca. This was followed by a much slower accumulation during the subsequent 30 min. In normal RE, the values for membrane-associated ^{45}Ca were always greater than those for cell-associated ^{45}Ca, particularly at the early time points. With A18-E cells, however, cell-associated ^{45}Ca exceeded membrane-associated ^{45}Ca after only a 45-sec exposure to this isotope. TPA induced a small (approximately 20%) but reproducible stimulation of uptake of cell-associated ^{45}Ca, which was apparent within 15 sec. This effect, however, was transient and persisted for only about 1 min. Because the stimulation was small and only transient, we are not certain that it explains the above described ability of TPA to enhance cell growth in low Ca^{2+} medium. Further studies are required to determine if TPA exerts other effects on Ca^{2+} metabolism, for example, by altering the intracellular distribution of Ca^{2+} or by altering the activity or synthesis of calmodulin or other Ca^{2+} receptors. In this regard, it is of interest that certain tumor cells can apparently contain higher levels of calmodulin than normal cells (21).

THE TUMOR-PROMOTING ACTIVITY OF POLYCYCLIC AROMATIC HYDROCARBONS MAY BE MEDIATED BY THE AROMATIC HYDROCARBON RECEPTOR

Although the application of a single low dose of benzo(a)pyrene (BP) or other polycyclic aromatic hydrocarbon (PAH) carcinogens to mouse skin does not induce tumors unless followed by repeated applications of a tumor promoter, repeated applications of a PAH carcinogen alone will induce skin tumors (3,8,46). It is not clear whether this is because in the latter case carcinogenesis proceeds by a mechanism that does not involve tumor promotion, or that PAH can act both as initiators and as promoters. For this reason, we have recently studied the possibility that BP and related PAH carcinogens might induce certain bio-chemical effects that are similar to those induced by the phorbol ester tumor promoters (25). Because of the evidence cited above—that the primary effects of the phorbol esters are exerted at the cell membrane—we thought that it would be particularly interesting to look at membrane-related effects. For this purpose, we examined possible effects of BP on the binding of ^{125}I-EGF to intact cells, since inhibition of this binding provides a sensitive marker for membrane-related effects of the phorbol ester and teleocidin tumor promoters (30,55).

Figure 4 indicates that, indeed, the exposure of C3H10T½ cells to a nontoxic dose of BP (1 μM) leads to a marked inhibition of ^{125}I-EGF binding. Although the inhibition of EGF-receptor binding obtained with the phorbol esters occurs within a few minutes (30,31), the inhibition obtained with BP was maximal only after about 24 hr (Fig. 4). This suggested that the effect obtained with

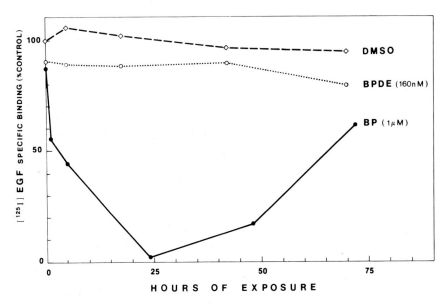

FIG. 4. The effects of BP, BP-7,8-dihydrodiol-9,10-oxide (BPDE), and the dimethylsulfoxide (DMSO) solvent (0.01%) on ^{125}I-EGF-receptor binding. The compounds were added at the indicated concentrations to confluent cultures of C3H10T½ cells, and ^{125}I-EGF binding measured at various time intervals thereafter. Binding assays were performed as previously described (32) for 50 min at 37°C.

BP was mediated by an indirect mechanism, perhaps related to a BP metabolite or as a consequence of DNA damage. We found, however, that the highly reactive metabolite and ultimate carcinogenic derivative of BP, BP-7,8-dihydro-diol-9,10-oxide, which reacts extensively with the DNA of these cells (6), did not inhibit ^{125}I-EGF binding (Fig. 4).

There is considerable evidence that the ability of BP and related PAH carcinogens to induce the cytochrome P_1-450 system and several other drug-metabolizing enzymes is mediated by binding to a specific cytosol receptor protein designated the Ah receptor (also called the TCDD receptor) (47,49). With a series of compounds, we found (25) a rather good correlation between their abilities to inhibit ^{125}I-EGF binding to 10T½ cells and published data (47,49) on their apparent affinities for the Ah receptor. Thus cholesterol, progesterone, and 17-β-estradiol had very little effect; nor was significant inhibition observed with phenobarbital, 2,2-di(p-chlorophenyl)-1,1,1-trichloroethane (pp′DDT), hexachlorobenzene, or pregnenolone-16α-carbonitrile. These compounds do not bind to the Ah receptor with high affinity, although some of them induce P-450's that are distinct from P_1-450 (47). On the other hand, several known inducers of P_1-450 that have a high affinity for the Ah receptor were very effective inhibitors of EGF binding, and these had the following order of potency: dimethylbenz(a)anthracene > BP > benz(a)anthracene > 3-methylcholanthrene

$> \beta$-naphthoflavone. With the active compounds, the time courses for inhibition of ^{125}I-EGF binding were similar to that obtained with BP.

The above findings lead us to propose that binding of certain compounds to the Ah receptor induces a pleiotropic program that includes not only increases in certain drug-metabolizing enzymes, but also changes in membrane structure and function and other biochemical effects that are similar to those induced by the phorbol ester tumor promoters. Consistent with this hypothesis are published data that, like the phorbol esters, PAH carcinogens can induce ornithine decarboxylase (ODC) (46) and also the release of arachidonic acid from membrane phospholipids (35). It is of interest that the effects of PAH on EGF-receptor binding (25), ODC induction (46), and arachidonic acid release (35) are much more delayed than those produced by TPA. Ultraviolet light and certain carcinogens also induce plasminogen activator, again with a much longer delay than seen with TPA (40). The authors attributed this effect to DNA damage (40), but other mechanisms were not excluded. The repeated application of PAH to mouse skin induces a generalized hyperplasia, metaplasia, and inflammation (46), histologic effects that also mimic those of the phorbol ester tumor promoters. The compound TCDD, which binds to the Ah receptor with an extremely high affinity (49), can induce disorders in epidermal cell growth and differentiation (28,49), and TCDD is an extremely potent tumor promoter in rat liver (48). When BP was used as a "complete" carcinogen for the induction of subcutaneous sarcomas or pulmonary tumors, the susceptibility of different genetic strains of mice to tumor formation correlated with aryl hydrocarbon hydroxylase (AHH) inducibility and the presence of high-affinity Ah receptors (1,47). On the other hand, no correlation between the Ah locus and skin tumor induction was found when BP was used as an initiator on mouse skin followed by promotion with TPA (1). Although other explanations have not been excluded, these results support our hypothesis that the Ah receptor system plays an important role in tumor promotion, if we assume that in the experiments in which BP was used as a complete carcinogen, BP was serving both as an initiator and a promoter.

Thus, whereas the effects of the phorbol esters appear to be mediated by binding to specific, high-affinity receptors in the plasma membrane (9,13,23, and Shoyab and Todaro, *this volume*), we suggest that certain PAH carcinogens achieve their tumor-promoting activity by binding to the Ah receptors in the cytosol, and that this binding induces a complex set of events, some of which overlap those induced via the phorbol ester receptors. The tissue and species specificities of certain complete carcinogens could, therefore, be a function of not only their ability to generate metabolites that bind covalently to cellular macromolecules, but also their ability to interact with specific protein receptors in target tissues and whether or not occupancy of these receptors induces in that target tissue biochemical events that contribute to the process of tumor promotion.

A UNIFIED THEORY OF INITIATION AND PROMOTION

The mechanism by which tumor promoters enhance the conversion of initiated cells to tumor cells must take into account the mechanism of action of initiating carcinogens. Although current evidence suggests that covalent binding of carcinogens like BP to cellular DNA is the critical event in initiation, the subsequent biochemical events that lead to establishment of the initiated cell are not known. Possible mechanisms have been discussed in detail elsewhere (See Table 1 and refs. 56,58,60).

The initiating event in chemical carcinogenesis is often described as a simple random point mutation resulting from errors in replicating the damaged DNA. Data from several laboratories, however, indicate that the frequency of transformation of rodent cell cultures induced by radiation or carcinogens can be 10 to several hundred times that obtained for the induction of mutations to specific markers such as drug resistance, even when both types of phenomena are scored in the same cell culture system (for review, see ref. 58). This discrepancy is even greater when one considers the likelihood that cell transformation occurs via a multistep process that is limited, therefore, by the joint probabilities of each of the successive steps. Thus the initial step induced by the carcinogen may occur with an even greater frequency than the net transformation frequency. Indeed, there is evidence that when exposure to chemical carcinogens (41) or radiation (26) occurs at low cell densities, almost 100% of the exposed cells are capable of giving rise to progeny that are transformed. The fact that the phorbol ester tumor promoters enhance the transformation frequency in cultures previously exposed to chemical carcinogens or radiation also provides evidence that we tend to underestimate the frequency of the initial event induced by chemical carcinogens or radiation.

Our laboratory has recently found that mutagenesis by BP-7,8-dihydrodiol-9,10-oxide in *E. coli* is mediated via "SOS" functions (24). It is not known if similar responses to DNA damage occur in eukaryotic cells, and if so, what the components of this response might be. Nevertheless, these results raise the possibility that DNA damage could induce host responses that mediate initiation of the carcinogenic process with high efficiency. Elsewhere (58), we have discussed the possibility that during normal development, the establishment of specific populations of stem cells involves gene transpositions (for evidence of

TABLE 1. *Possible molecular mechanisms of initiation of the carcinogenic process*

A. *With permanent changes in DNA sequence:*
1. Random point mutations
   a. Direct: base substitution, frame shift, deletion in structural or regulatory gene.
   b. Indirect: induction of "SOS-type," error-prone DNA synthesis.
2. Ordered gene rearrangements: transposition, amplification, deletion, integration of exogenous sequences, etc.
B. *Without permanent changes in DNA sequence:*
   Altered chromatin structure, altered DNA methylation, altered feedback loops, etc.

TABLE 2. *Mechanism of action of initiating carcinogens: Evidence against random mutation and favoring gene transposition*[a]

A. High frequency of cell transformation *in vitro* speaks against random mutation:
   1. This has been seen with chemical carcinogens or X-ray, in 10T½ mouse embryo or hamster embryo cultures.
   2. The transformation frequency >> frequency of mutation at specific loci, even in the same cell system.
   3. "Initiation" of transformation by chemical carcinogens or radiation can approach 100% at low cell density.
B. Certain characteristics of gene transposition suggest that it could play a role in carcinogenesis:
   1. Gene transposition occurs not only in prokaryotes but also in eukaryotes (i.e., cassette model in yeast, immunoglobulin synthesis in mammals).
   2. Gene transposition occurs with high specificity and efficiency.
C. Models suggested from the action of retroviruses:
   1. Multiple sarc genes exist in normal vertebrate cells.
   2. Transformation by retroviruses resembles gene transposition.

[a] For details related to points (1) and (2), see Weinstein et al. (58). For a review on sarc genes and retroviruses, see Bishop (2).

gene transpositions and their possible role in chemical carcinogenesis, see Table 2 and ref. 58). We have postulated that DNA damage by initiating carcinogens might induce aberrant forms of gene transposition, thus establishing aberrant stem cells (58). The subsequent role of tumor promoters could be to enhance the outgrowth of these cells, as well as "switch on" their aberrant programs of differentiation, just as normal growth factors might induce normal stem cells to grow and express their specialized functions. Presumably, the phorbol ester tumor promoters accomplish this by binding to and usurping the function of receptors normally occupied by endogenous factors that control stem cell replication and differentiation. Following repeated exposure of initiated cells to TPA, a neoplastic population might eventually emerge which grows autonomously in the absence of TPA, perhaps due to further changes in genome structure. Certain aspects of this hypothesis are currently being tested in our laboratory.

ACKNOWLEDGMENTS

This research was supported by NCI Grants CA-26056 and CA-21111 (to I. Bernard Weinstein), NCI Fellowship CA06747 (to Ellen Greenebaum), and an award from the Dupont Company.

REFERENCES

1. Benedict, W. F., Considine, N., and Nebert, D. W. (1973): Genetic differences in aryl hydrocarbon hydroxylase induction and benzo(a)pyrene-produced tumorigenesis in the mouse. *Mol. Pharmacol.,* 6:266–277.
2. Bishop, J. M. (1980): The molecular biology of RNA tumor viruses: A physician's guide. *N. Engl. J. Med.,* 303:675–682.

3. Boutwell, R. K. (1974): The function and mechanism of promoters of carcinogenesis. *CRC Crit. Rev. Toxicol.,* 2:419–443.

4. Boynton, A. L., and Whitfield, J. F. (1980): Stimulation of DNA synthesis in calcium-deprived T51B liver cells by the tumor promoters phenobarbitol, saccharin, and 12-O-tetradecanoylphorbol-13-acetate. *Cancer Res.,* 40:4,541–4,545.

5. Boynton, A. L., Whitfield, J. F., and Trembley, R. J. (1975): Calcium-dependent stimulation of BALB/c 3T3 mouse cell DNA synthesis by a tumor-promoting phorbol ester (PMA). *J. Cell. Physiol.,* 87:25–32.

6. Brown, H. S., Jeffrey, A. M., and Weinstein, I. B. (1979): Formation of DNA adducts in 10T½ mouse embryo fibroblasts incubated with benzo(a)pyrene or dihydrodiol derivatives. *Cancer Res.,* 39:1,673–1,677.

7. Brown, K. D., Dicker, P., and Rozengurt, E. (1979): Inhibition of epidermal growth factor binding to surface receptors by tumor promoters. *Biochem. Biophys. Res. Commun.,* 86:1,037–1,043.

8. Burns, F. J., and Albert, R. E. (1980): Mouse skin papillomas as an early marker of carcinogenesis. *J. Environ. Toxicol. Pathol. (in press).*

9. Delclos, K. B., Nagle, D. S., and Blumberg, P. M. (1980): Specific binding of phorbol ester tumor promoters to mouse skin. *Cell,* 19:1,025–1,032.

10. Diamond, L., O'Brien, T. G., and Rovera, G. (1977): Inhibition of adipose conversion of 3T3 fibroblasts by tumor promoters. *Nature,* 269:247–248.

11. Diamond, L., O'Brien, T. G., and Rovera, G. (1978): Tumor promoters: Effects on proliferation and differentiation of cells in culture. *Life Sci.,* 23:1,979–1,988.

12. Dicker, P., and Rozengurt, E. (1980): Phorbol esters and vasopressin stimulate DNA synthesis by a common mechanism. *Nature,* 280:607–612.

13. Driedger, P. E., and Blumberg, P. M. (1980): Specific binding of phorbol ester tumor promoters. *Proc. Natl. Acad. Sci. USA,* 77:567–571.

14. Fisher, P. B., Bozzone, J. H., and Weinstein, I. B. (1979): Tumor promoter and epidermal growth factor stimulate anchorage-independent growth of adenovirus-transformed rat embryo cells. *Cell,* 18:695–705.

15. Fisher, P. B., Goldstein, N. I., and Weinstein, I. B. (1979): Phenotypic properties and tumor promoter-induced alterations in rat embryo cells transformed by adenovirus. *Cancer Res.,* 39:3,051–3,057.

16. Fisher, P. B., and Weinstein, I. B. (1980a): Effects of tumor promoters and extracellular calcium on the growth of normal, transformed, and temperature-sensitive rat liver epithelial cells. *Cancer Letters,* 10:7–17.

17. Fisher, P. B., and Weinstein, I. B. (1980b): Enhancement of cell proliferation in low calcium medium by tumor promoters. *Carcinogenesis,* 2:89–95.

18. Fujiki, H., Mori, M., Nakayasu, M., Terada, M., and Sugimura, T. (1979): A possible naturally occurring tumor promoter, teleocidin B, from *streptomyces. Biochem. Biophys. Res. Commun.,* 90:976–983.

19. Fujiki, H., Mori, M., Nakayasu, M., Terada, M., Sugimura, T., and Moore, R. (1981): Indole alkaloids, dihydroteleocidin B, teleocidin, and lyngbyatoxi A: A new class of tumor promoters. (See also Fujiki et al., *this volume*). *Proc. Natl. Acad. Sci. USA,* 78:3872–3876.

20. Grunberger, D., and Weinstein, I. B. (1979): Conformational changes in nucleic acids modified by chemical carcinogens. In: *Chemical Carcinogens and DNA,* edited by P. L. Grover, pp. 59–93. CRC Press, Boca Raton, Florida.

21. Hard, G., Clarke, F. M., and Toh, B. H. (1980): Comparison of polypeptide profiles in normal and transformed kidney cell lines derived from control, dimethylnitrosamine-treated, and renal tumor-bearing rats, with particular reference to contractile proteins. *Cancer Res.,* 40:3,728–3,734.

22. Hirata, F., and Axelrod, J. (1980): Phospholipid methylation and biological signal transmission. *Science,* 209:1,082–1,090.

23. Horowitz, A. D., Greenebaum, E., and Weinstein, I. B. (1981): Identification of receptors for phorbol ester tumor promoters in intact mammalian cells and of an inhibitor of receptor binding in biologic fluids. *Proc. Natl. Acad. Sci. USA,* 78:2,315–2,319.

24. Ivanovic, V., and Weinstein, I. B. (1980): Genetic factors in *Escherichia coli* that affect cell killing and mutagenesis induced by benzo(a)pyrene-7,8-dihydrodiol-9,10-oxide. *Cancer Res.,* 40:3,508–3,511.

25. Ivanovic, V., and Weinstein, I. B. (1981): Benzo(a)pyrene and other inducers of cytochrome

P₁-450 inhibit binding of epidermal growth factor (EGF) to cell surface receptors. *J. Supramolec Structure* (Suppl.) S (abstr.) 232.

26. Kennedy, A. R., and Little, J. B. (1980): High efficiency, kinetics, and numerology of transformation by radiation *in vitro*. In: *Cancer 1980: Achievement, Challenges, Prospects. International Symposium on Cancer Proceedings (in press)*. (See also Little et al., *this volume*).

27. Kinzel, V., Kreibich, G., Hecker, E., and Suss, R. (1979): Stimulation of choline incorporation in cell cultures by phorbol derivatives and its correlation with their irritant and tumor-promoting activity. *Cancer Res.*, 39:2,743–2,750.

28. Knudson, J. C., and Poland, A. (1980): Keratinization of mouse teratoma cell line XB produced by 2,3,7,8-tetrachlorodibenzo-*p*-dioxin: An *in vitro* model of toxicity. *Cell*, 22:27–36.

29. Lechner, J. F., and Kaighn, M. D. (1979): Reduction of the calcium requirement of normal human epithelial cells by EGF. *Exp. Cell Res.*, 123:432–435.

30. Lee, L. S., and Weinstein, I. B. (1978*a*): Tumor-promoting phorbol esters inhibit binding of epidermal growth factor to cellular receptors. *Science*, 202:313–315.

31. Lee, L. S., and Weinstein, I. B. (1978*b*): Uptake of the tumor-promoting agent 12-O-tetradecanoylphorbol-13-acetate by HeLa cells. *J. Environ. Pathol. Toxicol.*, 1:627–639.

32. Lee, L. S., and Weinstein, I. B. (1979): Mechanism of tumor promoter inhibition of cellular binding of epidermal growth factor. *Proc. Natl. Acad. Sci. USA*, 76:5,168–5,172.

33. Lee, L. S., and Weinstein, I. B. (1980): Studies on the mechanism by which a tumor promoter inhibits binding of epidermal growth factor to cellular receptors. *Carcinogenesis*, 1:669–678.

34. Levine, L., and Hassid, A. (1977): Effects of phorbol-12,13-diesters on prostaglandin production and phospholipase activity in canine kidney (MDCK) cells. *Biochem. Biophys. Res. Commun.*, 79:477–483.

35. Levine, L., and Ohuchi, K. (1978): Stimulation by carcinogens and promoters of prostaglandin production by dog kidney (MDCK) cells in culture. *Cancer Res.*, 38:4,142–4,146.

36. Matthew, E., Laskin, J. D., Zimmerman, E. A., Weinstein, I. B., Hsu, K. C., and Engelhardt, D. L. (1981): Benzodiazepines have high-affinity binding sites and induce melanogenesis in B16 mouse melanoma cells. *Proc. Natl. Acad. Sci. USA*, 78:3,935–3,939.

37. McKeehan, W. L., and McKeehan, K. A. (1979): Epidermal growth factor modulates extracellular Ca²⁺ requirement for multiplication of normal human skin fibroblasts. *Exp. Cell. Res.*, 123:397–400.

38. Michell, R. H., Jafferji, S. S., and Jones, L. M. (1977): The possible involvement of phosphatidylinositol breakdown in the mechanism of stimulus-response coupling at receptors which control cell surface calcium gates. In: *Function and Biosynthesis of Lipids*, edited by N. G. Bazam, R. R. Brenner, and N. M. Guisto, pp. 447–464. Plenum Press, New York.

39. Miller, E. (1978): Some current perspectives on chemical carcinogenesis in human and experimental animals. Presidential address, *Cancer Res.*, 38:1,479–1,496.

40. Miskin, R., and Reich, E. (1980): Plasminogen activator: Induction of synthesis by DNA damage. *Cell*, 19:217–224.

41. Mondal, S., and Heidelberger, C. (1970): *In vitro* malignant transformation by methylcholanthrene of the progeny of single cells derived from C3H mouse prostate. *Proc. Natl. Acad. Sci. USA*, 65:219–225.

42. Mufson, R. A., DeFeo, D., and Weinstein, I. B. (1979): Effects of phorbol ester tumor promoters on arachidonic acid metabolism in chick embryo fibroblasts. *Mol. Pharmacol.*, 16:569–578.

43. Mufson, R. A., Fisher, P. B., and Weinstein, I. B. (1979): Effect of phorbol ester tumor promoters on the expression of melanogenesis in B-16 melanoma cells. *Cancer Res.*, 39:3,915–3,919.

44. Mufson, R. A., Laskin, J. D., Fisher, P. B., and Weinstein, I. B. (1979): Melittin shares certain cellular effects with phorbol ester tumor promoters. *Nature*, 280:72–74.

45. Mufson, R. A., and Weinstein, I. B. (1980): Phorbol esters stimulate the rapid release of choline from cellular phosphatidyl choline. *Proc. Am. Assoc. Cancer Res.*, (abstr.), 21:117.

46. O'Brien, T. G. (1976): The induction of ornithine decarboxylase as an early, possibly obligatory, event in mouse skin carcinogenesis. *Cancer Res.*, 36:2,644–2,653.

47. Okey, A. B., Bondy, G. P., Mason, M. E., Kahl, G. F., Eisen, H. J., Guenther, T. M., and Nebert, D. W. (1979): Regulatory gene product of the Ah locus. Characterization of the cytosolic inducer-receptor complex and evidence for its nuclear translocation. *J. Biol. Chem.*, 254:11,636–11,648.

48. Pitot, H. C., Goldsworthy, T., Campbell, H. A., and Poland, A. (1980): Quantitative evaluation of the promotion by 2,3,7,8-tetrachlorodibenzo-*p*-dioxin of hepatocarcinogenesis from diethylnitrosamine. *Cancer Res.*, 40:3,616–3,620.

49. Poland, A., Greenlee, W. F., and Kende, A. S. (1979): Studies on the mechanism of action of the chlorinated dibenzo-*p*-dioxins and related compounds. In: *Health Effects: Halogenated Aromatic Hydrocarbons*, edited by W. J. Nicholson and J. A. Moore. *Annals New York Academy of Sciences*, 320:214–230.

50. Rohrscheneider, L. R., and Boutwell, R. K. (1973): The early stimulation of phospholipid metabolism by 12-O-tetradecanoylphorbol-13-acetate and its specificity for tumor promotion. *Cancer Res.*, 33:1,945–1,952.

51. Schimmel, S. D., and Hallarn, T. (1980): Rapid alteration in Ca^{++} content and fluxes in phorbol-12-myristate-13-acetate-treated myoblasts. *Biochem. Biophys. Res. Commun.*, 92:624–630.

52. Shoyab, M., DeLarco, J. E., and Todaro, G. J. (1979): Biologically active phorbol esters specifically alter affinity of epidermal growth factor membrane receptors. *Nature*, 279:387–391.

53. Slaga, T. J., Fischer, S. M., Nelson, K., and Gleason, G. L. (1980): Studies on the mechanism of skin tumor promotion: Evidence for several stages in promotion. *Proc. Natl. Acad. Sci. USA*, 77:3,659–3,663.

54. Slaga, T. J., Sivak, A., and Boutwell, R. K., editors (1978): *Carcinogenesis, Vol. 2: Mechanisms of Tumor Promotion and Cocarcinogenesis*. Raven Press, New York.

55. Umezawa, K., Weinstein, I. B., Horowitz, A. D., Fujiki, H., Matsushima, T., and Sugimura, T. (1981): Teleocidin B and the phorbol ester tumor promoters produce similar effect on membranes and membrane receptors. *Nature*, 290:411–413.

56. Weinstein, I. B. (1981): Studies on the mechanism of tumor promoters and their relevance to mammary carcinogenesis. In: *Cell Biology of Breast Cancer*, edited by C. M. McGrath, J. J. Brennan, and M. A. Rich. Academic Press, New York, pp. 425–480.

57. Weinstein, I. B., Lee, L. S., Fisher, P. B., Mufson, R. A., and Yamasaki, H. (1979): Action of phorbol esters in cell culture: Mimicry of transformation, altered differentiation, and effects on cell membranes. *J. Supramol. Struct.*, 12:195–208.

58. Weinstein, I. B., Mufson, R. A., Lee, L. S., Fisher, P. B., Laskin, J., Horowitz, A., and Ivanovic, V. (1980): Membrane and other biochemical effects of the phorbol esters and their relevance to tumor promotion. In: *Carcinogenesis: Fundamental Mechanisms and Environmental Effects*, edited by B. Pullman, P. O. P. Ts'o, and H. Gelboin, pp. 543–563. R. Reidel Publishing Company, Amsterdam, Holland *(in press)*.

59. Weinstein, I. B., Wigler, M., and Pietropaolo, C. (1977): The action of tumor-promoting agents in cell culture. In: *Origins of Human Cancer*, edited by H. H. Hiatt, J. D. Watson, and J. A. Winston, pp. 751–772. Cold Spring Harbor Laboratories, New York.

60. Weinstein, I. B., Yamasaki, H., Wigler, M., Lee, L. S., Fisher, P. B., Jeffrey, A., and Grunberger, D. (1979): Molecular and cellular events associated with the action of initiating carcinogens and tumor promoters. In: *Carcinogens: Identification and Mechanisms of Action*, edited by A. C. Griffin and C. R. Shaw, pp. 399–418. Raven Press, New York.

61. Wertz, P. W., and Mueller, G. C. (1980): Activation of CTP:Phosphorylcholine citidyl transferase by 12-O-tetradecanoylphorbol-13-acetate (TPA). (Abstract). *Proc. Amer. Assoc. Cancer Res.*, 21:128. (See also Mueller, *this volume*).

62. Whitfield, J. F., MacManus, J. P., and Gillan, D. J. (1973): Calcium-dependent stimulation by a phorbol ester (PMA) of thymic lymphoblast DNA synthesis and proliferation. *J. Cell. Physiol.*, 82:151–156.

63. Yamasaki, H., Mufson, R. A., and Weinstein, I. B. (1979): Phorbol ester-induced prostaglandin synthesis and ^{3}H-TPA metabolism by TPA-resistant Friend erythroleukemia cells. *Biochem. Biophys. Res. Commun.*, 89:1,018–1,025.

Carcinogenesis, Vol. 7, edited by E. Hecker et al.
Raven Press, New York © 1982.

Virus Induction by Tumor Promoters

Harald zur Hausen, N. Yamamoto, and G. Bauer

Institut für Virologie, Zentrum für Hygiene, 7800 Freiburg, West Germany

This chapter intends to review data on induction of persisting viruses, Epstein-Barr virus (EBV) genomes, and additional oncogenic viruses by 12-O-tetradeca-noylphorbol-B-acetate (TPA) and related compounds. Some studies will be presented that attempt to analyze the mechanism of TPA induction. Finally, the effect of TPA on virus-induced cell transformation will be reviewed briefly.

EBV induction by TPA and related compounds was discovered in the course of experiments initiated to study polyploidization of human lymphoblasts by tumor promoters (30,31). Lymphoblastoid lines of B-cell origin are easily established from Burkitt's lymphomas, the peripheral blood of lymphomatous patients, but also from EBV-seroreactive adult donors (22). Cells of these lines harbor EBV-genomes in multiple copies, commonly between 20 to 80 genome equivalents per cell being present as large episomes. Cell lines derived from tumor patients often reveal spontaneous induction of EBV particle synthesis in a small percentage. Lines obtained from small children or after *in vitro* transformation of human umbilical cord blood are usually nonproducers, i.e., the cells express only the virus-specific nuclear antigen EBNA without synthesis of viral structural proteins and viral particles.

Studies on the molecular biology of EBV and virus-host cell interactions were greatly hampered in the past by the lack of a suitable tissue culture system for virus propagation and the limited amount of virus-specific components obtained from cells with a high spontaneous induction rate (8). Although synthesis of virus-specific proteins could be enhanced substantially by addition of bromo- and iododeoxyuridine (5,7) or *n*-butyric acid (11), the inhibition of deoxyribonucleic acid (DNA) synthesis exerted by these drugs did not permit recovery of increased yields of viral particles following purification procedures. Thus, an induction system with complete maturation of EBV particles would clearly benefit EBV research, particularly in view of the possible involvement of this virus in two human malignant tumors, Burkitt's lymphoma and nasopharyngeal carcinoma (22).

If induction of EBV by TPA and related compounds correlates with their tumor-promoting activity, this induction system may represent a convenient screening assay for certain promoters. Moreover, the limited genetic information encoded by a viral genome may offer a promising approach to study the mechanism of tumor promoter interaction with specific and relatively well-defined components of the host cell.

INDUCTION OF EBV BY TPA

Treatment of the EBV producer lines P3HR-1 and B95-8 resulted in highly efficient induction of viral antigen synthesis approximately 5 days following treatment (30,31). Five to 20 ng TPA induced more than 50% of cells from the respective lines to viral structural antigen synthesis, whereas spontaneous induction in control cultures reached approximately 5%. Concomitant with antigen synthesis, an increase in released infectious virus was noted, increasing by a factor of approximately 10 within 10 days after induction. Within this period the amount of intracellular viral DNA increased at least 10 to 20-fold (9) as determined by nucleic acid hybridizations. The latter value corresponded to the increase in viral particle yields obtained after virus purification procedures. Cleavage patterns with restriction endonucleases obtained from viral DNA isolated after induction did not differ from preparations collected from noninduced cultures, stressing again the induction of complete viral cycles by TPA.

In subsequent studies, a total of 27 EBV-transformed lymphoblastoid lines was tested for virus induction. Twenty-four of these lines responded well to the inducing drug; three, however, (all nonproducer lines) remained refractory to the inducer. The increase in viral antigen-positive cells amounted in responsive lines on average to a factor of approximately 10 (31).

It was of particular interest that one of the lines tested (Raji and its derivative NC 37) responded to TPA only by induction of early antigens without any evidence for viral structural antigen synthesis and viral DNA replication (2,9, 30,31). These cells contain an average of 50 EBV genome equivalents per cell. The reason for the abortive induction has not been clarified up to now. It may be due to a deletion within the persisting viral DNA. Raji cells and its subline NC 37 respond efficiently to TPA induction with early antigen (EA) synthesis, which can be visualized by indirect immunofluorescence. These antigens are synthesized prior to viral DNA replication (6). Since Raji cells reveal a very low (<0.1%) spontaneous induction rate of EA-positive cells, this system is especially suited to analyze requirements of DNA synthesis for EBV induction and to use it as a screening assay for induction by promoters. Indeed, induction of these cells under conditions of inhibition of DNA synthesis showed that DNA synthesis is not required for EA induction (29). Most of the subsequent studies were performed in the Raji or NC 37 cell system.

INDUCTION BY TPA IN ADDITIONAL VIRAL SYSTEMS

Initial experiments included studies on the inducing effect of TPA in cells transformed by additional oncogenic viruses. Efficient induction was noted in cells transformed by EBV-related old world primate herpesviruses, like baboon-

EBV (31) and African green monkey EBV (3). In addition, T-lymphoblasts transformed by herpesvirus saimiri (31) and Marek's virus of chicken (15) also responded to the inducing stimulus.

In contrast to persisting oncogenic herpesviruses, substantial difficulties were encountered in demonstrating significant induction of persisting papovavirus or retrovirus genomes. Analysis of SV 40 or BK virus-transformed hamster and monkey cells failed to provide clear-cut evidence for viral structural antigen synthesis (zur Hausen, *unpublished data*). A few laboratories, however, have been able to demonstrate small increases of intracellular viral DNA in SV 40-transformed cells (Männer and Brandner, *personal communication*) or HD-virus carrier cultures (Krieg and Sauer, *personal communication*).

A somewhat similar situation was encountered in the induction of endogenous retroviruses. In most systems analyzed thus far, no or only small increases of viral DNA have been noted after TPA treatment. Exceptionally efficient, however, has been the induction of mouse mammary tumor virus reported by Arya (1). In this system TPA effected an approximately 20-fold increase in virus particle synthesis, which closely correlates to the data obtained with oncogenic herpesviruses.

To summarize this part, TPA efficiently induces persistent genomes of oncogenic herpesviruses. Particularly in EBV-transformed systems, this induction permitted 10- to 20-fold increased yields of viral particles. The benefit of this system is revealed by yields of sufficient EBV DNA for strain comparison, physical genomic mapping, and cloning in bacterial vectors. In addition, analysis of early and late virus-induced proteins by immunoprecipitation procedures and the development of monoclonal antibodies to EBV surface components were greatly facilitated by this system (12,14).

INDUCTION BY ADDITIONAL DITERPENE ESTERS

A number of additional diterpene esters, as well as some tumor initiators, were analyzed for their inducing capacity of persisting EBV DNA. The results can be summarized as follows: all potent tumor promoters like TPA, 3-O-hexa-decanoylingenol and Pimelea factor P_2, induced EA in Raji cells at molarities ranging between 5×10^{-10} and 1×10^{-8}. The marginal promoter 4-O-methyl-TPA and the irritants 12-deoxyphorbol-B-decatrienoate and resiniferatoxin represented relatively weak inducers, being 100- to 500-fold less active than the potent promoters. Nonpromoters like 4αphorbol-12,13-didecanoate (4αPDD), phorbol, and ingenol did not induce EA production. Structurally unrelated compounds like anthralin and griseofulvin were inactive as inducers under the conditions of this test (30). It is interesting to note that the percentage of induced cells remained relatively constant over a wide range of concentrations for the potent inducers and did not differ from that of the weak inducers when the latter were applied at their optimal concentrations.

All tumor initiators tested thus far (7,12-dimethylbenz(α)anthracene, benzo(α)-pyrene, 1:2,5:6-dibenzanthracene, 20-methylcholanthrene, anthracene, 4-nitroquinoline-1-oxide, and N-acetoxy-N-2-acetylaminofluorene) failed to induce EA at biologically active concentrations.

Thus, this study shows that EBV induction is specifically restricted to diterpene esters and correlates to some extent with the promoting activity of the respective drugs. An interesting exception appears to be teleocidin and lyngbyatoxin (Sugimura et al., *this volume*) which are structurally unrelated to diterpene esters and have recently been reported to efficiently induce persisting EBV DNA (Hinuma, *personal communication*).

MECHANISM OF VIRUS INDUCTION BY TUMOR-PROMOTING DITERPENE ESTERS

Inhibition of Virus Induction

The reproducible increase in the activity of ornithine decarboxylase (ODC) after treatment of cells with tumor promoters has been reported (16,17). ODC induction is inhibited by feedback inhibition with putrescine (21). Colchicine has also been reported to inhibit TPA-induced ODC activity (16). In order to analyze a possible relationship between induction of ODC activity and virus induction, putrescine, or spermidine, and colchicine were added to Raji cells at various concentrations. No effect on virus induction was noted, which seems to dissociate virus induction from stimulation of ODC activity.

Retinoic acid has also been reported to inhibit ODC induction by tumor promoters (10,24). Moreover, retinoic acid acts, as well, as an inhibitor in experimental two-stage carcinogenesis models (19). The following experiments were therefore devised to analyze the effect of retinoic acid on virus induction by TPA and other inducers (25). Retinoic acid inhibits, indeed, EBV induction by all groups of inducing compounds tested thus far. Inhibition is particularly effective in TPA induction, but also in induction by anti-immunoglobulin M (IgM) which induces EBV in IgM-producing lymphoblasts (23). Iododeoxyuridine and *n*-butyric acid induction is less efficiently, though still significantly, inhibited. The active concentrations of retinoic acid range between 10^{-8} and 10^{-5} M. Even pretreatment of the cells with retinoic acid (10^{-6} M) for 12 hr, followed by subsequent washing and addition of TPA, still resulted in more than 90% inhibition of EA induction.

In marked contrast, superinfection of Raji cells with EBV was not influenced by retinoic acid, providing evidence for different molecular events leading to induction when compared to initiation of infection.

In additional experiments, an inhibitor of protein synthesis, L-canavanine, was applied to the induction system (26). L-canavanine represents an amino acid occurring in jack beans and is a structural analog of arginine. It has been noted as a potent inhibitor for the multiplication of bacteria, plants, and some viruses (4,18,20). The data revealed that L-canavanine inhibited at 0.3 mM more than 95% of EA induction by TPA, but also induction by anti-IgM, iododeoxy-uridine, and *n*-butyric acid. At this concentration, viral antigen induction by superinfection was not affected. Here an inhibition was only noted at more than 10-fold higher concentrations of L-canavanine. This observation stresses again the different pathway followed in antigen induction by promoters when compared to exogenous infection (26).

Attempts to Analyze the Mechanism of Viral Induction

The subsequent part will be devoted to a discussion of the possible mechanism of EBV induction by tumor-promoting diterpene esters.

As a working hypothesis, we speculated that these data would be compatible with the assumption that virus induction by the various groups of inducing agents would be effected by a cellular mediator synthesized in an initial response to the inducing event. This speculation seemed to receive additional support by sequential inhibition experiments performed with cycloheximide (CH) and actinomycine D (act. D) (29). If Raji cells were treated simultaneously with TPA and CH for 2 days, washed subsequently, and were treated thereafter with act. D, no induction of EA was noted. Superinfection experiments, however, performed under the same regimen by omitting TPA resulted in significant induction. These results seemed to support the view that a specific messenger ribonucleic acid (RNA) had to accumulate during CH treatment of TPA-induced cells, which, after translation and upon interaction with persisting EBV DNA, would initiate the derepression of the viral genomes.

Unfortunately, however, additional experiments did not support this interpretation. Treatment of EBV-negative lymphoblastoid B- or T-cell lines, as well as of various strains of human fibroblasts, with TPA, followed subsequently by fusion of these cells with genome-harboring Raji cells under conditions of CH and AD treatment or by treating the fused cells with rerinoic acid did not result in significant induction, although appropriate controls without inhibitors were clearly positive.

Despite the possibility of alternative interpretations, like an exclusive nuclear localization of the postulated cellular mediator and a possible failure of nuclear fusion, another interpretation may be more plausible: this implies that under conditions of latent infection, EBV and possibly other oncogenic herpesviruses would code for their own repressors. TPA and related promoters either block this repressor synthesis or interfere with its function. This, in turn, would enable the viral DNA to initiate its independent transcription and DNA replication.

It should be emphasized again that these are speculations, which contain however some testable predictions. If correct, this model could provide a valuable tool for our understanding of the regulation of specific genes by tumor-promoting diterpene esters.

TPA at very low concentrations stimulates transformation of B-lymphocytes by EBV between five- and eight-fold (28). This effect is to some extent opposed to the efficient induction that leads to cell lysis and virus release. There is not clear-cut evidence available indicating that enhancement of transformation and induction of persisting genomes are related events. Since enhancement of transformation occurs within a narrow dose range, this effect may be due to mitogenic stimulation and prolonged survival of the target cells for EBV transformation. There exists, however, no direct evidence to support this claim, and alternative mechanisms are certainly possible.

To summarize: tumor-promoting diterpene esters efficiently induce persisting genomes of oncogenic herpesviruses and a few other agents. The Raji cell system may represent a very convenient assay to screen for promoters in this group of compounds. Induction by tumor promoters provides a convenient tool to study the mechanism of virus restriction under conditions of latent infection.

ACKNOWLEDGMENT

Original observations cited in this chapter were supported by the Deutsche Forschungsgemeinschaft, SFB 31 (Medizinische Virologie, Tumorentstehung und -Entwicklung).

REFERENCES

1. Arya, S. K. (1980): Phorbol ester-mediated stimulation of the synthesis of mouse mammary tumour virus. *Nature,* 284:71–72.
2. Bister, K., Yamamoto, N., and zur Hausen, H. (1979): Differential inducibility of Epstein-Barr virus in cloned Raji cells. *Int. J. Cancer,* 23:818–825.
3. Böcker, J. F., Tiedemann, K. H., Bornkamm, G. W., and zur Hausen, H. (1980): Characterization of an EBV-like virus from African green monkey lymphoblasts. *Virology,* 101:291–295.
4. Cushing, R. T., and Morgan, H. R. (1952): Effect of some metabolic analogs on growth of mumps and influenza viruses in tissue cultures. *Proc. Soc. Exp. Biol. (N.Y.),* 79:497–500.
5. Gerber, P. (1972): Activation of Epstein-Barr virus by 5-bromodeoxyuridine in "virus-free" human cells. *Proc. Natl. Acad. Sci. USA,* 69:83–85.
6. Gergely, L., Klein, G., and Ernberg, Z. (1971): Appearance of Epstein-Barr virus-associated antigens in infected Raji cells. *Virology,* 45:10–21.
7. Hampar, B., Derge, J. G., Martos, L. M., and Walker, J. L. (1972): Synthesis of Epstein-Barr virus after activation of the viral genome in a "virus-negative" human lymphoblastoid cell (Raji) made resistant to 5-bromodeoxyuridine. *Proc. Natl. Acad. Sci. USA,* 69:78–82.
8. Hinuma, Y., Konn, M., Yamaguchi, J., Wudarski, D. J., Blakeslee, J. R., and Grace, J. T. (1967): Immunofluorescene and herpes-type virus particles in the P3HR-1 Burkitt lymphoma cell line. *J. Virol.,* 1:1,045–1,051.
9. Hudewentz, J., Bornkamm, G. W., and zur Hausen, H. (1980): Effect of the diterpene ester TPA on Epstein-Barr virus antigen and DNA synthesis in producer and nonproducer cell lines. *Virology,* 100:175–178.
10. Kensler, T. W., Verma, A. K., Boutwell, R. K., and Müller, G. C. (1978): Effects of retinoic acid and juvenile hormone on the induction of ornithine decarboxylase activity by 12-O-tetradecanoylphorbol-13-acetate. *Cancer Res.,* 38:2,896–2,899.
11. Luka, J., Kallin, B., and Klein, G. (1979): Induction of the Epstein-Barr virus (EBV) cycle in latently infected cells by *n*-butyrate. *Virology,* 94:228–231.
12. Müller-Lantzsch, N., Georg, B., Yamamoto, N., and zur Hausen, H. (1980): Epstein-Barr virus-induced proteins: II. Analysis of surface polypeptides from EBV-producing and -superinfected cells by immunoprecipitation. *Virology,* 102:401–411.
13. Müller-Lantzsch, N., Georg-Fries, B., Herbst, H., zur Hausen, H., and Braun, D. (1981):

Epstein-Barr virus strain and group-specific antigenic determinants detected by monoclonal antibodies. *Int. J. Cancer,* 28:321–327.

14. Müller-Lantzsch, N., Yamamoto, N., and zur Hausen, H. (1979): Analysis of early and late Epstein-Barr virus associated polypeptides by immunoprecipitation. *Virology,* 97:378–387.

15. Nazerian, K. (1979): Persistent infection of Marek's disease lymphoblastoid cell lines with Marek's disease virus and enhancement of virus expression with a tumor promoter. American Society of Microbiology, 79th Annual Meeting, May 4 to 8. Los Angeles, California.

16. O'Brien, T. G. (1976): The induction of ornithine decarboxylase as an early, possibly obligatory, event in mouse skin carcinogenesis. *Cancer Res.,* 36:2,644–2,653.

17. O'Brien, T. G., Simsiman, R. C., and Boutwell, R. K. (1975): Induction of the polyamine biosynthetic enzymes in mouse epidermis by tumor-promoting agents. *Cancer Res.,* 35:1,662–1,670.

18. Pearson, H. E., Lagerborg, D. L., and Winzler, R. J. (1952): Effects of certain amino acids and related compounds on propagation of mouse encephalomyelitis virus. *Proc. Soc. Exp. Biol. N.Y.,* 79:409–411.

19. Shamberger, R. J. J. (1971): Inhibitory effect of vitamin A on carcinogenesis. *J. Natl. Cancer Inst.,* 47:667–673.

20. Shive, W., and Skinner, C. G. (1963): Amino acid analogues. In: *Metabolic Inhibitors, Vol. I,* edited by R. M. Hochster and J. H. Quastel, pp. 2–73. Academic Press, New York.

21. Tabor, C. W., and Tabor, H. (1976): 1,4-Diaminobutane (putresine), spermidine, and spermine. *Annu. Rev. Biochem.,* 45:282–306.

22. Tooze, J. (1980): DNA tumor viruses. In: *Molecular Biology of Tumor Viruses, Part 2.* Cold Spring Harbor Laboratory Press, Cold Spring Harbor, New York.

23. Tovey, M. G., Lenoir, G., and Begon-Lours, J. (1978): Activation of latent Epstein-Barr virus by antibody to human IgM. *Nature,* 276:271–273.

24. Verma, A. K., and Boutwell, R. K. (1977): Vitamin A acid (retinoic acid), a potent inhibitor of 12-O-tetradecanoylphorbol-13-acetate-induced ornithine decarboxylase activity in mouse epidermis. *Cancer Res.,* 37:2,196–2,201.

25. Yamamoto, N., Bister, K., and zur Hausen, H. (1979): Retinoic acid inhibition of Epstein-Barr virus induction. *Nature,* 278:553–554.

26. Yamamoto, N., Müller-Lantzsch, N., and zur Hausen, H. (1980*a*): Differential inhibition of Epstein-Barr virus induction by the amino acid analogue L-canavanine. *Int. J. Cancer,* 25:439–443.

27. Yamamoto, N., Müller-Lantzsch, N., and zur Hausen, H. (1980*b*): Effect of actinomycin D and cycloheximide on Epstein-Barr virus early antigen induction in lymphoblastoid cells. *J. Gen. Virol.,* 51:255–261.

28. Yamamoto, N., and zur Hausen, H. (1979): Tumour promotor TPA enhances transformation of human leukocytes by Epstein-Barr virus. *Nature,* 280:244–245.

29. Yamamoto, N., and zur Hausen, H. (1980): Effect of inhibition of DNA synthesis on Epstein-Barr virus induction by tumor promoters. *Virology,* 101:104–110.

30. zur Hausen, H., Bornkamm, G. W., Schmidt, R., and Hecker, E. (1979): Tumor initiators and promoters in the induction of Epstein-Barr virus. *Proc. Natl. Acad. Sci. USA,* 76:782–785.

31. zur Hausen, H., O'Neill, F. J., Freese, U. K., and Hecker, E. (1978): Persisting oncogenic herpes virus induced by tumour promoter TPA. *Nature,* 272:373–375.

Carcinogenesis, Vol. 7, edited by E. Hecker et al.
Raven Press, New York © 1982.

Effect of Tumor Promoters in Immunological Systems—The Macrophage as a Target Cell for the Action of Phorbol Esters

Edgar Pick, Yona Keisari, Yael Bromberg, Maya Freund, and
Aniela Yakubowski

*Section of Immunology, Department of Human Microbiology, Sackler School of Medicine,
Tel-Aviv University, Ranat-Aviv, Tel-Aviv, Israel*

Our interest in the effects of phorbol myristate acetate (PMA) stems from the observation that low concentrations of this agent block macrophage (MP) motility *in vitro* (12). Thirty seconds of contact with 200 nM PMA was sufficient to induce prolonged but reversible inhibition of migration in guinea pig MPs. Similar to the effect of the lymphocyte-derived migration inhibitory factor (MIF), the PMA-induced reduction in MP motility was prevented by colchicine, suggesting that microtubules are involved in the intracellular mediation of the PMA effect. Indeed, we found that brief incubation of MPs with 200 nM PMA resulted in a marked increase in the density of cytoplasmic microtubules that paralleled the induction of cell spreading. Biochemical analysis of the state of tubulin polymerization in PMA-treated MPs seemed to indicate that the morphological change was not accompanied by a significant increase in the quantity of tubulin polymer (12). Recently we have reexamined this issue, however, and found that by using improved conditions of microtubule stabilization, a significant and reproducible elevation in the amount of tubulin in polymeric form can be detected (M. Seger and E. Pick, *in preparation*). It is significant that incubation of MPs with the weak tumor promoter 4-O-methyl-PMA did not alter the ratio of polymeric to dimeric tubulin.

In the light of these results and of findings reported by other authors indicating that PMA has a number of additional effects on MPs (including plasminogen activator production, stimulating prostaglandin release, enhancement of pinocytosis, induction of an oxidative burst), we decided to investigate the biochemical mechanism(s) by which PMA influences MP physiology.

EFFECT OF PMA ON CYCLIC GUANOSINE 3'5'-MONOPHOSPHATE LEVELS

Since it has been reported that microtubule generation was enhanced by agents increasing cyclic guanosine 3'5'-monophosphate (cyclic GMP) levels and since

PMA was found to elevate cyclic GMP in fibroblasts and platelets (5), we examined the effect of PMA on cyclic GMP levels in MPs. As seen in Table 1, incubation of MPs with 20 nM PMA for 10 min had no effect on the cellular content of cyclic GMP. No effect was found by varying the concentration of PMA from 20 nM to 10μM and the length of incubation from 15 sec to 30 min in media containing either 0.54 mM or 1.8 mM Ca^{2+} (1). Using the same methodology, marked increases in cyclic GMP were induced in MPs by incubation with a number of NO-generating agents, such as sodium nitroprusside (1). Exposure of MPs to PMA was found to reduce the extent of the cyclic GMP elevation induced by nitroprusside while 4-O-methyl-PMA was inactive in this respect (Table 2). It was therefore concluded that under the experimental conditions employed, PMA had no effect on the concentration of cyclic GMP in MPs and that it is unlikely that its effect on microtubules was mediated via cyclic nucleotides.

INDUCTION BY PMA OF AN OXIDATIVE BURST

We have recently demonstrated that mineral oil-elicited guinea pig peritoneal MPs respond by a rapid and marked production of superoxide anions (O_2^-) and hydrogen peroxide (H_2O_2) to incubation with minute concentrations of PMA (11). Equimolar concentrations of 4-O-methyl-PMA were without effect. The production of O_2^- by PMA-stimulated MPs was independent of extracellular Ca^{2+} and, in this respect, differed from the induction of an oxidative burst (OB) by the divalent cation ionophore A23187. The production of H_2O_2 by guinea pig MPs was partially inhibited by the superoxide dismutase blocking drug sodium diethyldithiocarbamate (DDC), indicating that at least part of the H_2O_2 was generated from O_2^- by enzymatic dismutation. PMA was reported in the past to stimulate O_2^- production by human peripheral blood and alveolar MPs as well as by mouse peritoneal MPs. It is generally found that MP activation, such as that induced by chronic infection, by the local injection of *Corynebacterium parvum*, by endotoxin, or by contact with lymphokines, results in a marked enhancement of PMA-elicted H_2O_2 production. There is considerable support for the idea that the heightened microbicidal capacity of activated MPs is medi-

TABLE 1. *PMA does not stimulate cyclic GMP generation in MPs*[a]

Stimulant	Concentration	No. of expts	pmole cyclic GMP per mg macrophage protein $\pm$ SEM	
			$-$	$+$ Stimulant
PMA	20 nM	4	0.74 ± 0.07	0.50 ± 0.16
4-O-methyl-PMA	20 nM	4	0.34 ± 0.15	0.23 ± 0.12

[a] The culture medium contained 0.54 mM Ca^{2+} and 1 mM isobutylmethylxanthine. Incubation with stimulants was for 10 min.

TABLE 2. *Inhibition by PMA on the cyclic GMP-elevating effect of Na-nitroprusside[a]*

Stimulant	Concentration	No. of expts	pmole cyclic GMP per mg macrophage protein $\pm$ SEM	
			$-$	+ Na nitroprusside (1 mM)
$-$	$-$		0.71 ± 0.09	4.75 ± 1.64
		3		
PMA	20 nM		0.44 ± 0.21	2.64 ± 0.82
$-$	$-$		0.61	3.87
		2		
4-O-methyl-PMA	20 nM		0.40	5.17

[a] The culture medium contained 0.54 mM Ca^{2+} and 1 mM isobutylmethylxanthine. Incubation with stimulants was for 10 min.

ated via their enhanced readiness to release H_2O_2 as a consequence of phagocytosis. Some continuous MP cell lines in the mouse (J774.1, P388D1) have been reported to produce usually small amounts O_2^- when cultured with PMA. Lymphocytes and fibroblasts were unresponsive.

PMA-STIMULATED MP CYTOTOXICITY

It has been reported that activated mouse MPs incubated with PMA become cytotoxic towards some tumoral target cells. The principal agent responsible for target cell killing appears to be H_2O_2 released by the MPs (9). We have recently found that oil-elicited guinea pig MPs stimulated by PMA cause rapid lysis of syngeneic erythrocytes in tissue culture (8). 4-O-methyl-PMA was active only at a 100-fold higher concentration. PMA-stimulated MP cytotoxicity was blocked by low concentrations of DDC and was partially inhibited by catalase. On the other hand, inhibition of catalase by 3-aminotriazole or the addition of exogenous peroxidase markedly enhanced erythrocyte lysis. Close cell contact among MPs and target erythrocytes was required for cytolysis to occur. Morphologically, the process could be observed under the microscope in a system consisting of a layer of erythrocytes on top of a MP monolayer, in the form of rapidly developing hemolytic plaques surrounding individual MPs. The final mediator(s) of the cytotoxic process has not been determined but the blocking effect of catalase indicates that H_2O_2 is either the toxic material itself or an intermediate in the formation of a different toxic oxygen metabolite, such as hydroxyl radicals (OH·) or singlet oxygen($^1O_2$). With the purpose of investigating the nature of the lytic process itself, we have analyzed the extent of lipid peroxidation in the target erythrocytes by the determination of malonyldialdehyde (MDA) formation in cultures of PMA-stimulated MPs and erythrocytes. As seen in Table 3, large quantities of MDA were detected when maximal red cell lysis was achieved by the inhibition of catalase by sodium azide. The molecular mechanism

TABLE 3. *Lipid peroxidation in target erythrocytes incubated with PMA-stimulated Mps[a]*

	nmole malonyldialdehyde per tube	
Content of tubes	−	+ NaN$_3$ (1 mM)
MPs	0.630	0.525
MPs + PMA	1.330	1.890
Erythrocytes + PMA	0.840	0.735
MPs + erythrocytes	0.735	0.770
MPs + erythrocytes + PMA	1.820	12.005[b]

[a] 45 μl packed guinea pig peritoneal exudate MPs + 125μl packed guinea pig erythrocytes + 20 nM PMA in 2.5 ml medium, and the adequate controls, were incubated for 4 hr at 37°C in closed tubes on a rotator. Malonyldialdehyde present in the deproteinized supernatants was determined by the thiobarbituric acid test.
[b] Complete lysis of erythrocytes.

of the MP-mediated damage to erythrocytes remains unknown and represents a challenging subject for further investigation.

PMA-INDUCED MP AUTOTOXICITY

It is generally accepted that the remarkable ability of MPs to inflict oxidative damage upon phagocytosed microorganisms or adjacent cells is coexistent with efficient mechanisms for protecting the MP itself from autotoxic damage. Part of this protection is offered by the fact that the bulk of oxygen metabolites is released from the cell membrane, where they are generated, to the exterior of the cell. In addition to this, O_2^-, which might have diffused into the cytoplasm, is degraded by superoxide dismutase, while H_2O_2 is eliminated by the actions of catalase and the glutathione peroxidase-reduced glutathione system. In spite of this, we found evidence for cytotoxic damage in MPs incubated with PMA under conditions resulting in the production of O_2^- and H_2O_2. Thus, MPs incubated for 24 hr with 200 nM PMA demonstrated modest but reproducible increases in the accumulation of MDA (Table 4). Another, more direct indicator for the presence of PMA-induced peroxides in the interior of the cell is the massive increase in oxidized glutathione (GSSG) detectable within 5 min in MPs incubated with PMA (Table 5). It seems likely that the recently described rapid (within 1 hr) stimulation of the hexose monophosphate shunt (HMPS) by PMA in MPs (6) serves as a compensatory mechanism for the regeneration of NADPH consumed in the course of O_2^- production and during the reduction of GSSG by glutathione reductase. It has been recently reported that polymorphonuclear leukocytes (PMN) incubated with PMA show clear evidence of autotoxic damage which can be quantitated by the release of ^{51}Cr from prelabeled

TABLE 4. *Induction of lipid peroxidation in MPs by PMA[a]*

Stimulant	Concentration	No. of expts	nmole malonyldialdehyde per 10⁶ MPs ± SEM	
			−	+ Stimulant
PMA	200 nм	9	0.078 ± 0.009	0.121 ± 0.010

[a] Oil-induced guinea pig peritoneal Mps were incubated in monolayer with the stimulants for 24 hr. Total malonyldialdehyde (cells + culture medium) was determined by the thiobarbituric acid test.

cells (16). Interestingly, the autotoxicity could be prevented by methionine and histidine, two scavengers which had no preventive effect on toxicity caused by exogenous H_2O_2.

We have recently suggested that limited and reversible toxicity caused by oxygen metabolites may offer an alternative explanation for the MP migration inhibitory action of PMA which has, so far, been attributed to the increase in the density of cytoplasmic microtubules (7). Such an effect could be mediated by a direct toxic action of a product of the OB on membrane lipids, on enzymes, or on cytoskeletal structures essential for cell motility. Alternatively, the positive feedback mechanism put in motion by the accumulation of GSSG could result in excessive activation of the HMPS-glutathione reductase tandem, with a consequent elevation in the reduced/oxidized glutathione ratio and the induction of tubulin polymerization and microtubule generation. Inhibition of MP motility and the induction of increased cell substrate adherence appear to be properties common to a number of unrelated agents sharing the capacity to stimulate an OB. We have therefore investigated if the migration inhibitory effect of PMA could be reversed by scavengers of specific oxygen metabolites. Our preliminary

TABLE 5. *Effect of PMA on levels of GSSG in MPs[a]*

Agent	Concentration	Length of incubation	No. of expts	% glutathione in oxidized form (GSSG)
−	−			2.1
		5 min	2	
PMA	2 μM			11.4
−	−			2.7 ± 0.9
		10 min	9	
PMA	2 μM			12.9 ± 1.8
−	−			7.8
Diamide 500 nmole/10⁶ cells				52.2
		10 min	1	
Tertiary-500 nmole/10⁶ cells butyl hydroperoxide				24.0

[a] Oil-elicited guinea pig peritoneal Mps were incubated with PMA or glutathione-oxidizing agents at 37°C in serum-free culture medium. The % of glutathione in oxidized form was determined by the method of Tietze (15).

results indicate that the effect of PMA can be partially reversed by superoxide dismutase and by high concentrations of catalase. The addition of exogenous peroxidase will intensify the migration inhibitory effect of PMA. These results support the involvement of H_2O_2 and/or of a product of the interaction between O_2^- and H_2O_2, such as OH·. The effect of PMA could not, however, be reversed by mannitol, sodium benzoate, or dihydroxybenzoic acid, which scavenge OH·. Partial reversal of PMA effects was caused by L-methionine. An alternative possibility explored by us was that PMA affects MP motility by inducing the formation of prostaglandin (PG) endoperoxides and thromboxane A_2, agents known to induce platelet aggregation and enhance leukocyte adhesiveness. PMA is a potent inducer of phospholipid deacylation (10) and PG synthesis in a number of cells, including MPs (3). PMA-induced MP migration inhibition was not modified by mepacrine (inhibitor of phospholipase A_2), indomethacin (inhibitor of cyclooxygenase), or 5,8,11,14-eicosatetraynoic acid (ETYA) (blocker of both cyclooxygenase and lipoxygenase). Reversal of the inhibitory effect of PMA was, however, induced by three thromboxane A_2 synthetase inhibitors: imidazole, (5Z, 9α, 11α, 13E)-9, 11-azoprosta-5,13-dienoic acid (U-51605), and (15S)-hydroxy-9α,11α-(epoxymethano)-prosta-5Z, 13E-dienoic acid (U-44069). These results suggest that the effects of PMA on cell motility may involve, at some stage, the action of thromboxane A_2. The relative importance of thromboxanes, oxygen radicals, and the cytoskeletal changes in the causation of PMA-induced changes in MP behavior is subject to further investigation.

We would like to suggest that the yet unexplained inhibition by PMA of the activation of guanylate cyclase by nitroprusside (Table 2) might also be the result of oxidative damage to the enzyme by oxygen radicals produced by the MPs. Studies are in progress on the effect of antioxidants and reductants as protective agents against PMA-induced "poisoning" of guanylate cyclase.

EFFECT OF PMA ON CYCLIC ADENOSINE 3',5'-MONOPHOSPHATE METABOLISM

In the course of studies on the effect of PMA on cyclic GMP levels, we performed parallel measurements of cyclic adenosine 3',5'-monophosphate (cyclic AMP) levels in MPs incubated with PMA. We found that exposure of MPs to 20 nM PMA results in a two- to fivefold elevation in cyclic AMP levels (2). 4-O-methyl-PMA elevated cyclic AMP only in the 2 to 20 μM concentration range. The PMA-elicited rise in cyclic AMP levels was evident at 10 min (but not at 30 sec) of incubation and was best expressed in the presence of the phosphodiesterase inhibitor 3-isobutylmethylxanthine and of low concentrations of extracellular Ca^{2+} (which are associated with low basal levels of cyclic AMP). In the light of the facts that PMA induces E-type PG synthesis in MPs (3) and that PGE_1 and PGE_2 stimulate MP adenylate cyclase, we examined the possibility that the PMA-elicited rise in cyclic AMP was PG mediated. We found that PMA caused an increase in cyclic AMP levels even in the presence of mapacrine, ETYA, indomethacin, and aspirin, demonstrating that the rise was independent of PG synthesis. The stimulation of cyclic AMP accumulation by PMA was also not influenced by superoxide dismutase, catalase, or α-tocopherol, indicating that it was not mediated by a product of the OB. On the contrary, we found that PMA-induced cyclic AMP elevation is enhanced by ETYA and α-tocopherol. The most likely explanation for this is that the two agents cause a lowering in the level of PG endoperoxides and possibly other peroxides that would normally act as feedback inhibitors of adenylate cyclase. All this indicates that the effect of PMA on cyclic AMP levels in MPs is independent of the two major processes normally associated with PMA action in these cells, namely, the OB and PG synthesis. The fact that PMA acts via the stimulation of adenylate cyclase and not the inhibition of phosphodiesterase is shown by the fact its effects on cyclic AMP develop optimally in the presence of an inhibitor of phosphodiesterase. Two main possibilities should therefore be considered: (a) activation of adenylate cyclase by the intermediary of the PMA receptor via a coupling mechanism to the catalytic component of the enzyme, or (b) mediation by an intracellular messenger, such as Ca^{2+}, possibly by the intermediary of calmodulin.

HYPOTHESIS: PIVOTAL ROLE OF Ca^{2+} IN THE MEDIATION OF PMA EFFECTS ON MPs

This hypothesis is based on the following experimental facts: (a) An OB can be induced in both MPs and PMNs by the Ca^{2+} ionophore A23187; (b) O_2^- production by human PMNs (4) and mouse MPs (E. Pick, *in preparation*) stimulated by PMA is inhibited by trifluoperazine, an inhibitor of calmodulin; (c) PMA-elicited release of granule-associated enzymes from PMNs is inhibited by the intracellular Ca^{2+} antagonist TMB-8 (13), which also blocks MP chemotaxis in a PMA gradient (14); (d) the basal level of cyclic AMP in MPs increases with increasing extracellular Ca^{2+} concentrations; (e) calmodulin was found to participate in the stimulation of adenylate cyclase by Ca^{2+} in a number of cells; (f) the arachidonic acid releasing enzymes phospholipase A_2 or the phospholipase C-diacylglycerol lipase sequence are Ca^{2+} dependent; and (g) there is evidence for the involvement of calmodulin in phospholipase A_2 action.

We are therefore proposing that the major biochemical sequences initiated by the binding of PMA to MPs are mediated by an elevation in the cytoplasmic Ca^{2+} concentration. This can be the consequence of either increased influx from outside the cell or liberation from intracellular stores. The latter mechanism appears more likely since both the induction of an OB and the activation of adenylate cyclase by PMA proceed normally in Ca^{2+}-free medium. The mechanism by which PMA affects Ca^{2+} transport is unknown, but stimulation of phospholipid methylation or increased phosphatidylinositol turnover in membranes appear likely possibilities. The multiple and complex consequences of the interaction of PMA with MPs are illustrated schematically in Fig. 1. The

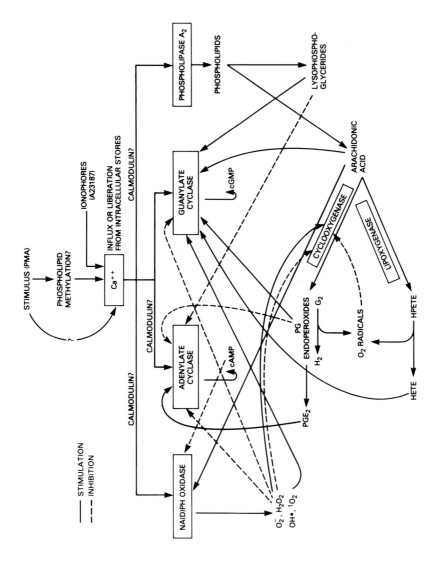

FIG. 1. Multiple consequences of the interaction of PMA with the MP.

three principal correlated events are the activation of the O_2^--producing enzyme, of adenylate cyclase, and of the enzyme(s) releasing arachidonic acid from phospholipids. While Ca^{2+} is offered as the common activator of all three systems, the nature and the quantity of the end products of these enzymatic reactions are determined by a complex set of positive and negative feedback mechanisms which are illustrated in the scheme. The intensity of a certain negative feedback mechanism can be such that the reaction becomes abortive. This is exemplified by the fact that while guanylate cyclase in MPs is exquisitely sensitive to a rise in Ca^{2+} levels, the enzyme is nevertheless not activated by PMA. As mentioned before, the stimulation of guanylate cyclase by nitroprusside is in fact blocked by PMA, most likely by oxidative damage to the enzyme by a product of the OB. The lack of guanylate cyclase activation in MPs by A23187 (1) is similarly explained by the ability of the ionophore to elicit a potent OB. Although the present scheme is essentially based on data derived from the study of the interaction of PMA with MPs, it seems likely that similar mechanisms form the basis for the pleiotropic effects of PMA on a variety of other cells.

INVOLVEMENT OF MPs IN TUMOR PROMOTION BY PMA

It is generally assumed that the tumor-promoting effect of PMA is the result of a direct interaction between the promoter and the target cells. In the light of the high responsiveness of MPs to PMA and the widespread repartition of MPs and MP-like cells in many tissues, including the skin, the possibility should be considered that MPs play a role in tumor promotion. Two such roles can be visualized: (a) MP-derived oxygen radicals or a product of arachidonic acid oxidation could be involved in some stage of tumor promotion themselves, reaching their target cells by diffusion from either local tissue MPs or exudative MPs derived from the circulation. (b) Oxygen radicals or a product of the arachidonic acid oxidation may have an opposite, protective effect, by eliminating transformed cells, in accordance with the results of Nathan et al. (9) and Grimm et al. (6), demonstrating the ability of PMA-treated MPs to be cytotoxic or cytostatic to tumor cells. In this second situation, PMA is seen acting at two levels: a direct tumor-promoting effect on a certain target cell, and an activating effect on tissue or blood-derived MPs which could result in the elimination of a certain proportion of the transformed cells. The final outcome of tumor promotion depends on the relative strengths of these two antagonistic processes. Of special relevance for this hypothesis is fact that the skin, the tissue on which most of the work on the tumor-promoting effects of phorbol esters was performed, contains as an integral component the Langerhans cells, which closely resemble MPs.

Finally, this approach to the mechanism of cocarcinogenesis offers new prospects in the search for drugs capable of antagonizing or preventing the effects of tumor promoters. There seems to be sufficient justification for investigating the effect of specific scavengers of oxygen-derived radicals on PMA-induced tumor promotion. For a number of these, the levels of toxicity *in vivo* have been worked out in the past, and, in the case of the skin, both topical and systemic administration are feasible. In addition to antioxidants, an ever increasing number of inhibitors for specific products of the arachidonic acid pathway (such as thromboxanes or hydroxyeicosatetraenoic acids) are becoming available and could be tested for possible modulation of the effects of phorbol esters. Both interference with and enhancement of the process of tumor promotion would provide us with valuable information on the mechanisms involved.

ACKNOWLEDGMENTS

The work described was supported by the National Council for Research and Development, Israel, and the Deutsches Krebsforschungszentrum, Heidelberg, and by grant No. 1505 from the U.S.-Israel Binational Science Foundation.

REFERENCES

1. Bromberg, Y., and Pick, E. (1980): Cyclic GMP metabolism in macrophages. I. Regulation of cyclic GMP levels by calcium and stimulation of cyclic GMP synthesis by NO-generating agents. *Cell. Immunol.,* 52:73–83.
2. Bromberg, Y., and Pick, E. (1981): Activation of macrophage adenylate cyclase by stimulants of the oxidative burst and by arachidonic acid—Two distinct mechanisms. *Cell Immunol.,* 61:90–103.
3. Brune, K., Kälin, H., Schmidt, R., and Hecker, E. (1978): Inflammatory, tumor-initiating, and promoting activities of polycyclic aromatic hydrocarbons and diterpene esters in mouse skin as compared with their prostaglandin releasing potency *in vitro. Cancer Letters,* 4:333–342.
4. Cohen, H. J., Chovaniec, M. E., and Ellis, S. E. (1980): Chlorpromazine inhibition of granulocyte. superoxide production. *Blood,* 56:23–29.
5. Estensen, R. D., Hadden, J. W., Hadden, E. M., Touraine, F., Touraine, J. L., Haddox, M. K., and Goldberg, N. S. (1974): Phorbol myristate acetate: Effects of a tumor promoter on intracellular cyclic GMP in mouse fibroblasts and as a mitogen on human lymphocytes. In: *Control of Proliferation in Animal Cells,* edited by B. Clarksman and R. Baserga, pp. 627–634. Cold Spring Harbor Press, Cold Spring Harbor, New York.
6. Grimm, W., Bärlin, E., Leser, H. G., Kramer, W., and Gemsa, D. (1980): Induction of tumor cytostatic macrophages by TPA. *Clin. Immunol. Immunopathol.,* 17:617–628.
7. Keisari, Y., and Pick, E. (1980): Lymphokine mimicry by phorbol myristate acetate and the ionophore A27187—A new hypothesis for explaining the action mechanism of migration inhibitory factor. In: *Biochemical Characterization of Lymphokines,* edited by A. deWeck, F. Kristensen, and M. Landy, pp. 113–121. Academic Press, New York.
8. Keisari, Y., and Pick, E. (1981): Macrophage-mediated cytolysis (MMC) of erythrocytes in the guinea pig. I. Activation by stimulators of the oxidative burst. *Cell Immunol.,* 62:172–186.
9. Nathan, C. F., Brukner, L. H., Silverstein, S. C., and Cohn, Z. A. (1979): Extracellular cytolysis by activated macrophages and granulocytes. I. Pharmacological triggering of effector cells and the release of hydrogen peroxide. *J. Exp. Med.,* 149:84–99.
10. Ohuchi, K., and Levine, L. (1978): Stimulation of prostaglandin synthesis by tumor-promoting phorbol-12,13-diesters in canine kidney (MDCK) cells. *J. Biol. Chem.,* 253:4,783–4,790.
11. Pick, E., and Keisari, Y. (1981): Superoxide and hydrogen peroxide production by chemically elicited peritoneal macrophages.—Induction by multiple stimuli. *Cell Immunol.,* 59:301–318.
12. Pick, E., Seger, M., Honig, S., and Griffel, B. (1979): Intracellular mediation of lymphokine action: Mimicry of migration inhibitory factor (MIF) action by phorbol myristate acetate (PMA) and the ionophore A23187. *Ann. N.Y. Acad. Sci.,* 332:378–394.

13. Smith, R. J., and Iden, S. S. (1979): Phorbol myristate acetate-induced release of granule enzymes from human neutrophils: Inhibition by the calcium antagonist 8-(N,N-diethyl-amino)-octyl-3,4,5-trimethoxybenzoate hydrochloride. *Biochem. Biophys. Res. Commun.,* 91:263–271.
14. Smith, B., Kessler, F. K., Carchman, S. H., and Carchman, R. A. (1981): The role of calcium in macrophage chemotaxis. *J. Reticuloendothel. Soc.* (abstract) *(in press).*
15. Tietze, F. (1969): Enzymic method for the quantitative determination of nanogram amounts of total and oxidized glutathione. Applications to mammalian blood and other tissues. *Anal. Biochem.,* 27:502–522.
16. Tsan, M. F., and Denison, R. C. (1980): Phorbol myristate acetate-induced neutrophil autotoxicity. A comparison with H_2O_2 toxicity. *Inflammation,* 4:371–380.

Carcinogenesis, Vol. 7, edited by E. Hecker et al.
Raven Press, New York © 1982.

Effects of Tumor-Promoting Agents on Cells of the Murine Immune System: Inhibition of Antibody Synthesis and of Macrophage-Mediated Tumor Cell Cytotoxicity

*C. Stuart Baxter, *Larry A. Fish, †Thomas A. Ferguson,
†J. Gabriel Michael, and *Jerry A. Bash

Departments of *Environmental Health and †Microbiology, University of Cincinnati
College of Medicine, Cincinnati, Ohio 45267

Recent studies have shown that the tumor-promoting phorbol diesters modify responsiveness of T lymphocytes (4), macrophages (2), and other cells of the immune system. Agents of this type are also known to have inflammatory activity by being chemotactic for immune cells. In light of these findings, active phorbol diesters may owe all or part of their activity to an ability to modulate the host immune response. In order to address this question, we set out to examine their effects on various *in vitro* manifestations of immune cell functions, specifically in the mouse, in which tumor promotion has been most thoroughly characterized.

MATERIALS AND METHODS

Phorbol and diesters were obtained from Dr. Peter Borchert, University of Minnesota, Minneapolis, Minnesota.

Measurement of Antibody Synthesis

Weanling female BDF_1 mice (Jackson Labs, Bar Harbor, Maine) were used for all experiments. Spleens were removed and dispersed by passage through a stainless steel mesh. 5×10^6 lymphocytes were incubated in 0.5 ml RPMI 1640 supplemented with antibiotics, 10% fetal calf serum, 5×10^{-5}M 2-mercaptoethanol, and bicarbonate buffer. Cultures were maintained on a rocking platform at 37°C under 10% Co_2, 7% O_2, and 83% N_2, and fed 0.05 ml of a

Dr. Fish's present address is Children's Hospital, Division of Haematology/Oncology, 4650 W. Sunset Boulevard, Los Angeles, California 90027.

Dr. Bash's present address is Division of Immunologic Oncology, Georgetown University School of Medicine, Washington, D.C. 20007.

nutritional cocktail daily for 4 days. Plaque-forming cells (PFC) were determined in all cases against sheep red blood cells (SRBC) by the slide modification of the Jerne plate method. *E. coli* lipopolysaccharide (LPS) was used at a concentration of 10 μg/ml; muramyl dipeptide (MDP), 100 μg/ml. SRBC cultures were immunized with 0.05 ml of a 1% solution of fresh SRBC.

Macrophage-Mediated Tumor Cell Lysis

Tumor cells used were the Meth A fibrosarcoma cell line (5) obtained from Dr. Ted Ball, Department of Microbiology, University of Cincinnati College of Medicine, Cincinnati, Ohio, and the TN8 transformed cell line, derived from methylcholanthrene transformation of a normal, contact-inhibited mouse epidermal cell line.

Activated peritoneal macrophages were obtained by washing the peritoneal cavity of Balb/c mice (Jackson Memorial Labs, Bar Harbor, Maine) 7 days after i.p. injection of a 0.7-mg suspension of killed *Corynebacterium parvum.*

Macrophage-mediated tumor cell cytotoxicity was measured by release of radiolabel from tumor cells preincubated with 40 μCi/ml ³H-thymidine for 48 hr, and subsequently overlaid onto activated macrophages previously treated for 4 hr with tumor promoters and thoroughly washed. Following incubation, the remaining intact cells were harvested using a semiautomatic harvester and the retained radioactivity was measured. Significance between treated and control values was obtained unless quoted otherwise (Student's *t* test, $p < 0.05$).

RESULTS

B Cell Maturation and Antibody Synthesis

The B lymphocyte response was of interest not only in an immunologic context, but also as a differentiating system, perturbation of which is a frequent response to tumor-promoting agents (6). When added to cultures within a few hours of antigen (SRBC) or polyclonal activator (LPS or MDP), 12-O-tetradecanoylphorbol-13-acetate (TPA) was found to enhance the mitogenic response to these agents without being mitogenic *per se,* in parallel to its activity on murine T lymphocytes (Baxter et al., *unpublished data*). Concurrent potent inhibition of the antibody-synthesizing response was found (Table 1). Other phorbol diesters were also active, paralleling their activities as tumor promoters (Baxter et al., *unpublished data*). If TPA addition was delayed after start of the culture, the inhibition was essentially lost with the elapse of more than 3 days (Fig. 1). These results supported the hypothesis that TPA inhibited cell differentiation, rather than antibody secretion, since it was only effective when few cells were differentiated.

TABLE 1. *Inhibition of B lymphocyte antibody synthesis by TPA*

Antigen	PFC/10^6 viable cells	% Inhibition[a]
SRBC	406 ± 26	—
SRBC + TPA (1.0 µg/ml)	15 ± 3	96.3[b]
LPS (*E. coli* 0127, 10 µg/ml)	191 ± 41	—
LPS + TPA (1.0 µg/ml)	110 ± 31	42.2[b]
MDP (100 µg/ml)	116 ± 37	—
MDP + TPA (1.0 µg/ml)	10 ± 3	91.4[b]
TPA (1.0 µg/ml) alone	11 ± 2	—
Media control	16 ± 6	—

[a] Expressed as $1 - \left(\dfrac{\text{experimental PFC/}10^6 \text{ cells}}{\text{control PFC/}10^6 \text{ cells}} \right) \times 100$.

[b] Significantly different from control as determined by Student's *t*-test, $p < 0.01$. 5×10^6 splenic lymphocytes were incubated with SRBC, LPS, or MDP, as described in Materials and Methods.

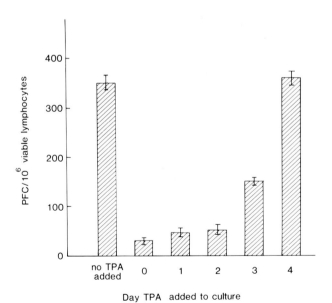

FIG. 1. Effect of delay of TPA addition on inhibition of antigen-specific antibody response. Cultures were immunized with SRBC on day 0 and TPA (1 µg/ml) was added on either day 0, 1, 2, 3, or 4. Results are expressed as mean number of PFC per 10^6 viable lymphocytes ± SEM. Determinations are from quadruplicate cultures.

Macrophage-Mediated Tumor Cell Lysis

When preincubated with phorbol diesters, the ability of macrophages to kill TN8 tumor cells was reduced, being approximately 50% in the case of TPA (Fig. 2). A similar effect was also found for Meth A cells (data not shown). Phorbol-12,13-didecanoate (PDD) was seen to have similar activity to TPA in this assay, phorbol-12,13-dibenzoate (PDB) much weaker, and phorbol to be without effect. A separate set of experiments, presented in Table 2, indicated the dose-dependent nature of the effects of phorbol esters on Meth A cells. It was observed that the most potent tumor-promoting agents exhibited the highest potential for interfering with the primary antitumor effector mechanism. Similar results were obtained for both target cell lines.

DISCUSSION

The results reported above show that active phorbol diesters inhibit essential functions of two major cell types of the normal immune system, which parallels their tumor-promoting activities *in vivo*. In the case of inhibition of B lymphocyte maturation and antibody synthesis, our findings are consistent with a previous report (1), and extend the studies reported therein to effects on polyclonal activators, as well as antigen-induced responses.

Our results for the activities of TPA and phorbol on macrophage-mediated cell cytolysis are analogous to those found by Keller (2) for rat peritoneal macro-

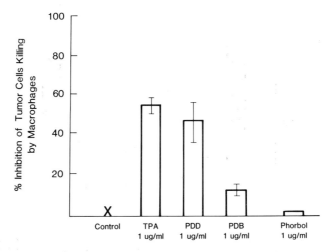

FIG. 2. Inhibition of the tumoricidal activity of activated macrophages against TN8 tumor cells by tumor promoters. Activated macrophages were treated with various phorbol esters for 4 hr, washed, and overlaid with ^{3}H-TdR-labeled TN8 tumor cells. Results are expressed as % inhibition of tumor cell killing by activated macrophages due to exposure to the phorbol esters. Cells were cultured for 72 hr at an effector:target (E:T) ratio of 10:1. Except for phorbol, the values for all agents were significantly different from the control ($p < 0.01$).

TABLE 2. *Inhibition of macrophage-mediated cytotoxicity by phorbol esters; Target: Meth A tumor cells[a]*

Agent	Dose (μg/ml)	CPM + SEM	% Inhibition of cytotoxicity[d]
[b]Target control	—	90,046 ± 8,675	—
[c]Control	—	41,081 ± 3,935	—
TPA	1	63,676 ± 5,087	46%
TPA	0.1	57,924 ± 4,673	34%
PDD	1	59,567 ± 5,296	38%
PDD	0.1	51,762 ± 4,235	22%
PDB	1	49,708 ± 4,556	18%
PDB	0.1	44,367 ± 4,054	7%
Phorbol	5.0	43,901 ± 5,475	5%

[a] Macrophages were harvested from the peritoneal cavity of mice injected 7 days previously with .7 mg killed *C. parvum*. Macrophages were exposed to tumor promoter for 4 hr at 37°C, washed 3×, and overlaid with radiolabeled Meth A tumor cells at a 10:1 E:T ratio. Phorbol diesters did not induce cell toxicity *per se*.

[b] Tumor cells incubated alone.

[c] Tumor cells and macrophages incubated without further additions.

[d] Calculated as $\dfrac{\text{cpm (treated)} - \text{cpm (control)}}{\text{cpm (target control)} - \text{cpm (control)}} \times 100$.

phages. The latter species, however, has proved largely resistant to tumor promotion by phorbol diesters. In concordance with the above author, however, we believe our studies are more relevant to considerations of macrophage activity in tumor promotion than others (3) in which TPA was found to have stimulatory effects. The short-term cytolytic activity of macrophages is mediated by hydrogen peroxide, an agent to which the target cells employed therein, a transformed macrophage line, were especially sensitive. The target cells used herein and in Keller's study in long-term tumoricidal studies were much more resistant, reflecting our and Keller's (2) inability to find promoter-induced cytotoxicity in the systems examined.

The reported findings may thus not only be valuable in understanding the mechanism of tumor promotion by phorbol diesters, but also in explaining the role of the immune response in chemical carcinogenesis in general.

ACKNOWLEDGMENT

This work was supported by NIH grants ES 07073 and CA 24022.

REFERENCES

1. Castagna, M., Yagello, M., Rabourdin-Combe, C., and Fridman, W. H. (1980): Tumor-promoting agents inhibit *in vitro* antibody synthesis. *Cancer Letters*, 8:365–371.
2. Keller, R. (1979): Suppression of natural antitumour defense mechanisms by phorbol esters. *Nature*, 282:729–731.

3. Laskin, D. L., Laskin, J. D., Weinstein, I. B., and Cachman, R. A. (1980): Modulation of phagocytosis in normal and transformed macrophages. *Cancer Res.,* 40:1,028–1,033.
4. Mastro, A. M., and Mueller, G. C. (1978): Inhibition of the mixed lymphocyte proliferative response by phorbol esters. *Biochim. Biophys. Acta,* 517:246–254.
5. Old, L., Boyse, E., Clarke, D., and Carswell, E. (1962): Antigenic properties of chemically induced tumors. *Ann. N.Y. Acad. Sci.,* 101:80–85.
6. Weinstein, I. B., Yamasaki, H., Wigler, M., Fisher, P., Lee, L. S., Jeffrey, A. M., and Grunberger, D. (1979): Molecular and cellular events associated with the action of initiating carcinogens and tumor promoters. In: *Carcinogens, Identification and Mechanisms of Action,* edited by A. C. Griffin and C. F. Shaw, pp. 399–418. Raven Press, New York.

Carcinogenesis, Vol. 7, edited by E. Hecker et al.
Raven Press, New York © 1982.

Suppression of Natural Tumor Resistance by Tumor Promoters

R. Keller, R. Keist, P. Köppel, and *E. Hecker

*Immunobiology Research Group, Institute for Immunology and Virology, University of
Zurich, CH-8032 Zurich, Switzerland; and *Institut für Biochemie, Deutsches
Krebsforschungszentrum, D-6900 Heidelberg, Federal Republic of Germany*

There is various experimental evidence suggesting that host resistance against initial tumor growth is based on natural defense mechanisms. Among these natural, noninduced mechanisms, cell-mediated cytotoxicity, manifested by mononuclear phagocytes and by "natural killer" (NK) cells, has been accorded special emphasis (1,2). Recent studies in this laboratory have shown that the potent tumor promoter 12-O-tetradecanoylphorbol-13-acetate (TPA) effectively suppressed the tumoricidal capacity of macrophages and of NK cells *in vitro* and, moreover, enhanced tumor growth *in vivo* when administered locally shortly before the tumor cell challenge (4,5). This chapter shows that TPA, quite apart from suppressing the manifestation of cytotoxicity by activated macrophages, is particularly effective in preventing the lymphokine-induced enhancement of natural cytolytic activity in resting macrophages.

MATERIAL AND METHODS

Effector Cells

Peritoneal washouts from normal, untreated controls ("resting" macrophages) or taken 7 days after i.p. injection of 3 mg heat-killed *Corynebacterium parvum* ("activated" macrophages) were seeded into plastic Petri dishes, and nonadherent cells removed after 120 min (3). Rat spleen cells and the mitogen concanavalin A (5 μg/ml) were cultured for 72 hr, and the cell-free supernatant utilized as a source of macrophage activating factor (MAF). In a final concentration of 20%, such supernatants enhanced the cytolytic activity of resting adherent peritoneal cells.

Assessment of Effector/Target Cell Interaction

Py-12 tumor cells labeled with [^{14}C]thymidine (6) were utilized as targets and interacted for 36 hr at 37°C with adherent effector cells. Afterwards, radioactivity was measured in sediments and supernatants, and net cytotoxicity calculated as described in (6).

RESULTS

Resting adherent peritoneal cells from untreated animals manifested low but consistently measurable tumoricidal activity (Table 1). Following 24-hr incubation with the MAF preparation, the cytolytic capacity of these effector cells had been enhanced considerably. The tumoricidal capacity of *C. parvum*-induced, *in vivo* activated macrophages, however, was even significantly higher than after activation *in vitro* (Table 1). In the presence of 10^{-7} (Table 1), 10^{-8}, and even 10^{-9} M TPA, the MAF-induced *in vitro* enhancement of the macrophage cytolytic activity was markedly suppressed. Phorbol was without such effect (Table 1).

In confirmation of our earlier work (4), TPA also suppressed the manifestation of the already acquired, stimulated tumoricidal potential of macrophages (Table 1).

SUMMARY

The findings of the present and other studies (4,7) show that TPA and other tumor-promoting esters suppress various *in vitro* manifestations of natural cell-mediated tumor resistance: (a) prevention of enhancement of macrophage cytocidal activity; (b) suppression of cytocidal capacity by activated macrophages; and (c) suppression of cytolytic activity of NK cells. Moreover, they abrogate host tumor resistance *in vivo*. These suppressive effects of tumor promoters on natural antitumor effector systems may constitute a fundamental mechanism in carcinogenesis.

ACKNOWLEDGMENT

R. Keller was supported by the Swiss National Science Foundation (grant 3.173.77) and the Canton of Zurich.

TABLE 1. *Effects of TPA and phorbol on the acquisition and/or the manifestation of natural cytotoxicity by macrophages*

Effector cells	% specific lysis of Py-12 tumor cells		
	Controls	TPA 10^{-7} M	Phorbol 10^{-7} M
Resting peritoneal macrophages[a]	10 ($\pm$7)	5 ($\pm$3)[b]	10 ($\pm$6)
Resting peritoneal macrophages + MAF 24 hr[a]	25 ($\pm$7)	8 ($\pm$8)[b]	21 ($\pm$7)
C. parvum-induced, activated macrophages[a]	56 ($\pm$14)	38 ($\pm$15)[b]	55 ($\pm$12)

[a] Adherent DA rat effector cells were interacted for 36 hr with Py-12 rat targets (ratio 10:1) prelabeled with [^{14}C]thymidine.
[b] Significantly ($p < 0.001$) different from controls; Student's *t*-test.

REFERENCES

1. Herberman, R. B. editor (1980): *Natural Cell-Mediated Immunity Against Tumors.* Academic Press, New York.
2. James, K., McBride, W. H., and Stuart, A. editors (1977): *The Macrophage and Cancer.* Econoprint, Edinburgh.
3. Keller, R. (1979a): Competition between foetal tissue and macrophage-dependent natural tumor resistance. *Br. J. Cancer,* 40:417–423.
4. Keller, R. (1979b): Suppression of natural antitumour defense mechanisms by phorbol esters. *Nature,* 282:729–731.
5. Keller, R. (1980): Distinctive characteristics of host tumor resistance in a rat fibrosarcoma model system. In: *Mononuclear Phagocytes. Functional Aspects,* edited by R. van Furth, pp. 1,725–1,740. Martinus Nijhoff Publishers, The Hague.
6. Keller, R., and Keist, R. (1978): Comparison of three isotope-release assays for spontaneous cytotoxicity of macrophages. *Br. J. Cancer,* 37:1,078–1,082.
7. Keller, R., Keist, R., Adolf, W., Operkuch, H. J., Schmidt, R., and Hecker, E. (1982): Tumor-promoting diterpene esters prevent macrophage activation and suppress macrophage tumoricidal capacity. *Exp. Cell. Biol.* (in press).

Conclusions and Perspectives

In this epilogue, I shall not try to review all the fascinating features of cocarcinogenesis, i.e., amplification of carcinogenesis by noncarcinogens, which have been presented in this volume. The subject is still much too obscure to be ready for an attempt at a total synthesis at the level of molecular biology. Instead, I shall consider how the study of promotion may prove to be an important part of the war against cancer and try to look ahead and guess what classes of discovery we may expect in the near future to come from the study of promoters.

In the 1940s, in pioneering experiments, especially by Rous and by Berenblum, it was shown that the production of experimental cancers does not occur in a single step but usually is the result of a long sequence of events. Shortly afterwards, a similar conclusion was reached by the epidemiologists, who saw that the steep relationship between age and the incidence of human cancer could most easily be interpreted in terms of a multistep process. For certain human cancers, the evidence is now rather strong. For example, the fact that risk of lung cancer, experienced by someone exposed to cigarette smoke and to asbestos, is the product (not the sum) of the risks due to each agent alone implies that the two agents are driving different steps in the sequence, i.e., there must be more than one step in the reaction. Similarly, the effect of stopping smoking on the incidence of lung cancer suggests that cigarette smoke must be catalyzing an early and a late step but not the last step in the sequence.

Of course, such matters are more easily investigated in experimental animals, and in several protocols of experimental carcinogenesis have now been shown to proceed by way of a rather rigorous sequence of events, each of which can be catalyzed by a different agent.

Some people may feel that this attempt to break down the entire process of carcinogenesis into its component parts is an exercise that tends to select for the most intricate sequences, and therefore make carcinogenesis more complicated than it really is. It is important to remember, however, that many varieties of human cancer are clearly determined by multiple factors, often acting in sequence; therefore, cocarcinogenesis, and particularly initiation/promotion, is not simply an artefact of the experimentalist.

The early experimentalists divided carcinogens into *initiators* and *promoters* (words first coined by Friedewald and Rous). Perhaps the most perfect example of this dichotomy is the case in which mice are initiated by a single feeding of urethane and are then made to produce skin cancers by the repeated application of croton oil. Here the cancers occur only if the agents are applied in that order, and neither agent alone will produce cancer even after repeated applications.

In the last few years, it has been possible to divide promotion into two stages. The first, like initiation, is apparently irreversible and can be brought about by one single application of TPA, whereas the second requires prolonged application of various weak promoters such as turpentine or mezerein. This separation of promotion into two distinct processes is supported by the observation that the protease inhibitor TPCK will block the first process but not the second, whereas retinoic acid will block the second but not the first. In these cases, therefore, carcinogenesis is occurring in at least three stages—initiation, followed by a first stage of promotion, followed by a second stage of promotion (actually, the last of these requires prolonged exposure to the second stage promoter and therefore seems to be itself a multihit process).

As the details of promotion become more and more complicated, it should, in principle, become easier to find what is the exact molecular biology of its various stages. Before discussing that aspect of promotion, however, I think it is worth considering what are the possible rewards that might come from the general study of promotion.

1. It is not unreasonable to suppose that most forms of human cancer arise as the result of a similar sequence, in which the key event initiation is followed by a prolonged period of promotion. This implies that most of the population will already have undergone initiation and they are now slowly progressing through the stage(s) of promotion. If, therefore, we want to prevent people from having cancer, we should be directing our attention more to the promoters in our environment than to the initiators, because it is only by removing the promoters that we can hope to benefit everyone. Therefore, we need to learn enough about the nature of promoters and about the underlying mechanism of promotion to identify the promoters of human cancer.

2. The main problem in implementing any program in cancer prevention is the difficulty in persuading people to alter their habits. In the affluent, industrialized countries of the world, people's habits and way of life are usually the result of choice rather than necessity, and so we should expect that the population will be reluctant to change its habits. There has been rather little success in persuading people to stop smoking, and I suspect that the same may be true for any other program of prevention that demands abstinence. The discovery, however, that there are not only promoters but also antipromoters may offer a much more promising form of cancer prevention, for, if it is generally true that retinoic acid and certain related compounds are capable of acting as antipromoters, then we could imagine a program of prevention in which people were merely asked to add such substances to their diet. At this point, the prevention of certain cancers could become rather like the prevention of goiter, the avitaminoses, and dental caries, which were achieved by additions to our diet.

3. Despite many years of intensive effort, the search for specific chemotherapeutic agents active against cancer cells has been unsuccessful. So far no such agents have been discovered for any of the common cancers. As the cells of most classes of cancer still retain some of the form and pattern of differentiation

of the tissues from which they have arisen, it seems clear that the cancer cells are still responding to some of the signals that normally determine cell behavior. Therefore, it might be possible to make this the point of attack by chemotherapy. Unfortunately, although some of the systemic signals (hormones) have been identified that control the overall growth of tissues such as bone marrow, liver, and the various endocrine organs, virtually nothing is known about the local signals that determine the precise architecture of tissues. However, it seems likely that certain promoters affect the progress of carcinogenesis because they are analogues of these local signaling substances, and so are able to inhibit the normal process of differentiation. Therefore, the study of promoters may prove to be the easiest way of learning about the signals that control differentiation, and it could eventually lead to the design of special agents for forcing cancer cells to undergo terminal differentiation.

Apart from such particular benefits that may or may not come to pass, it is usually true that once we understand any biological process we find we have learned how to manipulate it, so the study of promotion can be recommended on general grounds. And here we come to what I think is the most remarkable feature of the whole process of carcinogenesis, which is that we still know almost nothing about the molecular biology of any of the steps in the reaction. The salient feature of initiation is its irreversibility; once an animal has been exposed to an initiator it can be made to produce cancers by prolonged exposure to promoters at any time later. By contrast, promotion is somewhat reversible, at least in its early stages; for example, if too long an interval is left between each application of the promoter, the effect can be lost. Because initiators are usually agents that damage DNA, whereas promoters are agents that influence cell proliferation and differentiation, most people (myself included) have assumed that initiation is probably conventional mutagenesis and that promotion is some process affecting gene expression that displays the mutations present in the genome—for example, somatic recombination allowing the expression of recessive mutations, or some semipermanent derepression of certain genes as part of a process of dedifferentiation. Unfortunately, this picture of carcinogenesis is becoming less and less plausible. If initiation were the production of potentially carcinogenic mutations, it should be a rare event (unless, of course, we are prepared to believe that there are hundreds of "cancer" genes that can be the target for such mutagenesis); yet several experiments have shown that even a low dose of initiator can, in certain circumstances, convert every cell into a source for clones of cancer cells. Conversely, promotion, which one might have guessed to be an efficient reaction for any cell that had undergone initiation, proves to be a rather rare event. So neither initiation nor promotion is behaving exactly as we would have expected. Furthermore, it turns out that promotion can sometimes be divided into at least two separate stages. So we now have to conceive of some three-stage process in which each step has to occur in the correct order.

Several people have recently proposed that the critical event in carcinogenesis is not a local change in base sequence produced by a conventional mutagen, but is usually a genetic transposition. It has always been rather hard to see why the regulatory circuits of mammalian cells should be arranged in such a way that the whole pattern of cell behavior can be altered by minor changes in base sequence. It is easy to imagine, however, that there are many possible rearrangements that will radically alter the cell's phenotype. Furthermore, visible chromosomal translocations are commonly found both in experimental cancers and in "spontaneous" human cancers. We should therefore consider the possibility that carcinogenesis consists of a sequence of events that include the synthesis of appropriate transposases (perhaps triggered by certain kinds of DNA damage), the actual process of transposition, and, finally, the expression of the consequences of the transposition; these consequences could include alterations in the pattern of gene expression, or a destabilization of limited regions of the genome so that further rearrangements take place (as is known to happen in maize and yeast, for example).

In the present context, perhaps the most interesting feature of the model is simply that it has originated so recently (see Cairns, J. (1981): The origin of human cancer. *Nature* 289:353–357). The fact that we are still able to consider novel explanations for the process of carcinogenesis shows, all too clearly, how little we know about the molecular aspects of the subject. I believe, however, that this uncertainty is not going to last much longer. With some further refinement, the techniques of genetic engineering should, in principle, make it possible to itemize all the features that distinguish the genome of a mammalian cancer cell from its normal counterpart; this includes not only differences in base sequence but also differences in gene expression—and at that point, we should become much more certain about the molecular biology of initiation and of the subsequent steps of promotion.

There remains one other aspect of promotion that has to be discussed. To someone outside the field, the extraordinary feature of a promoter like TPA is that it interacts with so many facets of cell physiology. The response of the cell to signals like epidermal growth factor, the production of signals such as the prostaglandins, the synthesis and interactions of cell surface proteins and lipids, the balance between various intracellular substances such as cGMP and cAMP, the control of DNA replication and of events at the chromosomal level such as sister chromatid exchange—all these are direct or indirect targets for the action of TPA. Because the effects can be demonstrated with concentrations of TPA as low as 10^{-10} M (i.e., about 1000 molecules per cell), it seems likely that TPA must be acting as an analogue of some local signaling substance that determines cell behavior and tissue architecture. Here we come into an area that is poorly understood. Developmental biologists have found it very difficult to investigate the chemistry of the factors that operate during embryogenesis and regeneration because the absolute quantity of any substances that form the basis for "positional information" is presumably very small. Furthermore, there is no reason for thinking that these are fundamentally simple, easily analyzed systems. The great advances of molecular biology have, for the most part, been very simple. But that is the nature of the problem: the general principles of the one-dimensional organization of genetic information have to be simple. The way the structure of multicellular organisms has evolved is probably rather complicated. The different signaling substances may be few in number, but each of them can be expected to touch directly or indirectly upon the network of competing biochemical pathways at several points, and so we should expect the effects of any one of them (or of any particular analogue, such as TPA) to be almost uninterpretable until we understand the whole network that determines a cell's form and differentiation. I am drawing a perhaps unjustifiable distinction here between most of intermediary metabolism (which is nothing more than a matter of routine housekeeping) and the special functions that distinguish one cell from another in a multicellular organism. It seems much more likely, however, that it is these latter functions, rather than something like anaerobic glycolysis, that we shall find to be affected in cancer cells. And so we will have difficulty in piecing together the phenotype of the cancer cell until we understand much more about the network of reactions that is the basis for development and differentiation. As mentioned earlier, the study of the cell biological effects of promoters may be the easiest way of dissecting the network. In years to come we may judge that this was the main contribution to derive from such work.

John Cairns
Department of Microbiology,
Harvard School of Public Health
Boston, Massachusetts 02115

Subject Index

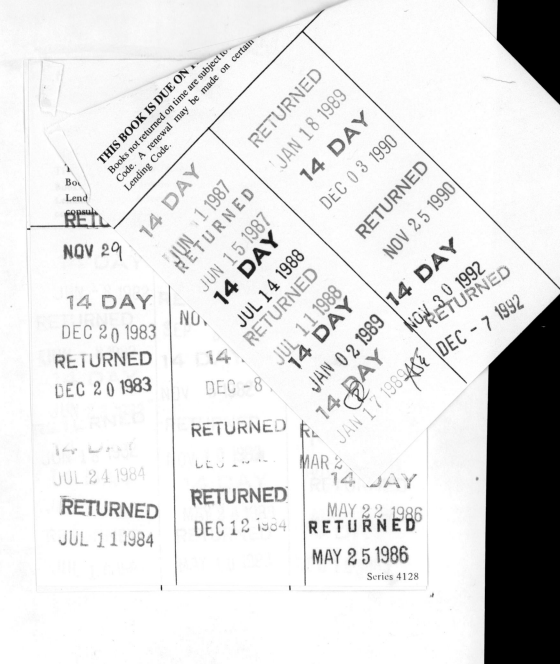

RETURNED
JAN 18 1989

14 DAY
DEC 0 3 1990

RETURNED
NOV 2 5 1990

14 DAY
JUN 1 1 1987

RETURNED
JUN 15 1987

14 DAY
JUL 14 1988

14 DAY
NOV 3 0 1992

RETURNED
DEC – 7 1992

RETURNED
JUL 1 1 1988

14 DAY
JAN 0 2 1989

14 DAY
JAN 17 1989

RETURNED
NOV 29

14 DAY
DEC 2 0 1983

RETURNED
DEC 2 0 1983

14 DAY
JUL 2 4 1984

RETURNED
JUL 1 1 1984

14 DAY
DEC – 8

RETURNED
DEC 1 2 1984

RETURNED
MAR 2

14 DAY
MAY 2 2 1986

RETURNED
MAY 2 5 1986

Series 4128